Immunotoxicology: Integrated Concepts and Clinical Theory

Immunotoxicology: Integrated Concepts and Clinical Theory

Editor: Jim Wang

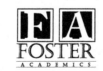

www.fosteracademics.com

www.fosteracademics.com

Cataloging-in-Publication Data

Immunotoxicology : integrated concepts and clinical theory / edited by Jim Wang.
 p. cm.
Includes bibliographical references and index.
ISBN 978-1-63242-487-7
1. Immunotoxicology. 2. Cellular immunity. 3. Immunologic diseases--Treatment. 4. Cell-mediated cytotoxicity.
I. Wang, Jim.
RC582.17 .I66 2017
616.079--dc23

© Foster Academics, 2017

Foster Academics,
118-35 Queens Blvd., Suite 400,
Forest Hills, NY 11375, USA

ISBN 978-1-63242-487-7 (Hardback)

This book contains information obtained from authentic and highly regarded sources. Copyright for all individual chapters remain with the respective authors as indicated. All chapters are published with permission under the Creative Commons Attribution License or equivalent. A wide variety of references are listed. Permission and sources are indicated; for detailed attributions, please refer to the permissions page and list of contributors. Reasonable efforts have been made to publish reliable data and information, but the authors, editors and publisher cannot assume any responsibility for the validity of all materials or the consequences of their use.

Trademark Notice: Registered trademark of products or corporate names are used only for explanation and identification without intent to infringe.

Printed and bound in the United States of America.

Contents

Preface IX

Chapter 1 **Characterization of a Novel Anti-Cancer Compound for Astrocytomas** 1
Sang Y. Lee, Becky Slagle-Webb, Elias Rizk, Akshal Patel, Patti A. Miller,
Shen-Shu Sung, James R. Connor

Chapter 2 **Sodium-Glucose Transporter-2 (SGLT2; SLC5A2) Enhances Cellular Uptake of Aminoglycosides** 12
Meiyan Jiang, Qi Wang, Takatoshi Karasawa, Ja-Won Koo, Hongzhe Li,
Peter S. Steyger

Chapter 3 **Gold(I) Complexes of 9-Deazahypoxanthine as Selective Antitumor and Anti-Inflammatory Agents** 26
Ján Vančo, Jana Gáliková, Jan Hošek, Zdeněk Dvořák, Lenka Paráková,
Zdeněk Trávníček

Chapter 4 **Integrated mRNA-MicroRNA Profiling of Human NK Cell Differentiation Identifies MiR-583 as a Negative Regulator of IL2Rγ Expression** 41
Sohyun Yun, Su Ui Lee, Jung Min Kim, Hyun-Jun Lee, Hae Young Song,
Young Kyeung Kim, Haiyoung Jung, Young-Jun Park, Suk Ran Yoon,
Sei-Ryang Oh, Tae-Don Kim, Inpyo Choi

Chapter 5 **Hydroxyapatite-Coated Sillicone Rubber Enhanced Cell Adhesion and It May Be through the Interaction of EF1β and γ-Actin** 55
Xiao-hua Shi, Shao-liang Wang, Yi-ming Zhang, Yi-cheng Wang, Zhi Yang,
Xin Zhou, Zeyuan Lei, Dong-li Fan

Chapter 6 **Cadmium Telluride Quantum Dots (CdTe-QDs) and Enhanced Ultraviolet-B (UV-B) Radiation Trigger Antioxidant Enzyme Metabolism and Programmed Cell Death in Wheat Seedlings** 66
Huize Chen, Yan Gong, Rong Han

Chapter 7 **Novel Positively Charged Nanoparticle Labeling for *In Vivo* Imaging of Adipose Tissue-Derived Stem Cells** 79
Hiroshi Yukawa, Shingo Nakagawa, Yasuma Yoshizumi, Masaki Watanabe,
Hiroaki Saito, Yoshitaka Miyamoto, Hirofumi Noguchi, Koichi Oishi, Kenji Ono,
Makoto Sawada, Ichiro Kato, Daisuke Onoshima, Momoko Obayashi,
Yumi Hayashi, Noritada Kaji, Tetsuya Ishikawa, Shuji Hayashi, Yoshinobu Baba

Chapter 8 **3-O-Galloylated Procyanidins from *Rumex acetosa* L. Inhibit the Attachment of Influenza A Virus** 91
Andrea Derksen, Andreas Hensel, Wali Hafezi, Fabian Herrmann,
Thomas J. Schmidt, Christina Ehrhardt, Stephan Ludwig, Joachim Kühn

Chapter 9   Lichen Secondary Metabolites in *Flavocetraria cucullata* Exhibit Anti-Cancer Effects on Human Cancer Cells through the Induction of Apoptosis and Suppression of Tumorigenic Potentials 104
Thanh Thi Nguyen, Somy Yoon, Yi Yang, Ho-Bin Lee, Soonok Oh, Min-Hye Jeong, Jong-Jin Kim, Sung-Tae Yee, Florin Crişan, Cheol Moon, Kwang Youl Lee, Kyung Keun Kim, Jae-Seoun Hur, Hangun Kim

Chapter 10   Fasting Enhances TRAIL-Mediated Liver Natural Killer Cell Activity via HSP70 Upregulation 118
Vu T. A. Dang, Kazuaki Tanabe, Yuka Tanaka, Noriaki Tokumoto, Toshihiro Misumi, Yoshihiro Saeki, Nobuaki Fujikuni, Hideki Ohdan

Chapter 11   Synergism between Basic Asp49 and Lys49 Phospholipase A_2 Myotoxins of Viperid Snake Venom *In Vitro* and *In Vivo* 131
Diana Mora-Obando, Julián Fernández, Cesare Montecucco, José María Gutiérrez, Bruno Lomonte

Chapter 12   The Protective Effect of Esculentoside A on Experimental Acute Liver Injury in Mice 142
Fang Zhang, Xingtong Wang, Xiaochen Qiu, Junjie Wang, He Fang, Zhihong Wang, Yu Sun, Zhaofan Xia

Chapter 13   PSMA Ligand Conjugated PCL-PEG Polymeric Micelles Targeted to Prostate Cancer Cells 155
Jian Jin, Bowen Sui, Jingxin Gou, Jingshuo Liu, Xing Tang, Hui Xu, Yu Zhang, Xiangqun Jin

Chapter 14   Structure-Activity Relationships of Novel Salicylaldehyde Isonicotinoyl Hydrazone (SIH) Analogs: Iron Chelation, Anti-Oxidant and Cytotoxic Properties 167
Eliška Potůčková, Kateřina Hrušková, Jan Bureš, Petra Kovaříkoví, Iva A. Špirková, Kateřina Pravdíková, Lucie Kolbabovà, Tereza Hergeselová, Pavlína Hašková, Hana Jansová, Miloslav Macháček, Anna Jirkovská, Vera Richardson, Darius J. R. Lane, Danuta S. Kalinowski, Des R. Richardson, Kateřina Vávrová, Tomáš Šimůnek

Chapter 15   Celastrol Stimulates Hypoxia-Inducible Factor-1 Activity in Tumor Cells by Initiating the ROS/Akt/p70S6K Signaling Pathway and Enhancing Hypoxia-Inducible Factor-1α Protein Synthesis 184
Xiaoxi Han, Shengkun Sun, Ming Zhao, Xiang Cheng, Guozhu Chen, Song Lin, Yifu Guan, Xiaodan Yu

Chapter 16   Mechanisms by Which Low Glucose Enhances the Cytotoxicity of Metformin to Cancer Cells Both *In Vitro* and *In Vivo* 199
Yongxian Zhuang, Daniel K. Chan, Allison B. Haugrud, W. Keith Miskimins

Chapter 17   Putrescine-Dependent Re-Localization of TvCP39, a Cysteine Proteinase Involved in *Trichomonas vaginalis* Cytotoxicity 211
Bertha Isabel Carvajal-Gamez, Laura Itzel Quintas-Granados, Rossana Arroyo, Laura Isabel Vázquez-Carrillo, Lucero De los Angeles Ramón-Luing, Eduardo Carrillo-Tapia, María Elizbeth Alvarez-Sánchez

Chapter 18 **Methyllycaconitine Alleviates Amyloid-β Peptides-Induced Cytotoxicity in SH-SY5Y Cells** 221
XiaoLei Zheng, ZhaoHong Xie, ZhengYu Zhu, Zhen Liu, Yun Wang, LiFei Wei, Hui Yang, HongNa Yang, YiQing Liu, JianZhong Bi

Permissions

List of Contributors

Index

Preface

This book aims to highlight the current researches and provides a platform to further the scope of innovations in this area. This book is a product of the combined efforts of many researchers and scientists from different parts of the world. The objective of this book is to provide the readers with the latest information in the field.

Immunotoxicology is the design and development of drugs that reduce the function of the immune system. Immunotoxicology medication and treatment are known as anti-rejection drugs for the role they play in transplantation and radiation treatment. The text elucidates the concepts and innovative models around prospective developments with respect to this field. Immunotoxiciology is an upcoming field of science that has undergone rapid development over the past few decades. This text aims to shed light on some of the unexplored aspects and the recent researches in this field. In this book, understanding of the difficult concepts of immunotoxicology as easy and informative as possible, for the readers.

I would like to express my sincere thanks to the authors for their dedicated efforts in the completion of this book. I acknowledge the efforts of the publisher for providing constant support. Lastly, I would like to thank my family for their support in all academic endeavors.

Editor

Characterization of a Novel Anti-Cancer Compound for Astrocytomas

Sang Y. Lee[1]*, Becky Slagle-Webb[1], Elias Rizk[1], Akshal Patel[1], Patti A. Miller[2], Shen-Shu Sung[3], James R. Connor[1]

[1] Department of Neurosurgery, Pennsylvania State University College of Medicine, Penn State M.S. Hershey Medical Center, Hershey, Pennsylvania, United States of America, [2] Department of Radiology, Pennsylvania State University College of Medicine, Penn State M.S. Hershey Medical Center, Hershey, Pennsylvania, United States of America, [3] Department of Pharmacology, Pennsylvania State University College of Medicine, Penn State M.S. Hershey Medical Center, Hershey, Pennsylvania, United States of America

Abstract

The standard chemotherapy for brain tumors is temozolomide (TMZ), however, as many as 50% of brain tumors are reportedly TMZ resistant leaving patients without a chemotherapeutic option. We performed serial screening of TMZ resistant astrocytoma cell lines, and identified compounds that are cytotoxic to these cells. The most cytotoxic compound was an analog of thiobarbituric acid that we refer to as CC-I. There is a dose-dependent cytotoxic effect of CC-I in TMZ resistant astrocytoma cells. Cell death appears to occur via apoptosis. Following CC-I exposure, there was an increase in astrocytoma cells in the S and G2/M phases. In *in vivo* athymic (*nu/nu*) nude mice subcutaneous and intracranial tumor models, CC-I completely inhibited tumor growth without liver or kidney toxicity. Molecular modeling and enzyme activity assays indicate that CC-I selectively inhibits topoisomerase IIα similar to other drugs in its class, but its cytotoxic effects on astrocytoma cells are stronger than these compounds. The cytotoxic effect of CC-I is stronger in cells expressing unmethylated O^6-methylguanine methyltransferase (MGMT) but is still toxic to cells with methylated MGMT. CC-I can also enhance the toxic effect of TMZ on astrocytoma when the two compounds are combined. In conclusion, we have identified a compound that is effective against astrocytomas including TMZ resistant astrocytomas in both cell culture and *in vivo* brain tumor models. The enhanced cytotoxicity of CC-I and the safety profile of this family of drugs could provide an interesting tool for broader evaluation against brain tumors.

Editor: Javier S. Castresana, University of Navarra, Spain

Funding: This project is funded, in part, by a grant with the National Cancer Institute of the National Institutes of Health under Award Number R21CA167406 to SL. The content is solely the responsibility of the authors and does not necessarily represent the official views of the National Institutes of Health. This study also supported in part by the Elsa U. Pardee Foundation and the Tara Leah Witmer Endowment. The funders had no role in study design, data collection and analysis, decision to publish, or preparation of the manuscript.

Competing Interests: Connor is partial owner of NuHope LLC which has a financial interest in development of compounds for treating brain tumors that were initially screened using cell lines chosen for HFE genotype. Lee has a royalty agreement with NuHope LLC.

* Email: SYL3@psu.edu

Introduction

Gliomas account for 28% of all primary brain and central nervous system (CNS) tumors, and 80% of gliomas are malignant [1]. Among gliomas, glioblastoma (glioblastoma multiforme, grade IV astrocytoma, GBM) is the most common malignant glioma. The mortality rate of primary malignant brain and CNS tumors is high; approximately 22,620 new adult cases of malignant brain and CNS cancers in 2013 [1] and 13,700 deaths occurred in 2012 [2]. The median survival for GBM patients was 14.6 months and the 2 year survival of patients with GBM was 10.4% for radiotherapy alone and only 26.5% undergoing combined therapy treatment of temozolomide (TMZ) and radiation [3].

The current standard treatment for GBM is total resection followed by radiotherapy alone or combination with TMZ chemotherapy [4,5]. TMZ is an oral alkylating agent used in the treatment of brain cancer, *e.g.*, GBM and oligodendroglioma [6]. It has also been used to treat melanoma, prostate cancer, pancreatic carcinoma, soft tissue sarcoma, and renal cell carcinoma [7–11]. TMZ inhibits cell reproduction by inhibiting DNA replication [12] and has unique characteristics compared with other alkylating agents. For example, it is administered orally, crosses the blood-brain barrier, is less toxic than other alkylating agents, and does not chemically cross-link DNA. However, although TMZ is the current chemotherapeutic standard for treating brain tumors and other cancers, as many as 50% of brain tumors are resistant to TMZ therapy [13,14]. In addition, almost all tumors eventually come back and the large majority of recurrent tumors are resistant to chemotherapy [15,16]. Therefore, the development of new treatment options including novel drugs for therapy resistant brain tumors is urgently needed.

In addition to the alkylation agents like TMZ, topoisomerase inhibitors are another group of anti-cancer drugs under evaluation. Topoisomerases are important nuclear enzymes that regulate the topology of DNA, maintain genomic integrity and are essential for DNA replication, recombination, transcription and chromosome segregation [17]. There are six human topoisomerase enzymes [18] and three of them, topoisomerase I, topoisomerase IIα and topoisomerase IIβ, have significant involvement in cancer and cancer chemotherapy [19]. The topoisomerase I enzyme nicks and rejoins one strand of the duplex DNA, and topoisomerase II enzyme transiently breaks and closes double-stranded DNA [20]. The topoisomerase I inhibitors (e.g., topotecan) have been used in patients with recurrent small-cell lung cancer, recurrent malignant gliomas, recurrent childhood brain tumors [21,22]. Although topoisomerase II inhibitors were studied in glioma cells [23–25], the topoisomerase II inhibitors haven't been widely used in adults with primary brain tumors due to their poor CNS penetrance. Therefore, small molecules with the capability to penetrate the brain would be highly desirable to treat gliomas *in vivo*.

We have previously reported that human neuroblastoma cells and human astrocytoma cells lines expressing commonly occurring polymorphisms in the HFE gene were resistant to chemotherapy and radiation [26]. The HFE gene product is involved in iron homeostasis and the common HFE polymorphisms, H63D and C282Y, lead to a number of changes in cells such as increased endoplasmic reticulum stress and increased oxidative stress [27–29]. In the present study, we used astrocytoma cell lines that we identified with the HFE gene variants and TMZ resistance to screen compounds from DIVERSet compound library from Chembridge (San Diego, CA) and found a number of effective compounds with a similar chemotype. We identified an analog of a thiobarbituric acid compound which has strong toxic effect on TMZ-resistant astrocytoma cells. We report here the characterization of the lead compound in *in vitro* cell culture and *in vivo* brain tumor models.

Materials and Methods

Materials

Dulbecco's Modified Eagle Medium (DMEM), fetal bovine serum (FBS) and other cell culture ingredients were purchased from Life Technologies (Grand Island, NY). All the PCR Array ingredients were supplied from SABiosciences (Frederick, MD). TMZ was purchased from Oakwood Products Inc. (West Columbia, SC) and was dissolved in cell culture medium or 100% DMSO. The lead chemotype compound–I (CC-I) was ordered from ChemBridge Corporation (San Diego, CA). The compound was dissolved in DMSO as a stock solution and diluted for the experiment. Topoisomerase enzymes I and IIα assay kits were ordered from TopoGen Inc. (Port Orange, FL). Merbarone was obtained from Calbiochem (San Diego, CA). All of the other chemicals used were purchased from Sigma Co. (St. Louis, MO).

Human astrocytoma cell culture, treatment and cytotoxicity assay

Human astrocytoma cells (SW1088-grade III, U87-MG-grade IV, CCF-STTG1-grade IV, T98G-grade IV, LN-18-grade IV) were ordered from American Type Culture Collection (ATCC, Manassas, VA) and maintained in DMEM (Gibco by Life Technologies, catalog 11885) supplemented with 100 U/mL penicillin, 100 μg/mL streptomycin, 0.29 mg/mL L-glutamine, and 10% FBS. All experiments were performed at 37°C in 5% CO_2 atmosphere cell culture conditions. For the cytotoxicity assays, the compounds tested were prepared by first diluting them from the stock solution in cell culture media. The compounds were exposed to the cells for 3–6 days. Cell cytotoxicity was performed by MTS [3-(4,5-dimethylthiazol-2-yl)-5-(3-carboxymethoxyphenyl)-2-(4-sulfophenyl)-2H-tetrazolium] cell proliferation assay (Pro-

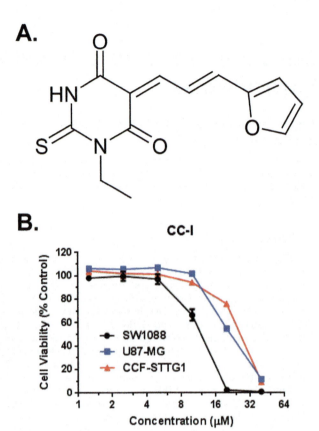

Figure 1. Chemical structure and cytotoxicity of CC-I in *in vitro*. (A) The structure of CC-I. (B) Cytotoxicity of CC-I in *in vitro*. Human astrocytoma cell lines were cultured with different doses of CC-I for 3 days and then the cytotoxicity was determined by SRB assay. The LC_{50} of CC-I to SW1088 cell lines (13.6 μM) are significantly different with the LC_{50} of CC-I to U87-MG and CCF-STTG1 cell lines (23.6 μM and 25.4 μM) ($p<0.001$).

mega, Madison, WI) or sulforhodamine B (SRB) assay at the end of the cell culture period.

Acute toxicity determination

Acute toxicity of CC-I was determined in athymic nude mice (strain 088 or 490, Charles River Laboratories, Wilmington, MA) according to the NIH drug development program's acute toxicity procedure with minor modification. To determine the acute toxicity, a total of six female mice (1–2 month old) were injected intraperitoneally with 3 different doses (e.g., 20 mg/kg, 37.5 mg/kg, 50 mg/kg) of CC-I or vehicle control once a week and then observed for a period of 7–14 days. The mice were observed daily for changes in body weight, visible and/or palpable dermal infection, presence of ascites, food consumption or nutrition status, and grooming or impaired mobility or death to determine acute toxicity. At 7–14 days after treatment, 0.5–1 ml of blood was collected through a cardiac heart puncture while the mice were under anesthesia (Ketamine 100 mg/kg body weight/xylazine 10 mg/kg body weight, intraperitoneally) for blood toxicity examination. All the animals in the study were housed in germ-free environmental rooms, and individual bubble systems. All the animal experiments were approved (IACUC #2011-062) by the Pennsylvania State University Institutional Animal Care and Use Committees.

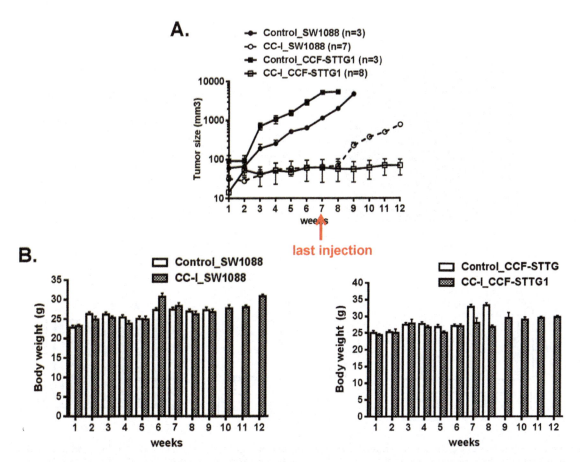

Figure 2. The anti-tumor effect of CC-I in a subcutaneous mouse tumor model. (A) Mice were implanted with ten million cells with the SW1088 or CCF-STTG1 cells. The starting tumor size for the CCF-STTG1 cells ranged from 80–100 mm³. The SW1088 cells grew more slowly so CC-I treatment was started when the tumors reached 30 mm³. CC-I was injected intraperitoneally at a concentration of 25 mg/kg body weight once a week for 7 weeks (n = 7~10). The control group was given PBS in the same volume and regimen (n = 3–8). The tumor slowly reoccurred in the TMZ-sensitive SW1088 astrocytoma injected nude mice but did not reoccur in the TMZ resistant CCF-STTG1 injected nude mice when CC-I was discontinued (beyond 7 weeks). CC-I inhibited the tumor growth and was not lethal in any of the treatment groups. Some error bars are too small to be visible. (B) Mean body weight of mice is presented in grams. Some error bars are too small to be visible.

Subcutaneous tumor model

To test the anti-tumor effect of CC-I against human astrocytoma tumor, one-two month old female immunodeficient (nu/nu) nude mice (strain 088, Charles River Laboratories, Wilmington, MA) were implanted 10×10^6 cells per mouse subcutaneously with TMZ sensitive SW1088 or TMZ resistant CCF-STTG1 astrocytoma cells. When the tumor reached approximately 32–100 mm³ in size, the mice (n = 10 or 11) were randomly divided into two groups. The CC-I was injected intraperitoneally at a concentration of 25 mg/kg body weight in a volume of 200–300 μL in 12.5% ethanol once a week for 7 weeks. The control group was given phosphate-buffered saline (PBS) in the same volume and regimen. Tumor size was measured weekly with a Vernier caliper for 7 weeks by an investigator blinded to experimental conditions. Tumor volume (V) was calculated according to the formula $V = a^2/2 \times b$, where a and b are minor and major axes of the tumor foci, respectively. The tumor size, health, and survival of the mice were visibly monitored daily and the tumor size measured weekly. We did not take pictures of the tumors. We will consider taking pictures for upcoming experiments. To monitor the toxicity of compounds, the animals were euthanized with ketamine/xylazine 100/10 mg/kg body weight intraperitoneally, and measured liver and kidney toxicity at the end of the experiment.

Intracranial xenograft model

Female immunodeficient nude mice (strain 088, Charles River Laboratories, Wilmington, MA) weighing 20–30 g were anesthetized by intraperitoneal injection of ketamine-xylazine 100 mg/kg–10 mg/kg body weight. Human U87-MG and CCF-STTG1 astrocytoma cell lines were implanted to create the brain tumor xenograft. In brief, the head was held in horizontal position and 1 million astrocytoma cells in a volume of 10 μL were injected slowly into the caudate putamen region using a small animal stereotactic apparatus. The stereotactic co-ordinates used for the xenografts are P = 0.5, L = 1.7, H = 3.8 mm. The astrocytoma cells were injected slowly for 10 minutes to avoid elevation in the intracranial pressure or upward cell suspension leakage through the track of the needle. The animals were given buprenorphine (0.05–0.1 mg/kg body weight subcutaneous) for pain during and after surgery. This was given every 8–12 hours for 24–48 hours after surgery. The animals were subjected to T1 weighted magnetic resonance imaging (MRI) twice; once to determine that a tumor is established in the brain (~3 weeks injection of astrocytoma cells) and at the end of the experiment. The animals were monitored on a daily basis and the body weight was recorded weekly. Once a tumor was observed, the mice (n = 12 or 15) were randomly divided into two groups. CC-I (25 mg/kg body weight) or PBS was injected once a week intraperitoneally. The overall

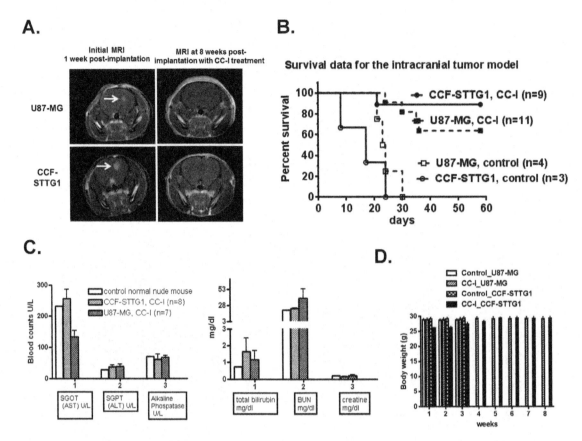

Figure 3. Anti-tumor effect of CC-I in an intracranial xenograft mouse model. (A) Representative MRI images taken with T1-weighted MRI contrast (7T MR imaging system) after intracranial tumor formation (one-three weeks post-implantation of astrocytoma cells) or after tumor formation followed by injection of CC-I (25 mg/kg body weight) for 7 weeks. CC-I completely inhibited tumor growth in both astrocytoma cell lines. (B) Kaplan-Meier survival graph of intracranial brain tumor mice after the administration of CC-I. CC-I extends the survival of the mice when compared to the untreated mice (n = 9 or 11) ($p<0.0001$). None of the mice which received PBS (control) survived after 30 days and median survival of all those animals was 20 days (n = 3 or 4). (C) Liver and kidney toxicity of CC-I. The liver and kidney toxicity (total bilirubin, blood urea nitrogen (BUN), creatine, aspartate aminotransferase (AST), alanine aminotransferase (ALT), and alkaline phosphatase) were determined using an automated chemistry analyzer machine (Roche Cobase MIRA) and kits manufactured by Thermo Electron. These data indicate no liver or kidney toxicity by CC-I in nude mice. Toxicity data displayed as means ± SEM. (D) Mean body weight of mice in grams.

survival of mice was performed by a Kaplan-Meier survival curve. The animals were euthanized according to acceptable method of euthanasia as defined by the American Veterinary Medical Association (AVMA) Guidelines on Euthanasia - Approved Euthanasia Methods, 2013. Once the animals receive a body condition score of less than 2, the animals were euthanized with ketamine/xylazine 100/10 mg/kg body weight intraperitoneally as well as a secondary method of cervical dislocation. At the termination of the experiment, plasma was collected for analysis of liver and kidney toxicity after euthanized with ketamine/xylazine 100/10 mg/kg body weight intraperitoneally.

T1 weighed MRI images

T1 weighted MRI contrast was used to visualize the tumor growth using 7T MRI system (Bruker, Biospec GmbH, Ettlingen, Germany). The imaging parameters of the T1 scan are TR/TE = 540 ms/11 ms, 8 averages, 192×192, 0.5 mm slice thickness, and 3.2 cm^2 FOV. The mice were anesthetized by inhalation of 1–2% isoflurane and placed in a position with brain located at the center of the coil. Intracranial tumor volume was estimated using Gadolinium enhanced T1 weighed multislice axial fast spin echo images. From these images the size of the tumor was calculated using the Region-of-Interest tool available on the Paravision software (Bruker Biospec, Ettlingen, Germany).

Liver and kidney toxicity

The liver and kidney toxicity (total bilirubin, blood urea nitrogen (BUN), creatine, aspartate aminotransferase (AST), alanine aminotransferase (ALT), and alkaline phosphatase) was assessed for both subcutaneous tumor model and intracranial xenograft model using an automated chemistry analyzer (Roche Cobase MIRA) and kits manufactured by Thermo Electron (Louisville, CO). The blood was obtained from the control or CC-I injected mice with astrocytoma cells at the termination of the experiment.

Apoptosis assay

For apoptosis assay, the 3×10^6 of CCF-STTG1 cells were cultured for 48 hr with several concentrations (~36 µM) of CC-I or actinomycin D (~80 nM) as a positive control. The cells were harvested following trypsine-EDTA exposure and washed in cold PBS. Then 100 µL of the cell suspension (~1×10^6 cells) was incubated with 1 µL of 100 µg/mL red-fluorescent propidium iodide nucleic acid binding dye and 5 µL Annexin V-FITC (Molecular Probes, Carlsbad, CA) for 15 minutes at room

A. Apoptotic cell death

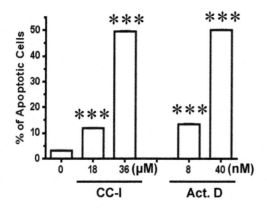

B. Necrotic cell death

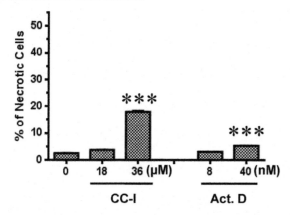

Figure 4. CC-I-induced cell death in CCF-STTG1 cells. Cell death was monitored with apoptotic and necrotic cell markers after 48 hours CC-I exposure in CCF-STTG1 cells. Cell death was determined with the recombinant annexin V conjugated to fluorescein, followed by flow cytometric analysis. Apoptotic cell death is shown in panel A. Panel B is necrotic cell death. Actinomycin D was used as a positive control to induce apoptotic cell death. The percentage of apoptotic cells following CC-I treatment was increased in a dose-dependent manner in CCF-STTG1 cells. There was not a pronounced dose dependent increase in necrotic cell death in the CCF-STTG1 cells until the higher concentration. Data assessed using Student t test and displayed as means ± SEM. Some error bars are too small to be visible. The symbols indicate a significant difference compared to the control. (***$p<0.001$).

temperature in the dark. The cells were analyzed by flow cytometry (Becton Dickinson, Franklin Lakes, NJ) of emission at 530 nm (e.g. FL1) and >575 nm (e.g. FL3). The cells that are bound by Annexin V illustrate early apoptotic cells. Cells that are reactive for both Annexin V and propidium iodide are necrotic cells.

Gene expression profiling

We used Apoptosis PCR Array (SABiosciences, Frederick, MD) to determine which genes are altered by CC-I in TMZ resistant CCF-STTG1 cells. The PCR Array was performed according to the manufacturer's instructions. In brief, total RNA was extracted from vehicle (0.1% DMSO) treated or CC-I treated CCF-STTG1 cell lines using qPCR-Grade RNA Isolation kit. One µg of RNA was used for first strand cDNA synthesis by reverse transcription with MMLV reverse transcriptase. Then real-time PCR was performed with diluted cDNA and master mix with ROX filter.

For signal detection, the ABI Prism 7900 Sequence Detector System was programmed with an initial sterilization step of 2 minutes at 50°C, followed by 10 minutes denaturation at 95°C and then 40 cycles for 15 second at 95°C, 1 minute at 60°C and 30 second at 72°C. Each reaction sample was performed in triplicate. PCR Array data was calculated by the ΔΔcycle threshold (ΔΔCt) method, then normalized against multiple housekeeping genes and expressed as mean fold changes in CC-I treated samples relative to vehicle treated control samples.

Cell cycle analysis

For cell cycle analysis, CCF-STTG1 cells were cultured overnight at a density of $2-5 \times 10^6$ cells per flask. The following day, the cells were treated with different concentrations of CC-I in fresh cell culture medium. After 24–48 hr later, the adherent cells were harvested and split (1×10^6 cells per tube) for washing with HANK's buffer, then fixed in ice-cold 70% ethanol overnight at −20°C. For DNA staining day, the cells were incubated with propidium iodide (100 µg/ml) and RNase A (20 µg/ml) for 15 min at 4°C (protect from light). Samples were analyzed using BD FACS Calibur Flow Cytometry Analyzer.

Topoisomerase relaxation and decatenation assay

DNA relaxation and kinetoplast DNA (kDNA) decatenation assay was performed using topoisomerase I or II drug screening kit or Topopoisomerase II assay kit (TopoGEN, Inc., Port Orange, FL) according to the manufacturer's instructions [30]. Topoisomerase IIα decatenates kDNA which consists of highly catenated networks of circular DNA in an ATP-dependent reaction to yield individual minicircles of DNA. In brief, for topoisomerase IIα mediated kDNA decatenation assay, the 20 µL reaction mixture contains following components; 50 mM Tris-HCl, pH 8.0, 150 mM NaCl, 10 mM $MgCl_2$, 0.5 mM dithiothreitol, 30 µg/mL bovine serum albumin, 2 mM ATP, 260 ng of kDNA, several concentrations of compounds, and 4 U of human topoisomerase IIα. The final concentration of 0.5% (v/v) DMSO was used because this concentration does not affect activity of topoisomerase IIα. The incubation of assay mixture was carried out at 37°C for 30 minutes and terminated by the addition of 4 µL stop loading dye. The kDNA decatenation products from the reaction mixture was resolved on a 1% agarose gel at 100 V for 40 minutes, then stained with 0.5 µg/mL ethidium bromide in TAE buffer (4 mM Tris base/glacial acetic acid [0.11% (v/v)]/2 mM Na_2EDTA).

Molecular modeling study

The molecular modeling studies were based on the X-ray crystal structure of human topoisomerase IIα bound to L-peptide at 1.50 Å resolution (PDB identification code: 2q5a) [31]. The position of the L-peptide was used to specify the dimensions of the CC-I binding site for the docking study. Docking between topoisomerase IIα protein and CC-I was carried out using the GLIDE program (Grid Based Ligand Docking from Energetics, from Schrödinger, L.L.C.) [32,33]. The Jorgensen OPLS-2005 force field was employed in the GLIDE program. The optimal binding geometry for each model was obtained with GLIDE, which relies upon Monte Carlo sampling techniques coupled with energy minimization. GLIDE SP (Standard Precision mode) was used to dock the compound CC-I followed by GLIDE XP (Extra Precision mode). Schrödinger's LigPrep was used to generate the 3D conformations of CC-I

Table 1. Gene expression profile of human Apoptosis PCR Array in CC-I treated CCF-STTG1 cells.

Gene Name (Gene Symbol)	GenBank Accession Number	Description	Fold (Compare to control)
BAG-3/BIS (BAG3)	NM_004281	BCL2-associated athanogene 3	up 8.2
BCL-B/Boo (BCL2L10)	NM_020396	BCL2-like 10 (apoptosis facilitator)	up 29.4
BIP1/BP4 (BIK)	NM_001197	BCL2-interacting killer (apoptosis-inducing)	up 9.9
AIP1/API2 (BIRC3)	NM_001165	Baculoviral IAP repeat-containing 3	up 10.4
ILP-2/ILP2 (BIRC8)	NM_033341	Baculoviral IAP repeat-containing 8	up 8.0
ALPS2/FLICE2 (CASP10)	NM_001230	Caspase 10, apoptosis-related cysteine peptidase	up 16.8
MGC119078 (CASP14)	NM_012114	Caspase 14, apoptosis-related cysteine peptidase	up 45.5
Bp50/CDW40 (CD40)	NM_001250	CD40 molecule, TNF receptor superfamily member 5	up 95.1
CD154/CD40L (CD40LG)	NM_000074	CD40 ligand (TNF superfamily, member 5, hyper-IgM syndrome)	up 52.2
CIDE-A (CIDEA)	NM_001279	Cell death-inducing DFFA-like effector a	up 27.3
APT1LG1/CD178 (FASLG)	NM_000639	Fas ligand (TNF superfamily, member 6)	up 33.3
DP5/HARAKIRI (HRK)	NM_003806	Harakiri, BCL2 interacting protein (contains only BH3 domain)	up 66.6
LT/TNFB (LTA)	NM_000595	Lymphotoxin alpha (TNF superfamily, member 1)	up 110.6
ASC/CARD5 (PYCARD)	NM_013258	PYD and CARD domain containing	up 6.3
DIF/TNF-alpha (TNF)	NM_000594	Tumor necrosis factor (TNF superfamily, member 2)	up 703.4
APO2/CD261 (TNFRSF10A)	NM_003844	Tumor necrosis factor receptor superfamily, member 10a	up 22.8
S152/T14 (CD27)	NM_001242	CD27 molecule	up 8.1
4-1BB/CD137 (TNFRSF9)	NM_001561	Tumor necrosis factor receptor superfamily, member 9	up 302.6
CD27L/CD27LG (CD70)	NM_001252	CD70 molecule	up 38.2
CD153/CD30L (TNFSF8)	NM_001244	Tumor necrosis factor (ligand) superfamily, member 8	up 22.3

Statistical Analysis

All of the data was subjected to statistical analysis by the student t-test when comparing two groups. We used one-way ANOVA followed by Tukey-Kramer test for more than two group comparisons to determine if the differences are significant. For comparisons of time course or concentration data we performed repeated measures two-way ANOVA followed by Tukey-Kramer test. Differences among means are considered statistically significant when the p value is less than 0.05. The LC_{50} (50% lethal concentration) of compounds was determined using statistical software (GraphPad Prism 6) as a general indicator of a chemical's toxicity. In the *in vivo* brain tumor model, the tumor volume data was summarized as the mean values with standard errors. The mice survival was compared between the groups using Kaplan-Meier survival analysis with logrank test.

Results

Identification of a cytotoxic compound against TMZ resistant astrocytoma cells

Our screening approach identified a thiobarbituric acid analog and given the identification tag of chemotype compound-I (CC-I). The structure of CC-I is shown in **Figure 1A**. CC-I was cytotoxic to both the TMZ-resistant human astrocytoma cell lines CCF-STTG1 and to TMZ-sensitive SW1088 (**Figure 1B**). The LC_{50} of CC-I to SW1088, U87-MG and CCF-STTG1 cell lines is 13.6 µM, 23.6 µM and 25.4 µM respectively.

Acute toxicity of CC-I in nude mice

Injections of CC-I once a week at 50 or 75 mg/kg body weight were lethal within 7 days. A once a week injection at 35 mg/kg body weight was tolerated. Therefore, we used approximately 70% of the tolerated dose (25 mg/kg body weight) of CC-I concentration for the *in vivo* tumor model study.

Anti-tumor effect of CC-I in the subcutaneous mouse tumor model

To establish the anti-tumor effect of CC-I on astrocytoma cells, we used the immunodeficient nude mouse subcutaneous tumor model injected with either TMZ sensitive SW1088 or TMZ resistant CCF-STTG1 cell lines. The mice with tumors from the CCF-STTG1 cell line showed no evidence of tumor progression following CC-I injections even after the injections ended (**Figure 2A**) whereas in the untreated control group the tumor volume dramatically increased over 7 weeks ($p<0.0001$). The tumors in mice from the SW1088 cell line also failed to progress during the injection period, but the tumor progressed when the CC-I injections were discontinued (**Figure 2A**). We did not take pictures of the tumors. We will consider taking pictures for upcoming experiments. The body weight for the control or CC-I treated mice did not decrease during course of the study (**Figure 2B**).

Anti-tumor effect of CC-I in intracranial brain tumor model

After establishing the *in vivo* efficacy and safety of CC-I against both TMZ sensitive and resistant cell lines in the subcutaneous brain tumor model, we examined the intracranial xenograft brain tumor model. U87-MG or CCF-STTG1 astrocytoma cells were injected into the mouse brain and formed tumors (verified by MRI) ~3 weeks post implantation (**Figure 3A**). None of the untreated control mice survived more than 30 days, and the

A. Cell cycle (day 1)

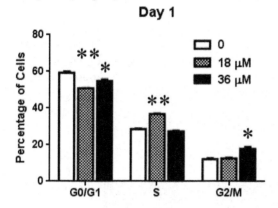

B. Cell cycle (day 2)

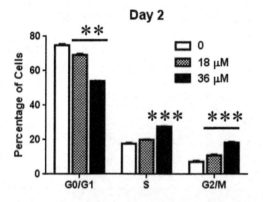

Figure 5. CC-I-induced cell cycle arrest in CCF-STTG1 cells. The CCF-STTG1 cells were treated with 18 or 36 μM of CC-I for 24 or 48 hours. The cells were stained with propidium iodide and then analyzed for cell cycle distribution using a FACScan analyzer. CC-I treatment significantly increased the S and G2/M cell population, but decreased in G0/G1 phase. The symbols indicate a significant difference compared to the control. (*$p<0.05$; **$p<0.01$; ***$p<0.001$).

median survival was 20 days. If the mice were being treated with CC-I, however 64% (7/11) of the U87-MG tumor bearing mice were still alive at 60 days and 89% (8/9) of the CCF-STTG1 tumor bearing mice were still live at 60 days ($p<0.0001$) (**Figure 3B**) and no tumor was visible on MRI (**Figure 3A**). Five mice in the U87-MG tumor group and six in the CCF-STTG1 tumor group receiving CC-I injections were alive 200 days after the tumor injection (137 days after the last CC-I injection). As with the systemic tumor model, there was no indication of liver or kidney toxicity from CC-I in intracranial xenograft mice (**Figure 3C**). The body weight of the animals did not decrease in the animals receiving CC-I (**Figure 3D**).

Apoptosis of CC-I in the TMZ resistant astrocytoma cells

Next we asked whether the cell death by CC-I to the TMZ resistant CCF-STTG1 astrocytoma cells is mediated through an apoptotic pathway. CC-I induced apoptosis in a dose dependent manner in CCF-STTG1 cell lines (**Figure 4A**). The amount of CCF-STTG1 apoptotic cell death at 36 μM was comparable to the positive control apoptosis inducer, actinomycin D. There is evidence of necrotic cell death in CCF-STTG1 following exposure to CC-I, but fewer cells were labeled and significance was not achieved until twice the concentration at which apoptosis was first observed (**Figure 4B**).

Apoptosis gene array in CC-I treated TMZ resistant CCF-STTG1 cells

To determine which apoptotic pathway was activated by CC-I treatment, we performed gene expression profiles using targeted arrays for apoptosis. The Human Apoptosis Microarray revealed that tumor necrosis factor (TNF) pathway genes have the greatest changes in gene expression in the CC-I treated cells compared to the vehicle treated cells. CC-I (36 μM) increased TNF superfamily member 1, 2, 5, 6, and 9 as well as TNF receptor superfamily 5, 9, 10a from 30 to 700 fold. Among caspase pathway genes, only caspase 10 and caspase 14 were induced. The fold ratio of the altered genes is summarized in **Table 1**.

Effect of CC-I on the cell cycle of TMZ resistant astrocytoma cells

To better understand the cytotoxic effect of CC-I, we performed a cell cycle analysis in CCF-STTG1 cells after CC-I treatment. CC-I treatment of CCF-STTG1 cells resulted in a significant decrease in the G0/G1 phase, and an increase in the S and G2/M phase compared to untreated cells (**Figure 5A & B**).

Topoisomerase IIα inhibition by CC-I

We determined whether CC-I can bind human topoisomerase IIα in a molecular modeling study. The molecular modeling data between human topoisomerase IIα and CC-I suggested that CC-I fits into the cavity of human topoisomerase IIα where it could function as an inhibitor (**Figure 6A**). Therefore, we performed DNA relaxation and kDNA decatenation assays to determine the ability of CC-I to inhibit topoisomerase IIα enzyme activity. CC-I inhibited topoisomerase IIα activity in a dose dependent manner. At concentrations greater than 23 μM, CC-I inhibited topoisomerase IIα catalyzed kDNA decatenation (**Figure 6B**). Etoposide (VP16), a known topoisomerase II poison, inhibited topoisomerase IIα at 1 mM but not at 0.1 mM concentration (**Figure 6B**). Next, we determined whether CC-I is a specific inhibitor of topoisomerase IIα using a supercoiled DNA relaxation assay. CC-I did not enhance topoisomerase I-mediated relaxation of supercoiled pHOT1 DNA (**Figure 6C**). Camptothecin, a topoisomerase I inhibitor, was used as a positive control for the assay and showed the expected inhibition of topoisomerase I mediated DNA relaxation. In contrast, CC-I exhibited a strong inhibitory effect on topoisomerase IIα-mediated relaxation of supercoiled pHOT1 DNA (**Figure 6D**). The effective concentration of CC-I on topoisomerase IIα mediated DNA relaxation was first seen at 11 μM.

Comparison of cytotoxicity between CC-I and topoisomerase inhibitors on the astrocytoma cells

We compared the relative toxicity of structurally similar topoisomerase inhibitors using TMZ resistant CCF-STTG1 and T98G cells (**Figure 7A**). The LC_{50} of CC-I for CCF-STTG1 and T98G astrocytomas was approximately 22.5 and 29.1 μM. The LC_{50} concentration for CC-I is significantly lower than that found for merbarone (LC_{50}: >40 μM, $p<0.01$). We observed similar relative toxicity of these compounds on SW1088 and U87-MG cell lines.

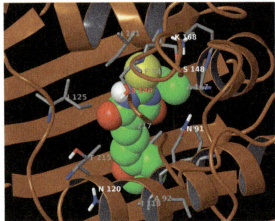
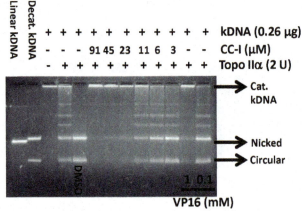
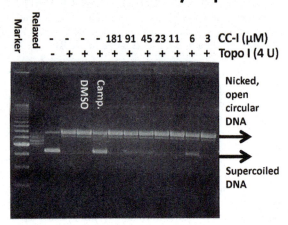
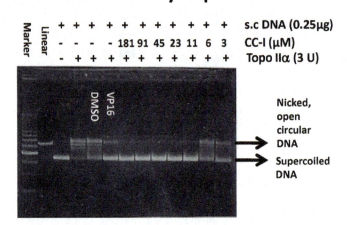

Figure 6. Topoisomerase IIα inhibition by CC-I. (A) Structure of CC-I docked into topoisomerase IIα (pdb code 1ZXM). Topoisomerase is shown as the brown-colored ribbon with residues on the binding site. Carbon atoms of CC-I are colored green, while those of topoisomerase is colored gray. Other atoms are colored according to atom types, i.e., nitrogen-blue, oxygen-red, sulfur-yellow, and polar hydrogen white. Non-polar hydrogen atoms are not shown. (B) The CC-I concentration-dependent inhibition of human topoisomerase IIα-mediated kDNA decatenation. All experiments were carried out according to instructions from the Topogen kit (Port Orange, FL). Reactions contained 4U of enzyme, 0.26 µg of DNA substrate, and different concentrations of the CC-I dissolved in DMSO (0.5% final concentration (v/v)). Different topological forms exhibited different mobility as indicated. Linear, linear kDNA; Decat., decatenated kDNA; Nicked, nicked decatenated kDNA; circular, circular decatenated kDNA; kDNA, kinetoplast DNA. VP16 was used as a positive control. (C) CC-I did not inhibit topo-I mediated supercoiled pHOT1 DNA relaxation. The procedures are described in method section. Camptothecin (camp.) was used as a positive control. (D) CC-I dose dependently inhibited topoisomerase IIα-mediated supercoiled pHOT1 DNA relaxation. VP16 was used as a positive control. s.c DNA, super-coiled DNA.

Cytotoxicity of CC-I on the MGMT promoter methylated and unmethylated GBM cells

We determined the effect of CC-I using several GBM cell lines that have different MGMT promoter methylation status and MGMT protein expression levels. The LN-18 cell line, which has unmethylated MGMT promoter and MGMT protein expression [26,34], is more sensitive to CC-I than CCF-STTG1 or T98G cells (LC_{50}: 9.03 µM, 14.8 µM, and 13.5 µM respectively; p< 0.05) (**Figure 7B**). The latter cells have methylated MGMT promoter [26].

Combination effect of CC-I and TMZ on the TMZ resistant astrocytoma cell line

To test whether CC-I can enhance cytotoxicity of TMZ in astrocytoma cell lines, we determined effect of combination of both drugs (CC-I & TMZ) on the survival of CC-I resistant T98G cell lines. Survival of cells was evaluated following treatment with concentrations of CC-I and TMZ around their respective the LC_{50}. There was an additive effect of both drugs. Cell survival which was significantly (p<0.001) reduced in the combined therapy group compared to single treatment in T98G cells after 3 days exposure (**Figure 8**).

Discussion

The present study investigated the development of anti-tumor compounds for TMZ resistant cancer cell lines. Using TMZ resistant cancer cell lines, we identified a lead compound CC-I which is an analog of thiobarbituric acid. The results of the *in vivo* study demonstrate that CC-I is a safe and effective anti-tumor compound against astrocytoma cell lines, including those shown to be resistant to chemotherapy and radiation. CC-I induced

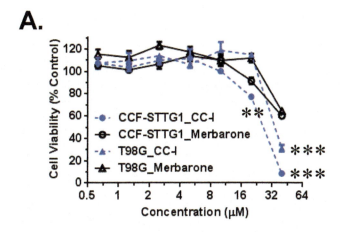

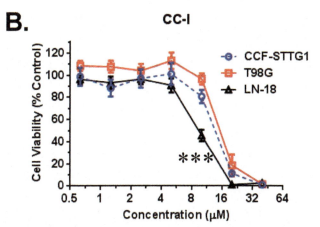

Figure 7. Cytotoxicity of CC-I, merbarone, and combination of CC-I and TMZ on the astrocytoma cells. (A) TMZ-resistant human CCF-STTG1 and T98G cell lines were cultured for 3 days with CC-I and other similar structure topoisomerase II inhibitor (merbarone) followed by cytotoxicity measurement by SRB assay. CC-I showed greater toxicity than merbarone on the astrocytomas. The symbols indicate a significant difference between the merbarone treated and CC-I treated groups (**$p<0.01$; ***$p<0.001$). (B) The MGMT methylated (T98G, CCF-STTG1) or un-methylated (LN-18) astrocytoma cell lines were cultured for 3 days with CC-I and determined cytotoxicity by SRB assay. T98G cells have methylated MGMT promoter, but show weak MGMT expression. CC-I is more cytotoxic to LN-18 cells which has un-methylated MGMT promoter and MGMT expression. The symbol (***) indicates the most difference between the cells ($p<0.001$).

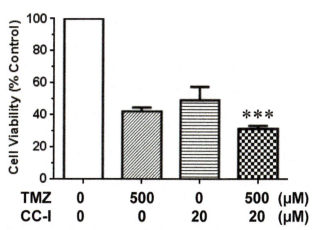

Figure 8. Combination effect of CC-I and TMZ on the T98G astrocytoma cells. T98G cells were cultured for 3 days with CC-I and TMZ, and cytotoxicity was evaluated by SRB assay. Both CC-I and TMZ treatment on the T98G cells showed much more cytotoxic effect than either single treatment. The symbol (***) indicates a significant difference between the control and single treatment groups ($p<0.001$).

apoptosis and cell cycle arrest in astrocytoma cells. Because of its structural similarity to topoisomerase inhibitors, we examined CC-I for topoisomerase inhibition and found it selective for topoisomerase IIα. The cytotoxicity of CC-I is greater than other compounds of similar structure.

We have previously reported that human neuroblastoma cells and human astrocytoma cells lines expressing commonly occurring polymorphisms in the HFE gene were resistant to chemotherapy and radiation [26]. The CCF-STTG1 astrocytoma cell lines that carry the HFE C282Y gene variant were even more resistant to TMZ than T98G or U343-MG cell lines, which are considered standards for TMZ resistance [26,35,36]. The CCF-STTG1 cells are also resistant to geldanamycin, its derivatives, and radiation [26] and less sensitive to merbarone; a compound chemotypically similar to our CC-I compound that reached Phase II clinical trials. Our approach using TMZ resistant astrocytoma cells was successful and identified a lead therapeutic agent, CC-I, with strong cytotoxicity to tumors, prevention of tumor recurrence, and an acceptable safety profile in *in vivo*. Tumors did not return in 45–66% (depending on cell line) of the mice for 151 days after the last injection and the mice were still alive at 200 days of age when the study was terminated.

CC-I belongs to the thiobarbituric acid family. Various barbituric acid derivatives have been studied as anti-inflammatory and anti-cancer compounds [37–39]. Thiobarbituric acid derivatives also have been studied as anti-tumor agents, uridine phosphorylase inhibitors, HIV-1 integrase inhibitors, and hepatitis C virus polymerase inhibitors [40–43]. An example of thiobarbituric acid derivative evaluated as a treatment for brain cancer is merbarone [5-(N-phenylcarboxamido)-2-thiobarbituric acid] which has a similar structure to CC-I. Merbarone is a non-sedating derivative of thiobarbituric acid and induces single strand breaks in DNA apparently without binding to DNA [44,45]. CC-I also shares structural similarity with ICRF-193 which is a bisdioxopiperazine derivative compound. It has been reported that merbarone and ICRF-193 inhibit topoisomerase [46]. The present study demonstrated that CC-I also inhibits topoisomerase activity within a similar concentration range to merbarone but CC-I is more cytotoxic to the TMZ resistant CCF-STTG1 astrocytoma cell lines than these two compounds. The reason for the differences in cytotoxicity may be due to a structural difference between CC-I which has diene motif linking the barbiturate C5 position with the terminal aromatic ring rather than a shorter amide linker as in merbarone. There is also a structure difference in the functional residue at N1 position; CC-I compound has N-ethyl group, but merbarone has a NH residue.

CC-I exposure resulted in S and G2/M arrest in CCF-STTG1 astrocytoma cell line. This observation is consistent with a number of anti-tumor agents such as 9-methoxycamptothecin, topoisomerase II poisons (doxorubicin, etoposide) [47,48]. For example, 9-methoxycamptothecin induced apoptosis through TNF and Fas/FasL pathway, oxidative stress, and G2/M cell cycle arrest in multiple cancer cell lines [47]. Camptothecin, a topoisomerase I poison, also triggers S and G2/M arrest in cancer cell lines [49]. Our PCR array data indicate that CC-I induces cell death through TNF signaling pathway and the Annexin V data indicate cells die via apoptosis. Therefore our present cell cycle analysis study indicates that CC-I has a similar impact on cell cycle and subsequent apoptosis as many anti-cancer compounds.

CC-I was identified by screening against TMZ resistant astrocytoma cells. However, CC-I was also toxic to TMZ sensitive astrocytoma cells (SW1088, U87-MG). In vivo, CC-I showed greater efficacy against TMZ resistant CCF-STTG1 subcutaneous and intracranial tumors than TMZ sensitive astrocytoma cells (**Figure 2A & 3B**). MGMT methylation status influenced CC-I cytotoxicity, but CC-I has a lower LC_{50} than regardless of methylation status compared to TMZ [26]. This finding is important because there is a correlation between MGMT promoter methylation and GBM patient survival [50]. Because of the relative differences in effect based on methylation status (and HFE genotype) we investigate CC-I in combination with TMZ and found the addition of CC-I improves TMZ efficacy in TMZ resistant astrocytoma cell lines. These findings are consistent with several studies reporting a combination effect with an anti-tumor compound and TMZ in TMZ resistant astrocytoma cell lines [51,52]. The data suggest that CC-I could be considered an adjuvant therapy with TMZ. There are many limitations in translating studies, such as ours, that find compounds that show efficacy in animal models to clinical application. Nonetheless, the results of the initial analyses of CC-I warrant further investigation.

In conclusion, we identified an anti-tumor compound for TMZ resistant and sensitive astrocytomas with strong *in vivo* efficacy and safety profiles in mouse tumor models. The cytotoxicity of CC-I is mediated by apoptosis, cell cycle arrest at S and G2/M phase. CC-I has a similar biological profile to other topoisomerase inhibitors but it is smaller and shows effects in orthotopic models, therefore we believe it has more attractive properties than most other topoisomerase inhibitors that allows it access the brain.

Acknowledgments

We thank to the Dr. Mohammed Alsaidi for technical help. We also thank to the Drug Discovery Core at Penn State Hershey for the compounds they provided. We further thank to Dr. Qing Yang for MRI imaging. We thank Dr. Mandy Snyder for her critical reading.

Author Contributions

Conceived and designed the experiments: SYL. Performed the experiments: SYL BS ER AP PAM SS. Analyzed the data: SYL JRC. Contributed to the writing of the manuscript: SYL BS PAM SS JRC.

References

1. Ostrom QT, Gittleman H, Farah P, Ondracek A, Chen Y, et al. (2013) CBTRUS Statistical Report: Primary brain and central nervous system tumors diagnosed in the United States in 2006–2010. Neuro Oncol 15 Suppl 2:ii1–56. doi:10.1093/neuonc/not151.
2. American Cancer Society (2012) Cancer Facts & Figures 2012. Atlanta: American Cancer Society. Available: http://www.cancer.org/research/cancerfactsstatistics/cancerfactsfigures2012/.
3. Stupp R, Mason WP, van den Bent MJ, Weller M, Fisher B, et al. (2005) Radiotherapy plus concomitant and adjuvant temozolomide for glioblastoma. N Engl J Med 352: 987–996.
4. Theeler BJ, Groves MD (2011) High-Grade Gliomas. Curr Treat Options Neurol 13: 386–399.
5. Nishikawa R (2010) Standard therapy for glioblastoma – a review of wehere we are. Neurol Med Chir (Tokyo) 50: 713–719.
6. Friedman HS, Kerby T, Calvert H (2000) TMZ and treatment of malignant glioma. Clin Cancer Res 6: 2585–2597.
7. Atallah E, Flaherty L (2005) Treatment of metastatic malignant melanoma. Curr Treat Options Oncol 6: 185–193.
8. van Brussel JP, Busstra MB, Lang MS, Catsburg T, Schröder FH, et al. (2000) A phase II study of TMZ in hormone-refractory prostate cancer. Cancer Chemother Pharmacol 45: 509–512.
9. Moore MJ, Feld R, Hedley D, Oza A, Siu LL (1998) A phase II study of TMZ in advanced untreated pancreatic cancer. Invest New drugs 16: 77–79.
10. Jakob J, Wenz F, Dinter DJ, Ströbel P, Hohenberger P (2009) Preoperative intensity-modulated radiotherapy combined with TMZ for locally advanced soft-tissue sarcoma. Int J Radiat Oncol Biol Phys 75: 810–816.
11. Park DK, Ryan CW, Dolan ME, Vogelzang NJ, Stadler WM (2007) A phase II trial of oral TMZ in patients with metastatic renal cell cancer. Cancer Chemother Pharmacol 50: 160–162.
12. Marchesi F (2007) Triazene compounds: mechanism of action and related DNA repair systems. Pharmacol Res 56: 275–287.
13. Friedman HS, McLendon RE, Kerby T, Dugan M, Bigner SH, et al. (1998) DNA mismatch repair and O6-alkylguanine-DNA alkyltransferase analysis and response to Temodal in newly diagnosed malignant glioma. J Clin Oncol 16: 3851–3857.
14. Hegi ME, Liu L, Herman JG, Stupp R, Wick W, et al. (2008) Correlation of O6-methylguanine methyltransferase (MGMT) promoter methylation with clinical outcomes in glioblastoma and clinical strategies to modulate MGMT activity. J Clin Oncol 26: 4189–4199.
15. Cahill DP, Levine KK, Betensky RA, Codd PJ, Romany CA, et al. (2007) Loss of the mismatch repair protein MSH6 in human glioblastomas is associated with tumor progression during temozolomide treatment. Clin Cancer Res 13: 2038–2045.
16. Yip S, Miao J, Cahill DP, Lafrate AJ, Aldape K, et al. (2009) MSH6 mutations arise in glioblastomas during temozolomide therapy and mediate temozolomide resistance. Clin Cancer Res 15: 4622–4629.
17. McClendon AK, Osheroff N (2007) DNA topoisomerase II, genotoxicity, and cancer. Mutat Res 623: 83–97.
18. Champoux JJ (2001) DNA topoisomerases: structure, function, and mechanism. Annu Rev Biochem 70: 369–413.
19. Beck WT (1996) DNA topoisomerases and tumor cell resistance to their inhibitors. In: Schilsky R, Milano G, Ratain M, editors. Principles of Antineoplastic Drug Development and Pharmacology (Basic and Clinical Oncology). CRC Press. 487–502.
20. Falaschi A, Abdurashidova G, Sandoval O, Radulescu S, Biamonti G, et al. (2007) Molecular and structural transactions at human DNA replication origins. Cell Cycle 6: 1705–1712.
21. Bruce JN, Fine RL, Canoll P, Yun J, Kennedy BC, et al. (2011) Regression of recurrent malignant gliomas with convection-enhanced delivery of topotecan. Neurosurgery 69: 1272–1279.
22. Minturn JE, Janss AJ, Fisher PG, Allen JC, Patti R, et al. (2011) A phase II study of metronomic oral topotecan for recurrent childhood brain tumors. Pediatr Blood Cancer 56: 39–44.
23. Matsumoto Y, Tamiya T, Nagao S (2005) Resistance to topoisomerase II inhibitors in human glioma cell lines overexpressing multidrug resistant associated protein (MRP) 2. J Med Invest 52: 41–48.
24. Chen Y, Su YH, Wang CH, Wu JM, Chen JC, et al. (2005) Induction of apoptosis and cell cycle arrest in glioma cells by GL331 (a topoisomerase II inhibitor). Anticancer Res 25: 4203–4208.
25. Schmidt F, Knobbe CB, Frank B, Wolburg H, Weller M (2008) The topoisomerase II inhibitor, genistein, induces G2/M arrest and apoptosis in human malignant glioma cell lines. Oncol Rep 19: 1061–1066.
26. Lee SY, Liu S, Mitchell RM, Slagle-Webb B, Hong Y-S, et al. (2011) HFE polymorphisms influence the response to chemotherapeutic agents via induction of p16INK4A. Int J Cancer 129: 2104–2114.
27. de Almeida SF, Picarote G, Fleming JV, Carmo-Fonseca M, Azevedo JE, et al. (2007) Chemical chaperones reduce endoplasmic reticulum stress and prevent mutant HFE aggregate formation. J Biol Chem 282: 27905–27912.
28. Liu Y, Lee SY, Neely E, Nandar W, Moyo M, et al. (2011) Mutant HFE H63D protein is associated with prolonged endoplasmic reticulum stress and increased neuronal vulnerability. J Biol Chem 286: 13161–13170.
29. Lee SY, Patton SM, Henderson RJ, Connor JR (2007) Consequences of expressing mutants of the hemochromatosis gene (HFE) into a human neuronal cell line lacking endogenous HFE. FASEB J 21: 564–576.
30. Gong Y, Firestone GL, Bjeldanes LF (2006) 3,3′-diindolylmethane is a novel topoisomerase IIalpha catalytic inhibitor that induces S-phase retardation and mitotic delay in human hepatoma HepG2 cells. Mol Pharmacol 69: 1320–1327.
31. Wendorff TJ, Schmidt BH, Heslop P, Austin CA, Berger JM (2012) The structure of DNA-bound human topoisomerase II alpha: conformational mechanisms for coordinating inter-subunit interactions with DNA cleavage. J Mol Biol 424: 109–124.
32. Friesner RA, Banks JL, Murphy RB, Halgren TA, Klicic JJ, et al. (2004) Glide: a new approach for rapid, accurate docking and scoring. 1. Method and assessment of docking accuracy. J Med Chem 47: 1739–1749.
33. Halgren TA, Murphy RB, Friesner RA, Beard HS, Frye LL, et al. (2004) Glide: a new approach for rapid, accurate docking and scoring. 2. Enrichment factors in database screening. J Med Chem 47: 1750–1759.
34. Mellai M, Monzeglio O, Piazzi A, Caldera V, Annovazzi L, et al. (2012) MGMT promoter hypermethylation and its associations with genetic alterations in a series of 350 brain tumors. J Neurooncol 107: 617–631.
35. Kanzawa T, Germano IM, Kondo Y, Ito H, Kyo S, et al. (2003) Inhibition of telomerase activity in malignant glioma cells correlates with their sensitivity to TMZ. Br J Cancer 89: 922–929.

36. Uzzaman M, Keller G, Germano IM (2007) Enhanced proapoptotic effects of tumor necrosis factor-related apoptosis-inducing ligand on TMZ-resistant glioma cells. J Neurosurg 106: 646–651.
37. Cebo B, Krupinska J, Mazur J, Piotrowicz J (1980) Antiinflammatory activity of the new aminomethyl derivatives of 1-cyclohexyl-5-alkyl and 1-cyclohexyl-5,5-dialklbarbituric acids. Farmaco Sci 35: 248–252.
38. Brewer AD, Minatelli JA, Plowman J, Paull KD, Narayanan VL (1985) 5-(N-phenylcarboxamido)-2-thiobarbituric acid (NSC 336628), a novel potential antitumor agent. Biochem Pharmacol 34: 2047–2050.
39. Singh P, Kaur M, Verma P (2009) Design, synthesis and anticancer activities of hybrids of indole and barbituric acids-identification of highly promising leads. Bioorg Med Chem Lett 19: 3054–3058.
40. Balas VI, Hadjikakou SK, Hadjiliadis N, Kourkoumelis N, Light ME, et al. (2008) Crystal structure and antitumor activity of the novel zwitterionic complex of tri-n-butyltin(IV) with 2-thiobarbituric acid. Bioinorg Chem Appl 654137. doi:10.1155/2008/654137.
41. Balas VI, Verginadis II, Geromichalos GD, Kourkoumelis N, Male L, et al. (2011) Synthesis, structural characterization and biological studies of the triphenyltin(IV) complex with 2-thiobarbituric acid. Eur J Med Chem 46: 2835–2844.
42. Rajamaki S, Innitzer A, Falciani C, Tintori C, Christ F, et al. (2009) Exploration of novel thiobarbituric acid-, rhodanine- and thiohydrantoin-based HIV-1 integrase inhibitors. Bioorg Med Chem Lett 19: 3615–3618.
43. Lee JH, Lee S, Park MY, Myung H (2011) Characterization of thiobarbituric acid derivatives as inhibitors of hepatitis C virus NS5B polymerase. Virol J 8: 18. doi:10.1186/1743-422X-8-18.
44. Warrell RP Jr, Muindi J, Stevens YW, Isaacs M, Young CW (1989) Induction of profound hypouricemia by a non-sedating thiobarbiturate. Metabolism 38: 550–554.
45. Glover A, Chun HG, Kleinman LM, Cooney DA, Plowman J, et al. (1987) Merbarone: an antitumor agent entering clinical trials. Invest New Drugs 5: 137–143.
46. Drake FH, Hofmann GA, Mong SM, Bartus JO, Hertzberg RP, et al. (1989) In vitro and intracellular inhibition of topoisomerase II by the antitumor agent merbarone. Cancer Res 49: 2578–2583.
47. Wang H, Ao M, Wu J, Yu L (2013) TNFα and Fas/FasL pathways are involved in 9-Methoxycamptothecin-induced apoptosis in cancer cells with oxidative stress and G2/M cell cycle arrest. Food Chem Toxicol 55: 396–410.
48. Kolb RH, Greer PM, Cao PT, Cowan KH, Yan Y (2012) ERK1/2 signaling plays an important role in topoisomerase II poison-induced G2/M checkpoint activation. PLoS One 7: e50281. doi:10.1371/journal.pone.0050281.
49. Bhonde MR, Hanski ML, Notter M, Gillissen BF, Daniel PT, et al. (2006) Equivalent effect of DNA damage-induced apoptotic cell death or long-term cell cycle arrest on colon carcinoma cell proliferation and tumour growth. Oncogene 25: 165–175.
50. Melguizo C, Prados J, González B, Ortiz R, Concha A, et al. (2012) MGMT promoter methylation status and MGMT and CD133 immunohistochemical expression as prognostic markers in glioblastoma patients treated with temozolomide plus radiotherapy. J Transl Med 10: 250. doi:10.1186/1479-5876-10-250.
51. Vlachostergios PJ, Hatzidaki E, Befani CD, Liakos P, Papandreou CN (2013) Bortezomib overcomes MGMT-related resistance of glioblastoma cell lines to temozolomide in a schedule-dependent manner. Invest New Drugs 31: 1169–1181.
52. Peigñan L, Garrido W, Segura R, Melo R, Rojas D, et al. (2011) Combined use of anticancer drugs and an inhibitor of multiple drug resistance-associated protein-1 increases sensitivity and decreases survival of glioblastoma multiforme cells in vitro. Neurochem Res 36: 1397–1406.

Sodium-Glucose Transporter-2 (SGLT2; SLC5A2) Enhances Cellular Uptake of Aminoglycosides

Meiyan Jiang[1], Qi Wang[1], Takatoshi Karasawa[1], Ja-Won Koo[1,2], Hongzhe Li[1], Peter S. Steyger[1]*

[1] Oregon Hearing Research Center, Oregon Health & Science University, Portland, Oregon, United States of America, [2] Department of Otorhinolaryngology, Seoul National University College of Medicine, Bundang Hospital, Seongnam, Gyeonggi, Republic of Korea

Abstract

Aminoglycoside antibiotics, like gentamicin, continue to be clinically essential worldwide to treat life-threatening bacterial infections. Yet, the ototoxic and nephrotoxic side-effects of these drugs remain serious complications. A major site of gentamicin uptake and toxicity resides within kidney proximal tubules that also heavily express electrogenic sodium-glucose transporter-2 (SGLT2; SLC5A2) in vivo. We hypothesized that SGLT2 traffics gentamicin, and promotes cellular toxicity. We confirmed in vitro expression of SGLT2 in proximal tubule-derived KPT2 cells, and absence in distal tubule-derived KDT3 cells. D-glucose competitively decreased the uptake of 2-(N-(7-nitrobenz-2-oxa-1,3-diazol-4-yl)amino)-2-deoxyglucose (2-NBDG), a fluorescent analog of glucose, and fluorescently-tagged gentamicin (GTTR) by KPT2 cells. Phlorizin, an SGLT2 antagonist, strongly inhibited uptake of 2-NBDG and GTTR by KPT2 cells in a dose- and time-dependent manner. GTTR uptake was elevated in KDT3 cells transfected with SGLT2 (compared to controls); and this enhanced uptake was attenuated by phlorizin. Knock-down of SGLT2 expression by siRNA reduced gentamicin-induced cytotoxicity. In vivo, SGLT2 was robustly expressed in kidney proximal tubule cells of heterozygous, but not null, mice. Phlorizin decreased GTTR uptake by kidney proximal tubule cells in $Sglt2^{+/-}$ mice, but not in $Sglt2^{-/-}$ mice. However, serum GTTR levels were elevated in $Sglt2^{-/-}$ mice compared to $Sglt2^{+/-}$ mice, and in phlorizin-treated $Sglt2^{+/-}$ mice compared to vehicle-treated $Sglt2^{+/-}$ mice. Loss of SGLT2 function by antagonism or by gene deletion did not affect gentamicin cochlear loading or auditory function. Phlorizin did not protect wild-type mice from kanamycin-induced ototoxicity. We conclude that SGLT2 can traffic gentamicin and contribute to gentamicin-induced cytotoxicity.

Editor: Ines Armando, Universtiy of Maryland School of Medicine, United States of America

Funding: The colony-founding Sglt2+/− mice were a gift of the Wellcome Trust Sanger Institute (Hinxton, Cambridge, UK). This work was supported by NIH-NDCD grants R01 DC004555, R01 DC012588 (PSS), R03 DC011622 (HL), and P30 DC005983 [URL: https://www.nidcd.nih.gov/]. The funding agencies had no role in study design, data collection and analysis, preparation of the manuscript, or decision to publish.

Competing Interests: The authors have declared that no competing interests exist.

* Email: steygerp@ohsu.edu

Introduction

Aminoglycoside antibiotics, like gentamicin, are essential important clinically for treating critical gram-negative bacterial infections, and are frequently used worldwide [1,2]. Both infants and adults receive gentamicin for bacterial meningitis, endocarditis, septicemia and for prophylaxis in premature births and surgical cases. Unfortunately, the nephrotoxic and ototoxic side-effects of gentamicin therapy remain serious complications, limiting the clinical use of gentamicin [3]. Gentamicin-induced nephrotoxicity, characterized by proximal tubular necrosis without morphological changes in glomerular structures, can cause acute kidney failure and increased morbidity [4,5]. Acute renal toxicity is largely reversible because kidney tubule cells can proliferate to replace cells lost to aminoglycoside toxicity [6].

The mechanism of gentamicin-induced cytotoxicity is incompletely understood. Gentamicin can induce cell death mechanisms via mitochondrial damage and caspase activation [7–9], as well as the generation of toxic levels of reactive oxygen species [10,11]. Since it is difficult to inhibit the wide variety of cell death mechanisms that may be induced by gentamicin, an alternative strategy to prevent gentamicin-induced cytotoxicity is to block drug entry into cells. Gentamicin and other aminoglycosides are known to enter cells via at least two mechanisms: endocytosis and permeation through non-selective cation channels. In the kidney, the best characterized entry route for lumenal gentamicin is apical endocytosis and trafficking of gentamicin-laden endosomes to the Golgi complex and endoplasmic reticulum (ER) prior to release into the cytosol from the ER [12,13]. A non-endocytotic entry route for gentamicin into kidney cells has been demonstrated in vitro – via permeation of non-selective cation channels, presumptively transient receptor potential (TRP) channels [14,15]. Proximal tubule cells are presumed to be more pharmacologically sensitive to gentamicin because these cells take up and retain the drug. Distal tubule cells, however, are more resistant to gentamicin, most likely because they do not readily take up or retain gentamicin in the cytoplasm [14,16]. Another distinguishing feature is the abundant expression of sodium-glucose transporter-2 (SGLT2; a.k.a. SLC5A2) in proximal, but not distal, tubule cells [17,18].

SGLT2 is a low affinity, high capacity sodium-glucose electrogenic transporter of glycosides expressed in proximal tubules, and is responsible for ~90% of glucose resorption from the renal ultrafiltrate [18,19]. Antagonism of SGLT2 activity induces glycosuria [20,21] and aminoaciduria [22]. Aminoglycosides also induce glycosuria [23,24], and nephrotoxicity, predominantly within the proximal tubules [25]. The structure of SGLT2 resembles the major facilitator superfamily of transporters with a large, hydrophilic, elastic vestibule, an internal pore diameter of ~3 nm, and an exit pore (into cytosol) of ~1.5–2.5 nm [26,27], sufficiently large to potentially allow permeation by gentamicin. Non-lethal mutations in SGLT2 occur in humans, with little impact on kidney function besides glucosuria and aminoaciduria, with no reported loss of hearing acuity [22,28,29]. Several SGLT2 antagonists have been identified, including phlorizin, a hydrolyzable O-glucoside, several non-hydrolyzable antagonists including O-glycosides (sergliflozin [30], remogliflozin [20]) and C-glycosides (dapagliflozin [31], canagliflozin [21,32]). These non-hydrolyzable antagonists are being, or have been tested, to reverse Type II diabetes in mice [21,30,33] and humans [34].

We hypothesized that SGLT2 can traffic gentamicin into cells, and tested whether SGLT2 expression and was required for accelerated onset of gentamicin-induced toxicity in cell lines. If this hypothesis is correct, then loss of the SGLT2 function *in vivo* should reduce cellular uptake of gentamicin and protect against cytotoxicity. If so, this could potentially prevent nephrotoxicity and ototoxicity during gentamicin therapy.

Materials and Methods

Ethics Statement

The care and use of all animals reported in this study were approved by the Animal Care and Use Committee of Oregon Health & Science University (IACUC approval #IS00001801).

Conjugation and purification of GTTR

Gentamicin-Texas Red conjugate (GTTR) was produced as previously described [15,35–37]. Briefly, an excess of gentamicin (Sigma, MO, USA) in 0.1 M potassium carbonate (pH 10) was mixed with Texas Red (TR) succinimidyl esters (Invitrogen, CA) to minimize the possibility of over-labeling individual gentamicin molecules with more than one TR molecule, and to preserve the polycationic nature of the conjugate [38]. After conjugation, reversed phase chromatography, using C-18 columns (Grace Discovery Sciences, IL), was used to purify GTTR from unconjugated gentamicin, and potential contamination by unreacted TR [39]. The purified GTTR conjugate was aliquoted, lyophilized, and stored desiccated, in the dark at $-20°C$ until required.

Cell culture

The mouse kidney proximal tubule (KPT2) and distal tubule (KDT3) cell lines were generated and characterized as previously described [14,40]. These cell lines were maintained in DMEM with 10% FBS, without streptomycin or penicillin, at 37°C.

Competition and inhibition experiments

Cells plated on 8-well chambered coverslips were washed with DMEM twice and incubated as described below. To establish appropriate competition experiments, KPT2 cells were incubated with 0.4 mM 2-(N-(7-nitrobenz-2-oxa-1,3-diazol-4-yl)amino)-2-deoxyglucose (2-NBDG) (Life Technologies, NY, USA) without or with 1:1, 1:50 or 1:1000 molar ratios of D-glucose (Sigma, MO, USA) in DMEM. 2-NBDG (0.4 mM) was also incubated without or with 1:1, 1:10 or 1:50 molar ratios of phlorizin (Pfaltz & Baue, CT, USA) at 37°C for 20 mins. Phlorizin was solubilized in Dimethyl sulfoxide (DMSO) (Final concentration of DMSO in buffer was <0.001%) prior to dilution in buffer to the required concentration. Cells were washed three times with PBS prior to fixation with 4% paraformaldehyde for 15 minutes.

To examine the effect of D-glucose on GTTR uptake by KPT2 cells, cells plated on chambered coverslips were washed with DMEM twice, co-incubated with GTTR (5 μg/mL, gentamicin base, gentamicin: ~450–477 g/mol; GTTR: ~1100 g/mol) and 1:40, 1:2000 or 1:40000 molar ratios of D-glucose for 20 minutes in DMEM at 37°C, with 5% CO_2, then washed with PBS three times to remove GTTR from extracellular media prior to fixation with 4% paraformaldehyde containing 0.5% Triton X-100 (FATX) for 15 minutes at room temperature. To examine the effect of phlorizin on the uptake of GTTR by KPT2 cells, cells were co-incubated with 5 μg/mL GTTR and 1:5, 1:10 or 1:20 molar ratios of phlorizin at 37°C for 20 mins respectively prior to washing and fixation.

To examine the effect of sodium on GTTR uptake by KPT2 cells, Na^+ free buffer was made up as follows: 140 mM choline chloride, 5 mM KCl, 2.5 mM $CaCl_2$, 1 mM $MgSO4$, 1 mM KH_2PO4, and 10 mM HEPES (pH 7.4); choline chloride was replaced 140 mM NaCl in Na^+ buffer. GTTR uptake experiments were performed described as above.

GTTR uptake and confocal microscopy

The cellular distribution of fluorescence was examined using a Bio-Rad 1024 ES scanning laser system. For each individual set of images to be compared, the same confocal settings were used, with two acquisition images per well, two wells per experimental condition, and each experiment performed at least three times to confirm consistency of experimental data. GTTR fluorescent pixel intensities were obtained by histogram function of the ImageJ software after removal of nuclei and intercellular pixels using Adobe Photoshop. Pixel intensities were statistically compared within each set of images per experiment, and not compared between replicate experiments due to varying acquisition settings to obtain the best dynamic range. To normalize data between experimental sets, the mean intensity was ratioed against the standard (e.g., GTTR only cells) and plotted [15].

Immunofluorescence

For immunolocalization of SGLT2, paraformaldehyde-fixed cells were washed in PBS, immunoblocked in 1% serum in PBS for 30 min and incubated with polyclonal anti-SGLT2 antisera (rabbit, Abcam, MA, USA; or goat, Santa Cruz Biotechnology, TX, USA) at room temperature for 1 hour. After washing with 1% serum in PBS, specimens were further incubated with 1:200 Alexa-488-conjugated goat-anti-rabbit or donkey anti-goat antisera (Invitrogen, CA) for 1 hour at room temperature, washed, post-fixed with 4% paraformaldehyde for 15 min, rinsed and mounted under coverslips with VectorShield (Vector Labs, CA). In vitro studies, when double-labeled for SGLT2 plus GTTR, cells were permeabilized by 0.5% Triton X-100 after immunolabeling.

Immunoblotting

Kidney and cochlear tissues were analyzed by immunoblot as described before [41–44]. Briefly, total protein extracts were prepared by homogenizing tissues in T-PER tissue protein extraction buffer (Thermo Scientific, IL, USA) with protease inhibitor (Sigma, MO, USA), and the total protein concentration determined using the bicinchoninic acid (BCA) assay. Protein samples (100 μg) were separated by 4–20% pre-cast polyacrylamide gel (Bio-Rad, CA, USA), transferred to polyvinylidene difluoride membranes (Millipore Corporation, MA, USA), blocked with 5% non-fat milk and then incubated at 4 C overnight with goat (1:50; Santa Cruz, CA, USA) or rabbit (1:50; Abcam, MA, USA) polyclonal antibodies against SGLT2 in 5% non-fat milk. Rabbit polyclonal antibodies against anti-actin (1:1000; Sigma, MO, USA) were also used as an internal standard. Peroxidase-conjugated anti-goat (1:1000) or anti-rabbit (1:2500) antisera were used to localize primary antisera and visualized using an ECL-Plus detection kit (Thermo Scientific, IL, USA), documented with a photoscanner and analyzed with the Fiji (freeware) program.

KDT3-SGLT2 cell line generation

Mouse SGLT2 cDNA from Open Biosystems (Clone ID: 4235707) was amplified by PCR, using primers 5'-TTT GAA TTC GCC ACC ATG GAG CAA CAC GTA GAG-3' and 5'-CCC GTC GAC TTA TGC ATA GAA GCC CCA GAG-3', digested with EcoRI/SalI, and subcloned into pBabe-puro vector. The resultant plasmid was transfected into Phoenix Eco packaging cell using Lipofectamine 2000. After 48 hours, the retrovirus-containing medium was collected, diluted (1:500) with growth medium and added to mouse kidney distal tubule KDT3 cells in DMEM with 10% FBS. Culture medium was changed again after 24 h and puromycin was added at 2.5 μg/ml to select for retrovirus-infected cells. From dozens of surviving cells after several days of puromycin treatment, several clones were selected, expanded and used for GTTR uptake experiments as described above. Puromycin was not applied during GTTR uptake experiments.

Transfection and cell viability measurement

Cell viability was determined by the reduction of 3-(4,5-dimethylthiazol-2-yl)-2,5-diphenyltetrazolium bromide (MTT), an indicator of mitochondrial dehydrogenase activity, as previously described [40,45]. Briefly, KPT2 cells were plated at 3000 cells per well in a 96-well plate. After incubation overnight to allow cells to attach to the plate, cells were treated with small interfering RNA (siRNA) and control for SGLT2 (Invitrogen, CA). Transfection of siRNA was performed using Lipofectamine RNAiMAX (Invitrogen, CA). After 48 hours, transfected cells were treated with gentamicin (5 or 10 mM) in DMEM (10% FBS) for 1, 2 or 3 days. Subsequently, 20 μl of 5 mg/ml MTT solution was added to each well, and cells incubated for 4 h at 37°C, 5% CO_2. Culture medium was then replaced with 200 μl DMSO in each well and the optical density recorded at 540 nm with background subtraction at 660 nm. Student's t-test was used for statistical analysis [40,45].

Mice

$Sglt2^{+/-}$ mice were obtained from the Wellcome Trust Sanger Institute (Hinxton, Cambridge, UK), and an in-house colony established from these founders. Homozygous mice were generated either by crossing heterozygotes together or by crossing heterozygotes with homozygotes. Littermates of wild-type and heterozygotes served as controls. A PCR-based genotyping method was used to identify mutant and wild-type alleles. The mutant allele was identified using primers Slc5a2_55706_F: 5'-AGC AGG AGG GTT CAG GCA GG -3' and CAS_R1_term_x: 5'-TCG TGG TAT CGT TAT GCG CC -3' (172-bp product). The wild type allele was identified using primers Slc5a2_55706_F and Slc5a2_55706_R: 5'-TTT TGC GCG TAC AGA CCA TC -3' (412-bp product).

Mice (21–28 days old) received an intra-peritoneal (i.p.) injection of 800 mg/kg phlorizin (200 μg/μl phlorizin in 40% DMSO, pH 7.4; 4 μl/g), or the vehicle alone. Thirty minutes later, mice received an i.p. injection of 2 mg/kg GTTR (in sterile PBS, pH 7.4). After a further 30 minutes, cardiac serum was collected from deeply-anesthetized mice prior to cardiac perfusion with PBS, then 4% paraformaldehyde. Kidneys and cochleae were excised and post-fixed in FATX, and processed for immunofluorescence [39].

Determination of gentamicin levels in serum and in cells

Serum levels of gentamicin and the gentamicin epitope of GTTR were determined via enzyme-linked immunosorbent assay (ELISA). Serum supernatant was further diluted, centrifuged and protein extracted as needed for ELISA. Measurement of total gentamicin levels in serum was determined according to the manufacturers' instructions (EuroProxima, Arnhem, the Netherlands).

For cellular levels of gentamicin or the gentamicin epitope of GTTR, KPT2 cells were plated in 60 mm dishes and incubated at 37°C, with 5% CO_2 overnight. After washing with DPBS, cells were incubated in 5 μg/mL GTTR or 1 mM gentamicin and 1:5, 1:10 or 1:20 molar ratios of phlorizin respectively, as described above. After 20 minutes, cells were washed with DPBS three times and proteins extracted. The quantity of cell protein was measured by BCA protein assay kit. Gentamicin ELISAs were performed described as above.

Auditory testing

ABR thresholds to pure tones were obtained to evaluate hearing function. Wild-type, $Sglt2^{+/-}$ and $Sglt2^{-/-}$ mice were anesthetized and placed on a heating pad in a sound-proof, electrically isolated chamber. Needle electrodes were placed subcutaneously below the test ear, at the vertex, and with a ground on the claw. Each ear was stimulated separately with a closed tube sound delivery system sealed into the ear canal. The auditory brain-stem response to a 1-ms rise-time tone burst at 4, 8, 16, 24, and 32 kHz was recorded. Threshold was defined as an evoked response of 0.2 mV [46,47]. ABR thresholds were obtained both before and 30 minutes after phlorizin treatment in wild-type mice, and in $Sglt2^{+/-}$ and $Sglt2^{-/-}$ mice 6 and 12 weeks of age. In addition, ABRs were also obtained before and after aminoglycoside treatment.

Toxicity studies

Since immunofluorescence may not detect SGLT2 in the cochlea, toxicity studies with aminoglycosides in the presence or absence of phlorizin were conducted. Dosing with gentamicin to induce ototoxicity *in vivo* causes systemic toxicity in mice, therefore wild-type mice were treated with a similar aminoglycoside - kanamycin in the presence or absence of phlorizin [48]. ABR thresholds were obtained before kanamycin dosing. Four groups of mice were used: group 1, sterile Dulbecco's PBS (DPBS) only in the same delivery routes as for subsequent groups; group 2, 800 mg/kg kanamycin in DPBS twice daily, subcutaneously, for 14 days; group 3, 800 mg/kg kanamycin in DPBS twice daily, subcutaneously, plus DMSO vehicle only, i.p., for 14 days; group 4, 800 mg/kg kanamycin in DPBS twice daily, subcutaneously, plus phlorizin (100 mg/kg in DMSO, i.p.) for 14 days. Phlorizin was injected twice daily 15 minutes prior to each kanamycin injection. Subsequently, mice were allowed to recover for 3 weeks before final ABR thresholds were obtained to determine any permanent ABR threshold shift and mice euthanized.

Statistics

All *in vitro* experiments were performed multiple times to validate the observations, with the data expressed as means ± SEM. Statistical analysis was conducted using the nonparametric *t* test for comparison of 2 groups or ANOVA for comparisons of 3 groups (GraphPad Prism). For *in vivo* experiments, cytoplasmic GTTR fluorescence in kidney proximal tubules was compared between phlorizin treatment and control group. ABR thresholds (or threshold shifts) at each tested frequency were compared between $Sglt2^{-/-}$ mice and control mice, or between treatment groups in the kanamycin toxicity study, by nonparametric t-test (GraphPad Prism). A confidence level of 95% was considered statistically significant. *$p<0.05$ and **$p<0.01$.

Results

Uptake of a fluorescent glucose analog, 2-NBDG, was inhibited by phlorizin, an SGLT2 antagonist

We verified the presence (or absence) of SGLT2 immunoexpression in previously-characterized murine KPT2 and KDT3 cell [14]. SGLT2 was specifically immunolocalized at the periphery of KPT2 cells, but not KDT3 cells (Fig. 1A, B, respectively), presumptively at the cell membrane. Cellular uptake of the fluorescent glucose analog, 2-NBDG, is mediated by both SGLTs and also by facilitated glucose transporters (GLUTs) [49]. In KPT2 cells, 2-NBDG fluorescence was primarily localized at the cell periphery (Fig. 1C). Increasing concentrations of D-glucose (Fig. 1 C–F, K), or the SGLT2 antagonist phlorizin (Fig. 1 G–J, L), dose-dependently reduced 2-NBDG fluorescence in KPT2 cells. This demonstrated the presence of robust SGLT2 activity in KPT2 cells.

SGLT2-mediated uptake of GTTR by KPT2 cells can be competitively inhibited

GTTR is a fluorescently-tagged gentamicin conjugate used to visually test for gentamicin permeation of non-selective cation channels into cells [15,50–53]. We used phlorizin, an SGLT2 antagonist [54] or D-glucose to test whether SGLT2 was potentially GTTR-permeation. Increasing doses of phlorizin (Fig. 2 A–E) and D-glucose (Fig. 2 F, Fig. S1) significantly decreased GTTR fluorescence in KPT2 cells. We then used ELISA technology to verify the imaging data, and found that phlorizin reduced both GTTR and native gentamicin uptake by KPT2 cells in a dose-dependent manner (Fig. 2 G, H), validating GTTR as a tracer for gentamicin studies. Thus, SGLT2-mediated uptake of GTTR by KPT2 cell can be antagonized or competitively-inhibited.

SGLT2-mediated uptake of GTTR by KPT2 cells can be inhibited by Na$^+$ free buffer

SGLT2 is a Na$^+$-ligand symporter [55]. We examined whether GTTR uptake by KPT2 cells was attenuated in Na$^+$-free buffer after 5, 10 or 20 minutes at 37°C. GTTR fluorescence in KPT2 cells in Na$^+$-free buffer was significantly attenuated (~20%) after 20 minutes (Fig. 3 A). We used phlorizin to further verify this data over time. Phlorizin also significantly inhibited ~20% GTTR uptake of KPT2 cells, most consistently at the 20 minute timepoint (Fig. 3 B), and this timepoint was chosen for the majority of subsequent experiments. Thus, SGLT2 accounts for ~20% of total GTTR uptake in SGLT2-expressing KPT2 cells.

Enhanced GTTR uptake by KDT3 cells heterologously expressing SGLT2

To test if SGLT2 can enhance cellular uptake of GTTR, stable cell lines expressing SGLT2 were generated using KDT3 cells that do not endogenously express SGLT2 (Fig. 1 B). KDT3-derived cell lines expressing SGLT2 (KDT3-SGLT2) and empty vector control cell lines (KDT3-pBabe) retained the parental KDT3 morphology (Fig. S2). Immunofluorescence revealed expression of SGLT2 in most KDT3-SGLT2 cells, with negligible immunofluorescence for SGLT2 in KDT3-pBabe cells (Fig. 4 A, G and D, J respectively).

Following a 20 minute incubation with GTTR, robust GTTR uptake was present in KDT3-SGLT2 cells immunolabeled for SGLT2, but not in control KDT3-pBabe cells lacking SGLT2 immunofluorescence (Fig. 4 B, E). Pixel intensity analysis revealed statistically significant increases in GTTR fluorescence within KDT3-SGLT2 cells compared to that of control KDT3-pBabe cells (Fig. 4 M). In the presence of phlorizin (100 μg/ml), GTTR fluorescence in KDT3-SGLT2 cells was significantly less than in KDT3-SGLT2 cells treated without phlorizin (Fig. 4 B, H, respectively). In addition, GTTR fluorescence in phlorizin-treated KDT3-SGLT2 cells was not significantly different to KDT3-pBabe cells with or without phlorizin treatment (Fig. 4 M), demonstrating the specificity of phlorizin for SGLT2 in these cells. Thus, exogenous expression of SGLT2 in KDT3 cells facilitated GTTR uptake.

Knock-down of SGLT2 reduced gentamicin-induced cytotoxicity

To test whether SGLT2 contributes to gentamicin-induced cytotoxicity, we transfected KPT2 cells with siRNA for SGLT2 to knock-down protein expression of SGLT2 prior to drug exposure. Immunofluorescence confirmed that SGLT2 siRNA reduced SGLT2 expression compared to control siRNA-transfected cells (Fig. 5 A–H). The effect of SGLT2 siRNA was apparent 1 day after transfection and further reduced SGLT2 expression 2 days after transfection (Fig. 5 A–D). This knock-down of SGLT2 expression lasted at least 5 days (Fig. 5 A–H). Two days after transfection with control or SGLT2 siRNA, KPT2 cells were treated with gentamicin (5 mM or 10 mM) for 1, 2 or 3 days, prior to MTT assay for cell viability [40,45]. Control and SGLT2 siRNA-transfected cells showed no difference in viability (Fig. S3), demonstrating that loss of SGLT2 did not affect cell viability. Although gentamicin reduced cell viability, SGLT2 knock-down attenuated the degree of gentamicin-induced toxicity, most significantly at 2 or 3 days of gentamicin treatment (Fig. 5 I). Thus, KPT2 cells with SGLT2 expression were more susceptible to gentamicin-induced cytotoxicity than KPT2 cells with SGLT2 knock-down, suggesting that SGLT2 trafficking of gentamicin contributed to gentamicin-induced cytotoxicity.

Immunoexpression of SGLT2 in renal and cochlear tissues *in vivo*

To determine if SGLT2 is appropriately located for gentamicin uptake *in vivo*, the immunoexpression of SGLT2 was characterized in fixed renal proximal tubules and cochleae *in situ* using two different antibodies. In the kidney, as previously described [17,18,56], SGLT2 was immunolocalized at the apical brush border membranes of wild-type renal proximal tubule cells, but not in adjacent distal tubule regions (Fig. 6 A, C), nor in the kidney of $Sglt2^{-/-}$ mice (Fig. 6 B, D). In the cochlea, the rabbit anti-SGLT2 antibody did not label wild-type marginal cells above background (Fig. 6 E), or exhibited non-specificity in marginal cells of $Sglt2^{-/-}$ mice (Fig. 6 F). The goat anti-SGLT2 antibody consistently exhibited non-specific fluorescence in marginal cells of $Sglt2^{-/-}$ mice (Fig. 6 H) similar to that observed in wild-type marginal cells (Fig. 6 G). Both SGLT2 antibodies consistently exhibited a punctate labeling pattern within the intra-stria vascularis (Fig. 6 I, K) that was not present in $Sglt2^{-/-}$ mice

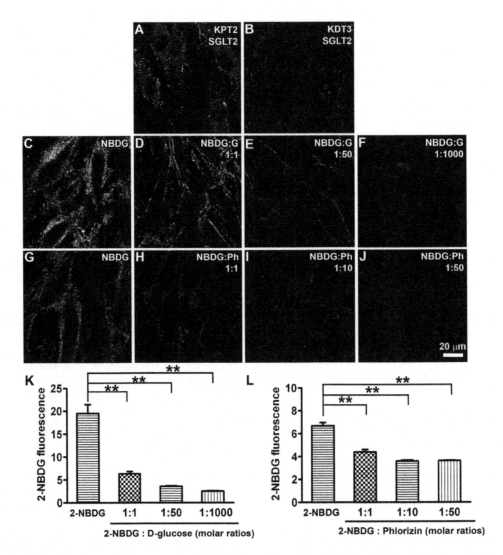

Figure 1. Uptake of the fluorescent glucose analog 2-NBDG is mediated by SGLT2 in KPT2 cells. KPT2 cells (A) had robust SGLT2 immunolabeling compared to KDT3 cells (B). Increasing doses of (C–F) D-glucose (molar ratios of 1:0, 1:1, 1:50 or 1:1000 [2-NBDG/D-glucose]), or (G–J) phlorizin (molar ratios of 1:0, 1:1, 1:10 or 1:50 [2-NBDG/phlorizin]) dose-dependently decreased 2-NBDG fluorescence in KPT2. Scale bar = 20 μm. (K, L). The fluorescence intensity of 2-NBDG in KPT2 cells was significantly decreased with increasing doses of D-glucose (K) or phlorizin (L; **$p<0.01$).

(Fig. 6 G, L). Immunoblotting revealed SGLT2 protein expression in kidneys of wild-type and $Sglt2^{+/-}$ mice, but not in $Sglt2^{-/-}$ mice (Fig. 6 M). Immunoblotting of wild-type cochlear tissues detected actin, but not SGLT2 (data not shown), indicative of the low level expression of SGLT2 protein in cochlear tissues. PCR-based genotyping demonstrated the absence of wild-type alleles in $Sglt2^{-/-}$ mice (Fig. 6 N).

Phlorizin decreased renal uptake and increased serum levels of GTTR *in vivo*

Since phlorizin had no effect on the bactericidal activity of gentamicin on *E. coli* by disk diffusion assay (Table S1), the *in vitro* data suggested that phlorizin may decrease cellular uptake of GTTR *in vivo* and potentially reduce aminoglycoside-induced cytotoxicity *in vivo*. To test whether phlorizin decreased cellular uptake of GTTR *in vivo*, the intensity of cytoplasmic GTTR fluorescence was determined in proximal tubule cells of $Sglt2^{+/-}$ and $Sglt2^{-/-}$ mice. In $Sglt2^{+/-}$ mice, rabbit anti-SGLT2 immunolabeling was co-localized with GTTR fluorescence in proximal, but not distal tubule cells (Fig. 7 A–C). GTTR fluorescence was diffusely distributed throughout the cytoplasm, and intensely localized at the brush border of proximal tubule cells of $Sglt2^{+/-}$ mice that received GTTR plus vehicle only *in vivo* (Fig. 7 D). Phlorizin pre-treatment visibly reduced cytoplasmic GTTR fluorescence within proximal tubule cells and at their brush border (Fig. 7 E, F). In $Sglt2^{-/-}$ mice, unexpectedly, GTTR fluorescence was diffusely distributed throughout the cytoplasm, and intense fluorescence at the brush border of proximal tubule cells (Fig. 7 G), as observed in untreated $Sglt2^{+/-}$ mice (Fig. 7 D). Phlorizin had no significant effect on the intensity (uptake) or distribution of GTTR fluorescence in proximal tubule cells of $Sglt2^{-/-}$ mice (Fig. 7 H, I). Thus, SGLT2 is not required for renal proximal tubule uptake of GTTR in $Sglt2^{-/-}$ mice, although GTTR uptake by these cells can be acutely inhibited by the SGLT2 antagonist, phlorizin, in $Sglt2^{+/-}$ mice.

In $Sglt2^{+/-}$ mice, phlorizin increased serum levels of both gentamicin and GTTR levels compared to vehicle-treated mice (Fig. 7 J, K). In $Sglt2^{-/-}$ mice, phlorizin had no effect on serum levels of gentamicin or GTTR (Fig. 7 J, K). Gentamicin and

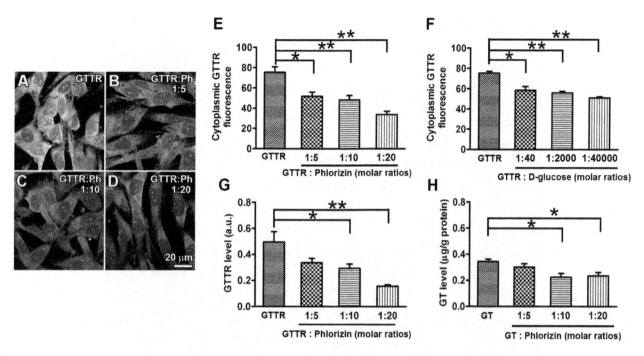

Figure 2. SGLT2-mediated uptake of GTTR can be competitively inhibited. (A–D) Cells were treated with 5 μg/ml GTTR for 20 minutes at 37°C with a dose-range of phlorizin (molar ratios of 1:0, 1:5, 1:10 or 1:20 [GTTR:phlorizin]) in DMEM buffer. Scale bar = 20 μm. Increasing doses of (E) phlorizin or (F) D-glucose (molar ratios of 1:0, 1:40, 1:2000 or 1:40000 [GTTR:D-glucose]) reduced GTTR fluorescence in KPT2 cells (*$p<0.05$; **$p<0.01$). Cell ELISAs demonstrated that (G) GTTR or (H) gentamicin levels in KPT2 cells are decreased by increasing doses of phlorizin.

GTTR serum levels in $Sglt2^{-/-}$ mice were significantly higher than in $Sglt2^{+/-}$ mice (Fig. 7 J, K). Thus, loss of SGLT2 function, by antagonism, or by gene deletion, increases serum levels of gentamicin.

Phlorizin did not affect cochlear uptake of GTTR or auditory function

To test whether the low levels of SGLT2 immunofluorescence in the cochlea (Fig. 6) were required for cochlear uptake of GTTR, we examined whether phlorizin modulated the distribution of GTTR in murine cochleae of $Sglt2^{+/-}$ and $Sglt2^{-/-}$ mice. Mice were injected with GTTR 30 minutes after phlorizin or vehicle injection. In the stria vascularis, GTTR was characteristically localized in marginal and intermediate cells (Fig. 8) as previously described [35]. The nucleoplasm of marginal cell nuclei displayed negligible fluorescence (Fig. 8 A, C, E, G), as expected. There were no significant differences in the uptake or distribution of GTTR fluorescence between phlorizin- and vehicle-treated groups of $Sglt2^{+/-}$ or $Sglt2^{-/-}$ mice (Fig. 8 A–H). As observed in the kidney, SGLT2 was not required for cochlear uptake of GTTR in $Sglt2^{-/-}$ mice, and this uptake could not be inhibited by acute exposure to phlorizin in either $Sglt2^{+/-}$ or $Sglt2^{-/-}$ mice.

In wild-type mice, no statistically significant changes in auditory brainstem response (ABR) thresholds were observed after intraperitoneal (i.p.) injection with 800 mg/kg phlorizin or vehicle [DMSO; Fig. S4]. Furthermore, $Sglt2^{-/-}$ mice displayed no significant differences in ABR thresholds at 6 or 12 weeks of age compared to wild-type or $Sglt2^{+/-}$ (Fig. 8 I, J), and gender differences were minimal (Fig. S5). Thus, auditory function was not affected by phlorizin antagonism, or genomic loss of functional SGLT2.

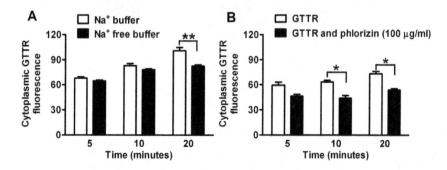

Figure 3. SGLT2-mediated uptake of GTTR by KPT2 cells was inhibited by Na⁺ free buffer. (A) KPT2 cells were incubated with GTTR for 5 minutes, 10 minutes or 20 minutes at 37°C in Na⁺ free buffer or Na⁺ buffer. GTTR fluorescence of KPT2 cell in Na⁺ buffer for 20 minutes was more intense than in Na⁺ free buffer (**$p<0.01$). (B) KPT2 cells were treated with GTTR and phlorizin in DMEM buffer. GTTR uptake by KPT2 cells was also inhibited by phlorizin (100 μg/ml) over time (*$p<0.05$).

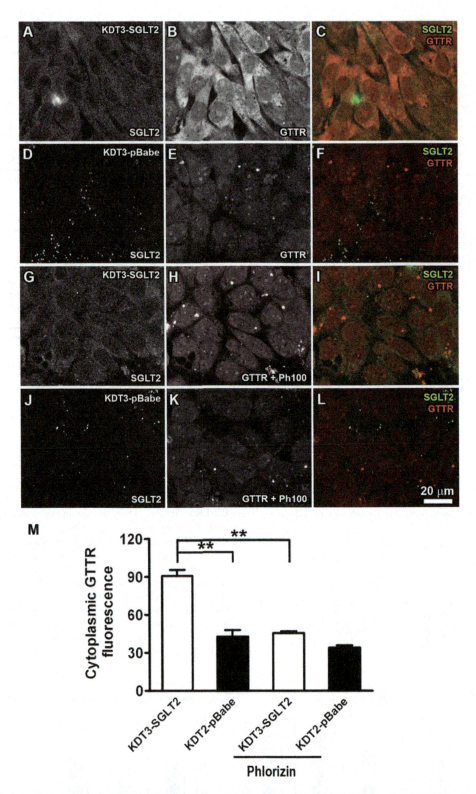

Figure 4. Heterologous expression of SGLT2 in KDT3 cells increased cellular uptake of GTTR. (A–C) KDT3-SGLT2 cells with positive SGLT2 immunofluorescence displayed robust GTTR uptake (B, C). (D–F) Empty vector control clones (KPT2-pBabe) showed negligible SGLT2 immunofluorescence (D) and weak, uniform levels of GTTR fluorescence (E, F) compared to (B, C). (H, I) GTTR fluorescence in KDT3-SGLT2 cells in the presence of phlorizin (100 μg/ml) was visibly less intense than in KDT3-SGLT2 cells without phlorizin treatment (B, C). (K, L) GTTR fluorescence in phlorizin-treated KDT3-pBabe cells showed weak levels of GTTR fluorescence as untreated in KDT3-pBabe cells (E, F). Scale bar = 20 μm. (M) Fluorescence intensities of GTTR in KDT3-SGLT2 or KDT3-pBabe cells in the presence or absence of phlorizin (100 μg/ml; **$p<0.01$).

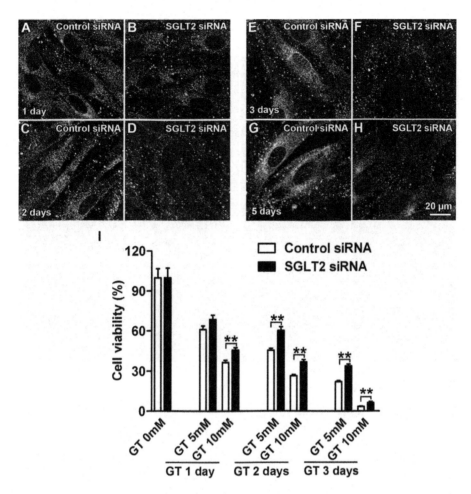

Figure 5. Knockdown of SGLT2 reduced gentamicin-induced cytotoxicity. (A–H) KPT2 cells transfected with siRNA for SGLT2 showed reduced immunoexpression of SGLT2 compared with cells transfected with control siRNA. (A–D) The effect of SGLT2 siRNA began within 1 day of transfection and was most apparent 2 days of transfection. (A–H) The effect SGLT2 siRNA tranfection lasted for at least 5 days. (I) MTT assay on cells (2-days post-transfection) treated with gentamicin for 1, 2 or 3 days revealed greater viability of SGLT2 siRNA-transfected KPT2 cells compared with KPT2 cells treated with control siRNA (**$p<0.01$).

Toxicity studies

Dosing wild-type mice with gentamicin *in vivo* causes systemic toxicity prior to induction of ototoxicity [48]. To test whether chronic phlorizin exposure ameliorates aminoglycoside cochleotoxicity as assessed by ABR threshold shifts, toxicity studies with another aminoglycoside, kanamycin, using a well-established protocol [48], in the presence or absence of phlorizin were conducted in wild-type mice. ABR threshold shifts were obtained before and after kanamycin dosing. In mice treated with just DPBS, insignificant threshold shifts were observed 3 weeks after dosing (Fig. 9; Fig. S6). In mice treated with kanamycin in DPBS, threshold shifts were observed at 32 kHz that were statistically significant compared with the DPBS-only group (Fig. 9; Fig. S6). In mice treated with kanamycin plus DMSO (vehicle for phlorizin), threshold shifts were observed at 16 and 32 kHz compared with the DPBS-only group, however, these thresholds shifts were significantly different only at 32 kHz (Fig. 9; Fig. S6). Mice treated with kanamycin plus phlorizin had statistically significant threshold shifts at 4, 8, 16 and 32 kHz compared with the DPBS-only group (Fig. 9; Fig. S6). The kanamycin plus phlorizin group also had threshold shifts were significantly different at 4, 8 and 16 kHz compared to the kanamycin in DPBS group (Fig. 9; Fig. S6). No significant differences in threshold shifts were observed between the kanamycin plus phlorizin and kanamycin plus DMSO groups (Fig. 9; Fig. S6). Thus, phlorizin did not protect auditory function from kanamycin-induced ototoxicity, and unexpectedly exacerbated drug-induced hearing loss at lower frequencies.

Discussion

Here we report evidence, for the first time, that the electrogenic sodium-glucose transporter SGLT2 contributes to the cellular uptake of aminoglycosides, particularly by proximal tubule cells that highly express SGLT2 [17,18,56]. *In vitro*, SGLT2-mediated uptake of 2-NBDG and GTTR was inhibited by phlorizin and D-glucose. Cellular uptake of GTTR was enhanced by heterologous expression of SGLT2 in KDT3 cells. Knock-down of SGLT2 expression by siRNA reduced gentamicin-induced cytotoxicity in KPT2 cells endogenously expressing SGLT2, further suggesting SGLT2 involvement in cellular uptake of gentamicin and subsequent cytotoxicity. *In vivo*, we observed SGLT2 immunoexpression at the apical brush border region of kidney proximal tubule cells, and phlorizin pre-treatment can acutely inhibit GTTR uptake by proximal tubules in *Sglt2*[+/−] mice. Loss of SGLT2 function increased serum levels of gentamicin and GTTR.

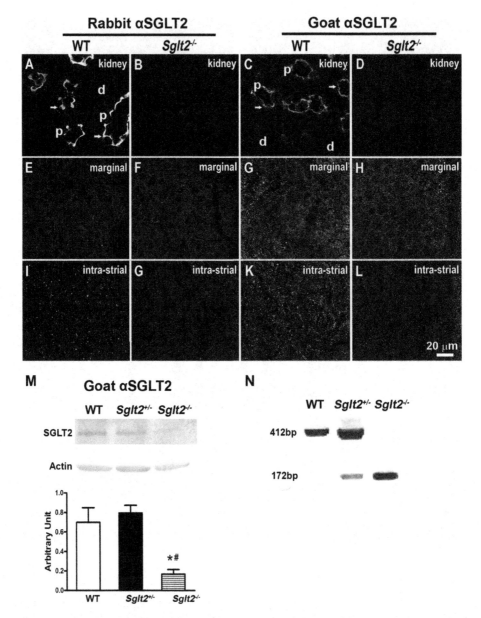

Figure 6. SGLT2 immunofluorescence in the kidney and cochlea. Two different SGLT2 antibodies were used, a rabbit polyclonal IgG to synthetic peptide derived from residues 250–350 of human SGLT2 and a goat polyclonal IgG against a murine peptide sequence within the N-terminal extracellular domain of SGLT2. (A, C) In wild-type mice, SGLT2 was immunolocalized at the apical membranes (arrows) of proximal tubules (p), but not in adjacent glomerular (not shown) or distal tubule (d) regions. (B, D) In $Sglt2^{-/-}$ mice, no immunoexpression for renal SGLT2 was observed with either antibody. (E, F) No labeling above background was observed in cochlear marginal cells of wild-type or $Sglt2^{-/-}$ mice with rabbit antisera for SGLT2. (G, H) Goat antisera for SGLT2 produced labeling patterns in cochlear marginal cells of both wild-type mice and $Sglt2^{-/-}$ mice, suggestive if substantial non-specificity in this cell type. (I, K) In the intra-strial layer of wild-type mice, predominantly composed of both marginal and intermediate cells, both antisera exhibited a punctate labeling pattern not observed in $Sglt2^{-/-}$ mice (J, L). Scale bar = 20 μm. (M) Immunoblotting with the goat antibody for SGLT2 revealed SGLT2 protein expression in wild-type and $Sglt2^{+/-}$ mice, but not $Sglt2^{-/-}$ mice. The ratio of SGLT2 to actin expression in kidney tissues of wild-type and $Sglt2^{+/-}$ mice were significantly higher than that in $Sglt2^{-/-}$ mice. There was no statistical difference in SGLT2 protein expression between wild-type and $Sglt2^{+/-}$ mice. (N) Genotyping demonstrated the absence of wild-type SGLT2 alleles in $Sglt2^{-/-}$ mice.

However, loss of SGLT2 function by phlorizin or gene knockout did not affect auditory function or cochlear uptake of GTTR. Phlorizin treatment exacerbated drug-induced hearing loss at lower frequencies.

Aminoglycosides enter cells, including kidney proximal tubule cells, via an endocytosis pathway [13,57–60]. However, aminoglycoside exposure also generates reactive oxygen species within seconds in euthermic cells at room temperature, precluding endocytosis [61,62]. Aminoglycosides also enter cells via non-selective cation channels, including TRP channels and the TRP-like mechanoelectrical transduction channels of sensory hair cells in the inner ear [15,35,51,53,63]. Identifying the molecular mechanisms by which aminoglycosides can enter cells, and particularly kidney proximal tubule and cochlear cells, is crucial

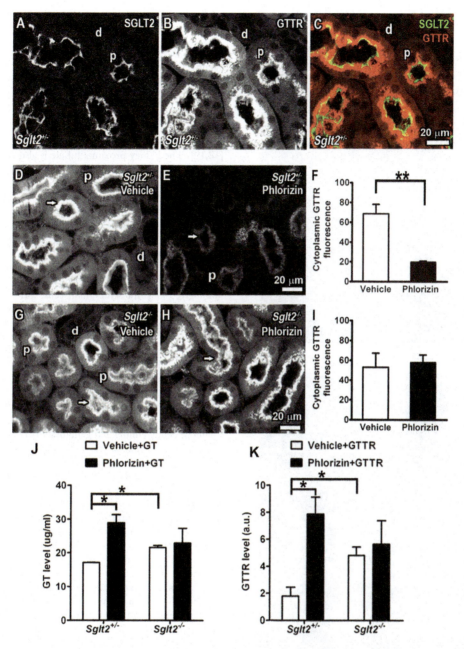

Figure 7. Phlorizin decreased renal GTTR uptake, and increased serum drug levels *in vivo*. (A) In $Sglt2^{+/-}$ mice, rabbit anti-SGLT2 immunolabeling was predominantly localized at the apical, lumenal region of proximal tubules (p), with negligible labeling in distal tubules (d). (B) GTTR fluorescence was most intense (as saturated puncta) in the apical region of proximal tubules (p), with less intense diffuse labeling in the cytoplasm of these same cells. Very weak and only diffuse GTTR fluorescence was observed in the cytoplasm of distal tubule cells (d). (C) Merged image showing colocalization of SGLT2 (green) and GTTR (red) in proximal tubules. (D–F) When $Sglt2^{+/-}$ mice were pre-treated with phlorizin, significantly reduced GTTR fluorescence was observed in the cytoplasm and apical brush border (arrows) of proximal tubule cells (E) compared to untreated mice (D, F; **$p<0.01$). (G, I) In $Sglt2^{-/-}$ mice, GTTR fluorescence was diffusely distributed throughout the cytoplasm of proximal tubule cells, with intense fluorescence at the apical brush border. (H, I) Phlorizin had no effect on the uptake, distribution or intensity of GTTR fluorescence in $Sglt2^{-/-}$ proximal tubule cells (**$p<0.01$). Scale bar = 20 µm. (J, K) In $Sglt2^{+/-}$ mice, phlorizin pre-treatment significantly increased both gentamicin and GTTR serum levels compared to vehicle treated control mice (*$p<0.05$). In $Sglt2^{-/-}$ mice, phlorizin did not significantly change gentamicin or GTTR serum levels. However, serum levels of gentamicin or GTTR serum level were significantly higher in $Sglt2^{-/-}$ mice than in $Sglt2^{+/-}$ mice in the absence of phlorizin treatment (*$p<0.05$).

to develop effective strategies to protect these pharmacologically-sensitive cells during clinically-essential gentamicin pharmacotherapy.

In the kidney, glomerular filtrate has ~150 mM Na^+ compared to intracellular levels of 12 mM, driving the inward electrogenic activity of Na^+-ligand symporters present on the lumenal (apical) membrane of proximal tubule cells [55]. Proximal tubule cells also express high levels of SGLT2, a Na^+-ligand symporter that traffics glycosides like glucose, facilitating the renal resorption of 90% of lumenal glucose from glomerular filtrate in promixal tubules

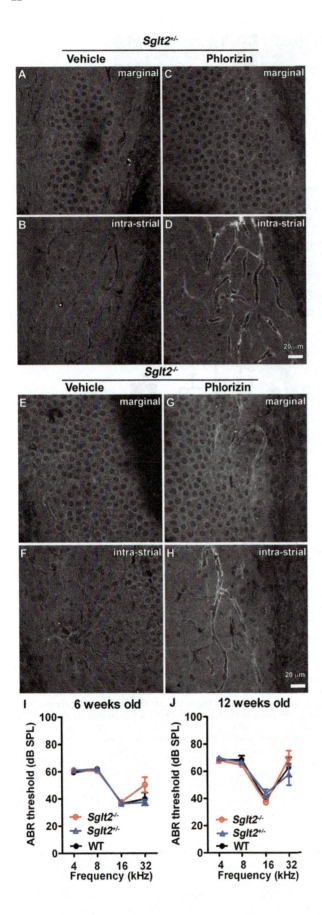

Figure 8. Loss of SGLT2 function had no effect on cochlear uptake of GTTR or auditory function. In the stria vascularis, GTTR was localized in marginal (A, E) and intermediate (B, F) cells of $Sglt2^{+/-}$ (A, B) and $Sglt2^{-/-}$ (E, F) mice. The nucleoplasm of marginal and intermediate cell nuclei displayed weak labeling. (C, D, G, H) Phlorizin had no effect on the uptake or distribution of GTTR fluorescence in the stria vascularis of $Sglt2^{+/-}$ or $Sglt2^{-/-}$ mice. Scale bar = 20 µm. (I, J) Wild-type, $Sglt2^{+/-}$ and $Sglt2^{-/-}$ mice, at 6 or 12 weeks of age, displayed no significant differences in ABR thresholds.

[18,19]. The kidney proximal tubule is also a primary location of aminoglycoside-induced nephrotoxicity [24,25,64].

In the cochlea, loop diuretics enhance the cochlear uptake of aminoglycosides [65]. Loop diuretics inhibit the $Na^+K^+Cl^-$ co-transporter (NKCC) [66], predominantly localized on the basolateral membrane of marginal cells [65,66], increasing the intra-strial concentration of Na^+ [65]. If SGLT2 is localized on the basolateral membrane of marginal cells, as implicated by the discrete, yet low level, of immunoexpression within the stria vascularis, SGLT2 may be appropriately located to traffic aminoglycosides into marginal cells, prior to clearance into endolymph, and uptake by hair cells as shown previously [36]. As noted above, SGLT2 has a large, hydrophilic, elastic vestibule, with an internal pore diameter of ~3 nm, and an exit pore (into cytosol) of ~1.5–2.5 nm [26,27] that is sufficiently large to potentially allow permeation by gentamicin. SGLT2 is blocked with high affinity by non-hydrolyzable glycoside derivatives that are generally well-tolerated acutely [30,33,67]. Thus, SGLT2 appeared to be rationally-identified candidate aminoglycoside transporter, and this hypothesis drove our experiments.

Fluorescently-conjugated gentamicin, GTTR, has been used to characterize the endocytotic trafficking of aminoglycosides to their intracellular domains in the kidney [12,13]. Although the relative molecular mass (g/mol) and minimum cross-sectional diameter (mcd) of GTTR is larger than that of untagged gentamicin (gentamicin, 440–470 g/mol, mcd, 0.81 nm, GTTR, ~1100 g/mol, mcd, ~1.47 nm), GTTR can also permeate non-selective cation channels, with a sufficiently large pore diameter, directly into cytoplasm [15,35,51]. Using GTTR, we have previously shown that cytoplasmic uptake of GTTR can occur rapidly at low temperatures, precluding endocytosis, and is regulated by cellular potential, pH, extracellular cations (Ca^{2+}, Gd^{3+}, La^{3+}), and non-specific cation channel blockers such as Ruthenium Red (RR), and verified using immunocytochemistry [15]. These properties are indicative of molecular permeation of ion channels, as for another fluorescent dye, FM 1–43 [68].

Using previously-described murine kidney cell lines [14], we observed specific SGLT2 immunofluorescence in proximal (KPT2), but not distal tubule (KDT3) cell lines, and in proximal tubules, but not distal tubules, *in vivo*. D-glucose is a primary substrate for SGLT2, which can also traffic the fluorescent glucose analog 2-NBDG. We found that a 1-fold molar excess of D-glucose competitively decreased 2-NBDG uptake by KPT2 cells. A 40-fold molar excess of D-glucose can also significantly decrease GTTR uptake of KPT2 cells. Thus, GTTR appears to have a greater affinity for SGLT2 than D-glucose and 2-NBDG. Uptake of 2-NBDG by KPT2 cells was also strongly inhibited by phlorizin, demonstrating robust SGLT2 activity in these cells, although not as efficaciously as D-glucose. Phlorizin also significantly decreased KPT2 uptake of GTTR and gentamicin in a dose-dependent manner by both immunofluorescence and ELISA. The uptake of GTTR was significantly attenuated ~20% by phlorizin or Na^+-free buffer, suggesting that this proportion of total GTTR uptake by KPT2 cells was mediated by SGLT2. Heterologous expression

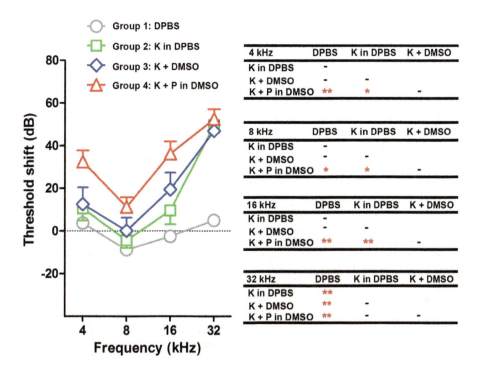

Figure 9. Phlorizin does not ameliorate kanamycin-induced ototoxicity. Three weeks after dosing, mice treated with kanamycin in DPBS or mice treated with kanamycin plus DMSO (vehicle for phlorizin) had significant ABR threshold shifts at 32 kHz only compared to mice treated with DPBS only (**$p<0.01$). The kanamycin plus phlorizin group had significantly different threshold shifts at 4, 8 and 16 kHz compared to the kanamycin in DPBS group; and significantly different threshold shifts at 4, 8, 16 and 32 kHz compared DPBS only group (*$p<0.05$; **$p<0.01$). However, no significant threshold shifts were observed between kanamycin plus phlorizin (in DMSO) and kanamycin plus DMSO groups.

of SGLT2 in distal tubule-derived KDT3 cells significantly enhanced GTTR uptake, and this enhanced uptake can be abolished by phlorizin. The residual uptake of GTTR in these cells after phlorizin treatment likely represents GTTR uptake via previously-identified gentamicin-permeant cation channels, as demonstrated previously [14,15,69]. Furthermore, siRNA knockdown of SGLT2 expression in KPT2 cells reduced cellular susceptibility to gentamicin-induced cytotoxicity. Phlorizin had no apparent effect on the bactericidal activity of gentamicin on *E. coli* by disk diffusion assay. These *in vitro* data suggested that phlorizin, or other SGLT2 antagonists, may decrease cellular uptake of GTTR *in vivo*, and protect cells against aminoglycoside-induced cytotoxicity *in vivo*.

In vivo, we used two antisera for SGLT2 to determine if SGLT2 was appropriately located to contribute to aminoglycoside trafficking in the kidney and cochlea. Both antisera provided specific localization for SGLT2 in renal proximal tubules, with weak, less defined immunoexpression for SGLT2 in the cochlear stria vascularis (Fig. 5), and negligible SGLT2 immunolabeling in the organ of Corti. Although the SGLT2 inhibitor – phlorizin – acutely decreased GTTR uptake in proximal tubules of $Sglt2^{+/-}$ mice (Fig. 7), phlorizin did not inhibit cochlear uptake of GTTR of $Sglt2^{+/-}$ and $Sglt2^{-/-}$ mice (Fig. 8). It is not known whether phlorizin crosses the blood-brain barrier or the blood-labyrinth barrier, which may have limited its efficacy of blocking cochlear SGLT2. We also speculate (Fig. S7) that phlorizin inhibition, if any, of low cochlear levels of SGLT2-mediated GTTR trafficking would be compensated by phlorizin-induced elevation of GTTR serum levels (Fig. 7). Elevated serum levels of GTTR would increase trafficking into the cochlea via other residual cellular mechanisms of aminoglycoside uptake, e.g., endocytosis [12,13] or ion channel permeation [14,15]. However, genomic loss of SGLT2 function, unexpectedly, did not reduce GTTR uptake by proximal tubules compared to $Sglt2^{+/-}$ mice. Phlorizin did not alter proximal tubule uptake of GTTR in $Sglt2^{-/-}$ mice (Fig. 7), indicating that phlorizin had negligible effects on the cellular uptake of aminoglycosides in $Sglt2^{-/-}$ mice, acting specifically on SGLT2 in $Sglt2^{+/-}$ mice. Thus, renal GTTR uptake by $Sglt2^{-/-}$ mice likely occurs via compensatory mechanisms such as endocytosis or aminoglycoside-permeant cation channels, as discussed above. In addition, genomic loss of SGLT2 function and phlorizin-pretreatment in $Sglt2^{+/-}$ mice elevated serum levels of gentamicin or GTTR (compared to control-treated heterozygous $Sglt2^{+/-}$ mice; Fig. 7). This may be the result of a reduced volume of distribution for these compounds, and/or by a reduced glomerular filtration rate (GFR) [70], providing an alternate explanation for the reduced GTTR cytoplasmic and punctate fluorescence in proximal tubule cells. However, phlorizin did not alter serum levels of gentamicin or GTTR in $Sglt2^{-/-}$ mice (Fig. 7) due to the absence of a binding partner (*i.e.*, SGLT2) that facilitates aminoglycoside trafficking, further indicating the specificity of phlorizin for SGLT2.

There is no demonstrable nephrotoxicity or renal damage following kanamycin treatment (at 700–900 mg/kg per dose twice daily for 14 days) to induce ototoxicity in mice [48], as used here. To test for permanent changes in auditory performance, a recovery period of three weeks is optimal [48]. In mice, gentamicin at doses to induce ototoxicity causes systemic toxicity and mortality [48,71]. Phlorizin or genomic loss of SGLT2 function did not affect auditory function, suggesting that SGLT2 activity is not required for cochlear function, and that glucose transport into the cochlea can be achieved by other transporters such as facilitated GLUTs [72,73]. Whether GLUTs are aminoglycoside-permeant remains uncertain, as crystal structures have yet to be determined. Phlorizin, and genomic loss of SGLT2, did not reduce cochlear uptake of GTTR. Phlorizin did not protect auditory function from kanamycin-induced ototoxicity in wild-type mice. Crucially, neither phlorizin nor genomic loss of SGLT2 increased serum levels of aminoglycosides. Thus, we did not attempt to repeat the ototoxicity studies with $Sglt2^{-/-}$ mice.

In summary, SGLT2 increased cellular uptake of gentamicin and exacerbated gentamicin-induced cytotoxicity *in vitro*. Acute inhibition of SGLT2 function reduced gentamicin-induced cytotoxicity in kidney proximal tubule cells, *in vitro*, and may reduce the risk of gentamicin-induced nephrotoxicity in the kidney *in vivo*. Acute inhibition, but not chronic loss, of SGLT2 function reduced GTTR uptake by kidney cells *in vivo*. Loss of SGLT2 function increased serum levels of gentamicin and GTTR, but did not prevent cochlear loading, and can increase the risk of aminoglycoside-induced ototoxicity. These data suggest that clinical antagonism of SGLT2 function by phlorizin, and phlorizin derivatives like O-glycosides and C-glycosides, may be contraindicated if patients are undergoing aminoglycoside therapy.

Supporting Information

Figure S1   SGLT2-mediated uptake of GTTR is attenuated by D-glucose. Cells were treated with 5 µg/ml GTTR for 20 minutes at 37°C with increasing doses of D-glucose (molar ratios of 1:0, 1:40, 1:2000 or 1:40000 [GTTR/D-glucose])). Increasing doses of D-glucose reduced GTTR fluorescence in KPT2 cells. Scale bar = 20 µm.

Figure S2   KDT3-SGLT2 cell line generation. Parental KDT3, KDT3-SGLT2 and KDT3-pBabe cell lines have similar epitheloid morphology. Scale bar = 50 µm.

Figure S3   Cell growth of control siRNA and SGLT2 siRNA transfected KPT2 cell. MTT assay showed there was no difference for cell growth between control siRNA and SGLT2 siRNA transfected KPT2 cell at 1, 2 or 3 days after transfection.

Figure S4   Phlorizin did not affect auditory function. The ABR thresholds of wild-type mice 30 minutes after injection with 800 mg/kg phlorizin or vehicle (DMSO) control i.p., displayed no significant differences.

Figure S5   Auditory function of $Sglt2^{-/-}$ mice. Wild-type, $Sglt2^{+/-}$ or $Sglt2^{-/-}$ mice displayed no significant differences in ABR thresholds at 6 or 12 weeks of age. Male (blue) and female (red) displayed no significance differences.

Figure S6   Auditory function by ABR before or 3 weeks after kanamycin treatment with or without phlorizin in wild-type mice. In mice treated with kanamycin in DPBS, threshold shifts at 32 kHz were observed 1 day, post-treatment, 1.5 weeks post-treatment and 3 weeks post-treatment with kanamycin. In mice treated with kanamycin plus DMSO (vehicle for phlorizin), further threshold shifts were observed at 16 and 32 kHz at these 3 post-treatment time points. In mice treated with kanamycin plus phlorizin (in DMSO), threshold shifts were observed at 4, 16 and 32 kHz. Male (blue) and female (red) mice have little difference.

Figure S7   Schematic representation of the effect of phlorizin on SGLT2-mediated GTTR uptake by the kidney or cochlea, as suggested by our data and interpretation.

Table S1   Phlorizin had no effect on bactericidal activity of gentamicin. In *E. coli* disk diffusion assay, gentamicin (0.4 µg or 1 µg) alone induced a colony-free halo around the drug-impregnated disk, indicating baseline bactericidal effect. The colony-free diameter or halo thickness was not attenuated by increasing doses of phlorizin, indicating that phlorizin had no effect on the bactericidal activity of gentamicin.

Author Contributions

Conceived and designed the experiments: PSS MJ QW. Performed the experiments: MJ QW TK JK HL PSS. Analyzed the data: MJ PSS QW. Contributed reagents/materials/analysis tools: MJ QW. Wrote the paper: MJ PSS.

References

1. Forge A, Schacht J (2000) Aminoglycoside antibiotics. Audiol Neurootol 5: 3–22.
2. Mwengee W, Butler T, Mgema S, Mhina G, Almasi Y, et al. (2006) Treatment of plague with gentamicin or doxycycline in a randomized clinical trial in Tanzania. Clin Infect Dis 42: 614–621.
3. Mohr PE, Feldman JJ, Dunbar JL, McConkey-Robbins A, Niparko JK, et al. (2000) The societal costs of severe to profound hearing loss in the United States. Int J Technol Assess Health Care 16: 1120–1135.
4. Karahan I, Atessahin A, Yilmaz S, Ceribasi AO, Sakin F (2005) Protective effect of lycopene on gentamicin-induced oxidative stress and nephrotoxicity in rats. Toxicology 215: 198–204.
5. Nagai J, Takano M (2004) Molecular aspects of renal handling of aminoglycosides and strategies for preventing the nephrotoxicity. Drug Metab Pharmacokinet 19: 159–170.
6. Mingeot-Leclercq MP, Tulkens PM (1999) Aminoglycosides: nephrotoxicity. Antimicrobial Agents and Chemotherapy 43: 1003–1012.
7. Dzhagalov IL, Chen KG, Herzmark P, Robey EA (2013) Elimination of self-reactive T cells in the thymus: a timeline for negative selection. PLoS Biology 11: e1001566.
8. Servais H, Van Der Smissen P, Thirion G, Van der Essen G, Van Bambeke F, et al. (2005) Gentamicin-induced apoptosis in LLC-PK1 cells: involvement of lysosomes and mitochondria. Toxicology and Applied Pharmacology 206: 321–333.
9. Karasawa T, Steyger PS (2011) Intracellular mechanisms of aminoglycoside-induced cytotoxicity. Integrative Biology 3: 879–886.
10. Cuzzocrea S, Mazzon E, Dugo L, Serraino I, Di Paola R, et al. (2002) A role for superoxide in gentamicin-mediated nephropathy in rats. Eur J Pharmacol 450: 67–76.
11. Kolodkin-Gal I, Sat B, Keshet A, Engelberg-Kulka H (2008) The communication factor EDF and the toxin-antitoxin module mazEF determine the mode of action of antibiotics. PLoS Biology 6: e319.
12. Sandoval RM, Molitoris BA (2004) Gentamicin traffics retrograde through the secretory pathway and is released in the cytosol via the endoplasmic reticulum. American Journal of Physiology Renal Physiology 286: F617–624.
13. Sandoval RM, Dunn KW, Molitoris BA (2000) Gentamicin traffics rapidly and directly to the Golgi complex in LLC-PK(1) cells. American Journal of Physiology Renal Physiology 279: F884–890.
14. Karasawa T, Wang Q, Fu Y, Cohen DM, Steyger PS (2008) TRPV4 enhances the cellular uptake of aminoglycoside antibiotics. Journal of Cell Science 121: 2871–2879.
15. Myrdal SE, Steyger PS (2005) TRPV1 regulators mediate gentamicin penetration of cultured kidney cells. Hearing Research 204: 170–182.
16. Dai CF, Steyger PS (2008) A systemic gentamicin pathway across the stria vascularis. Hearing Research 235: 114–124.
17. Sabolic I, Vrhovac I, Eror DB, Gerasimova M, Rose M, et al. (2012) Expression of Na+-D-glucose cotransporter SGLT2 in rodents is kidney-specific and exhibits sex and species differences. American Journal of Physiology Cell Physiology 302: C1174–1188.
18. You G, Lee WS, Barros EJ, Kanai Y, Huo TL, et al. (1995) Molecular characteristics of Na(+)-coupled glucose transporters in adult and embryonic rat kidney. Journal of Biological Chemistry 270: 29365–29371.
19. Kanai Y, Lee WS, You G, Brown D, Hediger MA (1994) The human kidney low affinity Na+/glucose cotransporter SGLT2. Delineation of the major renal reabsorptive mechanism for D-glucose. Journal of Clinical Investigation 93: 397–404.

20. Fujimori Y, Katsuno K, Nakashima I, Ishikawa-Takemura Y, Fujikura H, et al. (2008) Remogliflozin etabonate, in a novel category of selective low-affinity sodium glucose cotransporter (SGLT2) inhibitors, exhibits antidiabetic efficacy in rodent models. J Pharmacol Exp Ther 327: 268–276.
21. Nomura S, Sakamaki S, Hongu M, Kawanishi E, Koga Y, et al. (2010) Discovery of canagliflozin, a novel C-glucoside with thiophene ring, as sodium-dependent glucose cotransporter 2 inhibitor for the treatment of type 2 diabetes mellitus. J Med Chem 53: 6355–6360.
22. Magen D, Sprecher E, Zelikovic I, Skorecki K (2005) A novel missense mutation in SLC5A2 encoding SGLT2 underlies autosomal-recessive renal glucosuria and aminoaciduria. Kidney Int 67: 34–41.
23. Garry F, Chew DJ, Hoffsis GF (1990) Urinary indices of renal function in sheep with induced aminoglycoside nephrotoxicosis. Am J Vet Res 51: 420–427.
24. Banday AA, Farooq N, Priyamvada S, Yusufi AN, Khan F (2008) Time dependent effects of gentamicin on the enzymes of carbohydrate metabolism, brush border membrane and oxidative stress in rat kidney tissues. Life Sciences 82: 450–459.
25. Nonclercq D, Wrona S, Toubeau G, Zanen J, Heuson-Stiennon JA, et al. (1992) Tubular injury and regeneration in the rat kidney following acute exposure to gentamicin: a time-course study. Renal Failure 14: 507–521.
26. Naftalin RJ (2008) Osmotic water transport with glucose in GLUT2 and SGLT. Biophys J 94: 3912–3923.
27. Liu T, Speight P, Silverman M (2009) Reanalysis of structure/function correlations in the region of transmembrane segments 4 and 5 of the rabbit sodium/glucose cotransporter. Biochemical and Biophysical Research Communications 378: 133–138.
28. Santer R, Kinner M, Lassen CL, Schneppenheim R, Eggert P, et al. (2003) Molecular analysis of the SGLT2 gene in patients with renal glucosuria. J Am Soc Nephrol 14: 2873–2882.
29. van den Heuvel LP, Assink K, Willemsen M, Monnens L (2002) Autosomal recessive renal glucosuria attributable to a mutation in the sodium glucose cotransporter (SGLT2). Hum Genet 111: 544–547.
30. Katsuno K, Fujimori Y, Takemura Y, Hiratochi M, Itoh F, et al. (2007) Sergliflozin, a novel selective inhibitor of low-affinity sodium glucose cotransporter (SGLT2), validates the critical role of SGLT2 in renal glucose reabsorption and modulates plasma glucose level. J Pharmacol Exp Ther 320: 323–330.
31. Obermeier MT, Yao M, Khanna A, Koplowitz B, Zhu M, et al. (2009) In Vitro Characterization and Pharmacokinetics of Dapagliflozin (BMS-512148), a Potent Sodium-Glucose Cotransporter Type II (SGLT2) Inhibitor, in Animals and Humans. Drug Metab Dispos.
32. Sha S, Devineni D, Ghosh A, Polidori D, Chien S, et al. (2011) Canagliflozin, a novel inhibitor of sodium glucose co-transporter 2, dose dependently reduces calculated renal threshold for glucose excretion and increases urinary glucose excretion in healthy subjects. Diabetes Obes Metab 13: 669–672.
33. Han S, Hagan DL, Taylor JR, Xin L, Meng W, et al. (2008) Dapagliflozin, a selective SGLT2 inhibitor, improves glucose homeostasis in normal and diabetic rats. Diabetes 57: 1723–1729.
34. Nauck MA, Del Prato S, Meier JJ, Duran-Garcia S, Rohwedder K, et al. (2011) Dapagliflozin Versus Glipizide as Add-on Therapy in Patients With Type 2 Diabetes Who Have Inadequate Glycemic Control With Metformin: A randomized, 52-week, double-blind, active-controlled noninferiority trial. Diabetes Care 34: 2015–2022.
35. Wang Q, Steyger PS (2009) Trafficking of systemic fluorescent gentamicin into the cochlea and hair cells. Journal of the Association for Research in Otolaryngology 10: 205–219.
36. Li H, Steyger PS (2011) Systemic aminoglycosides are trafficked via endolymph into cochlear hair cells. Sci Rep 1: 159.
37. Li H, Wang Q, Steyger PS (2011) Acoustic trauma increases cochlear and hair cell uptake of gentamicin. PLoS One 6: e19130.
38. Sandoval R, Leiser J, Molitoris BA (1998) Aminoglycoside antibiotics traffic to the Golgi complex in LLC-PK1 cells. J Am Soc Nephrol 9: 167–174.
39. Myrdal SE, Johnson KC, Steyger PS (2005) Cytoplasmic and intra-nuclear binding of gentamicin does not require endocytosis. Hear Res 204: 156–169.
40. Karasawa T, Wang Q, David LL, Steyger PS (2011) Calreticulin binds to gentamicin and reduces drug-induced ototoxicity. Toxicological Sciences 124: 378–387.
41. Xiao F, Jiang M, Du D, Xia C, Wang J, et al. (2013) Orexin A regulates cardiovascular responses in stress-induced hypertensive rats. Neuropharmacology 67: 16–24.
42. Jiang MY, Chen J, Wang J, Xiao F, Zhang HH, et al. (2011) Nitric oxide modulates cardiovascular function in the rat by activating adenosine A2A receptors and inhibiting acetylcholine release in the rostral ventrolateral medulla. Clin Exp Pharmacol Physiol 38: 380–386.
43. Jiang M, Zhang C, Wang J, Chen J, Xia C, et al. (2011) Adenosine A(2A)R modulates cardiovascular function by activating ERK1/2 signal in the rostral ventrolateral medulla of acute myocardial ischemic rats. Life Sci 89: 182–187.
44. Zhang CR, Xia CM, Jiang MY, Zhu MX, Zhu JM, et al. (2013) Repeated electroacupuncture attenuating of apelin expression and function in the rostral ventrolateral medulla in stress-induced hypertensive rats. Brain Res Bull 97: 53–62.
45. Karasawa T, Sibrian-Vazquez M, Strongin RM, Steyger PS (2013) Identification of cisplatin-binding proteins using agarose conjugates of platinum compounds. PLoS ONE 8: e66220.
46. Zhang F, Dai M, Neng L, Zhang JH, Zhi Z, et al. (2013) Perivascular macrophage-like melanocyte responsiveness to acoustic trauma–a salient feature of strial barrier associated hearing loss. FASEB Journal 27: 3730–3740.
47. Mitchell C, Kempton JB, Creedon T, Trune D (1996) Rapid acquisition of auditory brainstem responses with multiple frequency and intensity tone-bursts. Hearing Research 99: 38–46.
48. Wu WJ, Sha SH, McLaren JD, Kawamoto K, Raphael Y, et al. (2001) Aminoglycoside ototoxicity in adult CBA, C57BL and BALB mice and the Sprague-Dawley rat. Hearing Research 158: 165–178.
49. Blodgett AB, Kothinti RK, Kamyshko I, Petering DH, Kumar S, et al. (2011) A fluorescence method for measurement of glucose transport in kidney cells. Diabetes Technology and Therapeutics 13: 743–751.
50. Stepanyan RS, Indzhykulian AA, Velez-Ortega AC, Boger ET, Steyger PS, et al. (2011) TRPA1-mediated accumulation of aminoglycosides in mouse cochlear outer hair cells. J Assoc Res Otolaryngol 12: 729–740.
51. Alharazneh A, Luk L, Huth M, Monfared A, Steyger PS, et al. (2011) Functional hair cell mechanotransducer channels are required for aminoglycoside ototoxicity. PLoS One 6: e22347.
52. Vu AA, Nadaraja GS, Huth ME, Luk L, Kim J, et al. (2013) Integrity and regeneration of mechanotransduction machinery regulate aminoglycoside entry and sensory cell death. PLoS ONE 8: e54794.
53. Marcotti W, van Netten SM, Kros CJ (2005) The aminoglycoside antibiotic dihydrostreptomycin rapidly enters mouse outer hair cells through the mechano-electrical transducer channels. Journal of Physiology 567: 505–521.
54. Ehrenkranz JR, Lewis NG, Kahn CR, Roth J (2005) Phlorizin: a review. Diabetes/Metabolism Research and Reviews 21: 31–38.
55. Wright EM (2001) Renal Na(+)-glucose cotransporters. American Journal of Physiology Renal Physiology 280: F10–18.
56. Santer R, Calado J (2010) Familial renal glucosuria and SGLT2: from a mendelian trait to a therapeutic target. Clinical Journal of the American Society of Nephrology 5: 133–141.
57. Hashino E, Shero M (1995) Endocytosis of aminoglycoside antibiotics in sensory hair cells. Brain Res 704: 135–140.
58. Hiel H, Schamel A, Erre JP, Hayashida T, Dulon D, et al. (1992) Cellular and subcellular localization of tritiated gentamicin in the guinea pig cochlea following combined treatment with ethacrynic acid. Hear Res 57: 157–165.
59. Nagai J, Komeda T, Yumoto R, Takano M (2013) Effect of protamine on the accumulation of gentamicin in opossum kidney epithelial cells. J Pharm Pharmacol 65: 441–446.
60. Raggi C, Fujiwara K, Leal T, Jouret F, Devuyst O, et al. (2011) Decreased renal accumulation of aminoglycoside reflects defective receptor-mediated endocytosis in cystic fibrosis and Dent's disease. Pflugers Arch 462: 851–860.
61. Hirose K, Hockenbery DM, Rubel EW (1997) Reactive oxygen species in chick hair cells after gentamicin exposure in vitro. Hear Res 104: 1–14.
62. Mamdouh Z, Giocondi MC, Laprade R, Le Grimellec C (1996) Temperature dependence of endocytosis in renal epithelial cells in culture. Biochim Biophys Acta 1282: 171–173.
63. Tanaka R, Muraki K, Ohya S, Yamamura H, Hatano N, et al. (2008) TRPV4-like non-selective cation currents in cultured aortic myocytes. Journal of Pharmacological Sciences 108: 179–189.
64. Humes HD (1999) Insights into ototoxicity. Analogies to nephrotoxicity. Annals of the New York Academy of Sciences 884: 15–18.
65. Higashiyama K, Takeuchi S, Azuma H, Sawada S, Yamakawa K, et al. (2003) Bumetanide-induced enlargement of the intercellular space in the stria vascularis critically depends on Na+ transport. Hearing Research 186: 1–9.
66. Crouch JJ, Sakaguchi N, Lytle C, Schulte BA (1997) Immunohistochemical localization of the Na-K-Cl co-transporter (NKCC1) in the gerbil inner ear. Journal of Histochemistry and Cytochemistry 45: 773–778.
67. Pajor AM, Randolph KM, Kerner SA, Smith CD (2008) Inhibitor binding in the human renal low- and high-affinity Na+/glucose cotransporters. J Pharmacol Exp Ther 324: 985–991.
68. Meyers JR, MacDonald RB, Duggan A, Lenzi D, Standaert DG, et al. (2003) Lighting up the senses: FM1-43 loading of sensory cells through nonselective ion channels. Journal of Neuroscience 23: 4054–4065.
69. Wang T, Yang YQ, Karasawa T, Wang Q, Phillips A, et al. (2013) Bumetanide hyperpolarizes madin-darby canine kidney cells and enhances cellular gentamicin uptake by elevating cytosolic Ca(2+) thus facilitating intermediate conductance Ca(2+)-activated potassium channels. Cell Biochemistry and Biophysics 65: 381–398.
70. Vallon V, Gerasimova M, Rose M, Masuda T, Satriano J, et al. (2013) SGLT2 Inhibitor Empagliflozin Reduces Renal Growth and Albuminuria in Proportion to Hyperglycemia and Prevents Glomerular Hyperfiltration in Diabetic Akita Mice. American Journal of Physiology Renal Physiology.
71. Fetoni AR, Sergi B, Ferraresi A, Paludetti G, Troiani D (2004) alpha-Tocopherol protective effects on gentamicin ototoxicity: an experimental study. International Journal of Audiology 43: 166–171.
72. Takeuchi S, Ando M (1997) Marginal cells of the stria vascularis of gerbils take up glucose via the facilitated transporter GLUT: application of autofluorescence. Hearing Research 114: 69–74.
73. Ando M, Edamatsu M, Fukuizumi S, Takeuchi S (2008) Cellular localization of facilitated glucose transporter 1 (GLUT-1) in the cochlear stria vascularis: its possible contribution to the transcellular glucose pathway. Cell and Tissue Research 331: 763–769.

Gold(I) Complexes of 9-Deazahypoxanthine as Selective Antitumor and Anti-Inflammatory Agents

Ján Vančo[1], Jana Gáliková[1], Jan Hošek[1], Zdeněk Dvořák[2], Lenka Paráková[3], Zdeněk Trávníček[1]*

[1] Regional Centre of Advanced Technologies and Materials & Department of Inorganic Chemistry, Faculty of Science, Palacký University, Olomouc, Czech Republic,
[2] Regional Centre of Advanced Technologies and Materials & Department of Cell Biology and Genetics, Faculty of Science, Palacký University, Olomouc, Czech Republic,
[3] Department of Human Pharmacology and Toxicology, Faculty of Pharmacy, University of Veterinary and Pharmaceutical Sciences Brno, Brno, Czech Republic

Abstract

The gold(I) mixed-ligand complexes involving O-substituted derivatives of 9-deazahypoxanthine (HL_n) and triphenylphosphine (PPh_3) with the general formula $[Au(L_n)(PPh_3)]$ (1–5) were prepared and thoroughly characterized by elemental analysis, FT-IR and multinuclear NMR spectroscopy, ESI+ mass spectrometry, single crystal X-ray (HL_5 and complex 2) and TG/DTA analyses. Complexes 1–5 were evaluated for their in vitro antitumor activity against nine human cancer lines, i.e. MCF7 (breast carcinoma), HOS (osteosarcoma), A549 (adenocarcinoma), G361 (melanoma), HeLa (cervical cancer), A2780 (ovarian carcinoma), A2780R (ovarian carcinoma resistant to cisplatin), 22Rv1 (prostate cancer) and THP-1 (monocytic leukaemia), for their in vitro anti-inflammatory activity using a model of LPS-activated macrophages, and for their in vivo antiedematous activity by λ-carrageenan-induced hind paw edema model on rats. The results showed that the complexes 1–5 exhibit selective in vitro cytotoxicity against MCF7, HOS, 22Rv1, A2780 and A2780R, with submicromolar IC_{50} values for 2 against the MCF7 (0.6 µM) and HOS (0.9 µM). The results of in vitro cytotoxicity screening on primary culture of human hepatocytes (HEP220) revealed up to 30-times lower toxicity of compounds against healthy cells as compared with cancer cells. Additionally, the complexes 1–5 significantly influence the secretion and expression of pro-inflammatory cytokines TNF-α and IL-1β by a similar manner as a commercially used anti-arthritic drug Auranofin. The tested complexes also significantly influence the rate and overall volume of the edema, caused by the intraplantar application of λ-carrageenan polysaccharide to rats. Based on these promising results, the presented compounds could qualify to become feasible candidates for advanced testing as potential antitumor and anti-inflammatory drug-like compounds.

Editor: Pedro V. Baptista, Universidade Nova de Lisboa, Portugal

Funding: The authors gratefully thank the Operational Program Research and Development for Innovations - European Regional Development Fund (CZ.1.05/2.1.00/03.0058), the National Program of Sustainability I (LO1305) of the Ministry of Education, Youth and Sports of the Czech Republic and Palacký University in Olomouc (IGA_PrF_2014009). The funders had no role in study design, data collection and analysis, decision to publish, or preparation of the manuscript.

Competing Interests: The authors have declared that no competing interests exist.

* Email: zdenek.travnicek@upol.cz

Introduction

Medicinal use of gold-based therapeutic agents can be traced back to 2500 BC in China [1,2]. Currently, the foremost clinical use of gold compounds is related to their application in the treatment of rheumatoid arthritis. The most important clinically used gold-based anti-arthritic drugs are various gold(I) thiolate salts, e.g. sodium aurothiomalate (Myochrysin, sodium ((2-carboxy-1-carboxylatoethyl)thiolato)gold(I), Figure 1A) and aurothioglucose (Solganol, {(2S,3R,4S,5S,6R)-3,4,5-trihydroxy-6-(hydroxymethyl)-oxane-2-thiolato}gold(I), Figure 1B) [3,4] belonging to the class of disease-modifying anti-rheumatic drugs so-called DMARDs, and an orally active gold(I) phosphine compound Auranofin (Ridaura, triethylphosphine-(2,3,4,6-tetra-O-acetyl-β-D-thiopyranosato)gold(I), Figure 1C) [5–7]. Over the past few years, research interests in medicinal chemistry of gold compounds have not been focused only on the development of gold-based drugs with better or comparable efficiency, and/or fewer negative side-effects than commercially clinically used anti-rheumatoid agents, but also on the study of the mode of action of gold compounds in the physiological environment with the aim to understand the relationship between the mechanism and anti-inflammatory activity as well as possible variety of their biological applications, e.g. anti-cancer, anti-microbial, anti-malarial and anti-HIV activities [8–15].

Deeper investigations of gold-based compounds as potential antitumor agents started when commercially used anti-arthritic drugs such as Auranofin and gold(I) thiolate salts showed promising results of cell growth inhibiting effects in vitro [16–18] and some efficacy in experimental in vivo models [19–20]. Accordingly, numerous Auranofin analogues, i.e. linear Au(I) phosphine complexes incorporating S-donor ligands [21–26] or heterocyclic N-donor ligands [27–30] as well as various analogues of tetrahedral gold(I) diphosphines e.g. of the type $[Au(DPPE)_2]Cl$, where DPPE represents a tetrasubstituted ethylene-1,2-diphosphine ligand [31–35] (for a representative example see Figure 1D) and Au(I) N-heterocyclic carbene (NHC) complexes of the type $[Au(NHC)_2]$ and $[Au(NHC)Cl]$, where NHC is a heterocyclic

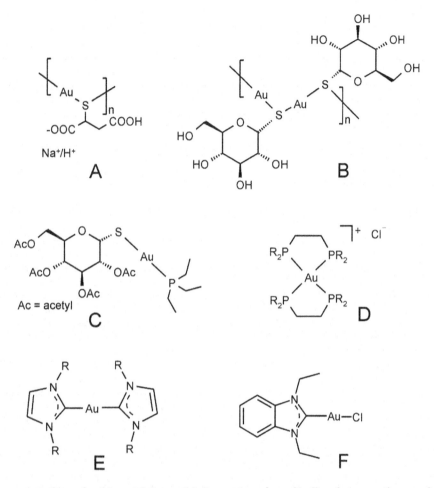

Figure 1. Schematic representations of gold-containing anti-inflammatory drugs (A–C) and some anticancer drug candidates (D–F).

carbene ligand derived from N,N'-disubstituted imidazole [36–37] (for representative examples see Figure 1E and 1F), have gained more attention due to their cytotoxicity and/or antitumor activity against several tumor cell lines/models, e.g. melanoma and leukaemia cell lines/leukaemia model.

Not surprisingly, the studies focusing on the class of gold(I) compounds containing triphenylphosphine and heterocyclic N-donor ligands (L), with the general composition [Au(L)(PPh₃)], described both anti-inflammatory and cytotoxic activities and also showed clinical potential of these compounds in the treatment of anti-inflammatory diseases or cancer. In relation, significant *in vitro* cytotoxicity against breast MCF7, lung A549, cervical (A431) colon (LoVo cell line and multi-drug resistant LoVo MDR cell line), ovarian (2008 and C13*) cancers was described for gold(I) complexes with triphenylphosphine and imidazoles [27]. Further, gold(I) complexes involving triphenylphosphine and 6-benzyladenine (HBap) derivatives, [Au(Bap)(PPh₃)], showed better anti-inflammatory effect and lower *in vitro* cytotoxicity as compared with the commercially used drug Auranofin [38].

9-Deazahypoxanthine derivatives (6-oxo-9-deazapurines) as inhibitors of purine nucleoside phoshorylase (PNP) [39], represent a novel class of prospective selective immunosuppressive agents with potential utilization in the treatment of autoimmune and T-cell proliferative diseases such as T-cell leukaemia and lymphomas [40]. The immucillin family (C9-substituted 9-deazahypoxanthines) represents the most powerful PNP inhibitors, with two members, immucillin-H and DADMe-immucillin-H, included in clinical trials for the treatment of T-cell and B-cell cancers [41–42].

One of the possible ways how to obtain metal-based drugs with improved biological activity is a coordination of suitable ligands to a proper metal. This general pathway, which is associated with a combination of suitable ligands with a proper transition metal (all these components being partly biologically active or even biologically inactive), may lead to the formation of biologically active compounds [e.g. 38, 43–45]. Despite the above-mentioned biological potential of 9-deazahypoxanthine derivatives in clinical applications, its coordination chemistry is still quite new. To date, only one work has been published in connection with the study of coordination compounds incorporating the molecule of 9-deazahypoxanthine [46].

In this work, we wish to present the preparation, characterization and evaluation of *in vitro* and *in vivo* antitumor and anti-inflammatory activities of a series of gold(I)-triphenylphosphine complexes with the general formula [Au(L$_n$)(PPh₃)], where HL$_n$ represents an O-substituted 9-deazahypoxanthine derivative.

As a model of *in vitro* inflammatory response, the expression of pro-inflammatory cytokine tumor necrosis factor α (TNF-α) and interleukin 1β (IL-1β) were determined in lipopolysaccharide (LPS)-stimulated macrophage-like cells THP-1. TNF-α plays an important role during inflammation, as it stimulates the expression of other cytokines and adhesion molecules, causes vasodilatation, participates on generation of reactive oxygen species (ROS), and also possesses other effects on inflamed tissues [47]. The IL-1β cytokine represents another key molecule involved in inflammation processes. It influences signalling pathways leading to fever, expression and activation of other inflammatory-related agents [48–49]. Both of these cytokines are under transcription control of the nuclear factor κB (NF-κB) since the LPS activation of NF-κB signalling pathway leads to the cleavage of its complex with the inhibitor of NF-κB (IκB), while the free NF-κB is translocated from cytoplasm to the nucleus and initiates the transcription of several hundreds of genes, including the TNF-α and IL-1β [50].

Overall positive results and findings related to biological activities are discussed within the framework of the following text.

Materials and Methods

Ethic Statement

This study was carried out in strict accordance with the recommendations in the Guide for the Care and Use of Laboratory Animals of the National Institute of Health [51]. The protocol was approved by the Expert Committee on the Protection of Animals Against Cruelty at the University of Veterinary and Pharmaceuticals Science in Brno (Permit Number: 73-2013). To minimize the suffering of laboratory animals, all pharmacological interventions were done under anaesthesia. The animal tissues for *ex vivo* experiments were taken *post mortem*, immediately after all animals were sacrificed by cervical dislocation.

Chemicals and Biochemicals

Chemicals and solvents used for the synthesis of *O*-substituted 9-deazahypoxanthine derivatives, HL_n ($n = 1$–5, HL_1 = 6-ethoxy-9-deazapurine, HL_2 = 6-isopropyloxy-9-deazapurine, HL_3 = 6-(tetrahydrofuran-2-yl-methyloxy)-9-deazapurine, HL_4 = 6-benzyloxy-9-deazapurine, HL_5 = 6-phenethyloxy-9-deazapurine), and gold(I) triphenylphosphine complexes **1–5** were purchased from Across Organics Co. (Pardubice, Czech Republic), Sigma-Aldrich Co. (Prague, Czech Republic) and Fisher-Scientific Co. (Pardubice, Czech Republic), and were used without any further purification. The precursor [AuCl(PPh$_3$)] was prepared by the synthetic procedure described in the literature [52–53].

The RPMI 1640 medium and penicillin-streptomycin mixture were purchased from Lonza (Verviers, Belgium). Phosphate-buffered saline (PBS), fetal bovine serum (FBS), phorbol myristate acetate (PMA), prednisone (≥98%), Auranofin (≥98%), erythrosin B, and *Escherichia coli* 0111:B4 lipopolysaccharide (LPS) were purchased from Sigma-Aldrich (Steinheim, Germany). Cell Proliferation Reagent WST-1, Cell Proliferation Kit I (MTT), cOmplete Proteinase Inhibitor Cocktail, and RealTime Ready Cell Lysis Kit used for the isolation of RNA from cells, and Transcriptor Universal cDNA Master used for reverse transcription of RNA to cDNA were obtained from Roche (Mannheim, Germany). Specific primers and probes (Gene Expression assays) for polymerase chain reaction (PCR) were obtained from Applied Biosystems (Foster City, CA, USA). The following assays were chosen for the quantification of gene expression: Hs00174128_m1 for TNF-α, Hs01555410_m1 for IL-1β, and 4326315E for β-actin, which served as an internal control of the gene expression. Quantitative PCR (qPCR) was performed with Fast Start Universal Probe Master from Roche (Mannheim, Germany). Instant ELISA Kits from eBioscience (Vienna, Austria) were used to evaluate the production of TNF-α and IL-1β by the enzyme linked immunosorbent assay (ELISA) method. The Immun-Blot PVDF (polyvinylidene fluoride) membrane 0.2 μm from Bio-Rad (Hercules, CA, USA) and albumin bovine fraction V (pH 7) (BSA) from Serva (Heidelberg, Germany) were used for Westernblot. Murine monoclonal anti-IκB-α from Cell Signaling (Danvers, MA, USA), murine monoclonal anti-β-actin from Abcam (Cambridge, UK) and goat polyclonal anti-mouse IgG (with conjugated peroxidase) antibodies from Sigma-Aldrich (Saint Louis, MO, USA) were applied for immunodetection. Conjugated peroxidase was detected by Opti-4CN Substrate Kit from Bio-Rad (Hercules, CA, USA).

Chemistry

The *O*-substituted 9-deazahypoxanthine derivatives, HL_n ($n = 1$–5, HL_1 = 6-ethoxy-9-deazapurine, HL_2 = 6-isopropyloxy-9-deazapurine, HL_3 = 6-(tetrahydrofuran-2-yl-methyloxy)-9-deazapurine, HL_4 = 6-benzyloxy-9-deazapurine, HL_5 = 6-phenethyloxy-9-deazapurine) were synthesized by a slight modification of the procedure involving the nucleophilic substitutions as published previously [54–55]. The purity and composition of the products were confirmed by elemental analysis (C, H, N), electrospray ionization (ESI+) mass spectrometry, FT-IR, ^{1}H and ^{13}C NMR spectroscopies, results of which are given in Information S1, including the detailed synthetic procedure of HL_{1-5}. The molecular structure of HL_5 was determined by single crystal X-ray analysis (for further details see Information S1).

Gold(I) complexes of the composition [Au(L$_{1-5}$)(PPh$_3$)] (**1–5**), where L$_{1-5}$ stands for the deprotonated form of the appropriate *O*-substituted 9-deazahypoxanthine derivative, were synthesized by a slightly modified procedure, as previously described in [38]. Accordingly, the acetone solutions of the appropriate *O*-substituted 9-deazahypoxanthine derivative (HL_{1-5}) (0.2 mmol in 10 mL) and [AuCl(PPh$_3$)] (0.2 mmol in 10 mL) were mixed. Then, an aqueous solution of 1 M NaOH (1 mL) was added and the reaction mixture was heated up to 50°C. The insoluble crystals of NaCl, formed during 2 hours of stirring, were filtered off. The colourless filtrate was evaporated to dryness by standing at room temperature. After a few days, the products **1–5** were precipitated by diethyl ether from the residue of gel-like consistency. The pale yellow powders were filtered off, washed with diethyl ether (5 mL) and dried at 40°C under an infrared lamp. The results of elemental analysis, ESI+ mass spectrometry, FT-IR spectroscopy, thermogravimetric (TG) and differential thermal (DTA) analyses are given in Information S1, including the selected crystallographic data and structure refinement of complex **2**.

Physical Measurements

Elemental analyses (C, H, N) were carried out using a Flash 2000 CHNO-S Analyzer (Thermo Scientific, USA). FT-IR spectra were measured on a Nexus 670 spectrometer (Thermo Nicolet, USA) in the 400–4000 cm^{-1} (ATR technique) and 150–600 cm^{-1} (Nujol technique) regions. Mass spectra of the methanol solutions (*ca* 10^{-5} *M*) of complexes **1–5** were obtained by an LCQ Fleet ion trap mass spectrometer by the positive mode electrospray ionization (ESI+) technique (Thermo Scientific, USA). All the observed isotopic distribution representations were compared with the theoretical ones (QualBrowser software, version 2.0.7, Thermo Fischer Scientific). Simultaneous TG/DTA analyses were performed using an Exstar TG/DTA 6200 thermal analyzer (Seiko Instruments Inc., Japan); ceramic crucible, 150 mL min^{-1} dynamic air atmosphere, 25–850°C temperature range and temperature gradient of 2.5°C min^{-1}. ^{1}H and ^{13}C NMR spectra and two dimensional correlation experiments (^{1}H–^{1}H gs-COSY, ^{1}H–^{13}C gs-HMQC, ^{1}H–^{13}C gs-HMBC; gs = gradient selected, COSY = correlation spectroscopy, HMQC = heteronuclear multiple quantum coherence, HMBC = heteronuclear multiple bond coherence) of the DMF-d_7 solutions were measured at 300 K on a Varian 400 device at 400.00 MHz (^{1}H) and 100.58 MHz (^{13}C). ^{1}H and ^{13}C spectra were adjusted against the signals of tetramethylsilane (Me$_4$Si). The splitting of proton resonances in the reported ^{1}H spectra is defined as s = singlet, d = doublet, t = triplet, br = broad band, dd = doublet of doublets, m = multiplet. The single crystal X-ray data of 6-phenethyloxy-9-deazapurine (HL$_5$) and [Au(L$_2$)(PPh$_3$)] (**2**) were collected on a Xcalibur2 diffractometer (Oxford Diffraction Ltd., UK) equipped with a Sapphire2 CCD detector using the MoKα radiation (monochromator Enhance, Oxford Diffraction Ltd.), and ω-scan technique at 120K. Data collection, data reduction and cell parameter refinements were performed by the CRYSALIS software package [56]. The molecular structures were solved by direct methods and all non-hydrogen atoms were refined anisotropically on F^2 with the full-matrix least-squares procedure (SHELX-97) [57]. H-atoms were located in difference maps and refined using the riding model. Molecular graphics were drawn and additional structural parameters were interpreted using DIAMOND [58].

Maintenance and Preparation of Macrophages

For the determination of biological activity, we used the human monocytic leukaemia cell line THP-1 (ECACC, Salisbury, UK). The cells were cultivated at 37°C in the RPMI 1640 medium supplemented with 2 mM L-glutamine, 10% FBS, 100 U/mL of penicillin and 100 µg/mL of streptomycin in a humidified atmosphere containing 5% CO$_2$. Stabilized cells (3rd–15th passage) were split into microtitration plates to get a concentration of 500 000 cells/mL and the differentiation to macrophages was induced by phorbol myristate acetate (PMA) dissolved in dimethyl sulfoxide (DMSO) at the final concentration of 50 ng/ml, and the cells were incubated for 24 h. In comparison with monocytes, differentiated macrophages tend to adhere to the bottoms of the cultivation plates. For next 24 h the cells were incubated with a fresh complete RPMI medium, i.e. containing antibiotics and FBS, without PMA. The medium was then aspirated, and the cells were washed with PBS and cultivated for next 24 hours in serum-free RPMI 1640 medium. These prepared macrophages were used for the detection of inflammatory response.

In Vitro Cytotoxicity Assay

In vitro cytotoxic activity was determined by the MTT assay in human breast adenocarcinoma (MCF7; ECACC no. 86012803), human osteosarcoma (HOS; ECACC no. 87070202), lung carcinoma (A549; ECACC no. 86012804), malignant melanoma (G361; ECACC no. 88030401), cervix epitheloid carcinoma (HeLa; ECACC no. 93021013), ovarian carcinoma (A2780; ECACC no. 93112519), *cisplatin*-resistant ovarian carcinoma (A2780R; ECACC no. 93112517) and prostate carcinoma (22Rv1; ECACC no 105092802) cancer cell lines, purchased from European Collection of Cell Cultures (ECACC). The cells were cultured according to the ECACC instructions and they were maintained at 37°C and 5% CO$_2$ in a humidified incubator. The primary culture of human hepatocytes (HEP220, batch number HEP220819) was obtained from Bioprodict International (France). The culture medium was Williams and HAM's F-12 (1:1) supplemented with penicillin, streptomycin, ascorbic acid, linoleic acid, holo-transferin, ethanolamine, glucagon, insulin, dexamethasone, pyruvate, glucose, glutamine, amphotericin. The medium was enriched for plating with 2% foetal calf serum (v/v). The medium was exchanged for a serum-free medium the day after and the culture was stabilized for additional 24 h. Thereafter, the cells were ready for treatments. The cultures were maintained at 37°C and 5% CO$_2$ in a humidified incubator. The cells were treated with complexes **1–5** (at the concentration levels of 0.01, 0.1, 1.0, 5.0, 25.0, and 50.0 µM), starting compounds e.g. HL$_{1-5}$, AuCl, and *cisplatin* (applied up to 50 µM) for 24 h, using multi-well culture plates of 96 wells. In parallel, the cells were treated with vehicle (DMF; 0.1%, v/v) and Triton X-100 (1%, v/v) to assess the minimal (i.e. the positive control), and maximal (i.e. the negative control) cell damage, respectively. The MTT assay [59] was performed spectrophotometrically at 540 nm (TECAN, Schoeller Instruments LLC).

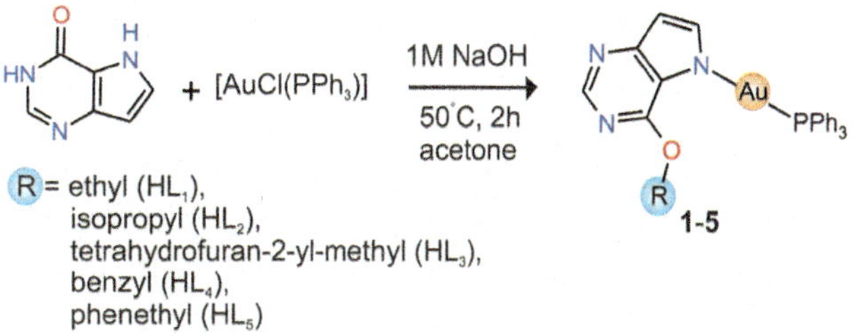

Before the *in vitro* anti-inflammatory testing, *in vitro* cytotoxicity on human monocytic leukaemia cells (THP-1, ECACC no. 88081201) was determined using the WST-1 assay. The THP-1 cells (floating monocytes, 500 000 cells/mL) were incubated in 100 µL of the serum-free RPMI 1640 medium and seeded into

Figure 3. A pathway for the preparation of complexes 1–5.

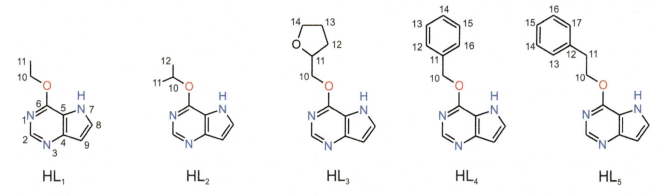

Figure 2. Schematic representations of *O*-substituted 9-deazahypoxanthine derivatives (HL$_{1-5}$) used as the ligands in complexes 1–5.

Table 1. ^1H and ^{13}C NMR coordination shifts ($\Delta\delta = \delta_{complex} - \delta_{ligand}$; ppm) of O-substituted 9-deazahypoxanthine moiety atoms in complexes **1–5**.

	^1H NMR			^{13}C NMR					
	C2H	C8H	C9H	C2	C8	C9	C4	C5	C6
1	−0.14	−0.10	−0.04	−2.17	10.10	−0.79	1.07	7.44	0.82
2	−0.16	−0.09	−0.03	−2.15	10.09	−0.76	1.07	7.64	0.86
3	−0.16	−0.10	−0.05	−2.16	10.16	−0.78	1.04	7.58	0.77
4	−0.16	−0.10	−0.02	−2.21	10.19	−0.72	1.14	7.65	0.74
5	−0.14	−0.08	−0.01	−2.20	10.13	−0.67	1.36	7.65	0.71

96-well plates in triplicate at 37°C. Measurements were taken 24 h after the treatment with the tested compounds dissolved in 0.1% DMSO in the concentration range of 0.16–10.00 μM. Viability was determined by the WST-1 test according to the manufacturer's manual. The amount of the formed formazan (which correlates to the number of metabolically active cells in the culture) was calculated as a percentage of the control cells, which were treated only with 0.1% DMSO and was set-up as 100%. The IC_{50} values of the tested compounds were calculated from the obtained data. The WST-1 assay was performed spectrophotometrically at 440 nm (FLUOstar Omega, BMG Labtech).

Drug Treatment and Induction of Inflammatory Response

Differentiated macrophages were pretreated with 300 nM solutions of the tested complexes, HL_n, AuCl, $[AuCl(PPh_3)]$, PPh_3 and Auranofin dissolved in DMSO (the final DMSO concentration was 0.1%) and with 0.1% DMSO solution itself (*vehicle*) for 1 h; the given concentrations of the tested compounds lack the cytotoxic effect (cell viability >94%) based on the results of WST-1 test. The inflammatory response in pretreated macrophages was triggered by the addition of 1.0 μg/mL lipopolysaccharide (LPS) dissolved in water, while the control cells (CTRL) remained without the LPS treatment.

RNA Isolation and Gene Expression Evaluation

In the order to evaluate the expression of TNF-α, IL-1β, and β-actin mRNA, total RNA was isolated directly from the LPS-stimulated THP-1 cells. THP-1 macrophages were pretreated with compounds **2**, **5**, and Auranofin at the concentration of 300 nM or the vehicle (0.1% DMSO) only. After 1 h of the incubation, the inflammatory response was induced by LPS [except for the control cells (CTRL)]. After 2 h of the incubation with LPS, the medium was aspirated and the total RNA was isolated directly from the cells in cultivation plates using a RealTime Ready Cell Lysis Kit (Roche), according to the manufacturer's instructions.

The gene expression was quantified by two-step reverse-transcription quantitative (real-time) PCR (RT-qPCR). The reverse transcription step was performed by Transcriptor Universal cDNA Master using cell lysate as a template. The reaction consists of 3 steps: (1) primer annealing 29°C for 10 min; (2) reverse transcription 55°C for 10 min; and (3) transcriptase inactivation 85°C for 5 min. A FastStart Universal Probe Master and Gene Expression assays were used for qPCR. These assays contain specific primers and TaqMan probes that bind to an exon-exon junction to avoid DNA contamination. The parameters for the qPCR work were adjusted according to the manufacturer's recommendations: 50°C for 2 min, then 95°C for 10 min, followed by 40 cycles at 95°C for 15 s and 60°C for 1 min. The results were normalized to the amount of ROX reference dye, and the change in gene expression was determined by the $2^{-\Delta\Delta CT}$ method [60]. A degree of transcription in the control cells (i.e. in the cells which were pretreated by vehicle only and not LPS stimulated) was set as 1 and other experimental groups were multiples of this value.

Evaluation of Cytokine Secretion

Macrophages, which were pretreated with the tested compounds (complexes **1–5**, HL_n, AuCl, $[AuCl(PPh_3)]$, PPh_3 and Auranofin) for 1 h, were incubated with LPS for next 24 h. After this period, the medium was collected and the concentration of TNF-α, and IL-1β was determined by the Instant ELISA Kit according to the manufactures' manual.

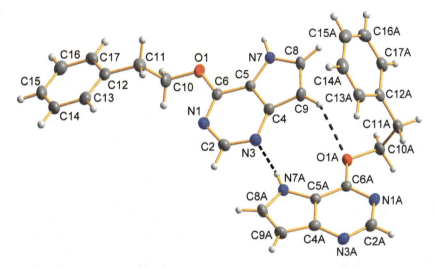

Figure 4. The molecular structure of 6-phenethyloxy-9-deazapurine (HL$_5$), showing the atom numbering scheme and N–H···N and C–H···O non-covalent bonding (dashed lines). Non-hydrogen atoms are displayed as ellipsoids at the 50% probability level.

Determination of IκB degradation

Macrophage-like THP-1 cells were pretreated with the tested compounds and stimulated by LPS as was describe above. Thirty minutes after the addition of LPS, the medium was aspirated and cells were washed by cold phosphate buffer solution (PBS). Subsequently, the cells were collected using the lysis buffer [50 mM Tris-HCl pH 7.5, 1 mM EGTA, 1 mM EDTA, 1 mM sodium orthovanadate, 50 mM sodium fluoride, 5 mM sodium pyrophosphate, 270 mM sucrose, 0.1% (v/v) Triton X-100, and cOmplete Protease Inhibitor Cocktail (Roche, Germany)] and scraper. The lysis of cells was facilitated by a short ($\approx$30 s) incubation in the ultrasonic water bath. The protein concentration was determined according to Bradford's method. For protein separation, 30 μg of protein was loaded onto the 12% polyacrylamide gel. Then, they were electrophoretically transferred on the PVDF membranes, which were subsequently blocked by 5% BSA dissolved in TBST buffer [150 mM NaCl, 10 mM Tris base pH 7.5, 0.1% (v/v) Tween-20]. The membranes were incubated with the primary anti-IκB-α antibody at the concentration ratio of 1:500, or with the primary anti-β-actin at the concentration ration of 1:5 000 at 4°C for 16 h. After washing, the secondary anti-mouse IgG antibody diluted 1:2 000 was applied on the membranes and incubated at laboratory temperature (22°C) for 1 h. The amount of the bound secondary antibody was detected colorimetrically by an Opti-4CN Kit according to the manufacturer's manual.

Animals

Wistar-SPF (6–8 weeks male) rats were obtained from AnLab, Ltd. (Prague, Czech Republic). The animals were kept in plexiglass cages at the constant temperature of 22±1°C and relative humidity of 55±5% for at least 1 week before the experiment. They were given food and water *ad libitum*. All the experimental procedures were performed according to the National Institutes of Health (NIH) Guide for the Care and Use of Laboratory Animals [51]. In addition, all the tests were conducted under the guidelines of the International Association for the Study of Pain [61]. After a one-week adaptation period, male Wistar-SPF rats (200–250 g) were randomly assigned to five groups (n = 7) of the animals in the study. The first, control group, received 25% DMSO (v/v in water, intraperitoneal; *i.p.*). The next three groups were pretreated with complexes **2**, **4** and **5**, and involved into the carrageenan-treatment. The fifth group was treated with a non-steroidal anti-inflammatory drug Indomethacin (5 mg/kg), which served as a positive control group (Indomethacin + carrageenan).

Carrageenan-Induced Hind Paw Edema

The carrageenan-induced hind paw edema model was used for the determination of anti-inflammatory activity [62]. Animals were *i.p.* pretreated with complexes **2**, **4**, and **5** (the dosages of the individual complexes were adjusted to contain the same amount of gold as in 10 mg/kg dose of Auranofin), Indomethacin (5 mg/kg), or 25% DMSO (v/v in water) 30 min prior to the injection of 1% λ-carrageenan solution (50 μL) into the plantar side of right hind paws of the rats. The paw volume was measured immediately after the carrageenan injection (this value was set-up as baseline value

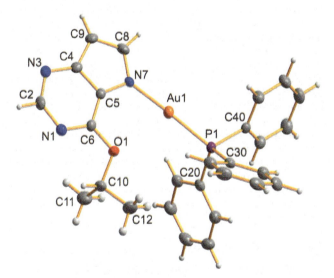

Figure 5. The molecular structure of [Au(L$_2$)(PPh$_3$)] (2), showing the atom numbering scheme. Non-hydrogen atoms are displayed as ellipsoids at the 50% probability level.

Table 2. The results of *in vitro* cytotoxicity of complexes 1–5 and *cisplatin* against variety of human cancer and healthy cell lines.

Compound	Human Cell Line								
	MCF7	HOS	A549	G361	HeLa	A2780	A2780R	22Rv1	THP-1	HEP220
1	3.1±0.2*	3.3±0.1*	20.7±0.1	3.5±0.2*	22.0±0.6	4.8±0.1*	5.2±0.3*	3.5±0.1*	0.8±0.1	24.0±1.9
2	0.6±0.1*	0.9±0.2*	17.2±0.7	3.4±0.1*	16.0±0.2	4.0±0.2*	5.3±0.4*	4.0±0.1*	0.8±0.1	18.5±1.5
3	2.2±0.2*	4.0±0.6*	21.4±0.2	3.4±0.2*	20.7±0.2	4.6±0.3*	5.3±0.4*	21.0±0.7	1.0±0.1	24.1±2.4
4	4.0±0.9*	1.8±0.3*	>20	3.5±0.2*	14.3±0.2	4.6±0.2*	5.1±0.3*	3.5±0.2*	1.7±0.1	23.7±2.1
5	>50	2.9±0.1*	18.3±0.5	3.5±0.2*	22.8±0.5	4.4±0.3*	5.0±0.3*	3.7±0.1*	1.4±0.1	19.0±1.8
cisplatin	17.9±1.2	20.5±0.1	>50	5.3±0.2	>50	11.5±0.5	27.0±1.5	26.9±1.2	n.d.	>50

Cells were treated with the tested compounds for 24 h; measurements were performed in triplicate, and cytotoxicity experiments were repeated on three different cell passages; data are expressed as IC$_{50}$±S.E. (μM). n.d. – not determined; asterisk (*) symbolizes significant difference (p<0.05) in vitro cytotoxicity of **1–5** as compared with *cisplatin*.

for the hind paw volume) and during the next 6 h after the administration of the edematogenic agent using a plethysmometer (model 7159, Ugo Basile, Varese, Italy). The degree of swelling was evaluated as a percentage of the change of the volume of the right hind paw after the carrageenan treatment from the baseline volume. A non-steroidal anti-inflammatory drug Indomethacin was used as a positive control and the obtained data were also compared with the previously reported profile of antiedematous activity for Auranofin [38]. After 6 h, the animals were sacrificed and the edematous feet were dissected, the tissue from the plantar parts was extracted, fixed and stained by a standard hematoxylin/eosin (HE) staining for cytological evaluation of polymorphonuclear cells infiltration.

Statistical Evaluations

The cytotoxicity data were expressed as the percentage of viability, where 100% represented the treatments with vehicle (0.1% DMF or 0.1% DMSO). The cytotoxicity data from the cancer cell lines were acquired from three independent experiments (conducted in triplicate) using cells from different passages. The IC$_{50}$ values were calculated from viability curves. The results are presented as arithmetic means±standard error of the mean (S.E.). The significance of the differences between the results was assessed by the ANOVA analysis with p<0.05 considered to be significant (QC Expert 3.2, Statistical software, TriloByte Ltd., Pardubice, Czech Republic).

The statistically significant differences between individual groups during anti- inflammatory testing were evaluated using a one-way ANOVA test for statistical analysis, followed by Tukey's *post-hoc* test for multiple comparisons. GraphPad Prism 5.02 (GraphPad Software Inc., San Diego, CA, USA) was used to perform the analysis. The results are presented as arithmetic means±S.E. values.

Interactions of the Complexes with Sulfur-containing Biomolecules

The interactions of selected gold(I) complexes **2** and **4**, involving the isopropyloxy and benzyloxy substituent on C6 of 9-deazapurine, with the sulfur-containing biomolecules (i.e. L-cysteine and reduced glutathione) were studied by ESI+ mass spectrometry (ESI+ MS). The experiments were carried out using a Thermo Scientific LTQ Fleet Ion-Trap mass spectrometer, in positive ionization mode. The reactions of the representative complexes **2** and **4** were performed in methanol/water mixture (1:1, v/v) containing the physiological concentrations of L-cysteine and glutathione (at the final concentrations of 290 μM, and 6 μM [63], respectively). The reference system consisted of the solutions of complexes (20 μM) in methanol/water mixture (1:1, v/v). The flow injection analysis (FIA) method was utilized to introduce the reaction system (5 μL spikes) into the mass spectrometer and pure acetonitrile was used as a mobile phase. The ESI-source was set-up as follows: source voltage (5 kV), the vaporizer temperature (160°C), the capillary temperature (250°C), the sheath gas flow (30 L/min), and auxiliary gas flow rate (10 L/min). The system was calibrated as stated in the manufactured specifications and no further tuning was needed.

Results and Discussion

General Properties of Gold(I) Complexes 1–5

The pale yellow gold(I) complexes of the composition [Au(L$_n$)(PPh$_3$)] (**1–5**), where L$_n$ stands for a deprotonated form of the appropriate *O*-substituted 9-deazahypoxanthine derivative (HL$_{1-5}$, Figure 2), were prepared in relatively high yields of

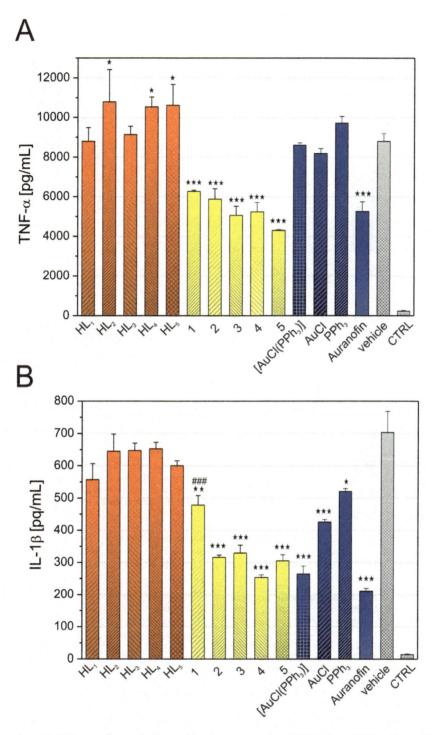

Figure 6. Effects of complexes 1–5, Auranofin, and other relevant compounds on LPS-induced TNF-α (A) and IL-1β (B) secretion. The cells were pretreated with the tested compounds (300 nM) or the vehicle (0.1% DMSO) only. After 1 h of the incubation, the inflammatory response was induced by LPS [except for the control cells (CTRL)]. The secretion was measured 24 h after the LPS addition. The results are expressed as means±S.E. of three independent experiments. Significant difference in comparison to: * vehicle-treated cells ($p<0.05$), ** vehicle-treated cells ($p<0.01$), *** vehicle-treated cells ($p<0.001$), ### Auranofin-treated cells ($p<0.001$) (determined only for complexes **1–5**).

60–75%, as shown in Figure 3. The complexes **1–5** are very soluble in N,N'-dimethylformamide, dimethyl sulfoxide and acetone, soluble in alcohols and very slightly soluble in water. Their composition and structure were proved using a variety of physical techniques, mainly by single crystal X-ray analysis in the case of [Au(L$_2$)(PPh$_3$)] (**2**). Moreover, their thermal stability was determined by TG/DTA techniques, using complexes **2** and **4** as representative samples (see Figure S1 in Information S1). ESI+ MS spectra of **1–5** in methanol solutions (10^{-5} M) showed the [Au(L$_n$)(PPh$_3$) + H]$^+$ molecular peaks of all the studied complexes at m/z 622.2 (**1**), 636.2 (**2**), 678.1 (**3**), 684.2 (**4**) and 698.1 (**5**). The sodium adducts of [Au(L$_n$)(PPh$_3$) + Na]$^+$ with usually lower

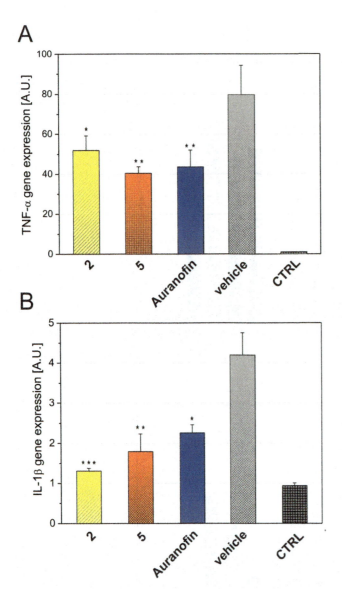

Figure 7. Effects of complexes 2 and 5, and Auranofin on gene expression of TNF-α (A) and IL-1β (B). THP-1 macrophages were pretreated with compounds **2**, **5**, and Auranofin at the concentration of 300 nM or the vehicle (0.1% DMSO) only. After 1 h of the incubation, the inflammatory response was induced by LPS [except for the control cells (CTRL)]. After 2 h, the level of TNF-α and IL-1β mRNA was evaluated by RT-qPCR. The amount of cytokines mRNA was normalised to β-actin mRNA. The results are expressed as means ± S.E. of three independent experiments. A.U. = arbitrary unit. * significant difference in comparison to vehicle-treated cells ($p<0.05$), ** significant difference in comparison to vehicle-treated cells ($p<0.01$), *** significant difference in comparison to vehicle-treated cells ($p<0.001$).

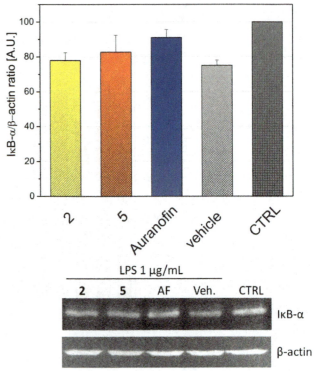

Figure 8. Effects of complexes 2 and 5, and Auranofin on the LPS-induced degradation of IκB-α. The cells were pretreated with tested compounds (300 nM) or the vehicle (Veh., DMSO) only. After 1 h of incubation, the inflammatory response was induced by LPS [except for the control cells (CTRL)]. The levels of IκB-α and β-actin were measured 30 min after LPS treatment. The graph indicates the IκB-α/β-actin ratio. The results are expressed as means ± S.E. of three independent experiments. The blots show the representative results from three independent experiments.

intensity than the molecular peaks were also observed in the mass spectra (for more detailed information about ESI+ mass spectra see Figure S2 in Information S1). The mid-IR spectra confirmed the presence of both types of the ligands in the complexes, as may be demonstrated by peaks observed at 3077–3018, 1593–1589 and 1545–1470 cm^{-1}, which could correspond to the ν(C–H)$_{ar}$, ν(C–N)$_{ring}$, and ν(C–C)$_{ring}$ stretching vibrations, respectively. In the far-IR spectra, the bands detected at ca. 509–502 cm^{-1} and 310–289 cm^{-1} can be assigned to the ν(Au–N), and ν(Au–P) stretching vibrations, respectively, [64–65] (for more detailed information about FT-IR spectra see Information S1).

The ^{1}H and ^{13}C spectra were obtained for all the complexes **1–5** and free ligands HL$_n$. The interpretation of the spectra clearly confirmed the presence of the organic molecules, i.e. deprotonated O-substituted 9-deazahypoxanthine derivatives (L$_n$) and triphenylphosphine (PPh$_3$), in the presented complexes (see Figure S3 and S4 in Information S1) and the comparison of chemical shifts (δ) in the NMR spectra of free compounds HL$_n$ and complexes **1–5**, which are further discussed as coordination shifts, $\Delta\delta = \delta_{complex} - \delta_{ligand}$; ppm, provided information about the possible coordination mode of these ligands to the metal centre (Table 1). In general, parts of NMR spectra regarding the HL$_n$ ligands in the complexes were qualitatively similar to the spectra of the corresponding free HL$_n$, except for the signals of the atoms lying in the vicinity of the coordination site, i.e. the N7 atom, whose chemical shifts changed significantly. Accordingly, the greatest changes were detected for the C5 and C8 atoms, adjacent to the N7 coordination site and shifted by 7.44–7.65 ppm, and 10.09–10.19 ppm downfield, respectively. In the proton NMR spectra, the most shifted signals were found for the C2H and C8H atoms (0.14–0.16 ppm, and 0.08–0.10 ppm upfield, respectively). It is noteworthy to mention that the ^{1}H NMR spectra of **1–5** also showed the absence of the signal corresponding to the N7H proton with respect to NMR spectra of free HL$_n$. Further, the signals of triphenylphosphine ligand in **1–5** were detected in the region around 7.70 ppm and 130 ppm in the proton, and carbon spectra,

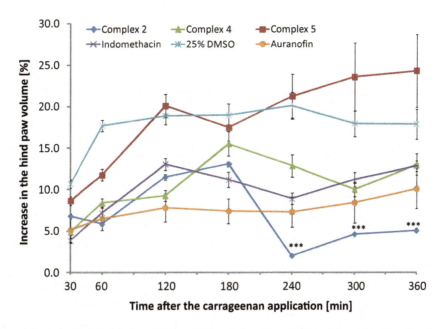

Figure 9. The time-dependent profile of antiedematous activity of complexes 2, 4 and 5, and Indomethacin.

respectively, with relative integral intensity corresponding to 15 protons of this compound. All the above mentioned chemical shifts of the signals observed in the NMR spectra of the herein reported complexes indirectly confirmed the presence of one molecule of PPh$_3$ and deprotonated L$_n$ molecule in **1–5**, and the coordination of L$_n$ through the N7 atom to the metal centre as it was determined using X-ray analysis of **2**.

Crystal Structures of 6-phenethyloxy-9-deazapurine (HL$_5$) and [Au(L$_2$)(PPh$_3$)] (2)

The crystals of 6-phenethyloxy-9-deazapurine (HL$_5$) and [Au(L$_2$)(PPh$_3$)] (**2**), where HL$_2$ = 6-isopropyloxy-9-deazapurine, suitable for the single crystal X-ray analysis were obtained by slow evaporation of the saturated acetonitrile, and acetone solution, respectively. The molecular structures of HL$_5$ and **2** are depicted in Figures 4, and 5, respectively. The crystal data and structure refinements (see Table S1 in Information S1), selected bond lengths and angles (see Tables S2 and S3 in Information S1) and parameters of selected non-covalent contacts (see Tables S4 and S5 in Information S1) are listed in Information S1. The molecular structure of HL$_5$ consists of two crystallographically independent molecules within the asymmetric unit (discussed as HL$_5$ and HL$_{5A}$), which are mutually connected through the N7–H···N3 and C9–H···O1 non-covalent contacts connecting also both individual molecules into one dimensional supramolecular chains (see Figure S5 in Information S1), which are mutually connected through C–H···C, C–H···N and C···C interactions. Parameters of selected non-covalent contacts are given in Table S4 in Information S1.

Single crystal X-ray analysis of **2** confirmed coordination mode of 6-isopropyloxy-9-deazapurine (HL$_2$) to the gold(I) centre in the complexes **1–5**, as suggested by ^{1}H and ^{13}C NMR spectrometry. As shown in Figure 5, the gold(I) atom of **2** is two-coordinated in a slightly distorted linear fashion [N7–Au1–P1 = 176.35(6)°], with the {NP} donor set formed by the N7 atom of 6-isopropyloxy-9-deazapurine and P1 atom of triphenylphosphine. The Au1–N7 and Au1–P1 bond lengths of **2**, i.e. 2.041(2) Å, and 2.2272(7) Å, respectively, are comparable with those found in the compounds involving the same N–Au–P structural motif deposited in Cambridge Structural Database (CSD, ver. 5.35, February 2014 update), which were found to lie in the range of 1.91–2.32, and 2.17–2.29 Å, respectively [66]. Based on the search within CSD, the mean N–Au–P angle is around 175° in about 260 gold(I) complexes. Further, the crystal structure of **2** is stabilized by C–H···C and C–H···N non-covalent interactions (see Table S5 in Information S1).

In Vitro Cytotoxicity

In order to analyse the potential of the gold(I) compounds as anticancer agents, complexes **1–5** were studied by the MTT assay for their *in vitro* cytotoxic activity against a variety of human cancer cell lines, i.e. MCF7 breast carcinoma, HOS osteosarcoma, A549 lung carcinoma, G361 malignant melanoma, HeLa cervix epitheloid carcinoma, A2780 ovarian carcinoma, A2780R ovarian carcinoma resistant to *cisplatin* and 22Rv1 prostate carcinoma. For comparison purposes, the cytotoxic activity of the commercially used drug *cisplatin* and other relevant compounds, i.e. AuCl, HAuCl$_4$ and free HL$_n$, was evaluated by using the same experimental conditions. As for the obtained results regarding the relevant compounds they were found as inactive up to the concentration of 50 µM, except for HAuCl$_4$ which showed a moderate effect only on G361 (IC$_{50}$ = 38.1±2.3 µM). *In vitro* anticancer activity data are summarized in Table 2.

As can be seen from Table 2, the complexes **1–5** were found to be anticancer effective against all the cancer cell lines tested, with IC$_{50}$≈0.6–22.8 µM. However, the complexes revealed selectively and significantly higher anticancer activity on MCF7, HOS, G361, A2780, A2780R and 22Rv1 as compared to *cisplatin*, with IC$_{50}$≈0.6–5.3 µM, except for complex **5** on MCF7 (IC$_{50}$ > 50 µM) and complex **3** on 22Rv1 (IC$_{50}$ = 21.0±0.7 µM). Moreover, the *in vitro* cytotoxicity testing of **1–5** evaluated against the A2780 and A2780R cell lines showed a similar pattern of response across the parental and resistant sub-lines and allowed the calculation of resistance factor (RF) values (defined as the ratio between the IC$_{50}$ values calculated for the resistant cells and those arising from the sensitive ones; IC$_{50}$(A2780R)/IC$_{50}$(A2780))

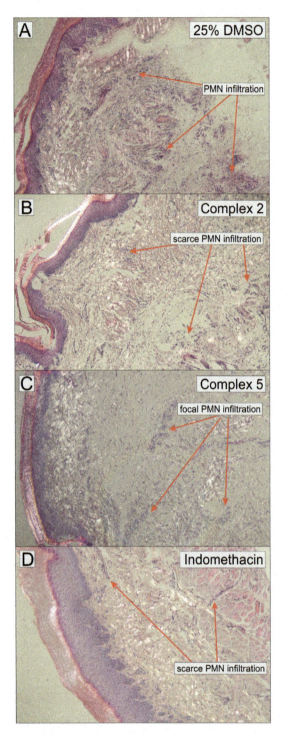

Figure 10. Histological evaluation of inflammatory response in tissue sections of the hind paw, stained with Hematoxylin – eosin (40x magnification). Tissue exposed to 25% DMSO (control; **A**) and complex **5** (**C**) with the acute inflammatory reaction dermis and hypodermis with a massive infiltrate of neurophils (PMN); tissue exposed to complex **2** (**B**) and Indomethacin (**D**) with the inflammatory reaction in the hypodermis with scarce PMN infiltrate.

ranging from 1.1 to 1.3 in comparison with the value obtained for *cisplatin*, which equals to 2.4.

All the gold(I) complexes **1–5** were also evaluated for *in vitro* cytotoxicity against the THP-1 cells (Table 2). The complexes showed a strong *in vitro* cytotoxic action with the IC_{50} values in the range of 0.8–1.7 μM, comparable to Auranofin ($IC_{50} = 0.9 \pm 0.1$ μM). An interesting finding is the fact that all the complexes showed the hormetic effect at very low concentrations of ca. 0.3 μM. This is in accordance with the behaviour of the previously reported gold(I) complexes containing derivatives 6-benzylaminopurines (HBap) of the composition [Au(Bap)(PPh$_3$)] [38,67].

With the aim to reveal the influence of complexes **1–5** on healthy tissues, the *in vitro* cytotoxicity against primary culture of human hepatocytes was evaluated. It has been found that the complexes **1–5** reached up to 30-times lower cytotoxicity (complex **2** on MCF7 *vs.* HEP220) against human healthy cells in comparison to cancer cell lines. A relatively broad concentration range between anti-proliferative and cytotoxicity on healthy cells shows on real applicability of the complexes, although we are aware of the fact that next deeper biological studies are needed. The respective data are included in Table 2.

In Vitro Anti-inflammatory Activity

For the evaluation of *in vitro* anti-inflammatory activity, the ability of the complexes **1–5** to decrease the production of pro-inflammatory cytokines TNF-α and IL-1β in LPS-stimulated macrophage-like cells was determined. The results showed that all the tested complexes significantly decreased the production of both pro-inflammatory cytokines (Figure 6), however the discrepancy was found between the abilities of complexes to influence the secretion of IL-1β in comparison with TNF-α. This observation is in accordance with our previous results regarding the anti-inflammatory activities of gold(I) complexes of the type [Au(L)(PPh$_3$)], where L represents other types of *N*-donor ligands, e.g. different adenine derivatives [38,67]. Concretely, the effect of complexes **1–5** on the secretion of pro-inflammatory cytokine TNF-α was comparable with Auranofin (Figure 6A), while none of the reference compounds, such as AuCl, HL$_n$, [AuCl(PPh$_3$)] and PPh$_3$, exhibited any expected effect. Moreover, the compounds HL$_2$, HL$_4$, and HL$_5$ were found to stimulate the production of this cytokine. This indicates that only the whole complexes are able to diminish the production of TNF-α. More complicated situation was found in the case of evaluation of secretion of pro-inflammatory cytokine IL-1β influenced by complexes **1–5**. Although complexes **1–5** significantly attenuated the secretion of this cytokine, only **2–5** had a similar effect as Auranofin with the secretion level decreased to 50–70% (Figure 6B). Further, compound **1** diminished the level of IL-1β only by 32%, similarly as free triphenylphosphine. To understand the role of individual constituent as a part of complexes in vanquished production of IL-1β, the other reference compounds, as free molecules of HL$_n$, PPh$_3$, AuCl and [AuCl(PPh$_3$)], were also evaluated. It can be pointed out that the compounds PPh$_3$ and AuCl decreased the production of IL-1β by a manner comparable to free ligands.

To evaluate whether the secretion of TNF-α and IL-1β is attenuated by post-translation or by pre-translation mechanism, the influence of selected complexes **2** and **5** (these were chosen in connection with their structural diversity in *O*-substitution at the C6 atom of the ligand) on gene expression was assessed on the level of mRNA [68]. Both the complexes as well as Auranofin were able to significantly reduce the transcription of these cytokines (Figure 7). Pro-inflammatory cytokines TNF-α and IL-1β are under the transcription control of the transcription factor NF-κB, therefore the effect of the complexes on this signalling pathway was examined. Particularly, the effect on IκB degradation was evaluated. As shown in Figure 8, the complexes **2** and **5** were able to block moderately the IκB degradation as effectively as

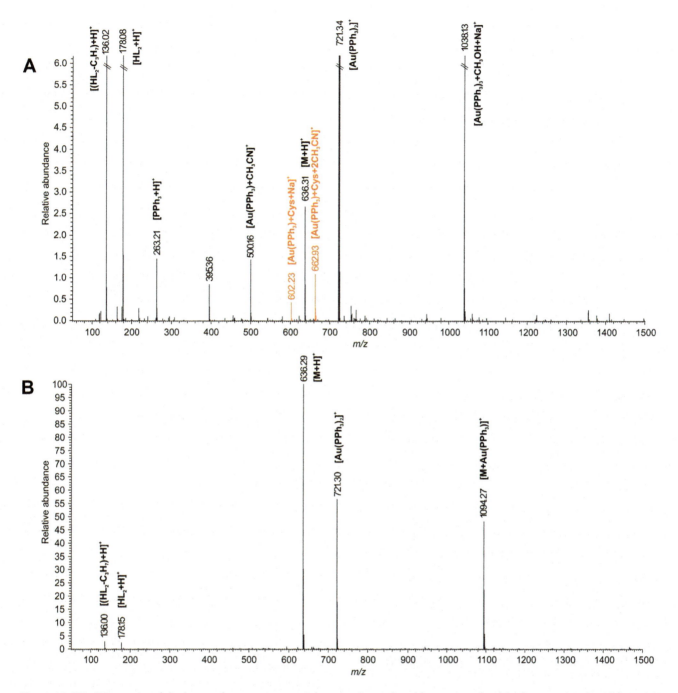

Figure 11. ESI+ MS spectra of the interacting system containing cysteine + glutathione + complex 2 in the water/methanol (1:1 v/v) mixture (A), and the solution of complex 2 in the water/methanol (1:1 v/v) mixture (B).

Auranofin. These results indicate that the tested complexes attenuate the pro-inflammatory cytokine production, at least in part, due to the blocking of the NF-κB signalling pathway through the inhibition of IκB degradation. This observation is in the concordance with previous findings, in which Auranofin and other gold-containing complexes are able to bind to cysteine residues of IκB kinase (IKK) and thus block its function [69].

In Vivo Anti-inflammatory Activity and Ex Vivo Histological Evaluation

Based on the promising results of *in vitro* experiments, the complexes **2**, **4** and **5** were subjected to *in vivo* tests of anti-inflammatory activity using the carrageenan-induced hind paw edema model. This model evaluates the effect of the tested complexes on the acute inflammatory process induced by the polysaccharide carrageenan injection. The main symptom of this process is the formation of edema, which is assessed plethysmometrically. The clinically used non-steroidal anti-inflammatory drug Indomethacin was used as a primary standard for anti-inflammatory activity, and pharmacological profiles of the tested complexes were compared to the previously published results of gold-containing drug Auranofin [38]. In the experiments, we used the dosages of the tested compounds equivalent by the content of gold to 10 mg/kg dosage of Auranofin. The complexes were applied intraperitoneally in the form of the fine suspension in 25% DMSO (v/v in water) 30 min before the intraplantar injection of carrageenan. A reference standard of Indomethacin was applied in the dose of 5 mg/kg [70]. The comprehensive overview of antiedematous activity profiles of the tested compounds is summarized in Figure 9.

The results of antiedematous activity showed very similar pharmacological profiles of complexes **2** and **4** with the reference drug Indomethacin up to the 180 min after the application of carrageenan. After this time point, the complex **2** showed significant increase in biological activity, leading to the amelioration of the inflammatory response, which resulted in elimination of hind paw swelling. In this time period, the antiedematous effect of complex **2** was found to be even better than that of gold-containing metallodrug Auranofin and showed a significant difference at the probability level $p<0.001$. With respect to the structural similarity of all tested complexes and expected similar mechanism of action, their efficacy is probably dependent on the bioavailability, while the molecular weight might be a key parameter in this matter. This hypothesis is supported by the results of antiedematous activity of complex **5** (having the highest molecular weight) that was identified as inactive.

To assess the tissue consequences connected with the reduction of inflammation caused by the tested compounds after the intraplantar injection of carrageenan, the histopathological observations were made on the tissue sections obtained from the laboratory animals after the plethysmometric experiments were finished. All animals were sacrificed by cervical dislocation, and immediately after that, the tissue samples were taken from the plantar area of hind paws. The histopathological changes in tissues, stained by the standard HE staining (see Figure 10), were evaluated by the presence of the inflammation infiltrate, which contained mainly neutrophils (polymorphonuclear cells - PMN). These changes provided evidence of the acute inflammation, which were manifested by the massive presence of PMN cells, in the samples from the control group (see Figure 10A) and the group pretreated with complex **5** (see Figure 10C), which showed the lowest antiedematous effect in plethysmometrical evaluation. On the other hand, the PMN distribution was mainly scarce and diffuse in samples obtained from the Indomethacin (see Figure 10D) and complex **2** (see Figure 10B) treated groups. Both these substances significantly decreased the inflammatory reaction.

Interactions with Cysteine and Reduced Glutathione Analysed by ESI MS

The gold(I) species prefer to form the strong coordination bonds with soft Lewis base ligands, i.e. thiolate or selenolate ions, or phosphine derivatives. It is a well known fact, that Au(I) complexes bind to selanyl- and sulfanyl- groups of biomolecules, such as amino acid cysteine (Cys), small proteins, such as glutathione (GSH), and high molecular weight proteins (e.g. selenium flavoproteins, serum albumin or globulins [71]) by the ligand exchange mechanism. The exchange of *N*-ligands for *S*-ligands occurs relatively fast (within 20 minutes when interacting with albumin and globulins in the blood [72]), while the *P*-ligand exchange proceeds much more slowly, involving a much more complicated mechanism. It seems that in this mechanism the cooperative effects of adjacent thiolato or selenolato ligands in the neighbourhood of the interaction site play an important role. As such, the described ligand exchange is interpreted as one of the molecular mechanisms of incorporation of gold into the active site of selenium-containing flavoreductases, such as thioredoxin reductase [73]. In the scope of this work, we strived to uncover the molecular behaviour of anti-inflammatory active complex **2** (applied in the concentration of 20 µM, corresponding approximately to the highest therapeutic blood levels of gold during chrysotherapy [74]) in biologically relevant conditions using a mixture of cysteine (at 290 µM concentration) and reduced glutathione (at the 6 µM concentration) [63].

Based on the results of the ESI-MS experiments, we confirmed that complex **2** is able to react with the used sulfhydryl-containing substances quite rapidly (the interaction intermediates were detected within 1 h) by the ligand-exchange mechanism associated with the substitution of the *N*-ligand (L_n) by the cysteine or glutathione molecule. This mechanism was confirmed by the emergence of the signals at 602.23 *m/z*, and 662.93 *m/z*, corresponding to the $[Au(PPh_3)+Cys+Na]^+$, and $[Au(PPh_3)+Cys+2CH_3CN]^+$ intermediates, respectively (see Figure 11).

In concordance with the above mentioned suggestion and in accordance with the previously reported behaviour of some Au(I) complexes in water-containing solutions [26], the mass spectra of the reacting systems involving sulfur-containing molecules and also the reference solutions of complexes revealed a considerable instability of the complexes demonstrated by the appearance of the intensive ion at 721.34 *m/z*, corresponding to the $[Au(PPh_3)_2]^+$ intermediate, and other ionic species involving the residue Au-PPh$_3$ (i.e. $[Au(PPh_3)_3+CH_3OH+Na]^+$ at 1038.30 *m/z*, and $[Au(PPh_3)+CH_3CN]^+$ at 500.16 *m/z*, the free HL$_n$ molecules ($[HL_2+H]^+$ at 178.08 *m/z*, or the free triphenylphosphine residue (i.e. $[PPh_3+H]^+$ at 263.24 *m/z*.

Conclusions

A series of gold(I) complexes of the general formula $[Au(L_n)(PPh_3)]$ (**1–5**) (involving *O*-substituted 9-deazahypoxanthine derivatives; HL$_n$) is reported. The complexes were thoroughly structurally characterized and their anticancer (*in vitro*) and anti-inflammatory (*in vitro* and *in vivo*) activities were evaluated. The cytotoxicity results revealed that the complexes are significantly anticancer effective against MCF7, HOS, A2780, A2780R and 22Rv1, with IC$_{50}$≈0.6–5.3 µM, whereas the complex **2** was identified as the most active, being at least 20-times more efficient as *cisplatin* on the MCF7 and HOS cell lines. On the other hand, the complexes showed up to 30-times lower cytotoxicity against healthy cells (human hepatocytes, HEP220) as compared with cancer cells. The results of *in vitro* and *in vivo* anti-inflammatory activity screening indicated that complexes **2** and **4** show significant anti-inflammatory effects on both levels, comparable with the commercially used drug Auranofin. It may be concluded, in connection with the overall positive findings regarding the biological testing, that the $[Au(L_n)(PPh_3)]$ **1–5** complexes could represent usable alternatives to anticancer (*cisplatin*) as well as anti-inflammatory (Auranofin) metallodrugs of major diseases negatively affecting humankind.

Supporting Information

Information S1 Synthesis, elemental analysis and ESI MS, FT-IR, ^{1}H and ^{13}C NMR data for HL$_{1-5}$ as well as the results of elemental analysis, TG/DTA, ESI MS, FT-IR, ^{1}H and ^{13}C NMR experiments assigned to complexes **1–5** are given in Information S1. **Figure S1**. TG/DTA curves of the complexes **2** and **4**. **Figure S2**. ESI+ MS spectrum of **4**. **Figure S3**. ^{1}H and ^{13}C

NMR spectra of **2**. **Figure S4**. ^{1}H–^{13}C HMQC NMR spectra of **2**. **Figure S5**. A part of the crystal structure of HL$_5$. **Table S1**. Crystal data and structure refinements for HL$_5$ and **2**. **Table S2**. Selected bond lengths and angles in HL$_5$. **Table S3**. Selected bond lengths and angles in complex **2**. **Table S4**. Selected non-covalent contacts in the crystal structure of HL$_5$. **Table S5**. Selected non-covalent contacts in the crystal structure complex **2**.

Acknowledgments

The authors would like to thank Mgr. Kateřina Kubešová for help with *in vitro* cytotoxicity testing, and assoc. prof. Pavel Suchý, Jr., for fruitful consultations regarding the *in vivo* testing.

Author Contributions

Conceived and designed the experiments: ZT JG JH ZD JV. Performed the experiments: ZT JG JH ZD LP JV. Analyzed the data: ZT JG JH ZD JV. Wrote the paper: ZT JG JH ZD JV.

References

1. Gielen M, Tiekink ERT (2005) Metallotherapeutic Drugs and Metal-based Diagnostic Agents: The Use of Metals in Medicine. London: John Wiley and Sons, Ltd., Chichester, England.
2. Farrer NJ, Sadler PJ (2011) Bioinorganic Medicinal Chemistry. In: Alessio E, editors. Weinheim: Wiley-VCH, Germany, pp. 1–48.
3. Sigler JW, Bluhm GB, Duncan H, Sharp JT, Ensign DC, McCrum WR (1974) Gold Salts in the Treatment of Rheumatoid Arthritis: A Double-Blind Study. Ann Intern Med 80: 21–26.
4. Williams HJ, Ward JR, Reading JC, Brooks RH, Clegg DO, et al. (1992) Comparison of Auranofin, methotreaxate, and the combination of both in the treatment of rheumatoid arthritis. A controlled clinical trial. Arthritis Rheum 35: 259–269.
5. Kean WF, Kean IRL (2008) Review: Clinical pharmacology of gold. Inflammopharmacology 16: 112–125.
6. Kean WF, Hart L, Buchanan WW (1997) Auranofin. Br J Rheumatol 36: 560–572.
7. Eisler R (2003) Chrysotherapy: a synoptic review. Inflamm Res 52: 487–501.
8. Bruijnincx PCA, Sadler PJ (2008) New trends for metal complexes with anticancer activity. Curr Opin Chem Biol 12: 197–206.
9. Berners-Price SJ, Filipovska A (2008) The Design of Gold-Based, Mitochondria-Targeted Chemotherapeutics. Aust J Chem 61: 661–668.
10. Hambley TW (2007) Metal-Based Therapeutics. Science 318: 1392–1393.
11. Ott I (2009) On the medicinal chemistry of gold complexes as anticancer drugs. Coord Chem Rev 253: 1670–1681.
12. Milacic V, Dou QP (2009) The tumor proteasome as a novel target for gold(III) complexes: implications for breast cancer therapy. Coord Chem Rev 253: 1649–1660.
13. Nardon C, Boscutti G, Fregona D (2014) Beyond platinums: gold complexes as anticancer agents. Anticancer Res 34: 487–492.
14. Casini A, Messori L (2011) Molecular mechanisms and proposed targets for selected anticancer gold compounds. Curr Top Med Chem 11: 2647–2660.
15. Che CM, Sun RW (2011) Therapeutic applications of gold complexes: lipophilic gold(III) cations and gold(I) complexes for anti-cancer treatment. Chem Commun (Camb). 47: 9554–9560.
16. Madeira JM, Gibson DL, Kean WF, Klegeris A (2012) The biological activity of auranofin: implications for novel treatment of diseases. Inflammopharmacology 20: 297–306.
17. Mirabelli CK, Johnson RK, Sung CM, Faucette L, Muirhead K, et al. (1985) Evaluation of the *in vivo* antitumor activity and *in vitro* cytotoxic properties of auranofin, a coordinated gold compound, in murine tumor models. Cancer Res 45: 32–39.
18. Simon TM, Kunishima DH, Vibert GJ, Lorber A (1979) Inhibitory effects of a new oral gold compound on HeLa cells. Cancer 44: 1965–1975.
19. Mirabelli CK, Johnson RK, Hill DT, Faucette L, Girard GR, et al. (1986) Correlation of the *in vitro* cytotoxic and *in vivo* antitumor activities of gold(I) coordination complexes. J Med Chem 29: 218–223.
20. Stallings-Mann M, Jamieson L, Regala RP, Weems C, Murray NR, et al. (2006) A novel small-molecule inhibitor of protein kinase Ciota blocks transformed growth of non-small-cell lung cancer cells. Cancer Res 66: 1767–1774.
21. Tiekink ERT (2008) Anti-cancer potential of gold complexes. Inflammopharmacology 16: 138–142.
22. Tiekink ERT (2002) Gold derivatives for the treatment of cancer. Crit Rev Hematol Oncol 42: 225–248.
23. Barreiro E, Casas JS, Couce MD, Sanchez-Gonzalez A, Sordo J, et al. (2008) Synthesis, structure and cytotoxicity of triphenylphosphinegold(I) sulfanylpropenoates. J Inorg Biochem 102: 184–192.
24. Casas JS, Castellano EE, Couce MD, Ellena J, Sánchez A, et al. (2006) A gold(I) complex with a vitamin K3 derivative: characterization and antitumoral activity. J Inorg Biochem 100: 1858–1860.
25. Casas JS, Castellano EE, Couce MD, Crespo O, Ellena J, et al. (2007) Novel Gold(I) 7-Azacoumarin Complex: Synthesis, Structure, Optical Properties, and Cytotoxic Effects. Inorg Chem 46: 6236–6238.
26. Ott I, Qian X, Xu Y, Kubutat D, Will J, et al. (2009) A gold(I) phosphine complex containing naphthalimide ligand functions as a TrxR inhibiting antiproliferative agent and angiogenesis inhibitor. J Med Chem 52, 763–770.
27. Gallassi R, Burini A, Ricci S, Pellei M, Rigobello MP, et al. (2012) Synthesis and characterization of azolate gold(I) phosphane complexes as thioredoxin reductase inhibiting antitumor agents. Dalton Trans 41: 5307–5318.
28. Serratrice M, Cinellu MA, Maiore L, Pilo M, Zucca A, et al. (2012) Synthesis, Structural Characterization, Solution Behavior, and *in Vitro* Antiproliferative Properties of a Series of Gold Complexes with 2-(2′-Pyridyl)benzimidazole as Ligand: Comparisons of Gold(III) versus Gold(I) and Mononuclear versus Binuclear Derivatives. Inorg Chem 51: 3161–3171.
29. Abbehausen C, Peterson EJ, de Paiva RE, Corbi PP, Formiga AL, et al. (2013) Gold(I)-phosphine-N-heterocycles: biological activity and specific (ligand) interactions on the C-terminal HIVNCp7 zinc finger. Inorg Chem 52: 11280–11287.
30. Illán-Cabeza NA, García-García AR, Martínez-Martos JM, Ramírez-Expósito MJ, Pena-Riuz T, et al. (2013) A potential antitumor agent, (6-amino-1-methyl-5-nitrosouracilato-N3)-triphenylphosphine-gold(I): Structural studies and *in vivo* biological effects against experimental glioma Eur. J. Med. Chem. 64, 2013, 260–272.
31. Berners-Price SJ, Mirabelli CK, Johnson RK, Mattern MR., McCabe FL, et al. (1986) *In Vivo* Antitumor Activity and *in Vitro* Cytotoxic Properties of Bis[1,2-bis(diphenylphosphino)ethane]gold(I) Chloride. Cancer Res 46: 5486–5493.
32. Mirabelli CK, Hill DT, Faucette LF, McCabe FL, Girard GR, et al. (1987) Antitumor activity of bis(diphenylphosphino)alkanes, their gold(I) coordination complexes, and related compounds. J Med Chem 30: 2181–2190.
33. Berners-Price SJ, Jarrett PS, Sadler PJ, et al. (1987) ^{31}P NMR Studies of [Au$_2$(μ-dppe)$^{2+}$)] Antitumor Complexes. Conversion into [Au(dppe)$_2$]$^+$ Induced by Thiols and Blood Plasma. Inorg Chem 26: 3074–3077.
34. Berners-Price SJ, Sadler PJ (1988) Phosphine and metal phosphine complexes: Relationship of chemistry to anticancer and other biological activity. Struct Bonding (Berlin) 70: 27–102.
35. Berners-Price SJ, Girard GR, Hill DT, Sutton BM, Jarrett PS, et al. (1990) Cytotoxicity and antitumor activity of some tetrahedral bis(diphosphino)gold(I) chelates. J Med Chem 33: 1386–1392.
36. Hickey JL, Ruhayel RA, Barnard PJ, Baker MV, Berners-Price SJ, et al. (2008) Mitochondria-targeted chemotherapeutics: the rational design of gold(I) N-heterocyclic carbene complexes that are selectively toxic to cancer cells and target protein selenols in preference to thiols. J Am Chem Soc 130: 12570–12571.
37. Rubbiani R, Kitanovic I, Alborzinia H, Can S, Kitanovic A, et al. (2010) Benzimidazol-2-ylidene gold(I) complexes are thioredoxin reductase inhibitors with multiple antitumor properties. J Med Chem 53: 8608–8618.
38. Trávníček Z, Štarha P, Vančo J, Šilha T, Hošek J, et al. (2012) Anti-inflammatory Active Gold(I) Complexes Involving 6-Substituted-Purine Derivatives. J Med Chem 55: 4568–4579.
39. Bzowska A, Kulikowska E Shugar D (2000) Purine nucleoside phosphorylase: properties, functions, and clinical aspects. Pharmacol Ther 88: 349–425.
40. Bantia S, Miller PJ, Parker CD, Ananth SL, Horn LL, et al. (2001) Purine phosphorylase inhibitor BCX-1777 (Immucillin-H) – a novel potent and orally active immunosuppressive agent. Int Immunopharmacol 1: 1199–1210.
41. Clinch K, Evans GB, Fröhlich RFG, Furneaux RH, Kelly PM, et al. (2009) Third-Generation Immucillins: Syntheses and Bioactivities of Acyclic Immucillin Inhibitors of Human Purine Nucleoside Phosphorylase. J Med Chem 52: 1126–1143.
42. Balakrishnan K, Verma D, O'Brien S, Kilpatrick JM Chen Y, et al.(2010) Phase 2 and pharmacodynamic study of oral forodesine in patients with advanced, fludarabine-treated chronic lymphocytic leukemia. Blood 116: 886–892.
43. Vrzal R, Štarha P, Dvořák Z, Trávníček Z (2010) Evaluation of in vitro cytotoxicity and hepatotoxicity of platinum(II) and palladium(II) oxalato complexes with adenine derivatives as carrier ligands. J Inorg Biochem 104: 1130–1132.
44. Horvat UEI, Dobrzańska L, Strasser CE, Bouwer (neé Potgieter) W, Joone G, et al. (2012) Amides of gold(I) diphosphines prepared from N-heterocyclic sources and their *in vitro* and *in vivo* screening for anticancer activity. J Inorg Biochem 111: 80–90.
45. Štarha P, Trávníček Z, Popa A, Popa I, Muchová T., et al. (2012) Highly in vitro anticancer effective cisplatin derivatives involving halogeno-substituted 7-azaindole. J Inorg Biochem 115: 57–63.
46. Gáliková J, Trávníček Z (2014) Effect of different reaction conditions on the structural diversity of zinc(II) complexes with 9-deazahypoxanthine. Polyhedron 79: 269–276.
47. Zelová H, Hošek J (2013) TNF-alpha signalling and inflammation: interactions between old acquaintances. Inflamm Res 62: 641–651.

48. Dinarello CA (2011) A clinical perspective of IL-1 beta as the gatekeeper of inflammation. Eur J Immunol 41: 1203–1217.
49. Sims JE, Smith DE (2010) The IL-1 family: regulators of immunity. Nature Rev Immunol 10: 89–102.
50. Hayden MS, Ghosh S (2008) Shared principles in NF-kappa B signaling. Cell 132: 344–362.
51. Garber JC, Barbee RW, Bielitzki JT, Clayton LA, Donovan JC, et al. (2011) Guide for the Care and Use of Laboratory Animals, 8th ed., Washington: The National Academies Press, USA.
52. Mann FG, Wells AF, Purdie D (1937) The constitution of complex metalic salts: Part IV. The constitution of the phosphine and arsine derivatives of silver and aurous halides. The coordination of the coordinated argentous and aurous complex. J Chem Soc 1828–1836.
53. Bruce MI, Nicholson BK Bin Shawkataly O (1989) Synthesis of gold-containing mixed-metal cluster complexes. Inorg Synth 26: 324–328.
54. Kamath VP, Juarez-Brambila JJ, Morris CB, Winslow CD Morris Jr PE (2009) Development of a Practical Synthesis of a Purine Nucleoside Phosphorylase Inhibitor: BCX-4208. Org Process Res Dev 13: 928–932.
55. Gibson AE, Arris CE, Bentley J, Boyle FT, Curtin NJ, et al. (2002) Probing the ATP Ribose-Binding Domain of Cyclin-Dependent Kinases 1 and 2 with O6-Substituted Guanine Derivatives. J Med Chem 45: 3381–3393.
56. Oxford Diffraction, CrysAlis RED and CrysAlis CCD Software (Ver. 1.171.33.52), Oxford Diffraction Ltd., Abingdon, Oxfordshire, UK.
57. Sheldrick GM (2008) A short history of SHELX. Acta Crystallogr Sect A 64: 112–122.
58. Brandenburg K (2011) DIAMOND, Release 3.2i, Crystal Impact GbR, Bonn, Germany.
59. Rode HJ (2008) Apoptosis, Cytotoxicity and Cell Proliferation. 4th edition. Mannheim: Roche Diagnostics GmbH., Germany, 178 p.
60. Livak KJ, Schmittgen TD (2001) Analysis of relative gene expression data using real-time quantitative PCR and the 2(T)(-Delta Delta C) method. Methods 25: 402–408.
61. Zimmermann M (1983) Ethical guidelines for investigations of experimental pain in conscious animals. Pain 16: 109–110.
62. Chang HY, Sheu MJ, Yang CH, Leu ZC, Chang YS, et al. (2011) Analgesic effects and the mechanisms of anti-inflammation of hispolon in mice. Evid Based Complement Alternat Med (Article ID 478246) DOI: 10.1093/ecam/nep027.
63. Salemi G, Gueli MC, D'Amelio M, Saia V, Mangiapane P, et al. (2009) Blood levels of homocysteine, cysteine, glutathione, folic acid, and vitamin B12 in the acute phase of atherothrombotic stroke. Neurol Sci 30: 361–364.
64. Nakamoto K (1997) Infrared and Raman Spectra of Inorganic and Coordination Compounds, Part B: Applications in Coordination, Orgametallic and Bioinorganic Chemistry. fifth ed. New York: Wiley.
65. Faggianhi R, Howard-Locck HE, Lock CJL, Turner MA (1987) The reaction of chloro(triphenylphosphine)gold(I) with 1-methylthymine, Can J Chem 65: 1568–1575.
66. Allen FH (2002) The Cambridge Structural Database: a quarter of a million crystal structures and rising. Acta Crystallogr Sect B Struct Sci 58: 380–388.
67. Hošek J, Vančo J, Štarha P, Paraková L, Trávníček Z (2013) Effect of 2-Chloro-Substitution of Adenine Moiety in Mixed-Ligand Gold(I) Triphenylphosphine Complexes on Anti-Inflammatory Activity: The Discrepancy between the In Vivo and In Vitro Models. Plos One 8: e82441.
68. Seitz M, Valbracht J, Quach J, Lotz M (2003) Gold sodium thiomalate and chloroquine inhibit cytokine production in monocytic THP-1 cells through distinct transcriptional and posttranslational mechanisms. Journal of Clinical Immunology 23: 477–484.
69. Jeon KI, Jeong JY, Jue DM (2000) Thiol-reactive metal compounds inhibit NF-kappa B activation by blocking I kappa B kinase. Journal of Immunology 164: 5981–5989.
70. Abdel-Salam OME, Baiuomy AR, El-Shenawy SM, Arbid MS (2003) The anti-inflammatory effects of the phosphodiesterase inhibitor pentoxifylline in the rat. Pharmacol Res 47: 331–340.
71. Shaw CF, Coffer MT, Klingbeil J, Mirabelli CK (1988) Application of phosphorus-31 NMR chemical shift: gold affinity correlation to hemoglobin-gold binding and the first inter-protein gold transfer reaction. J Am Chem Soc 110: 729–734.
72. Iqbal MS, Taqi SG, Arif M, Wasim M, Sher M (2009) In vitro distribution of gold in serum proteins after incubation of sodium aurothiomalate and auranofin with human blood and its pharmacological significance. Biol Trace Elem Res 130: 204–209.
73. Saccoccia F, Angelucci F, Boumis G, Brunori M, Miele AE, et al. (2012) On the mechanism and rate of gold incorporation into thiol-dependent flavoreductases. J Inorg Biochem 108: 105–111.
74. Lewis D, Capell HA, McNeil CJ, Iqbal MS, Brown DH, et al. (1983) Gold levels produced by treatment with auranofin and sodium aurothiomalate. Ann Rheum Dis 42: 566–570.

Integrated mRNA-MicroRNA Profiling of Human NK Cell Differentiation Identifies MiR-583 as a Negative Regulator of IL2Rγ Expression

Sohyun Yun[1☯], Su Ui Lee[2☯], Jung Min Kim[3], Hyun-Jun Lee[2], Hae Young Song[1], Young Kyeung Kim[1], Haiyoung Jung[1], Young-Jun Park[1], Suk Ran Yoon[1], Sei-Ryang Oh[2], Tae-Don Kim[1,4]*, Inpyo Choi[1,4]*

[1] Immunotherapy Research Center, Korea Research Institute of Bioscience and Biotechnology, Daejeon, Republic of Korea, [2] Natural Medicine Research Center, Korea Research Institute of Bioscience and Biotechnology, Ochang-eup, Republic of Korea, [3] NAR Center, Inc., Daejeon Oriental Hospital of Daejeon University, Daejeon, Republic of Korea, [4] Department of Functional Genomics, Korea University of Science and Technology, Daejeon, Republic of Korea

Abstract

Natural killer (NK) cells are innate immune effector cells that protect against cancer and some viral infections. Until recently, most studies have investigated the molecular signatures of human or mouse NK cells to identify genes that are specifically expressed during NK cell development. However, the mechanism regulating NK cell development remains unclear. Here, we report a regulatory network of potential interactions during *in vitro* differentiation of human NK cells, identified using genome-wide mRNA and miRNA databases through hierarchical clustering analysis, gene ontology analysis and a miRNA target prediction program. The microRNA (miR)-583, which demonstrated the largest ratio change in mature NK cells, was highly correlated with IL2 receptor gamma (IL2Rγ) expression. The overexpression of miR-583 had an inhibitory effect on NK cell differentiation. In a reporter assay, the suppressive effect of miR-583 was ablated by mutating the putative miR-583 binding site of the IL2Rγ 3′ UTR. Therefore, we show that miR-583 acts as a negative regulator of NK cell differentiation by silencing IL2Rγ. Additionally, we provide a comprehensive database of genome-wide mRNA and miRNA expression during human NK cell differentiation, offering a better understanding of basic human NK cell biology for the application of human NK cells in immunotherapy.

Editor: Pedro Gonzalez, Duke University, United States of America

Funding: This work was supported in part by grants from the GRL project (FGM1401223), the Ministry of Science, ICT & Future Planning, KRIBB Research Initiative Program, the Korean Health Technology R&D Project (A121934), and Basic Science Research Program through the National Research Foundation of Korea (RBM0261312). The funders had no role in study design, data collection and analysis, decision to publish, or preparation of the manuscript.

Competing Interests: The authors have declared that no competing interests exist.

* Email: tdkim@kribb.re.kr (TDK); ipchoi@kribb.re.kr (IC)

☯ These authors contributed equally to this work.

Introduction

Natural killer (NK) cells are lymphocytes that can eliminate cancer and some viral infections without prior sensitization by targeting major histocompatibility complex (MHC) antigens on target cells through their effector functions, such as cytotoxicity and cytokine secretion [1]. Human NK cells, granular CD56+CD3− lymphocytes, are derived from CD34+ hematopoietic stem cells (HSCs) in the bone marrow (BM) and are subsequently differentiate into fully functional mature NK cells (mNK) in peripheral tissue microenvironments, such as the fetal thymus [1,2]. During NK cell development process, these cells acquire optimal cytolytic and effector abilities depending on the balance between activating and inhibitory receptors. The determination of intermediates in the development of NK cells is primarily dependent on NK cell surface markers, including CD56 and killer inhibitory receptors (KIRs) in humans and NK1.1, DX5, and Ly49 in mice [1]. Although developmental intermediates in human T and B cells have been reasonably well defined, our knowledge about the *in vivo* stages of human NK cell development is very limited [3]. Recently, Aharon G. Freud *et al.* suggested that NK cells differentiate through four discrete intermediate stages in secondary lymphoid tissue: stage 1, CD34+CD117−CD94−, stage 2, CD34+CD117+CD94−, stage 3, CD34−CD117+CD94−, and stage4, CD34−CD117+/−CD94+ [4].

Most studies have identified genes that are closely related to NK cell development and function using mouse knockout (KO) models of the transcription factors (TFs) that modulate cell surface marker expression during NK cell differentiation. The TFs Ikaros [5], Ets-1 [6], PU.1 [7] and Id2 [8] are essential for the proliferation and differentiation of mature NK cells. Additionally, TFs such as GATA-3 [9], T-bet [10] and IRF-2 [11] appear to be involved in NK cell maturation. Furthermore, since the advent of *in vitro* protocols that analyze cytokine-mediated NK differentiation from HSCs, recent studies have demonstrated that important genes such as TOX [12] and IGF-1 [13] regulate human NK cell development. In these processes, interleukin-15 (IL-15) is an

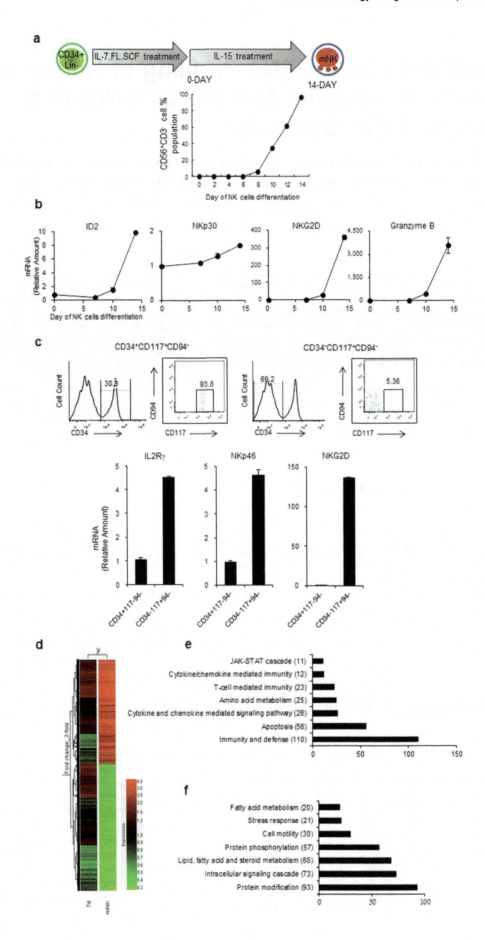

Figure 1. Genome-wide mRNA expression. (a) Isolated HPC (CD34⁺Lin⁻) cells were cultured in IL-15-supplemented media, and the culture media was replaced every 48 h. The expression of CD56 as an NK cell surface marker was analyzed using FACS. (b) The kinetics of the mRNA expression of Id2, NKp30, NKG2D and Granzyme B were analyzed by real-time qPCR. (c) Stage 2 progenitors (CD34⁺CD117⁺CD94⁻) and stage 3 progenitors (CD34⁻CD117⁺CD94⁻) were isolated from UCB by flow sorting. The mRNA expression of IL2Rγ, NKp46 and NKG2D were analyzed by real-time qPCR. (d) A dendrogram of hierarchical clustering revealed genes that were altered more than 2-fold in 7d- and 14-d (mNK) cultured NK cell compared with 1 d-cultured cells. (E-F) The bar graphs represent the top seven functional categories of upregulated (e) or downregulated (f) genes according to the gene ontology analysis (as determined by DAVID, as described in the Methods). The data are representative of three independent experiments performed using three different UCB samples and represent the mean values ± S.E.M. of duplicates.

essential cytokine that stimulates the development and expansion of NK cells in humans and mice. Interestingly, IL-15 KO mice failed to develop functional, mature NK cells [14]. In addition, mice with impaired STAT5 or Jak3, which can modulate IL-15 signaling, showed defects in NK cell development [14].

MicroRNAs (miRNAs) are endogenous short non-coding RNAs (19–22 nt) that inhibit the expression of target genes by binding to the 3′ UTR of specific target mRNAs in eukaryotic cells. Recently, the involvement of miRNAs in immune responses and the development of immune cells from HSCs have been widely investigated manipulating specific miRNAs levels [15,16] or disrupting molecules involved in the biogenesis/activity of all miRNAs, such as Argonaute [17], Drosha [18] and Dicer [19–22]. These genetic studies have demonstrated that miRNAs play essential roles in immune cell development and function [15,23,24]. In a previous study, miR-150 was reported to regulate the development of NK cell using miR-150 KO mice [25]. MiR-155 transgenic (tg) mice had increased numbers of NK cell and enhanced survival of NK cells; however, miR-155-deficient mice showed defects in NK cell maintenance and maturation at steady state [26,27].

In humans, miR-483-3p has been validated as a negative regulator of human NK cell development and cytotoxicity by targeting IGF-1 [13]. Moreover, miR-27a* has been shown to negatively regulate NK cell cytotoxicity by silencing the expression of Prf1 and GzmB, which are essential effector molecules for human NK cell cytotoxicity [28]. Despite evidence for a broad role in regulating immune function, the molecular mechanisms regulated by miRNAs during the development of human NK cells remains poorly understood [24,29,30].

Here, we performed genome-wide mRNA and miRNA arrays and analyzed the resulting data through hierarchical clustering analysis, gene ontology analysis and miRNA target prediction programs. Our data show the highly correlated target mRNAs for predicted miRNAs and identify miR-583 as a negative regulator of NK cell differentiation through its ability to silence IL2Rγ.

Materials and Methods

Cell preparation and culture

Umbilical cord blood (UCB) samples were provided by Chungnam National University Hospital (Daejeon, Republic of Korea). Samples of human CB were obtained from umbilical veins of normal and full-term infants after written informed consent by their mothers, and the protocol was approved by the guidance of the Korea Research Institute of Bioscience and Biotechnology (KRIBB) Institutional Review Board (KRIBB-IRB-20051216-05). *In vitro* NK cell differentiation from CD34⁺Lin⁻ was performed as previously described [31]. Briefly, the isolated CD34⁺Lin⁻ were maintained in MyeloCult H5100 supplemented with stem cell factor (SCF, 30 ng/ml) and flt-3 ligand (FL, 50 ng/ml) for 14 days at 37°C, 5% CO2. The culture medium was refreshed every 3 days. Then, the medium was changed to differentiation medium containing human IL-15 (30 ng/ml, R&D Systems) and cultured for another 14 days. Every 3–4 days, half of the medium was discarded and replenished by fresh medium containing freshly added cytokines. MyeloCult H5100 (Stem Cell Technologies) supplemented with 10^{-6} M freshly dissolved hydrocortisone (HC, Sigma) and 50 μg/ml gentamicin was used as culture medium.

RNA isolation

Total RNA from each sample was extracted using TRIZOL reagent (GibcoBRL, Rockville, MD, USA) according to the protocol of the manufacturer. RNA was treated with the RNase-free DNase I (Promega, Madison, WI, USA) to reduce DNA contamination. Total RNA concentration and purity were determined spectrophotometrically by the absorbance ratio at 260:280 nm 1.8 or more. The integrity of RNA samples was also confirmed by appearance of distinct 28S and 18S bands of ribosomal RNA using Bioanalyzer 2100 system (Agilent Technology, Santa Clara, CA, USA).

Flow cytometry and Ab used

Cell sorting was performed on the FACSAria (BD Bioscience), and phenotypic analysis was performed on the FACS Canto II (BD Bioscience) using CellQuest Pro Software (BD bioscience and FlowJo software. For cell-surface staining, collected cells were washed twice with ice-cold PBS followed by incubation with saturating concentrations of the appropriate mAbs for 15 min at 4°C and then, were washed twice in ice-cold PBS. For intracellular staining, cells were fixed and rendered permeable using the Fix and Perm kit (BD biosciences), according to the manufacturer's instructions. The antibodies used in this study were FITC-conjugated CD34, CD3 and NKp46, PE-conjugated CD56, NKG2D, NKp30, CD3, CD117, CD132, CD107a and p-STAT5, APC-conjugated CD56, CD94, and APC-Cy7 conjugated CD56 (BD bioscience).

Gene expression microarray

For control and test RNAs, the synthesis of target cRNAs and hybridization were performed using Agilent's Low RNA Input Linear Amplification Kit PLUS (Agilent Technology) according to the manufacturer's instructions. Briefly, each 0.5 μg total RNA was mixed with the diluted Spike mix and T7 promoter primer mix and incubated at 65°C for 10 min. cDNA master mix (5× First strand buffer, 0.1 M DTT, 10 mM dNTP mix, RNase-Out, and MMLV-RT) was prepared and added to the reaction mixer. The samples were incubated at 40°C for 2 h and then the RT and dsDNA synthesis was terminated by incubating at 65°C for 15 min. The transcription master mix was prepared as the manufacturer's protocol (4× Transcription buffer, 0.1 M DTT, NTP mix, 50% PEG, RNase-Out, inorganic pyrophosphatase, T7-RNA polymerase, and Cyanine 3/5-CTP). Transcription of dsDNA was performed by adding the transcription master mix to the dsDNA reaction samples and incubating at 40°C for 2 h. Amplified and labeled cRNA was purified on RNase Mini Spin Columns (Qiagen, Hilden, Germany) according to the manufacturer's protocol. Labeled cRNA target was quantified using ND-1000 spectrophotometer (NanoDrop Technologies, Wilmington,

Table 1. The signaling genes related to immune system changed between 7 d- and 14d-cultured (mNK) cells.

Category	Gene symbol	Gene Name	24 h vs. 7 d	24 h vs. mNK	ratio	Genbank Acc. No.
Receptor	LAIR2	leukocyte-associated immunoglobulin-like receptor 2	1.61	45.94	28.6	NM_002288
	NCR3	natural cytotoxicity triggering receptor 3	1.43	20.4	14.3	NM_147130
	MARCO	macrophage receptor with collagenous structure	0.6	7.79	12.9	NM_006770
	ITGB7	integrin, beta 7	1.07	10.56	9.9	NM_000889
	SLAMF6	SLAM family member 6	1.16	9.92	8.6	NM_052931
	IL2RA	interleukin 2 receptor, alpha	1.12	9.35	8.3	NM_000417
	CD69	CD69 molecule	1.02	8.04	7.9	NM_001781
	IFNAR2	interferon (alpha, beta and omega) receptor 2	1.39	9.75	7	NM_207585
	CR1	complement component (3b/4b) receptor 1	1.26	6.79	5.4	NM_000651
	CLECL1	C-type lectin-like 1	0.58	3.05	5.3	NM_172004
	EDNRB	**endothelin receptor type B**	**1.35**	**0.07**	**20**	**NM_003991**
	SPSB1	**splA/ryanodine receptor domain**	**1.84**	**0.25**	**7.3**	**NM_025106**
	CXCR2	**chemokine (C-X-C motif) receptor 2**	**1.16**	**0.21**	**5.6**	**NM_001557**
Cytokines	C1QTNF6	C1q and tumor necrosis factor related protein 6	0.59	4.38	7.4	NM_031910
	TNF	tumor necrosis factor (TNF superfamily, member 2)	0.54	3.49	6.5	NM_000594
	CCL1	chemokine (C-C motif) ligand 1	1.84	11.57	6.3	NM_002981
	IFNG	interferon, gamma	1.6	9.46	5.9	NM_000619
	IL24	interleukin 24	1.52	8.97	5.9	NM_006850
	CCL22	chemokine (C-C motif) ligand 22	0.57	2.97	5.2	NM_002990
Adaptor protein	TIRAP	toll-interleukin 1 receptor (TIR) domain	1.34	16.53	12.3	NM_001039661
	LGALS3BP	lectin, galactoside-binding, soluble, 3 binding protein	0.95	11.39	12	NM_005567
	EDA	ectodysplasin A	1.08	6.15	5.7	NM_001399
	RALGPS2	**Ral GEF with PH domain and SH3 binding motif 2**	**1.4**	**0.16**	**8.8**	**NM_152663**
	RAB3C	**RAB3C, member RAS oncogene family**	**1.2**	**0.16**	**7.6**	**NM_138453**
	SH3PXD2A	**SH3 and PX domains 2A**	**1.28**	**0.17**	**7.5**	**NM_014631**
Kinases	ZAP70	zeta-chain (TCR) associated protein kinase 70 kDa	1.18	10.54	8.9	NM_001079
	CSNK2A2	casein kinase 2, alpha prime polypeptide	1.09	6.09	5.6	NM_001896
	DGKG	**diacylglycerol kinase, gamma 90 kDa**	**1.68**	**0.16**	**10.8**	**NM_001346**
	PLK2	**polo-like kinase 2 (Drosophila)**	**1.42**	**0.24**	**5.8**	**NM_006622**
	SGK2	**serum/glucocorticoid regulated kinase 2**	**0.64**	**0.12**	**5.1**	**NM_170693**
Phosphatase	**PPM1A**	**protein phosphatase, Mg2+/Mn2+ dependent, 1A**	**0.95**	**0.18**	**5.2**	**NM_177951**
TF	ETS1	v-ets erythroblastosis virus E26 oncogene homolog 1	0.51	4.7	9.2	NM_005238
	STAT2	**signal transducer and activator of transcription 2**	**0.53**	**0.05**	**10.9**	**NM_005419**

DE, USA). After checking labeling efficiency, each 750 ng of cyanine 3-labeled and cyanine 5-labeled cRNA target were mixed and the fragmentation of cRNA was performed by adding 10X blocking agent and 25X fragmentation buffer and incubating at 60°C for 30 min. The fragmented cRNA was resuspended with 2X hybridization buffer and directly pipetted onto assembled

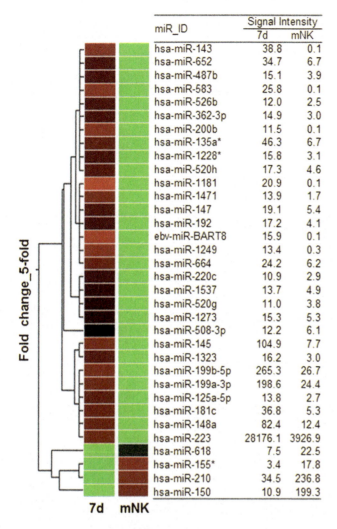

Figure 2. Genome-wide miRNAs expression profiles. A dendrogram showing hierarchical clustering for the miRNAs altered more than 5-fold in 7d-cultured cells compared with 14d-cultured (mNK) cells. The results are shown as the mean values of duplicate experiments.

Agilent Whole Human Genome Oligo Microarray (44K). The arrays hybridized at 65°C for 17 h with 10 rpm rotating in Agilent Hybridization Oven. The hybridized microarrays were washed as the manufacturer's washing protocol (Agilent Technology). The mRNA microarray data have been submitted to the Gene Expression Omnibus [5] database (GEO accession numbers: GSE47521).

MiRNAs expression microarray

For control and test RNAs, the labeling of target miRNAs and hybridization were performed using Agilent's miRNAs Labeling Reagent and Hybridization Kit (Agilent Technology) according to the manufacturer's instructions. Briefly, each 100 ng of total RNA were dephosphorylated with 15 units of calf intestine alkaline phosphatase (CIP), followed by RNA denaturation with 40% DMSO and 10 min incubation at 100°C. Dephosphorylated RNA were ligated with pCp-Cy3 mononucleotide and purified with Micro Bio-Spin 6 Columns (Bio-Rad, Hercules, CA, USA). After purification, labeled samples were resuspended with Gene Expression Blocking Reagent and Hi-RPM Hybridization buffer, followed by boiling for 5 min at 100°C and 5 min chilled on ice.

Finally, denatured labeled probes were pipetted onto assembled Agilent's Human miRNAs Microarray (15K) and hybridized at 55°C for 20 h with 20 rpm rotating in Agilent Hybridization Oven. The hybridized microarrays were washed as the manufacturer's washing protocol (Agilent Technology). The miRNAs microarray data have deposited as an Excel file in Table S3.

Data acquisition and analysis

The hybridization images were analyzed by Agilent DNA microarray Scanner and the data quantification was performed using Agilent Feature Extraction software. The average fluorescence intensity for each spot was calculated and local background was subtracted. All data normalization and selection of fold-changed genes were performed using GeneSpring GX 7.3 (Agilent Technology). For gene expression microarray data, genes were filtered with removing flag-out genes in each experiment. In the gene expression microarray, intensity-dependent normalization (LOWESS) was performed, where the ratio was reduced to the residual of the Lowess fit of the intensity vs. ratio curve. The averages of normalized ratios were calculated by dividing the average of normalized signal channel intensity by the average of normalized control channel intensity. Functional annotation of genes was performed according to Gene Ontology Consortium (http://www.geneontology.org/index.shtml) by GeneSpring GX 7.3. Gene classification was based on searches done by GeneCards (http://www.genecards.org/), miRanda (http://www.microrna.org/), DAVID (http://david. abcc.ncifcrf.gov/), and Medline databases (http://www.ncbi.nlm.nih.gov/).

MiRNA transfection

MiRNA mimic control, and miRNA mimics were purchased from Dharmacon RNA Technologies. Transfections of differentiating NK cell with miRNA mimic control, and miRNA mimics were performed by nucleofection using an Amaxa Human CD34 Cell Nucleofector kit (Lonza). In brief, 100 μL of one nucleofection sample contained 3×10^6 cells and 100 nM (final concentration) miRNA mimic control, and miRNA mimics. These cells were subjected to nucleofection using program U-08 according to the manufacturer's instructions (Amaxa).

NK cell functional assays

Cytotoxicity was examined using a standard 4-h ^{51}Cr-release assay. ^{51}Cr-labeled target cells (1×10^4 cells/well) and serial dilution cells were used in triplicates. Radioactivity of the supernatant containing ^{51}Cr was measured using a γ-counter. The percentage of specific lysis was calculated using the formula: (experimental release-spontaneous release)/(maximum release-spontaneous release) ×100. To evaluate cytokine secretion, differentiating NK cell (1×10^5 cells/well) were stimulated in duplicate for 16 h with IL-18 (30 ng/ml), or PMA (phorbol 12-myristate 13-acetate)/IO (ionomycin) (1 or 2 ng/ml, 0.1 or 0.2 μg/ml). The secretion of IFN-γ (eBioscience), into the supernatant was measured by ELISA.

Quantitative RT-PCR

For miR quantitative RT-PCR (qRT-PCR), cDNA was synthesized with the TaqMan MicroRNA Reverse Transcription Kit (Applied Biosystems, Carlsbad, CA), and primer/probe sets for miR-143, miR-223, miR-583, and miR-150, were purchased from Applied Biosystems. For quantitative real-time polymerase chain reaction (RT-PCR), total RNA was extracted using TRIzol (Invitrogen) and reverse transcribed into cDNA using M-MLV reverse transcriptase (Promega) with random primers (Takara Bio).

Table 2. The list of highly correlated genes between miRNA and mRNA expression between early (7 d) and mNK cells.

Gene Symbol	7d	mNK	Genbank Acc. No.	Predicted miRNA
NDFIP2	0.86	10.43	NM_019080	hsa-miR-583, has-miR-143
YTL3	0.88	7.01	NM_001009991	hsa-miR-583
MYBL1	0.74	6.36	NM_001080416	hsa-miR-200b,has-miR-143
SYTL3	0.70	6.35	NM_001009991	hsa-miR-583
AREG	0.67	5.51	NM_001657	hsa-miR-583
FUT8	0.92	4.92	NM_178155	hsa-miR-583
PPP4R2	0.98	4.76	NM_174907	hsa-miR-200b
KDELC1	0.82	4.72	NM_024089	hsa-miR-200b
NFATC2	0.36	4.66	AK025758	has-miR-143
RSAD2	0.85	4.38	NM_080657	hsa-miR-200b
LPIN1	0.69	3.89	NM_145693	hsa-miR-200b
PPP4R2	0.98	3.82	NM_174907	hsa-miR-200b
MLL5	0.62	3.78	NM_182931	hsa-miR-200b,has-miR-143
NSMCE1	0.85	3.66	NM_145080	hsa-miR-583
MYBL1	0.40	3.53	NM_001144755	hsa-miR-200b,has-miR-143
TTC19	0.66	3.15	NM_017775	hsa-miR-583,hsa-miR-200b
ELMO2	0.98	3.15	NM_182764	hsa-miR-200b
CACNG7	0.74	3.11	NM_031896	hsa-miR-583
XPNPEP1	0.82	3.01	NM_020383	hsa-miR-583
HDAC4	1.00	2.96	NM_006037	hsa-miR-200b,hsa-miR-1181
DIDO1	0.97	2.82	NM_022105	hsa-miR-200b
CAPRIN2	0.91	2.69	NM_001002259	hsa-miR-200b
FN1	0.96	2.66	NM_212482	hsa-miR-583
FYN	0.29	2.64	NM_002037	hsa-miR-583,hsa-miR-200b
CASK	0.98	2.64	NM_001126054	hsa-miR-583,hsa-miR-200b,has-miR-143
SHMT2	0.79	2.63	NM_005412	hsa-miR-583
CCDC50	0.61	2.60	NM_174908	hsa-miR-200b
C1orf97	0.97	2.60	NR_026761	hsa-miR-583,hsa-miR-200b
IL2RG	0.83	2.58	NM_000206	hsa-miR-583,has-miR-143
TBC1D22A	0.54	2.54	NM_014346	hsa-miR-583
XPNPEP1	0.83	2.49	NM_020383	hsa-miR-583
MSI2	0.94	2.43	NM_138962	hsa-miR-583has-miR-143
ASB4	0.89	2.41	NM_016116	hsa-miR-583,hsa-miR-200b
FAM127A	0.95	2.40	NM_001078171	hsa-miR-200b
SLC39A8	0.91	2.28	NM_022154	hsa-miR-200b
SLFNL1	0.72	2.27	NM_144990	has-miR-143
CTSC	0.99	2.26	NM_148170	hsa-miR-583,hsa-miR-200b
CLASP2	0.49	2.23	AJ288059	hsa-miR-200b
POLH	0.72	2.23	NM_006502	hsa-miR-583hsa-miR-200bhsa-miR-1181
CLDND1	0.90	2.22	NM_001040199	hsa-miR-583,hsa-miR-200b
SLC25A15	0.54	2.20	NM_014252	has-miR-143
TMEM14A	0.78	2.18	NM_014051	hsa-miR-200b
MCTP2	0.65	2.17	AL832717	hsa-miR-583,hsa-miR-200b,hsa-miR-1181
MYC	0.81	2.15	NM_002467	hsa-miR-200b
NEUROD2	0.97	2.09	NM_006160	hsa-miR-583,hsa-miR-1181
GPR18	0.73	2.01	NM_005292	hsa-miR-583,has-miR-143
YTHDC1	0.48	2.01	NM_001031732	hsa-miR-583,hsa-miR-200b

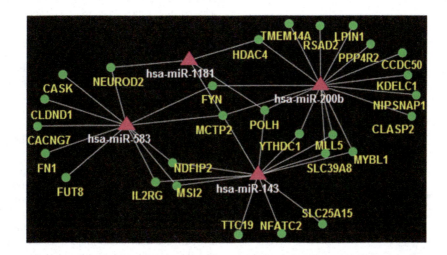

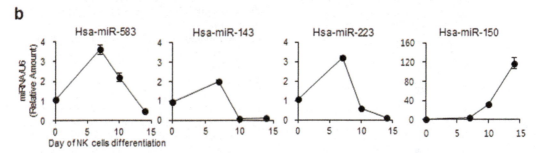

Figure 3. A regulatory network of NK cell differentiation derived from an integrated analysis of miRNAs-mRNA microarray data. (a) Negatively correlated miRNA-mRNA interactions were visualized as a network using Magia (miRNAs and genes integrated analysis web-based tool). This network provides for the first time a theoretical outline of the concerted action of regulating miRNAs (red triangles) and their potential target mRNAs (green circles). (b) Isolated HPC (CD34$^+$Lin$^-$) cells were cultured as described in the Materials and Methods. After being cultured in IL-15-supplemented media, the cells were collected at the indicated time intervals. The expression of miR-143, miR-223, miR-150 and miR-583 was analyzed by real-time qPCR. The data are representative of five independent experiments performed using two different UCB samples and represent the mean values ± S.E.M. of duplicates.

Real-time PCR was performed using a Dice TP 800 Thermal Cycler and the SYBR Premix Ex Taq (Takara Bio). The data were normalized to the amount of glyceraldehyde 3-phosphate dehydrogenase (GAPDH) transcript. The primer sequences were as follows: 5′-cagcctcaagatcatcagca-3′ and 5′-gtcttctgggtggcagtgat-3′ for IL2Rγ, 5′-cagcctcaagatcatcagca-3′ and 5′-gtcttctgggtggcagtgat-3′ for GAPDH, 5′-cgtgaggtccgttaggaaaa-3′ and 5′-atagtggatgcgagtccag-3′ for ID2, 5′-aaccaatcctgcttctgc-3′ and 5′-actgtcgtaataatggcgta-3′ for Granzyme B, 5′-catctgcctcttgggacct-3′ and 5′-agctctggacacagggtgag-3′ for AANAT, 5′-atgactgggcacaacagaca-3′ and 5′-agtgacaacgtcgagcacag-3′ for neomycin gene (Neo). 5′-gcagcagactctcccaaaac-3′ and 5′-tggcaacagatggtcacttg-3′ for NKp46, 5′-aggaggtgaggaatggaacc-3′ and 5′-tccactctgcacacgtagatg-3′ for NKp30, and 5′-tcggtcaagggaatttgaac-3′ and 5′-ttttcaacacgatggcaaaa-3′ for NKG2D.

Immunoblot analysis

Cells were washed twice with ice-cold PBS and lysed in RIPA (50 mM Tris–HCl, pH 7.4, 150 mM NaCl, 0.25% SDS, 1% NP-40, and 1 mM EDTA, supplemented with a protease inhibitor cocktail tablet from Roche). The cell lysates were resolved on 8 or 12% SDS PAGE gels and transferred to PVDF membranes (Millipore). The membranes were probed with antibodies specific for AANAT (Cell Signaling) and GAPDH (Assay Designs). After incubation with peroxide-conjugated anti-rabbit IgG (Jackson Immuno-Research), signals were detected using SuperSignal West Pico Chemiluminescent Substrate.

Results

Differential expression profiling of mRNAs during *in vitro* differentiation of human NK cells

Thus far, IL-15 has been known as an important cytokine for the differentiation of NK cells from HSCs *in vitro* [31]. We noted from previous work that the NK cell marker CD56 was detectable approximately 7 days (7d) after IL-15 supplementation during NK cell differentiation *in vitro* (Fig. 1a) [31]. To identify differentially expressed genes during human NK cell development, we performed mRNA arrays using total RNA isolated from 1-, 7- or 14-d (mNK) cultured cells that had been grown in media supplemented with IL-15 to induce their differentiation into NK cells. Next, we analyzed the expression kinetics of previously known NK cell markers that are induced during NK differentiation using real-time qPCR (Fig. 1b). The expression patterns of the NK cell related genes, Id2, NKp30, NKG2D, and GzmB were consistent with the CD 56 expression patterns; thus the time points used in our study could be considered suitable to explore the expression patterns of NK cell markers during NK cell development [1]. Additionally, we compared freshly isolated stage 2 progenitors (CD34$^+$CD117$^+$CD94$^-$) and stage 3

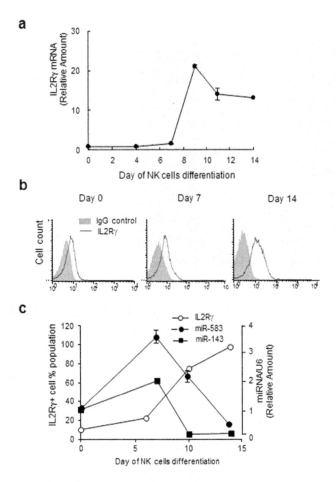

Figure 4. Possible involvement of microRNAs in IL2Rγ expression during human NK cell differentiation. Isolated CB HPCs (CD34⁺Lin⁻ cells) were cultured as described in the Materials and Methods. After being cultured in IL-15-supplemented media, the cells were collected at 48 h intervals. (a) The expression of the IL2Rγ gene was analyzed by real-time quantitative RT-PCR. (b) The expression of IL2Rγ protein was analyzed by FACS. (c) Expression profiling of IL2Rγ, miR-583 and miR-143 after IL-15 treatment. The data are representative of three independent experiments performed using five different UCB samples and represent the mean values ± S.E.M. of duplicates.

progenitors (CD34⁻CD117⁺CD94⁻) from UCB for their relative mRNA expression of genes important for NK cell differentiation and activity. Consistent with the mRNA array data (Table 1 and Fig. 1b), we observed that the expressions of NKp46, NKG2D and IL2Rγ were up-regulated throughout the NK cell developmental stages *in vivo* (Fig. 1c). As shown in Fig. 1d, the expressions of 2920 total genes was altered more than 2-fold in the 7- and 14-d (mNK) cultured NK cells compared with the 1-d cultured cells using hierarchical clustering, on the other hand, 1335 genes were upregulated and 1585 genes were downregulated. All the microarray data are available in the Gene Expression Omnibus under accession GSE47521.

Next, to define the functional properties of those genes that were altered more than 2-fold according to the mRNA array data, the upregulated (Fig. 1e) and downregulated (Fig. 1f) genes were categorized using gene ontology classifications. Following these analyses, the major categories of upregulated genes were classified as "immunity and defense" genes, whereas the downregulated genes were identified as "protein modification" and "intracellular and signaling cascade" genes. To better understand the expression of signaling molecules during human NK cell development, we selected the genes that were categorized as "immunity and defense" and "intracellular and signaling cascade" genes and listed them in Table 1 according to their functional properties. As shown in Table 1, the list of 33 genes, which includes 22 upregulated genes and 11 downregulated genes (in bold), that had intensity ratio changes in excess of 5-fold contained receptors (NCR1 and NCR3), cytokines (IFN-γ and CCL1) and TFs (Ets-1) known to be involved in NK cell development and activity.

Differential miRNA expression profiling during *in vitro* differentiation of human NK cells

Next, to investigate the relationship between miRNAs and their target mRNAs during NK cell development, we performed miRNA arrays using total RNA isolated from 7- or 14-d (mNK) cultured cells and deposited the summarized data in Table S3. As shown in Fig. 2, the expression of 34 miRNAs was found to be altered more than 5-fold in 14-d (mNK) cultured cells compared with the 7-d cultured cells using hierarchical clustering analysis. Of these 34 miRNAs, 4 miRNAs were upregulated and 30 were downregulated. In these results, we confirmed that the expression of miR-150 and miR-155* were strongly increased in mNK cells. Importantly, miR-150 was previously identified as a regulator of mouse NK cell development and cytotoxicity [25,32], and miR-155 was critically required for NK cell maturation and maintenance at steady state [27]. Additionally, the downregulation of miR-223 in human mNK cells was previously reported to regulate GzmB translation during murine NK cell activation [33]. Thus, we hypothesized that individual miRNAs could be evaluated as biomarkers that regulate the expression of key molecular signatures during NK cell development.

Based on the data presented in Fig. 2, we chose the 4 miRNAs (miR-583, miR-143, miR-200b and miR-1181) that were significantly downregulated in mNK cell, which suggested an inhibition of target genes by the predicted miRNAs. As shown in Table 2, we have summarized the highly correlated target proteins for the 4 selected miRNAs using the miRNAs target prediction program miRanda. However, it should be noted that individual miRNAs interact with the conserved sites of multiple target genes and that most miRNAs and their potential target mRNAs do not necessarily match. To demonstrate the relationship between the four selected the miRNAs and their target mRNAs during NK cell differentiation, we next attempted to construct a regulatory network of potential interactions between the miRNAs and mRNAs identified during the expression analysis.

A regulatory network of NK cell differentiation using the integrated analysis of miRNA-mRNA microarray data

Recently, a study on the epigenetic regulation of gene expression reported that specific miRNA expression changes might contribute to distinct mRNA expression profiles, suggesting that miRNAs inhibit the expression of target genes via a negative relationship [34,35]. Thus, we showed that negatively correlated miRNA-mRNA interactions could be visualized as a network; in this study, we used Magia (miRNA and genes integrated analysis web-based tool). As shown in Fig. 3a, this network gives information on the regulatory mechanisms between the largely suppressed four miRNAs (red triangles) in mNK cell and their potential target mRNAs (green circles). Importantly, both miR-583 and miR-143 were highly correlated with subunit IL2Rγ of the IL2 receptor, related to the IL-15 signaling pathway. In fact, IL2Rγ is essential for NK cell development, and it has been shown

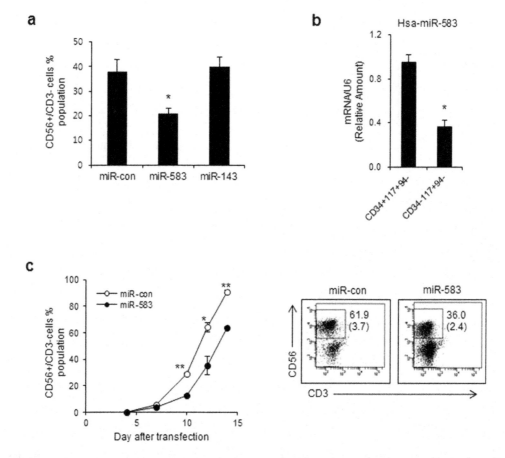

Figure 5. Human miR-583 downregulates NK cell differentiation. (a) Differentiating cells were transfected with miR-143, a miR-583 mimic or negative control miRNA. NK cell populations (CD56$^+$CD3$^-$ cells) were analyzed by FACS 10 days after transfection. *, $p<0.1$. (b) The expression level of miR-583 was decreased during NK cell development as shown by qRT-PCR. The results are shown as the mean expression values normalized against stage 2 (CD34$^+$CD117$^+$CD94$^-$). *, $p<0.1$. (c) NK cell populations (CD56$^+$CD3$^-$ cells) were analyzed by FACS after miR-583 transfection at regular intervals during NK cell differentiation. The absolute numbers of differentiated NK cells are shown in the parentheses ($\times 10^5$). *, $p<0.01$ **, $p<0.001$. The data are representative of three independent experiments performed using three different UCB samples and represent the mean values ± S.E.M. of duplicates.

that IL2Rγ-deficient mice were completely devoid of NK cells [36].

Prior to validating whether miR-583 and miR-143 contributed to targeted suppression of IL2Rγ expression, we analyzed the expression kinetics of miR-583 and miR-143, as well as the well-known miRNAs miR-223 and miR-150, during NK cell differentiation using real-time qPCR (Fig. 3b). Our results were consistent with the microarray data presented in Fig. 2 showing that the expression of miR-583, miR-143 and miR-223 were decreased; however, the expression of miR-150 was increased during NK cell differentiation. Given these collective data, we hypothesized that miR-583 or miR-143 may play a role in NK cell differentiation through the regulation of IL2Rγ expression.

Involvement of microRNA in IL2Rγ expression in human NK cells

To determine whether IL2Rγ expression is regulated by the miR-583 and miR-143 miRNAs as predicted, we examined the mRNA and protein expression of IL2Rγ during NK cell differentiation. IL2Rγ mRNA expression was dramatically increased after 7d of IL-15 treatment, after which it was slightly downregulated during the final maturation into mNK cells (Fig. 4a and 4b). IL2Rγ mRNA transcript expression increased during NK cell differentiation and peaked at 9 d after IL-15 treatment. By contrast, miR-583 expression peaked at 7d after IL-15 treatment but was dramatically reduced during NK differentiation, implying that posttranscriptional regulation is involved in the expression of this receptor molecule (Fig. 4c). Although IL-15–related NK cell differentiation is closely associated with the expression of the IL2R complex, little is known about the mechanism regulating receptor expression on NK cells.

Effects of miR-583 on differentiation and functional activity of NK cells

To investigate the biological effects of miRNAs on NK cell development, miR-583 and miR-143 were validated as regulators of NK cell differentiation by targeting IL2Rγ. Although IL-15 receptor-mediated signaling is important for NK cell differentiation, it is not known whether miRNAs regulate IL-15 receptor expression during NK cell differentiation. To evaluate whether overexpression of miRNAs caused the selective reduction of IL2Rγ we transfected synthetic miRNA mimics into differentiating NK cells (0 day). We transfected synthetic miR-583 mimics into differentiating NK cells (0 day). Then, the medium was changed to differentiation medium containing human IL-15 (30 ng/ml). The introduction of miR-583 mimics led to an approximately 2-fold

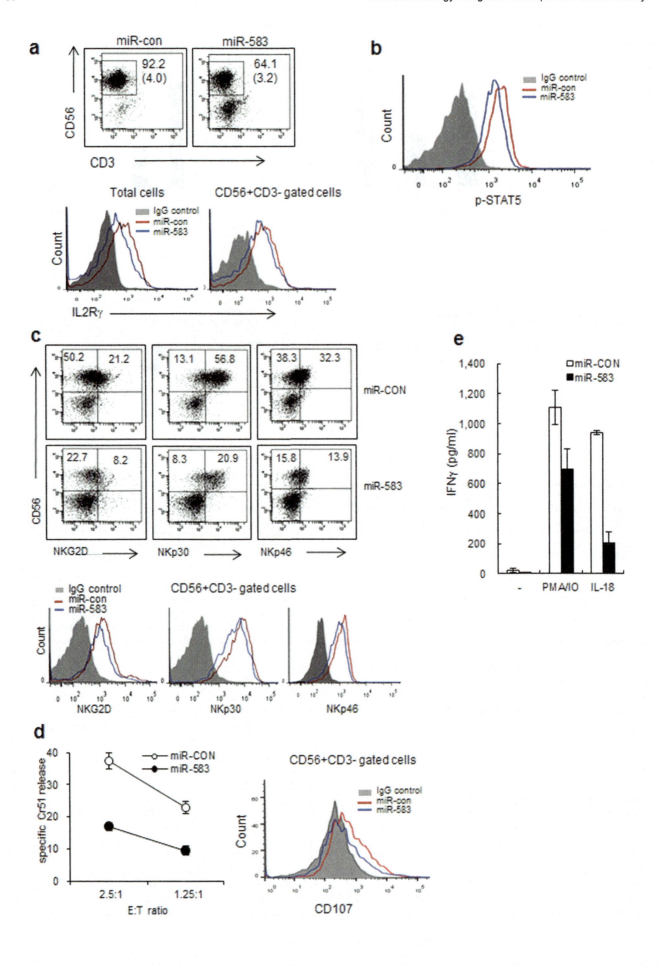

Figure 6. Human miR-583 downregulates NK cell activation by silencing IL2Rγ during NK cell differentiation. (a) The expression of IL2Rγ was analyzed by FACS 14 days after miR-control or miR-583 transfection in differentiating NK cells and CD56⁺CD3⁻ gated NK cells. Gray, IgG control; blue, miR-control; red, miR-583. The absolute numbers of differentiated NK cells are shown in the parentheses (×10⁵). (b) The expression of p-STAT5 was analyzed by FACS 7 days after miR-control or miR-583 transfection in differentiating NK cells. Gray, IgG control; blue, miR-control; red, miR-583. (c) The expression levels of NK cell activation receptors in differentiating NK cells and CD56⁺CD3⁻ gated NK cells were analyzed by FACS 14 days after miR-control or miR-583 transfection. Gray, IgG control; blue, miR-control; red, miR-583. (d). Cytotoxicity of differentiating NK cells was determined by ^{51}Cr release assay against K562 cells at the indicated effector/target (E:T) ratios. *, $p<0.1$. The expression levels of CD107a in differentiating NK cells and CD56⁺CD3⁻ gated NK cells were analyzed by FACS. Gray, IgG control; blue, miR-control; red, miR-583. (e) Differentiating NK cells were stimulated with PMA/IO or IL-18. After 16 h, the supernatants were assayed for IFN-γ production by ELISA. *, $p<0.1$. Values represent the mean % of positive cells ± S.E.M. of triplicates. The data are representative of three independent experiments performed using three different UCB samples and represent the mean values ± S.E.M. of duplicates.

decrease in the percentage of mature CD56⁺CD3⁻ NK cell by the 10 d after transfection compared with the mimic control (Fig. 5a and 5c). In contrast, the introduction of a miR-143 mimic resulted in similar percentages of mature CD56⁺CD3⁻ NK cells and mimic controls (Fig. 5a). Thus, we focused on miR-583 as a regulator of NK cell differentiation *via* the IL-15 signaling pathway.

Next, we compared freshly isolated stage 2 progenitors (CD34⁺CD117⁺CD94⁻) and stage 3 progenitors (CD34⁻CD117⁺CD94⁻) from UCB for their relative miR-583 expression. Consistent with the miRNAs array data (Fig. 2), we observed that the miR-583 transcript level was decreased throughout the primary NK cell developmental stage *in vivo* (Fig. 5b).

To determine whether the expression of IL2Rγ protein was suppressed by miR-583, we investigated the expression level of IL2Rγ on transfected differentiating NK cell by FACS. Differentiating NK cells transfected with miR-583 mimics showed decreases in IL2Rγ protein levels in both total cells and CD56⁺CD3⁻ gated cells (Fig. 6a). The signal transduction initiated by IL-15 involves tyrosine phosphorylation of STAT5, an essential transcription factor that mediates IL2R, by JAK3 in NK cells [37]. Therefore, we analyzed the expression level of p-STAT5 in differentiating NK cells by FACS 7 days after miR-control or miR-583 transfection. As shown in Fig. 6b, differentiating NK cell transfected with miR-583 mimics showed decreased levels of STAT5 phospholylation, compared with the differentiating NK cells transfected with the miR-control. We next considered the possibility that differentiating NK cell transfected with miR-583 mimics may have decreased expression of IL-15 dependent activation receptors because of reduced expression of p-STAT5 [38]. The expression levels of NK cell activation receptors decreased in differentiating NK cells transfected with miR-583 and in CD56⁺CD3⁻ gated NK cells (Fig. 6c).

Next, to confirm whether the differentiating NK cells transfected with miR-583 had full functional activity, we examined their functions such as cytolytic activity or production of cytokines. The miR-583-treated differentiating NK cells showed a markedly decreased capacity to kill K562 and produce IFN-γ. The reduced functional activities in miR-583 treated differentiating NK cells may reflect a relatively small population of NK cells by treatment

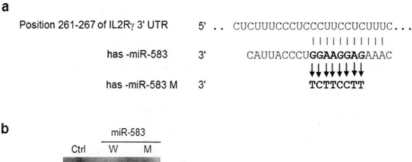

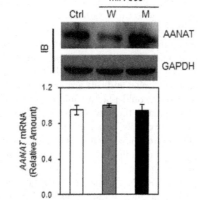

Figure 7. Human miR-583 specifically targets IL2Rγ 3′ UTR sequences. (a) Predicted miR-583 binding sites. Mutants (M). Point mutations are in bold. Numbers indicate the positions of nucleotides in the 3′ UTR. (b) Reporter assay using immunoblotting (IB) analysis. HEK-293FT cells were cotransfected with combinations of reporter plasmids containing IL2Rγ 3′ UTRs and miR-583 or mutant miR-583 (miR-583 M). Reporter AANAT mRNA levels were normalized to Neo mRNA levels as an internal control for the vector. The net amount of translated AANAT protein was determined by IB. GAPDH served as a loading control. The data are representative of two independent experiments (mean values ± S.E.M. of triplicates).

of miR-583 compared with controls (Fig. 6d and 6e). Lysosomal-associated membrane protein-1 (LAMP-1 or CD107a) lines the membrane of cytolytic granules and is used as a marker of NK cell degranulation [39]. The expression of activating receptors is also crucial for NK-mediated killing of various target cells [40]. Thus, to investigate single cell–based assay for NK cytolytic activity, we analyzed the expression level of CD107a, and activating receptors in differentiating NK cells transfected with miR-583 or control miR. The $CD56^+CD3^-$ gated NK cell population showed the expression levels of CD107a and activating receptors, including NKG2D, NKp30 and NKp46, were decreased in miR-583-overexpressed NK cells compared with those of the miR-control (Fig. 6c and 6d). Taken together, these results suggest that the decreased expression of miR-583 plays an important role in the differentiation and function of human NK cell through the de-repression of IL2Rγ expression.

Human miR-583 serves as a regulator of IL2Rγ protein expression in differentiating NK cells

To further test whether miR-583 specifically targets the IL2Rγ, we performed reporter assays in cell cultures as described previously [28]. Although the overexpression of miR-583 in HEK-293FT cells dramatically reduced the expression of an AANAT reporter gene construct containing the wild-type IL2Rγ 3′ UTR (Fig. 7a and 7b), the ectopic expression of a control miRNA (Ctrl_miR) had no significant effect on the expression of these reporters (Fig. 7b). Moreover, point mutations in miR-583 induced the recovery of reporter gene expression without changing the AANAT mRNA levels (Fig. 7b). For these experiments, the reporter AANAT mRNA levels were normalized to neomycin resistance (Neo) gene mRNA as an internal control and showed little difference among the samples. These data suggest that miR-583 downregulates IL2Rγ expression by specifically targeting its 3′ UTR sequences.

Discussion

In this study, we demonstrated a regulatory network of potential interactions between miRNA and mRNA expression during NK cell development induced by IL-15 treatment. First, we summarized the gene ontology classifications for the mRNA microarray expression profiles during the development of human NK cell. In these studies, we identified well-known marker genes, including cytokines, receptors and TFs (Table 2 and Table S1). Additionally, we found several key components of the cytotoxic NK cell machinery, including Prf1, GzmA, GzmB and CTSW. The KIR or KLR family members, IL2 receptor subunits (IL2Rα, IL2Rβ and IL2Rγ), NCR1 and CXCR3 are known as activating receptors that send activating signals to NK cells. The chemokines XCL1 and CCL3 (also known as MIP-1α) induce immune responses against pathogen infection.

In previous study, developmental process of mouse NK cells appears to be the transcriptional changes of genes associated with proliferation and effector function according to surface density of CD11b/CD27 [41]. As shown in Table S1, the expression of cyclin-dependent kinase (CDK) 14 that regulates cell cycle progression and cell proliferation [42] was decreased in mature NK cells whereas expressions of effector proteins such as GzmB and Prf1 were increased according to increment of CD56 expression. Furthermore, the expression of dual-specificity phosphatase (DUSP) family, controlling MAPKs, which is associated with cellular proliferation and differentiation increased in mature NK cells [43]. In these results, we suggest that maturation of NK cell in both mouse and human is accompanied by transcriptional changes of genes related to cell proliferation and acquisition of effector function.

For greater insight into the data, we performed signal pathway analysis using the KEGG pathway mapping tool (Table S2) based on the gene ontology classifications presented in Fig. 1d. These results suggested that 64 total genes (28 upregulated and 27 downregulated genes) are related to the PI3K-Akt signaling pathway, which regulates the balance between survival and apoptosis. Additionally, we showed that 138 total genes (19 upregulated and 3 downregulated genes) related to NK cell-mediated cytotoxicity pathways were altered. Thus, these data suggest that there were important changes in the expression of genes involved in cell proliferation and differentiation rather than genes involved in NK cell activation during NK cell development. Genome-wide mRNA array data examining key molecular signatures during human NK cell differentiation could provide additional important information.

Interestingly, human peripheral blood derived $CD56^{dim}CD16^+$ cells revealed more cytotoxicity than $CD56^{bright}CD16^-$ cells due to higher expression of GzmB and KIR3DL2, which are involved in regulation of cytotoxicity [44]. However, in vitro differentiated $CD56^+CD3^-$ NK cells by cytokines in mesenchymal stem cells derived umbilical cord blood indicate reduction of CD16 expression, but have potent cytotoxicity with upregulated expressions of NKG2D, Prf1, NCR44 and GzmB [45]. Similarly, our results showed that CD16 expression was decreased during in vitro differentiation of NK cells by IL-15 (data not shown), but expression of genes related to cytotoxicity such as GzmB, Prf1, NCR3 and KIR2DL4 was increased according to increment of CD56 expression (Table 1 and Table S1). Furthermore, PI3K/AKT pathway activated by IL-15 revealed critical pathway to enhance NK cell effector function in KEGG pathway (Table S2) [46]. Therefore, we suggest that in vitro differentiated-NK cells may have potent cytotoxicity ability due to induction of cytotoxicity-related genes.

Recently, miRNAs have been widely investigated as master regulators of gene expression during the development and activation of immune cells [15,16]. In addition, it was reported that changes in specific miRNAs contribute to distinct mRNA expression profiles when rescued tolerant $CD8^+$ T cells were preprogrammed to reestablish the tolerant state [34,35]. Furthermore, we have previously reported that human miR-27a* acts as a negative regulator of NK cell cytotoxicity by silencing Prf1 and GzmB expression. Thus, we focused on miRNAs that regulate marker gene expression during human NK cell differentiation.

As shown in Fig. 2, we found that the expression of miR-150 was strongly increased in mNK cells. Notably, miR-150 was previously identified as a regulator of NK cell development by targeting c-Myb in mice [25]. The mature miR-150 sequence in humans, mice and rats are identical [47]. Thus, we assumed that miR-150 could play an important role in humans and in mice. Additionally, the downregulation of miR-223 in human mNK cells was previously reported to regulate GzmB translation [33]. Therefore, these results suggest that genome-wide miRNA array data could offer important information on the regulation of marker genes related to human NK cell development. However, most miRNAs are novel candidates, the functions of which are unknown in immune cells, including NK cells. Despite the development of various target prediction algorithms, most miRNAs do not necessarily target their predicted target proteins. For this reason, new experimental strategies are required to explore target genes regulated by predicted miRNAs during NK cell differentiation. To identify highly correlated target genes of the four predicted miRNAs in this study, we illustrated a potential network between the four selected miRNAs and their highly correlated target mRNAs using Magia. Following this process, miR-583 showed the largest fold change in mNK cells, and this miRNA was correlated with IL2Rγ, which is a common subunit present in both the IL2 receptor and the IL-15 receptor that stimulates the differentiation and expansion of NK cells. Importantly, IL2Rγ-deficient mice showed a defect in mature T- and B-cell development, as well as a complete lack of NK cell development [36]. Thus, we suggest that miR-583 could act as an essential regulator of IL2Rγ expression during human NK cell development.

Recently, several miRNAs have been closely associated with NK cell development [22]. Bezman et al. examined the expression profile of miRNAs in mouse and human NK cells using microarrays. In mouse NK cells, miR-150 regulated NK cell development by targeting c-Myb [25]. Additionally, miR-155 Tg mice have an increased number of total NK cell and an excess of the $CD11b^{low}CD27^{high}$ NK cell subset, which is indicative of a halt in terminal NK cell differentiation; this occurrence proved to be intrinsic to the cell itself, in part via the diminished expression of the inositol phosphatase SHIP-1 [26]. In contrast, miR-155 deficient mice showed a defect in the homeostasis and activation in NK cells [27].

In addition, it has been reported that miR-181 promotes the development of NK cells from $CD34^+$ hematopoietic progenitor cells and IFN-γ production in primary human $CD56^+CD3^-$ NK cell, at least in part through the suppression of nemo-like kinase (NLK), an inhibitor of Notch signaling [48]. Thus, miRNAs have been implicated in human NK cell development and activation through their ability to regulate the expression of signature molecules involved in NK cell development. Here, for the first time, we have defined the expression profiles of genome-wide mRNA and miRNAs during human NK cell differentiation. The miR-583 is known to be involved in ZHENG differentiation during chronic Hepatitis B infection through the regulation of the MAPK signaling pathway in liver cells [49], but the effect of this miRNA on immune cell differentiation, including that of NK cells, has not been studied. In this study, we demonstrate that miR-583 regulates the NK cell developmental process by targeting IL2Rγ.

NK cell development requires the acquisition of NK cell-specific receptors and ultimately the acquisition of functional capacities that can act through these receptors, which will be required for NK cells to mediate therapeutic effects in human clinical trials. However, efforts to modulate the cytolytic activities of NK cells against human cancers have not been successful, suggesting that novel targets regulating NK cell development and cytotoxicity must be identified and targeted. The molecular insights into the role of the miRNAs that specifically regulate NK cell differentiation provided by our study suggest that it also may be possible to enhance NK cell–based immunotherapy against human cancers by modulating miRNAs expression during NK cell development.

Collectively, our results provide a comprehensive database of genome-wide mRNA and miRNA expression during human NK cell differentiation, furthering our understanding of basic human NK cell biology for the application of human NK cells in immunotherapy.

Supporting Information

Table S1 The molecular signatures involved in human NK cell differentiation. Genes showing altered more than 2-fold expression in 7d- and 14-d cultured mNK cells compared to 1 d-cultured (24 h) cells. Blue represents down-regulated genes in mNK cells.

Table S2 Canonical pathway in NK cell differentiation. KEGG pathway mapping was performed based on the gene ontology classification in Figure 1c.

Table S3 The list of miRNA expression during human NK cell differentiation. The miRNA microarray was performed using total RNA isolated from 7- or 14- d (mNK) culture cells after differentiation induction. The results are presented from duplicate experiments and deposited in supplemental materials as an Excel file named 'miRNA profile in human NK differentiation'.

Author Contributions

Conceived and designed the experiments: TDK IC. Performed the experiments: SY SUL. Analyzed the data: SY SUL JMK HJL HJ YJP SRY SRO. Contributed reagents/materials/analysis tools: HYS YKK. Wrote the paper: SY SUL IC TDK.

References

1. Di Santo JP (2006) Natural killer cell developmental pathways: a question of balance. Annu Rev Immunol 24: 257–286.
2. Galy A, Travis M, Cen D, Chen B (1995) Human T, B, natural killer, and dendritic cells arise from a common bone marrow progenitor cell subset. Immunity 3: 459–473.
3. Blom B, Spits H (2006) Development of human lymphoid cells. Annu Rev Immunol 24: 287–320.
4. Freud AG, Yokohama A, Becknell B, Lee MT, Mao HC, et al. (2006) Evidence for discrete stages of human natural killer cell differentiation in vivo. J Exp Med 203: 1033–1043.
5. Boggs SS, Trevisan M, Patrene K, Geogopoulos K (1998) Lack of natural killer cell precursors in fetal liver of Ikaros knockout mutant mice. Nat Immun 16: 137–145.
6. Barton K, Muthusamy N, Fischer C, Ting CN, Walunas TL, et al. (1998) The Ets-1 transcription factor is required for the development of natural killer cells in mice. Immunity 9: 555–563.
7. Colucci F, Samson SI, DeKoter RP, Lantz O, Singh H, et al. (2001) Differential requirement for the transcription factor PU.1 in the generation of natural killer cells versus B and T cells. Blood 97: 2625–2632.
8. Boos MD, Yokota Y, Eberl G, Kee BL (2007) Mature natural killer cell and lymphoid tissue-inducing cell development requires Id2-mediated suppression of E protein activity. J Exp Med 204: 1119–1130.
9. Samson SI, Richard O, Tavian M, Ranson T, Vosshenrich CA, et al. (2003) GATA-3 promotes maturation, IFN-gamma production, and liver-specific homing of NK cells. Immunity 19: 701–711.
10. Townsend MJ, Weinmann AS, Matsuda JL, Salomon R, Farnham PJ, et al. (2004) T-bet regulates the terminal maturation and homeostasis of NK and Valpha14i NKT cells. Immunity 20: 477–494.
11. Kaisho T, Tsutsui H, Tanaka T, Tsujimura T, Takeda K, et al. (1999) Impairment of natural killer cytotoxic activity and interferon gamma production in CCAAT/enhancer binding protein gamma-deficient mice. J Exp Med 190: 1573–1582.
12. Yun S, Lee SH, Yoon SR, Kim MS, Piao ZH, et al. (2011) TOX regulates the differentiation of human natural killer cells from hematopoietic stem cells in vitro. Immunol Lett 136: 29–36.
13. Ni F, Sun R, Fu B, Wang F, Guo C, et al. (2013) IGF-1 promotes the development and cytotoxic activity of human NK cells. Nat Commun 4: 1479.
14. Kennedy MK, Glaccum M, Brown SN, Butz EA, Viney JL, et al. (2000) Reversible defects in natural killer and memory CD8 T cell lineages in interleukin 15-deficient mice. J Exp Med 191: 771–780.
15. Lodish HF, Zhou B, Liu G, Chen CZ (2008) Micromanagement of the immune system by microRNAs. Nat Rev Immunol 8: 120–130.
16. Xiao C, Calado DP, Galler G, Thai TH, Patterson HC, et al. (2007) MiR-150 controls B cell differentiation by targeting the transcription factor c-Myb. Cell 131: 146–159.
17. O'Carroll D, Mecklenbrauker I, Das PP, Santana A, Koenig U, et al. (2007) A Slicer-independent role for Argonaute 2 in hematopoiesis and the microRNA pathway. Genes Dev 21: 1999–2004.

18. Chong MM, Rasmussen JP, Rudensky AY, Littman DR (2008) The RNAseIII enzyme Drosha is critical in T cells for preventing lethal inflammatory disease. J Exp Med 205: 2005–2017.
19. Cobb BS, Hertweck A, Smith J, O'Connor E, Graf D, et al. (2006) A role for Dicer in immune regulation. J Exp Med 203: 2519–2527.
20. Muljo SA, Ansel KM, Kanellopoulou C, Livingston DM, Rao A, et al. (2005) Aberrant T cell differentiation in the absence of Dicer. J Exp Med 202: 261–269.
21. Liston A, Lu LF, O'Carroll D, Tarakhovsky A, Rudensky AY (2008) Dicer-dependent microRNA pathway safeguards regulatory T cell function. J Exp Med 205: 1993–2004.
22. Bezman NA, Cedars E, Steiner DF, Blelloch R, Hesslein DG, et al. (2010) Distinct requirements of microRNAs in NK cell activation, survival, and function. J Immunol 185: 3835–3846.
23. Xiao C, Rajewsky K (2009) MicroRNA control in the immune system: basic principles. Cell 136: 26–36.
24. Baltimore D, Boldin MP, O'Connell RM, Rao DS, Taganov KD (2008) MicroRNAs: new regulators of immune cell development and function. Nat Immunol 9: 839–845.
25. Bezman NA, Chakraborty T, Bender T, Lanier LL (2011) miR-150 regulates the development of NK and iNKT cells. J Exp Med 208: 2717–2731.
26. Trotta R, Chen L, Costinean S, Josyula S, Mundy-Bosse BL, et al. (2013) Overexpression of miR-155 causes expansion, arrest in terminal differentiation and functional activation of mouse natural killer cells. Blood.
27. Zawislak CL, Beaulieu AM, Loeb GB, Karo J, Canner D, et al. (2013) Stage-specific regulation of natural killer cell homeostasis and response against viral infection by microRNA-155. Proc Natl Acad Sci U S A 110: 6967–6972.
28. Kim TD, Lee SU, Yun S, Sun HN, Lee SH, et al. (2011) Human microRNA-27a* targets Prf1 and GzmB expression to regulate NK-cell cytotoxicity. Blood 118: 5476–5486.
29. Sonkoly E, Stahle M, Pivarcsi A (2008) MicroRNAs and immunity: novel players in the regulation of normal immune function and inflammation. Semin Cancer Biol 18: 131–140.
30. Kim TD, Park JY, Choi I (2009) Post-transcriptional Regulation of NK Cell Activation. Immune Netw 9: 115–121.
31. Yun S, Lee SH, Kang YH, Jeong M, Kim MJ, et al. (2010) YC-1 enhances natural killer cell differentiation from hematopoietic stem cells. Int Immunopharmacol 10: 481–486.
32. Kim N, Kim M, Yun S, Doh J, Greenberg PD, et al. (2014) MicroRNA-150 regulates the cytotoxicity of natural killers by targeting perforin-1. Journal of Allergy and Clinical Immunology 134: 195–203.
33. Fehniger TA, Wylie T, Germino E, Leong JW, Magrini VJ, et al. (2010) Next-generation sequencing identifies the natural killer cell microRNA transcriptome. Genome Res 20: 1590–1604.
34. Schietinger A, Delrow JJ, Basom RS, Blattman JN, Greenberg PD (2012) Rescued tolerant CD8 T cells are preprogrammed to reestablish the tolerant state. Science 335: 723–727.
35. Guo H, Ingolia NT, Weissman JS, Bartel DP (2010) Mammalian microRNAs predominantly act to decrease target mRNA levels. Nature 466: 835–840.
36. DiSanto JP, Muller W, Guy-Grand D, Fischer A, Rajewsky K (1995) Lymphoid development in mice with a targeted deletion of the interleukin 2 receptor gamma chain. Proc Natl Acad Sci U S A 92: 377–381.
37. Becknell B, Caligiuri MA (2005) Interleukin-2, interleukin-15, and their roles in human natural killer cells. Adv Immunol 86: 209–239.
38. Horng T, Bezbradica JS, Medzhitov R (2007) NKG2D signaling is coupled to the interleukin 15 receptor signaling pathway. Nat Immunol 8: 1345–1352.
39. Winchester BG (2001) Lysosomal membrane proteins. European Journal of Paediatric Neurology 5: 11–19.
40. Moretta A, Bottino C, Vitale M, Pende D, Cantoni C, et al. (2001) Activating receptors and coreceptors involved in human natural killer cell-mediated cytolysis. Annual review of immunology 19: 197–223.
41. Chiossone L, Chaix J, Fuseri N, Roth C, Vivier E, et al. (2009) Maturation of mouse NK cells is a 4-stage developmental program. Blood 113: 5488–5496.
42. Shu F, Lv S, Qin Y, Ma X, Wang X, et al. (2007) Functional characterization of human PFTK1 as a cyclin-dependent kinase. Proceedings of the National Academy of Sciences 104: 9248–9253.
43. Jeffrey KL, Camps M, Rommel C, Mackay CR (2007) Targeting dual-specificity phosphatases: manipulating MAP kinase signalling and immune responses. Nature Reviews Drug Discovery 6: 391–403.
44. Hanna J, Bechtel P, Zhai Y, Youssef F, McLachlan K, et al. (2004) Novel insights on human NK cells' immunological modalities revealed by gene expression profiling. The Journal of Immunology 173: 6547–6563.
45. Wang J, Sun Z, Cao L, Li Q (2012) [Biological characteristics of cord blood natural killer cells induced and amplified with IL-2 and IL-15]. Zhongguo shi yan xue ye xue za zhi/Zhongguo bing li sheng li xue hui = Journal of experimental hematology/Chinese Association of Pathophysiology 20: 731–735.
46. Nandagopal N, Ali AK, Komal AK, Lee S-H (2014) The critical role of IL-15-PI3K-mTOR pathway in natural killer cell effector functions. Frontiers in immunology 5.
47. Griffiths-Jones S, Grocock RJ, van Dongen S, Bateman A, Enright AJ (2006) miRBase: microRNA sequences, targets and gene nomenclature. Nucleic Acids Res 34: D140–144.
48. Cichocki F, Felices M, McCullar V, Presnell SR, Al-Attar A, et al. (2011) Cutting edge: microRNA-181 promotes human NK cell development by regulating Notch signaling. J Immunol 187: 6171–6175.
49. Hosomi S, Chen Z, Baker K, Chen L, Huang YH, et al. (2013) CEACAM1 on activated NK cells inhibits NKG2D-mediated cytolytic function and signaling. Eur J Immunol 43: 2473–2483.

Hydroxyapatite-Coated Sillicone Rubber Enhanced Cell Adhesion and It May Be through the Interaction of EF1β and γ-Actin

Xiao-hua Shi[1,9], Shao-liang Wang[1,9], Yi-ming Zhang[1], Yi-cheng Wang[2], Zhi Yang[3], Xin Zhou[1], Ze-yuan Lei[1], Dong-li Fan[1]*

[1] Department of Plastic and Cosmetic Surgery, Xinqiao Hospital, the Third Military Medical University, Chongqing, 400037, People's Republic of China, [2] Department of Plastic and Cosmetic Surgery, Chongqing Armed Police Corps Hospital, Chongqing, 400061, People's Republic of China, [3] Department of War Trauma care, Hainan branch of PLA General Hospital, Sanya, Hainan, 572013, People's Republic of China

Abstract

Silicone rubber (SR) is a common soft tissue filler material used in plastic surgery. However, it presents a poor surface for cellular adhesion and suffers from poor biocompatibility. In contrast, hydroxyapatite (HA), a prominent component of animal bone and teeth, can promote improved cell compatibility, but HA is an unsuitable filler material because of the brittleness in mechanism. In this study, using a simple and economical method, two sizes of HA was applied to coat on SR to counteract the poor biocompatibility of SR. Surface and mechanical properties of SR and HA/SRs confirmed that coating with HA changes the surface topology and material properties. Analysis of cell proliferation and adhesion as well as measurement of the expression levels of adhesion related molecules indicated that HA-coated SR significantly increased cell compatibility. Furthermore, mass spectrometry proved that the biocompatibility improvement may be related to elongation factor 1-beta (EF1β)/γ-actin adjusted cytoskeletal rearrangement.

Editor: Jie Zheng, University of Akron, United States of America

Funding: This work was funded by a grant from National Natural Science Foundation of China (81372075) (http://www.nsfc.gov.cn/publish/portal0/default.htm), and a grant for Transformation of Scientific and Technological Achievements from Third Military Medical University (2012XZH05) (http://www.tmmu.edu.cn/). The funders had no role in study design, data collection and analysis, decision to publish, or preparation of the manuscript.

Competing Interests: The authors have declared that no competing interests exist.

* Email: fdltmmu@sina.com

9 These authors contributed equally to this work.

Introduction

From its first use as an augmented rhinoplasty material in 1955, silicone rubber (SR) has become a common biological implantation material in plastic surgery [1]. According to clinicians, SR is easily processed into various shapes for medical devices, soft tissue filler, and even artificial organs [2,3]. However, because of its compact structure and hydrophobicity, surrounding tissue cells cannot grow into the surface of the SR material, so it is easily to form capsule around the implant what is more to form capsular contracture [4]. The deposition of the collagenous structures onto the filler surface may lead to disfigurement as the implant bodies harden, shrink, or displaced, even greater harm, such as the implant bodies puncture the skin and lead to further complications including infection [5].

Hydroxyapatite (HA) is a naturally form of calcium apatite and is a key component of animal bones and teeth. By weight, it constitutes more than 96% of human teeth enamel and approximately 60% of human bone [6]. HA performs well in biocompatibility and corrosion resistance; furthermore, it has no toxic side effects. It can also integrates with the surrounding tissue and avoid the occurrence of rejection. For instance, when used for implantation in bone reconstruction, HA exhibits biocompatible properties but as a bulk material it suffers limitation because of its brittleness [7]. To counteract these difficulties, HA has been coated on to the surface of metallic implants, e.g. Citeau, Thian, Nelea, etc. [8–10] tried to blasting HA onto Titanium alloy (Ti6Al4V) and Magnetron *et al.* metallic materials found that HA coating can acquire both the mechanism properties and biocompatibility. The coating process can be made via several different methods including electro deposition plasma spraying, sputtering, and laser ablation *etc.* [11–13]. When implanted into bodies, the HA coating can help avoid the occurrence of rejection and encourages the integration of the implant with the surrounding tissue [14]. Thus, the implant is able to acquire both the desired mechanical properties and the required biocompatibility when HA is coated onto the surface of metal or other medical implants.

When HA was coated on to the surface of Ti6Al4 V, the material showed better bioabsorbability [15]. Using CoBlast to deposition HA onto a titanium substrate, Dunne *et al.* found a significant change to the surface properties of titanium [16]. Similarly, for nanostructured hydroxyapatite (nHA)/poly (lactic-co-glycolic acid) (PLGA) composite coatings on Mg-based substrates, the researchers observed synergistic properties that controlled the degradation of Mg-based substrates and improved bone-implant integration [17]. In addition to coating metal materials, HA is also used in composite with several types of polymers. For example, when HA was coated onto the surface of

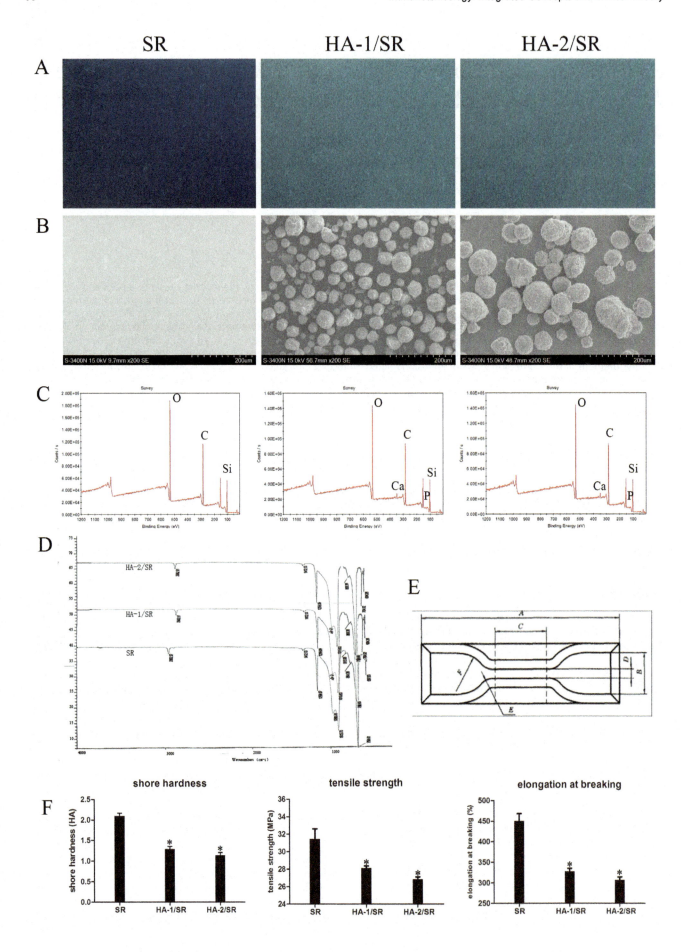

Figure 1. Characterization of HA coated SR. A, Optical microscopy pictures of the three kinds of samples (Left, SR; Middle, HA-1/SR; Right, HA-2/SR); B, SEM pictures of the three samples(Left, SR; Middle, HA-1/SR; Right, HA-2/SR); C, X-ray photoelectron spectroscopy of the three samples; D, FTIR of the three samples; E, Dumbbell shape of the sample for the mechanical properties study; F, Mechanical properties of the three samples (Shore hardness; elongation at breaking; tensile stress). Each number has six repeat, the average and stander standard error of the mean was used.

Poly L-lactic acid (PLLA) micro-fibers, that were implanted into Beagle dogs, histological and radiographic analysis showed that HA/PLLA screws induced significant increases in HA bone content from 36 months onward, and a burr hole was closed by 60 months [18].

In this study, we applied the HA coating process to SR, a material highly suitable for soft tissue implants, and measured the altered mechanical and cellular interaction properties of the SR. Our data indicate that we successfully produced HA coated SR materials, and the coating materials showed improved biocompatibility. Moreover, we developed a useful process for its production. In addition, through mass spectra we studied the molecular mechanism of cell adhesion.

Materials and Methods

Preparation of SR and HA coated SR

At temperature of 20°C and humidity of 50%, a mixture of equal proportions (A:B = 1:1) of the two-component liquid SR (Chenguang Research Institute of Chemical Engineering, Chengdu, China) was slowly injected into a metal plate mold (100 mm × 100 mm × 2 mm) and placed into a vacuum chamber at −0.1 MPa for 30 min, then, cure at room temperature for 5.5 h. To coat the SR with HA, using custom-made spray painting equipment [19] with two sizes of HA (particle diameter of 40 μm, named HA-1, and particle diameter of 100 μm, named HA-2). The HA (National Engineering Research Center for Biomaterials, Sichuan University, China) was spread onto the surface of the SR mold after 5 h temperature curing, and it was left to cure for 0.5 h.

Surface Characterization of HA coated SR

For SEM (scanning electron microscope, AMRAY 1000-B, Amray Inc, Bedford, Mass, USA) observations, SR and HA-SRs were cut into 10 mm × 10 mm squares and dried in 37°C. Before observation, these squares were put into a vacuum pump to spray painting gold coat on the surface. X-ray photoelectron spectroscopy (XPS) was conducted on a Physical Electronics PHI 5802 equipped with a monochromatic Al Kα source to determine the surface chemical composition and elemental depth profiles. The sputtering rate was estimated to be approximately 5.67 nm•min^{-1} based on that calculated from a SiO_2 standard sputtered under similar conditions, and the binding energies were referenced to the C 1s line at 285.0 eV. For Fourier transform infrared spectroscopy (FTIR) each material was cut into 10 mm × 10 mm squares and cleaned with dehydrated alcohol. After the alcohol volatilated, the material surface composition was studied by FTIR (Ni-colet 470 spectrometer); wave number is 4 cm^{-1}; the scan extent is 4000~400 cm^{-1}. The water contact angles of SR and two kinds of HA/SRs were measured with a drop shape analysis system (DSA100, Krü ss). Test was in the sessile mode at room temperature. The roughness of the three kinds of SR was tested by LEXT OLS4100 laser confocal microscope (Olympus, Janpan), using 20x objective and the scan size is 13352 μm, each sample repeats 6 times.

Mechanical Properties

An A-Type Shore hardness meter (Harbin Measuring & Cutting Tool Group Co. Ltd, China) was used to test the Shore hardness of the coated and non-coated SR. The samples were soaked in 75% medical alcohol for 3 min, then sonicated for 15 min in deionized water, and dried at 50°C. Three pieces of overlapping samples in thickness of 5 mm were placed on a smooth, flat metal plate to test the Shore hardness. The spacing between the two test points was greater than 6 mm, and the distance from the test point to the sample edge was 20 mm. Each sample test more than six times. In order to detect tensile stress-strain properties, vulcanized SR were cut into a dumbbell shape (Figure 1E), fixed on an electronic universal testing machine (Exceed, E44 MTS, USA). Following three times of pre-stretching at a speed of 30 mm/min and an intensity of less than 2 N, measurements were taken of tensile strength and elongation until breakage.

Cell Culture

Dermis fibroblasts (Homo sapiens) were employed to investigate the effects of HA coated SR on cell behavior. All cells were cultivated in a complete cell culture medium consisting of a mixture of Dulbecco's modified Eagle medium (DMEM, Gibco, USA) and 10% fetal bovine serum (FBS, Gibco, USA) in a humidified atmosphere of 5% CO_2 at 37°C.

Cell Adhesion and Cytotoxicity

Prior to cell cultivation, the samples were sterilized by immersion in 75% (v/v) ethanol for 30 min and subsequently rinsed three times with sterile phosphate buffered saline (PBS). The dermis fibroblasts were seeded on each sample in 24 well tissue culture plates at a density of 1×10^4 cells per well and cultured for 24 h. Afterwards, the seeded samples were rinsed twice with sterile PBS, fixed with 4% polyoxymethylene solution, and stained with fluorescein isothiocyanate (FITC)-labeled actin tracker (Beyotime Institute of Biotechnology, China) sequentially. Cell adhesion was determined from three random fields using a fluorescence microscope (Leica TCS SP5, Germany). For cytotoxicity detection, propidium iodide (PI) and Hoechst 33342 double staining was used. The final concentration of Hoechst 33342 solution was 1μM, and the final concentration of PI was 10μg/ml. Cells were cultured on the material surface for 24 h, rinsed two times with PBS, and incubated with Hoechst 33342 at 37 °C in darkness for 15 min. The Hoechst 33342 solution was then removed with a PBS rinse, and PI dye was added and incubated at 4°C for 15 min in darkness, followed by PBS rinse. Laser scanning confocal microscope (Leica TCS SP5, Germany) was used to observe the staining. Hoechst 33342 krypton laser excitation with a UV fluorescence excitation wavelength of 352nm and an emission wavelength of 400~500 nm, produces blue fluorescence. PI fluorescence with an argon ion laser excitation, excitation wavelength of 488 nm and emission wavelength greater than 630 nm, produces red fluorescence.

Cell Proliferation Assay and Cell morphology observation by SEM

A Cell Count Kit-8 (CCK-8, Dojindo, Japan) assay was used to determine the cell viability and cell proliferation. Fibroblasts were seeded at a density of 5×10^3 cells/well on the samples in 96-well tissue culture plates and cultured for 2 days. At the end of the incubation period, the samples were rinsed twice with sterile PBS

Table 1. Water contact angle of the three kinds of SR surface (n = 6, $\bar{x} \pm s$).

Group	SR	HA-1/SR	HA-2/SR
Water contact angle	111.4±2.7	107.7±1.1	106.3±1.5

and transferred to a new 96-well tissue culture plate. The attached cells were incubated in DMEM containing 5 mg/mL CCK-8 for 2 h. The optical density (OD) values were recorded by a Power Wave Microplate Spectrophotometer (Thermo, USA) at 450 nm to determine the cell viability. The cytoskeleton was stained with FITC-labeled actin Tracker probes (Beyotime Institute of Biotechnology, China). The results of the *in vitro* cell experiments were statistically analyzed using one-way analysis of variance (ANOVA) and a *p* value of less than 0.05 was considered to indicate statistical significance. As described previously [20], after cultured as monolayer on SR or HA/SR surface, human dermal fibroblasts were rinsed with PBS and fixed with 3% buffered glutaraldehyde for 20 min at 4°C. Then aqueous ethanol (30–100%) was used for dehydration step by step. Samples were lyophilized and coated with platinum. Cell morphology was observed by SEM (AMRAY 1000-B, Amray Inc, Bedford, Mass, USA).

Detection of cell adhesion molecules

Western blot was used to detect the expression of adhesion related molecules with a mouse anti-human vinculin monoclonal IgG (Sigma-Aldrich, USA) at a dilution of 1:1000. Horse radish peroxidase (HRP) labeled goat anti-mouse IgG (Santa Cruz, USA) was used at a dilution 1:1000; rabbit anti-human zyxin polyclonal IgG (Millipore, USA) was diluted to 1:1000, rabbit anti-human talin polyclonal IgG (Millipore, USA) diluted into 1:1000, rabbit anti-human OPN polyclonal IgG (Santa Cruz, USA) was diluted to 1:300, and HRP labeled goat anti-rabbit IgG (Santa Cruze, USA) was diluted to 1:1000. Antibody binding was detected using an enhanced chemiluminescence (ECL) detection system (Advanstar, USA). The intensity of each blot was quantified by Quantity one software, and was normalized to the loading control (GAPDH). Each experiment was repeated at least three times. For immuno-fluorescence experiments, human dermal fibroblasts were cultured on SR or HA-SR surfaces as a monolayer were washed three times with PBS, and fixed in cold paraformaldehyde (4%) for 15 min at 4°C. Cells were then blocked with 5% bovine serum albumin in PBS (pH 7.5) for 30 min, followed by overnight incubation with the primary antibody as following: rabbit anti-talin (Abcam, USA, 1:500), rabbit anti-zyxin (Cell Signaling, USA, 1:500), rabbit anti-OPN (Santa Cruz, USA, 1:100), or mouse anti-vinculin (Sigma-Aldrich, St. Louis, MO, USA, 1:500). The corresponding Cy3 or FITC-tagged secondary antibody (Invitrogen, Shanghai, China) was then added, and incubated for 1h at room temperature. The cell nuclei were stained with 4′, 6′-diamidino-2-phenylindole (DAPI; 0.5 μg/ml; Sigma-Aldrich, St. Louis, MO, USA). Cells were visualized by using a Leica confocal microscope (Leica TCS SP5, Germany) with the appropriate filters. All measurements were repeated six times for each condition.

Total RNA isolation and real-time reverse transcriptase polymerase chain reaction (RT-PCR)

The expression of talin, zyxin, OPN, vinculin mRNA was analyzed by real-time reverse transcription-polymerase chain reaction (RT-PCR), GAPDH mRNA expression was as control. Total RNA was prepared from cultured cells using TRIzol reagent (Invitrogen, CA, USA) according to the manufacturer's introduction. Spectrophotometrically at A260 and A280 were hired to measure the concentration and purity of RNA. ReverTra Ace RT-PCR kit (TOYOBO, Janpan) according to the manufacturer's instruction was used for RT-PCR. The resulting cDNA was used as a template for PCR with specific primer pairs using Primer Premier 5.0 software (Premier Biosoft, International, Palo Alto, CA, USA). The results were analyzed using delta Ct. All real-time PCRs were performed three times at least.

The primers used in the experiment are as bellows:
homo zyxin sense: GACCCAGGACCCAACAT,
homo zyxin antisense: CCTCCGCAAGCAGAGTA;
homo vinculin sense: ACAGATAAACGGATTAGAAC,
homo vinculin antisense: GCATTGTGAACCAGCA;
homo talin sense: CTGACAACAACCCTCAAC,
homo talin antisense: CCATTGGTCCTTCATCTA;
homo OPN sense: CAGCCAGGACTCCATT,
homo OPN antisense: TGTCAGGTCTGCGAAA;
homo GAPDH sense: ACCACAGTCCATGCCATCAC,
homo GAPDH antisense: TCCACCACCCTGTTGCTGTA.

Mass Spectrometry Analyses

Total cellular protein was extracted from SR and HA-coated SR surfaces after 48 h of culture. The protein was extracted and separated in 8% SDS-PAGE and stained with Coomassie blue. Protein bands were cut out of the gel for analysis by mass spectrometry (VG Auto Spec 3000). The mass spectrometry results were then analyzed using the tools of the NCBI and EMBL databases.

Generation of EF1β knockdown stable dermal fibroblasts by lentiviral infection and cytoskeleton stain

The dermal fibroblasts were seeded in a 6-well plate with 60% confluence in growth medium with polybrene,the EF1β knockdown stable dermal fibroblasts was constructed as before mentioned [20], using the EF1β shRNA lentiviral. The cytoskel-

Table 2. Surface roughness of the three kinds of SR surface (n = 6, $\bar{x} \pm s$, * $P<0.05$).

Group	SR (μm)	HA-1/SR (μm)	HA-2/SR (μm)
Surface roughness	3.808±0.165	6.856±0.066*	8.094±0.1342*

Table 3. Chemical composition (%) according to XPS analysis.

Group	%/binding energy) C	%/binding energy Si	%/binding energy O	%/binding energy Ca	%/binding energy P
SR	45.52/285.01	29.45/102.52	25.02/532.65		
HA-1/SR	43.86/285.02	28.33/102.55	26.33/532.7	0.77/348.19	0.71/133.94
HA-2/SR	42.65/285.01	27.46/102.7	24.54/532.65	2.69/347.91	2.61/134.26

eton was stained with FITC-labeled actin Tracker probes (Beyotime, Shanghai, China).

Statistical analysis

The data presented in this study were expressed as means ± standard error of the mean (SE). Statistical differences were analyzed by one-way ANOVA followed by multiple comparisons performed with post hoc Bonferroni tests (SPSS version 16.0). The standard value of $p<0.05$ was considered statistically significant. The significance of any differences between two groups was tested using the paired-samples t-test, when appropriate.

Results

HA coated SR Preparation and Physicochemical properties

Optical microscopy shows that SR was colorless and transparent (Figure 1A). In contrast, large amounts of white HA particles were clearly visible on HA coated SR (Figure 1A). Additionally, SR surface was flat and smooth without any impurities, while the HA-coated SR surface is uneven with a large number of uniformly sized HA particles tightly adhered to the surface (Figure 1A). In addition, the water contact angle of HA-coated SRs decreased a little compare to SR, but not significantly (Table 1).

SEM results showed that hydroxyapatite particles firm adhesion on the surface of SR (Figure 1B), the surface roughness of the material increased after hydroxyapatite coating, and HA/SR surface roughness also increased with hydroxyapatite particle size increase (Table 2).

The main components of SR are carbon, silicon, and oxygen (C, Si, and O). Thus, analysis of C, Si, O content with the HA modified surfaces can determine if there is any change in chemical composition. X-ray photoelectron spectroscopy (XPS) (Figure 1C, Table 3) showed that in HA-1/SR, there was a small amount of C reduction relative to the standard. XPS spectra of pure SR, C1s, Si2p, and O1s peak and peaks as well as of HA-1/SR and HA-2/SR showed a fluctuation range <0.1 eV, and they were not significantly different. While the corresponding calcium and phosphorus (Ca, P) corresponding peaks of HA-1/SR and HA-2/SR were observed (Table 3).

FTIR (Figure 1D) measurements detected the following bonds: -CH3 anti-symmetric stretching vibration absorption peaks at 2962 ± 1 cm^{-1}; Si-O (-C) diffraction peak at 1080 ± 1 cm^{-1}; -OH bending vibration wave at 680 ± 10 cm^{-1}; diffraction peak of CO_3^{2-} is at 1412 ± 1 cm^{-1}. In the spectra of HA-1/SR and HA-2/SR, HA was only sprayed onto the surface of SR, and thus its total content is very little, so the peak of PO_4^{3-} at $950 \sim 1200$ cm^{-1} was not significantly different between HA-1/SR and HA-2/SR.

The mechanical property data (Figure 1F) show that compare to SR, HA-1/SR and HA-2/SR had statistically significant ($p<0.05$) differences in terms of Shore hardness, tensile strength, and elongation. While between HA-1/SR and HA-2/SR there was no statistically significant difference ($p>0.05$).

Cell Compatibility

As shown by the double staining of Hoechst 33342 with PI test for cytotoxicity of materials shown in Figure 2A, the cells suffered no significant toxic effects from either SR or HA/SRs. The results of the FITC-labeled actin-tracker, used to label actin and hence the cellular cytoskeletal structure, showed that in cells on the non-coated SR group, actin staining was less, the protrusion of edges was shrink, and filaments were sparsely arranged, compared to the HA-coated materials. In contrast, cells on the HA/SR surface showed greater green fluorescence, outward expansion of edge protrusions, greater filament increased, a rearranged cytoskeleton into fiber bundles, and fibroblasts cells with irregular long spindle protruding edges but with regularly arranged and evenly distributed filaments along the projections. The HA-1/SR surface had more obvious cytoskeletal rearrangement than that of HA-2/SR, suggesting that its surface is more conducive to cell adhesion (Figure 2A). Cell proliferation was detected with CCK-8 (Figure 2B). Both HA coated surfaces, showed OD values significantly higher than that of uncoated surface groups ($p<0.05$).

According to the evaluation standard of ISO 10993-5:1999 (Table 4), we determined the cytotoxicity of the material (Table 5), the relative growth rate (RGR) was calculated from the OD values using the following Calculation formula: RGR = (OD value of test sample group - OD value of blank)/(OD value of control group - OD value of blank) ×100%. According to the standard of ISO 1093-5:1999 and the people's Republic of China GB/T 16886.5-2003, in biological evaluation of medical devices in vitro cytotoxicity test, high density polyethylene used as a negative control reaction materials. Both the HA coated materials, HA-1/SR and HA-2/SR, had RGR values >100%, indicating a toxicity level of 0. The pure SR had an RGR value between 75% and 99%, indicating a toxicity level of 1 (Table 5). Therefore, HA coated SR has no toxic effects to cells and is in fact safer than SR.

Cell proliferation analysis (Table 5, Figure 2B) showed that the proliferation of cells in the HA-1/SR and HA-2/SR groups showed cell growth greater than that of the SR group ($p<0.05$); while the SR group shows a slower cell growth rate with significantly fewer cells ($p<0.05$).

SEM image results further demonstrated a more fibroblastic appearance of fibroblasts cultured on HA/SRs (Figure 2A). We also quantified the morphology of fibroblasts on different substrates. The cell area depicted higher values for cells on HA coated SRs than those on SR (Figure 2C), But there was no statistically significant difference between HA-1/SR and HA-2/SR ($p>0.05$).

Cell Adhesion Molecules

Human dermal fibroblast cells were cultured on the surface of the SR, HA-1/SR, and HA-2/SR for 48 h, total cellular protein was extracted. Western blot analysis of the cell extracts that there

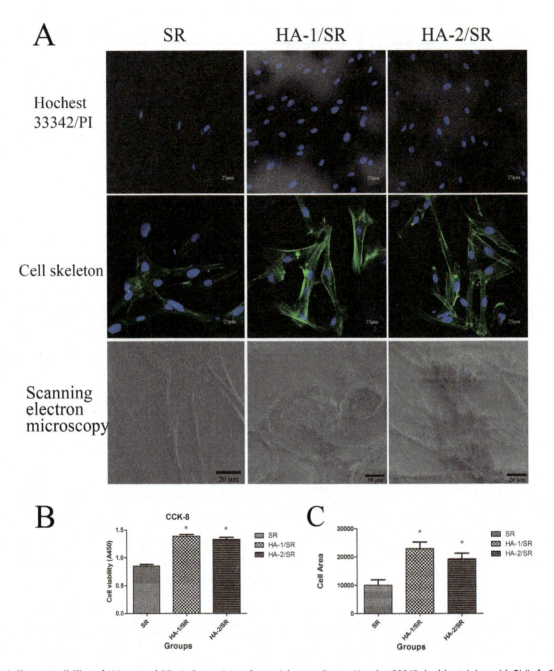

Figure 2. Cell compatibility of HA coated SR. A, Cytotoxicity of materials according to Hoechst 33342 double staining with PI (Left, SR; Middle, HA-1/SR; Right, HA-2/SR); Cell skeleton structure staining of each group (Left, SR; Middle, HA-1/SR; Right, HA-2/SR) (the scale bar is 25 μm); SEM images further demonstrated a more fibroblastic appearance of fibroblasts cultured on HA/SR (the scale bar is 20 μm); B, Cell proliferation of each group studied by CCK-8 (n = 6, *$p<0.05$); C, Cell area of each group studied by IPP6 (n = 6, *$p<0.05$).

were significant vinculin expression changes among the HA-1/SR and HA-2/SR groups compared with the SR group ($p<0.05$). The HA-1/SR and HA-2/SR groups showed greater expression, which may also indicate that the cell adhesion had improved with HA coating. Osteopontin (OPN) protein expression of the HA-1/SR and HA-2/SR groups was also significantly stronger than in the SR group ($p<0.05$). These results collectively indicate that without HA coating, SR is a poorer substrate for cells than with the HA coating SR, which improved the SR material properties to the extent that it became a better surface to support cell adhesion. In addition, zyxin and talin were also selected as candidate proteins; their protein expression levels were also greater in the HA-coated groups than in the noncoated group, the results both in Western-blot and realtime PCR are all the same (Figure 3C).

Mass spectrometry analysis of cellular protein expression on the surface of HA coated SR

As the results presented above, the compatibility to cells imparted by HA coating to SR implant materials was significantly increased. To better understand the signaling mechanisms behind this phenomenon, the cells cultured on the surface of the three

Table 4. ISO 10993-5:1999 standard of cytotoxicity evaluation of biomaterials according to RGR.

Cytotoxicity level	RGR(%)
Level 0	≥100
Level 1	75–99
Level 2	50–74
Level 3	25–49
Level 4	1–24
Level 5	0

kinds of SR were harvested after 48 h and total protein was extracted. Protein bands were isolated and identified by mass spectrometry. As shown in Figure 4B, the total protein SDS-PAGE points of difference 1, 2, and 3 were selected and identified by mass spectrometry. The results were analyzed on the website of SRS@EMBL-EBI. According to the references and bioinformatics analysis, elongation factor 1-beta (EF1β) may play an important role in cell adhesion. Furthermore, we hypothesized that EF1β may mediate γ-actin gene expression, leading to cytoskeletal rearrangements. To test this hypothesis, anti EF1β and anti γ-actin IgG were used for western blot analysis (shown in Figure 4C) to analyze EF1β and γ-actin expression levels. The results showed that EF1β expression was greater and γ-actin expression was less in the HA-coated SR compared to the noncoated SR, thus confirming our conjecture. We further analyzed the veracity of this hypothesis by using bioinformatics via the websites of EMBL, Genebank, protsite Documentation etc. We found that EF1β may regulate γ-actin rearrangements and induce increased cell adhesion. In order to confirm this speculation, we reduced the expression of EF1B by RNA interference, found that cytoskeleton in arrangement and the morphology of the cells on the surface of silicone rubber and HA/SR changed, and control to EF1B normal expression, cytoskeleton staining is more shallow, cell area decreased, and cell adhesion decreased (Figure 4D). This confirms that EF1β may regulate γ-actin, affect cytoskeleton arrangement and affect cell adhesion on material surface.

Discussion

SR is commonly used in plastic surgery. The molecular structure of SR is $(SiOR_2)_n$, in the absence of a double bond; it has stable physical and chemical properties while maintaining good flexibility. Because of its spatial configuration, SR has a relatively low intermolecular force, so it can easily be processed and shaped. Since the SR surface has strong hydrophobicity, it is a poor substrate for cells adhesion. Previous investigators have carried out surface modification or copolymerization with other substances and have achieved remarkable results [4,21].

HA, being chemically similar to the inorganic component of bone is one of the most popularly used bioactive ceramics in the surgical repair of hard tissue trauma and disease. Successful applications of HA have been witnessed in a range of surgical specialties: bone substitute in bony defects restoration in orthopedic surgery [22], sinus obliteration [23], and ossicular chain reconstruction in otolaryngological surgery, and craniofacial augmentation in plastic surgery [24]. However, HA is fragile and with a low mechanical property witch hamper it clinic using. So coating HA onto the surface of SR can assure the advantage of these two materials and improve the clinic using.

Currently, the common coating methods are aerosol deposition[25], laser cladding [26], plasma spraying [15], and sol–gel [26] methods etc.. Although plasma spraying of metal materials is commonly used, in our study, it has been proven to be difficult to apply on SR. The main reason might be the elastic and soft properties of SR, which surface is difficult for HA plasma spraying coating. Electrochemical reaction pulsed-laser-deposited HA coatings, which are usually used in alloy substrates, have been proven stable and can maintain the bioactivity of HA. But this method requires special equipment and the substrate must be heated to almost 600°C, under which SR will burn. In this study, we coated SR with HA via simple spray painting equipment at the vulcanization stage, and the surface coating was verified by SEM observation. The adhesion of HA to SR is tightly, which was confirmed by surface mechanical challenge (adhesive tape) experiments.

In this research, compare to the mechanical properties such as the Shore hardness, tensile strength, and elongation at breakage of HA-SR decreased. Even so, the HA-coated SR can still meet clinical demands as the Shore hardness ranges from 25 to 35 units in ideal filling materials [27]. The coating materials of HA-1/SR and HA-2/SR had Shore hardness values of 28.14±1.83 and 26.85±1.26 respectively, which are both in line with the soft tissue filling material hardness requirements. According to clinical experience, HA-1/SR and HA-2/SR can be used in the clinic as a soft tissue filling material [28].

Through FTIR analysis, the physical and chemical structures of pure SR, HA-1/SR, and HA-2/SR are similar. From XPS results, we can observe that HA coating significantly changed the surface elemental composition; Ca and P were detected on the surface of HA-1/SR and HA-2/SR, revealing that HA is attached on the SR, possibly facilitating cell adhesion.

In the present study, the dermal fibroblasts cultured on HA/SR grew faster and had a higher mobility and better viability than those cultured on pure SR. The cytoskeleton alignment was improved, and we observed increased expressions of adhesion-associated proteins, including talin-1, zyxin and vinculin in fibroblasts cultured on HA/SR, compared to those on SR. As is known, these proteins are involved in the formation of focal adhesion complexes, acting as a conjugation site for both cytoskeletal organization and intracellular signaling transduction, playing a vital role for cell adhesion and migration. The results

Table 5. Cell growth condition of SR and HA/SR (n = 6, $\bar{x}\pm s$, * P<0.05).

group	OD value	RGR (%)	Cytotoxicity level
SR	0.8511±0.0191	76.39	Level 1
HA-1/SR	1.3877±0.0119*	138.86	Level 0
HA-2/SR	1.3280±0.0183*	131.91	Level 0

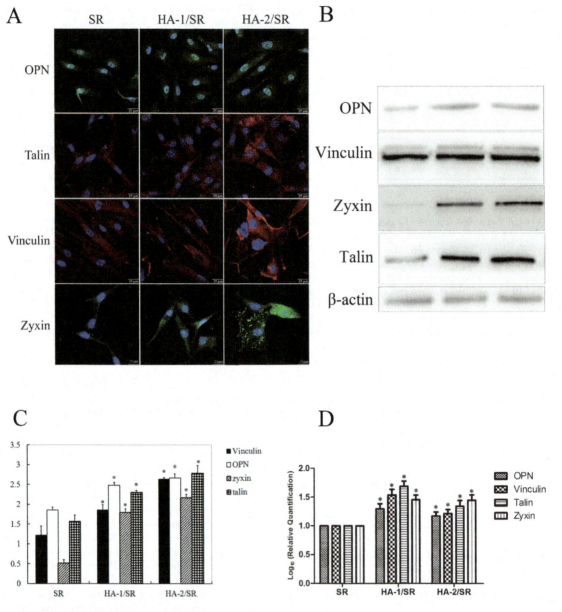

Figure 3. Detection of cell adhesion molecules. A, Immuno-fluorescence of the cells on the three kinds of SR (the scale bar is 20 μm); B, Western-blot of the cells on the three kinds of SR; C, Optical density ratio of Western-blot; D, Realtime PCR of the cells on the three kinds of SR (n = 6, *p<0.05).

indicated that the cell adhesion on HA/SR was significantly improved.

The roughness of materials surface can influence cell adhesion. We selected different particle sizes of hydroxyapatite to coat the surface of SR to prepare HA-coated SR of different roughnesses. To determine if two different particle sizes showed a significant difference, we used HA coating with 40 and 150 μm diameters because they were the only sizes available from the Materials College of Sichuan University. Through the roughness measurement of material surface we found material surface roughness between SR and HA/SR, and the two kinds of HA/SR has remarkable difference. However, using atomic force microscope we did not observed significant difference among the materials surface, the reason maybe that atomic force microscope detection range is too small to detect the difference. Between the two kinds of HA/SR, although the surface roughness is different, but there is no significant difference cytological behavior difference.

In the study presented here, it was interesting to find increased expression of OPN, which is thought to be an important extracellular matrix protein, mediates cell adhesion onto the surface of implants [20]. OPN exists both as a component of the extracellular matrix and as a soluble cytokine, interacting with cells by binding multiple integrins via two major domains that are conserved among species. The ligand-receptor interaction forms a focal adhesion complex, activating signal transduction and provoking recombination of the cytoskeleton. What is known is that this process involves adhesion-associated proteins including talin-1, vinculin, zyxin and others, but the molecular mechanism is still not well understand.

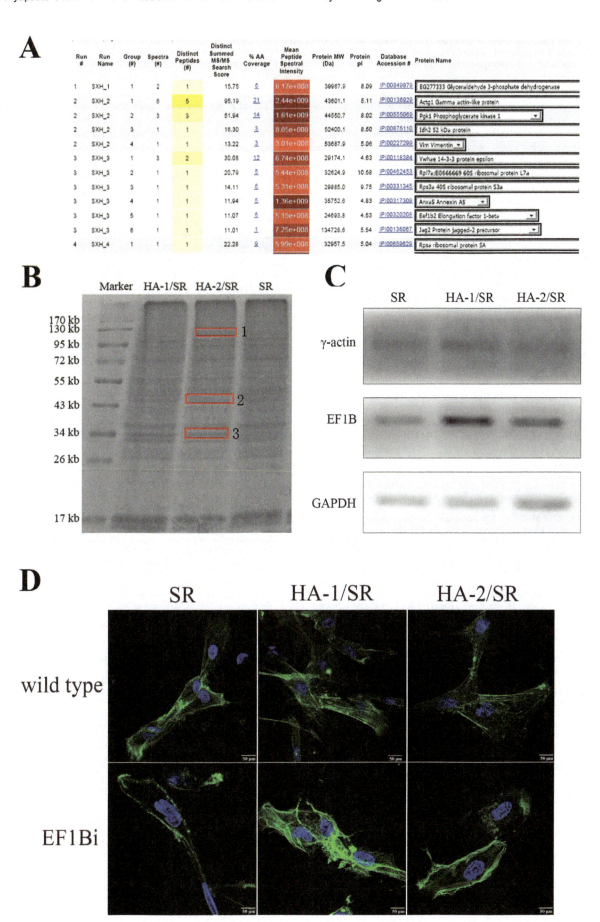

Figure 4. The mechanism of improved cell adhesion on the HA coated surface of SR. A, mass result; B, SDS-PAGE picture (1, 2, 3 represent the selected protein points); C, western-blot verification; D, Cell morphology of EF1β interference human dermal fibroblasts on the three kinds of SR (the scale bar is 50 μm) (wild type means common human dermal fibroblasts, EF1Bi means EF1β interference human dermal fibroblasts).

In order to clarify the intracellular cytoskeleton organization and the corresponding regulation mechanism, we utilized gel electrophoresis (SDS-PAGE) and mass spectrometry analysis to identify the proteins that associated with the HA coating. This approach allowed the identification of γ-actin as the major cytoskeletal protein that was expressed at a higher level by dermal fibroblasts cultured on HA-SR, compared with SR. In vertebrates, three main groups of actin isoforms, alpha, beta, and gamma, have been identified. The beta and gamma actins coexist in most cell types as components of the cytoskeleton and mediators of internal cell motility. Whereas the alpha actins are a major constituent of the contractile apparatus, mostly found in muscle tissues. Recent studies have shown that the interaction among adhesion-associated proteins and these proteins are essential to connect extracellular matrix-bound integrins to the cytoskeleton. For example, talin can bind to the cytoskeleton either directly, through its actin-binding motifs, or indirectly, by recruiting other actin-binding proteins [29]. In the current study, we found a significantly increased expression level of γ-actin in HA-coated SR compared to SR, as well as adhesion-associated proteins, including talin-1, vinculin and zyxin, which suggesting that γ-actin is involved in the cytoskeletal rearrangement that regulated by adhesion-associated proteins.

Moreover, we found that eEF1Bα was expressed to a higher level by dermal fibroblasts cultured on HA-SR compared to on SR. The eEF1Bα protein is highly conserved, and has been shown to support the canonical function of GTP/GDP exchange on the eEF1A protein [30]. In addition, eEF1Bα is essential for cellular growth and plays a critical role in translational fidelity [31,32]. More importantly, eEF1Bα has been proposed as a regulator of eEF1A dependent actin bundling [33]. In the presence of eEF1Bα, eEF1A may lose its ability to bind and cross-link F-actin in vitro. Mutant eEF1Bα, which weakly binds to eEF1A, exhibits remarkable changes in cellular morphology and F-actin organization [33]. In a previous study, eEF1Bα has also been implicated in directly binding to actin and exhibited a concentration-dependent negative effect on actin assembly [34].

In summary, we found significantly increased expression levels of eEF1Bα, γ-actin, and adhesion-associated proteins along with enhanced cell adhesion in HA-coated SR compared to noncoated SR. These findings suggest that improved cell adhesion by HA coating on SR may be mediated by eEF1Bα and γ-actin. However, the challenges that remains to determine the mechanism underlying these phenomenons.

Author Contributions

Conceived and designed the experiments: DF SW. Performed the experiments: XS YW ZY. Analyzed the data: XS YZ. Wrote the paper: XS YZ XZ. Analyzed the surface property of materials: XS ZL.

References

1. Zhang Y, Wang S, Lei Z, Fan D (2009) Mechanical and Biological Evaluations of β-Tricalcium Phosphate/Silicone Rubber Composite as a Novel Soft-Tissue Implant. Aesthetic plastic surgery 33: 760–769.
2. van NOORT R MMBBH (1979) Developments in the biomedical evaluation of silicone rubber.Journal of Materials Science 14: 197–204.
3. van der Houwen E, Kuiper L, Burgerhof J, van der Laan B, Verkerke G (2013) Functional buckling behavior of silicone rubber shells for biomedical use. Journal of the mechanical behavior of biomedical materials 28: 47–54.
4. Puskas JE, Luebbers MT (2012) Breast implants: the good, the bad and the ugly. Can nanotechnology improve implants? Wiley Interdisciplinary Reviews: Nanomedicine and Nanobiotechnology 4: 153–168.
5. Siggelkow W, Gescher D, Siggelkow A, Klee D, Malik E, et al. (2004) In vitro analysis of modified surfaces of silicone breast implants. The International journal of artificial organs 27: 1100–1108.
6. Chandanshive BB, Rai P, Rossi AL, Ersen O, Khushalani D (2013) Synthesis of hydroxyapatite nanotubes for biomedical applications. Mater Sci Eng C Mater Biol Appl 33: 2981–2986.
7. Kim BS, Kang HJ, Lee J (2013) Improvement of the compressive strength of a cuttlefish bone-derived porous hydroxyapatite scaffold via polycaprolactone coating. J Biomed Mater Res B Appl Biomater 101: 1302–1309.
8. Citeau A, Guicheux J, Vinatier C, Layrolle P, Nguyen TP, et al. (2005) In vitro biological effects of titanium rough surface obtained by calcium phosphate grid blasting. Biomaterials 26: 157–165.
9. Thian ES, Huang J, Best SM, Barber ZH, Bonfield W (2005) Magnetron co-sputtered silicon-containing hydroxyapatite thin films—an in vitro study. Biomaterials 26: 2947–2956.
10. Nelea V, Morosanu C, Iliescu M, Mihailescu IN (2004) Hydroxyapatite thin films grown by pulsed laser deposition and radio-frequency magnetron sputtering: comparative study. Applied Surface Science 228: 346–356.
11. Sisti KE, Piattelli A, Guastaldi AC, Queiroz TP, de Rossi R (2013) Nondecalcified histologic study of bone response to titanium implants topographically modified by laser with and without hydroxyapatite coating. Int J Periodontics Restorative Dent 33: 689–696.
12. Thanh DT, Nam PT, Phuong NT, Que le X, Anh NV, et al. (2013) Controlling the electrodeposition, morphology and structure of hydroxyapatite coating on 316L stainless steel. Mater Sci Eng C Mater Biol Appl 33: 2037–2045.
13. Peng F, Shaw MT, Olson JR, Wei M (2013) Influence of surface treatment and biomimetic hydroxyapatite coating on the mechanical properties of hydroxyapatite/poly(L-lactic acid) fibers. J Biomater Appl 27: 641–649.
14. Iskandar ME, Aslani A, Liu H (2013) The effects of nanostructured hydroxyapatite coating on the biodegradation and cytocompatibility of magnesium implants. J Biomed Mater Res A 101A (8):2340–2354.
15. Dunne CF, Twomey B, O'Neill L, Stanton KT (2014) Co-blasting of titanium surfaces with an abrasive and hydroxyapatite to produce bioactive coatings: Substrate and coating characterisation. J Biomater Appl 28: 767–778.
16. Bryington MS, Hayashi M, Kozai Y, Vandeweghe S, Andersson M, et al. (2013) The influence of nano hydroxyapatite coating on osseointegration after extended healing periods. Dent Mater 29: 514–520.
17. Johnson I, Akari K, Liu H (2013) Nanostructured hydroxyapatite/poly(lactic-co-glycolic acid) composite coating for controlling magnesium degradation in simulated body fluid. Nanotechnology 24: 375103.
18. Ruan H, Fan C, Liu S, Zheng X (2011) In vivo experimental study on antibacterial and osteogenic capabilities of hydroxyapatite antimicrobial coating with silver. Zhongguo Xiu Fu Chong Jian Wai Ke Za Zhi 25: 668–672.
19. Yang Z, Donli F, Zhang Y, Shi X, Wang S, Lei Z (2012) A spray painting equipment for silicone rubber surface modifiaction. In: Office SIP, editor. China.
20. Wang S, Shi X, Yang Z, Zhang Y, Shen L,et al. (2014) Osteopontin (OPN) Is an Important Protein to Mediate Improvements in the Biocompatibility of C Ion-Implanted Silicone Rubber. PLOS ONE 9: e98320.
21. Zeplin PH, Larena-Avellaneda A, Schmidt K (2010) Surface modification of silicone breast implants by binding the antifibrotic drug halofuginone reduces capsular fibrosis. Plast Reconstr Surg 126: 266–274.
22. Koshino T, Murase T, Takagi T, Saito T (2001) New bone formation around porous hydroxyapatite wedge implanted in opening wedge high tibial osteotomy in patients with osteoarthritis. Biomaterials 22: 1579–1582.
23. Moeller CW, Petruzzelli GJ, Stankiewicz JA (2010) Hydroxyapatite-based frontal sinus obliteration. Operative Techniques in Otolaryngology-Head and Neck Surgery 21: 147–149.
24. Tan F, Naciri M, Dowling D, Al-Rubeai M (2012) In vitro and in vivo bioactivity of CoBlast hydroxyapatite coating and the effect of impaction on its osteoconductivity. Biotechnol Adv 30: 352–362.
25. Park YJ, Choi KH, Hahn BD, Lee YC, Song JY, et al. (2013) New bone formation between bare titanium surface and hydroxyapatite coating by the aerosol deposition technique in the nasal mucosal penetration model. J Craniofac Surg 24: 632–635.
26. Rojaee R, Fathi M, Raeissi K (2013) Controlling the degradation rate of AZ91 magnesium alloy via sol-gel derived nanostructured hydroxyapatite coating. Mater Sci Eng C Mater Biol Appl 33: 3817–3825.

27. Hauser J, Zietlow J, Köller M, Esenwein S, Halfmann H, et al. (2009) Enhanced cell adhesion to silicone implant material through plasma surface modification. Journal of Materials Science: Materials in Medicine 20: 2541–2548.
28. Lewis D, Castleberry D (1980) An assessment of recent advances in external maxillofacial materials. The Journal of Prosthetic Dentistry 43: 426–432.
29. Franco-Cea A, Ellis SJ, Fairchild MJ, Yuan L, Cheung TY, et al. (2010) Distinct developmental roles for direct and indirect talin-mediated linkage to actin. Dev Biol 345: 64–77.
30. Le Sourd F, Boulben S, Le Bouffant R, Cormier P, Morales J, et al. (2006) eEF1B: At the dawn of the 21st century. Biochimica et Biophysica Acta (BBA) - Gene Structure and Expression 1759: 13–31.
31. Hiraga K, Suzuki K, Tsuchiya E, Miyakawa T (1993) Cloning and characterization of the elongation factor EF-1β homologue of Saccharomyces cerevisiae: EF-1β is essential for growth. FEBS Letters 316: 165–169.
32. Carr-Schmid A, Valente L, Loik VI, Williams T, Starita LM, et al. (1999) Mutations in elongation factor 1beta, a guanine nucleotide exchange factor, enhance translational fidelity. Mol Cell Biol 19: 5257–5266.
33. Pittman YR, Kandl K, Lewis M, Valente L, Kinzy TG (2009) Coordination of eukaryotic translation elongation factor 1A (eEF1A) function in actin organization and translation elongation by the guanine nucleotide exchange factor eEF1Balpha. J Biol Chem 284: 4739–4747.
34. Furukawa R, Jinks TM, Tishgarten T, Mazzawi M, Morris DR, et al. (2001) Elongation factor 1beta is an actin-binding protein. Biochim Biophys Acta 1527: 130–140.

Cadmium Telluride Quantum Dots (CdTe-QDs) and Enhanced Ultraviolet-B (UV-B) Radiation Trigger Antioxidant Enzyme Metabolism and Programmed Cell Death in Wheat Seedlings

Huize Chen[1,2,9], Yan Gong[1,3,9], Rong Han[1,2]*

[1] Higher Education Key Laboratory of Plant Molecular and Environmental Stress Response (Shanxi Normal University) in Shanxi Province, Linfen, China, [2] School of Life Science, Shanxi Normal University, Linfen, China, [3] School of Chemistry and Material Science, Shanxi Normal University, Linfen, China

Abstract

Nanoparticles (NPs) are becoming increasingly widespread in the environment. Free cadmium ions released from commonly used NPs under ultraviolet-B (UV-B) radiation are potentially toxic to living organisms. With increasing levels of UV-B radiation at the Earth's surface due to the depletion of the ozone layer, the potential additive effect of NPs and UV-B radiation on plants is of concern. In this study, we investigated the synergistic effect of CdTe quantum dots (CdTe-QDs), a common form of NP, and UV-B radiation on wheat seedlings. Graded doses of CdTe-QDs and UV-B radiation were tested, either alone or in combination, based on physical characteristics of 5-day-old seedlings. Treatments of wheat seedlings with either CdTe-QDs (200 mg/L) or UV-B radiation (10 KJ/m^2/d) induced the activation of wheat antioxidant enzymes. CdTe-QDs accumulation in plant root cells resulted in programmed cell death as detected by DNA laddering. CdTe-QDs and UV-B radiation inhibited root and shoot growth, respectively. Additive inhibitory effects were observed in the combined treatment group. This research described the effects of UV-B and CdTe-QDs on plant growth. Furthermore, the finding that CdTe-QDs accumulate during the life cycle of plants highlights the need for sustained assessments of these interactions.

Editor: Jin-Song Zhang, Institute of Genetics and Developmental Biology, Chinese Academy of Sciences, China

Funding: R.H. received funding from the National Natural Science Foundation of China No. 30671061 (http://www.nsfc.gov.cn/). The funders had no role in study design, data collection and analysis, decision to publish, or preparation of the manuscript.

Competing Interests: The authors have declared that no competing interests exist.

* Email: hhwrsl@163.com

9 These authors contributed equally to this work.

Introduction

Quantum dots are semiconductor nanoparticles (NPs) that are increasingly used in industrial and biological applications [1–5]. The considerable amount of QDs released into the ecosystem raised concern due to their possible toxic effects in living organisms, particularly crop plants [6–8].

Cadmium telluride QDs (CdTe-QDs) are the most frequently used QDs [9–13]. However, the toxicity of CdTe-QDs is of increasing concern due to their small size (2–10 nm) and heavy metal formulation [14]. The cytotoxicity of CdTe-QDs was shown to be associated with their concentration and the duration of exposure [15]. CdTe-QDs release free cadmium ions (Cd^{2+}) under UV-B irradiation, leading to the disruption of DNA replication, the displacement of Zn^{2+} in Zn finger structures, and the generation of reactive oxygen species (ROS) [16,17]. Furthermore, the toxicity of CdTe-QDs has been shown to be much higher than that of Cd^{2+} [12] and that the cytotoxicity was not solely due to free Cd^{2+} [13]. Cellular toxicity was found to be closely related to the size of quantum dots, with smaller diameter QDs (2 nm) demonstrating more toxic effects than larger QDs (5 nm) [18]. These studies demonstrated the potential toxic effects of QDs on inducing antioxidative enzyme activity and DNA replication processes in plants.

Owing to their unique sedentary lifestyle, plants are predicted to be most affected by the accumulation of CdTe-QDs in the environment. This effect is likely to be further exacerbated by the increasing levels of solar UV-B radiation (290–320 nm) at the Earth's surface due to the depletion of stratospheric ozone. Current levels of UV-B during the cropping season are somewhere between 2–12 kJ/m^2/d on the Earth's surface, which exhibits an increase of 6–14% of UV-B radiation over the pre-1980 levels [19]. Based on the UV-B dose per 10 min, the computative calculation of the erythermal UV-B doses range from 2 kJ/m^2 to 9 kJ/m^2 on a clear-sky day on 31 August 2014 (themis.nl). It has been estimated that a 1% decrease in ozone will lead to an increase in UV-B for about 2%. GISS (Goddard Institute for Space Studies) modeling showed a springtime enhancement of erythemal UV doses of up to 14% in the Northern hemisphere and 40% in the Southern hemisphere [20]. Plants are continuously exposed to solar UV-B radiation as a result of their sessile lifestyle [21]. UV-B has the highest energy of any part of the daylight spectrum and has the potential to damage macromolecules including DNA [22], generate ROS, and impair cellular processes

Table 1. Light/dark cycles and treatment regimens with UV-B and CdTe-QDs.

Group	Treatment	Light	UV-B irradiation	Dark	CdTe-QDs treatment
CK	Control	8 h/d	-	16 h/d	dH$_2$O
B	UV-B	8 h/d	8 h/d	16 h/d	dH$_2$O
C	CdTe-QDs	8 h/d	-	16 h/d	CdTe-QDs solution
B+C	UV-B+CdTe-QDs	8 h/d	8 h/d	16 h/d	CdTe-QDs solution

[23–25]. Recently, UV-B radiation was found to act as a key environmental signal that initiated diverse responses in plants affecting metabolism, development and viability [26].

The impact of the environmental accumulation of CdTe-QDs in the presence of enhanced UV-B radiation on living organisms in particular plants is largely unknown. Further studies are needed to understand the interactions of plants, QDs, and enhanced UV-B radiation at the biochemical and molecular levels.

In this study, we investigated the individual and combined effects of QDs and UV-B radiation on an important crop, wheat. We assessed the effect of QDs and UV-B radiation, either alone or in combination, on seedling growth, the activation of antioxidant enzymes, the distribution of CdTe-QDs in root cells, and the induction of programmed cell death.

Materials and Methods

Synthesis of CdTe-QDs

Water-soluble CdTe-QDs were prepared as described [27]. Millipore water (100 mL) was degassed with argon for approximately 1 hour. Cd(ClO$_4$)$_2$·6H$_2$O and 3-mercaptopropanoic acid were added and the pH adjusted to 11.3 with 1 M NaOH. The solution was gassed under argon for additional 30 min. H$_2$Te gas, generated from Al$_2$Te$_3$ by adding 0.5 M H$_2$SO$_4$ dropwise, was bubbled under a slow argon flow for approximately 10 min. The solution was subsequently refluxed for 2 hours. Samples were vacuum dried and stored in darkness before use.

QDs characterization

QDs were characterized using a JEM-2100 (JEOL, Japan) transmission electron microscope (TEM), and a D8 Advance (Bruker, Germany) X-ray diffractometer (Cu K$_\alpha$). Samples were prepared by drying sample droplets from water dispersion onto a 100-mesh Cu grid coated with a lacey carbon film, which was dried prior to imaging by TEM. Absorption and emission spectra were collected using fluorescence spectroscopy (JASCO FP-8000).

Seedling cultivation and chlorophyll content

Wheat seeds (*Triticum aestivum* L. *cv.* JIN-8) were sterilised for 10 min with 1% NaClO and then washed for 10 min in running distilled water. Thirty seeds were cultured per Petri dish in a growth chamber at 25°C with 60% relative humidity and were watered daily. Four treatments, each with three replicates, were applied, starting on the day of seed germination as outlined in Table 1. Briefly, seeds were soaked with either QDs [8] or water for the control group all day long. UV-B radiation was applied 8 h/day during the light cycle. Five graded doses of UV-B radiation intensities were tested: (B1) 2.5 KJ/m^2/d; (B2) 5 KJ/m^2/d; (B3) 7.5 KJ/m^2/d; (B4) 10 KJ/m^2/d and (B5) 12.5 J/m^2/d. CdTe-QDs were applied at five different concentrations: (C1) 25 mg/L; (C2) 50 mg/L; (C3) 100 mg/L; (C4) 200 mg/L and (C5) 400 mg/L. The effect of UV-B and QDs doses on seedling growth were determined by assessing height, root length, and the concentrations of malondialdehyde (MDA), soluble sugar and soluble protein. Five-day-old wheat seedlings were subsequently treated with the doses showing the most inhibitory effect and more detailed analyse including plant height, root length, biomass, and chlorophyll content were performed. After 5 d of growth, the plant height and root length were measured with a ruler. Twenty seedlings per replicate per treatment were randomly selected for analysis. A total of 90 seedlings were assessed for height, fresh weight (FW), and dry weight (DW). Fresh and dry weights were

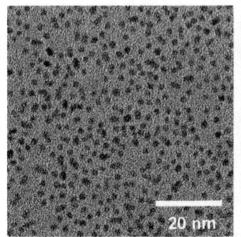
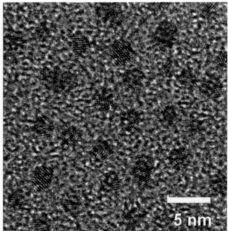

Figure 1. TEM image of synthesized CdTe-QDs.

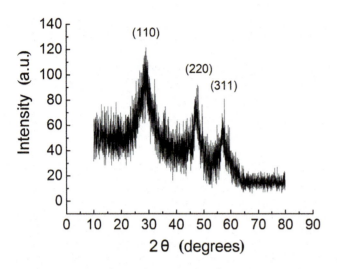

Figure 2. X-ray diffraction spectrum of CdTe-QDs.

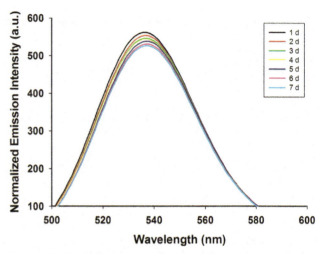

Figure 3. Emission spectra of QDs in H_2O over 7 days.

detected with an analytical balance. Chlorophyll content was measured as described [28].

Measurement of malondialdehyde (MDA), soluble sugar, and soluble protein concentrations

MDA concentration was determined using the trichloroacetic acid (TCA) method. Fresh tissues (1.0 g) were ground with SiO_2 in 2 mL 10% TCA. After centrifugation at 4000 rpm for 10 min, supernatants were removed, added to 2 mL 0.6% (w/v) thiobarbituric acid, and incubated in a 100°C water bath for 15 min. Reactions were stopped on ice. After centrifugation at 4000 rpm for 15 min, supernatants were assayed at 532 and 450 nm.

Total sugar concentration was determined using anthrone colorimetry. Dry plant tissues (50 mg) were triturated with 4 mL 80% ethyl alcohol. Supernatants were collected after 40 min continuous stirring in a water bath at 80°C. Activated carbon (10 mg) was used to decolorize the solution for 30 min, after which 5 mL anthrone were added and samples were incubated in a water bath at 100°C for 10 min. Samples were then cooled for 5 min before spectrophometric absorbance assessment at 625 nm. Concentrations were determined using standard curves.

Soluble protein was extracted according to Zhao [29], using bovine serum albumin as a calibration standard. Fresh tissues (1.0 g) were ground in 6 mL distilled water and then centrifuged at 4000 rpm for 15 min. After centrifugation, supernatants were added to 5 mL Coomassie brilliant blue G-250 and incubated at room temperature for 15 min before spectroscopic assessment at 595 nm.

Cd^{2+} Accumulation

The concentration of Cd^{2+} within shoots and roots was analyzed using Inductively Coupled Plasma Mass Spectrometry (ICP-MS) [30]. After exposure to CdTe-QDs for 5 days, 4–7 plants were recovered and roots were rinsed thoroughly with deionized water to remove material that was neither adsorbed nor

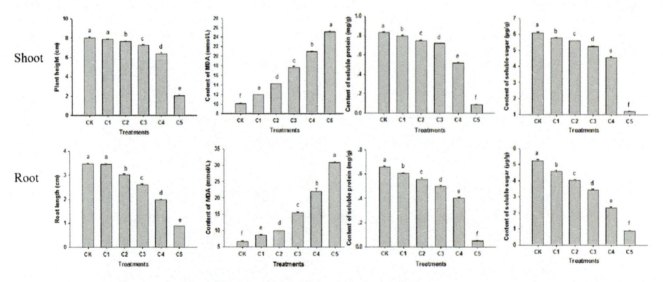

Figure 4. Effects of different CdTe-QDs concentrations on 5-day-old wheat seedlings. CK, control group; C, treatment groups with different concentrations of CdTe-QDs (C1, 25 mg/L; C2, 50 mg/L; C3, 100 mg/L; C4, 200 mg/L; C5, 400 mg/L). Data are means±SD (n = 3). Means with the same letter are not significantly different at Tukey's test (p≤0.05).

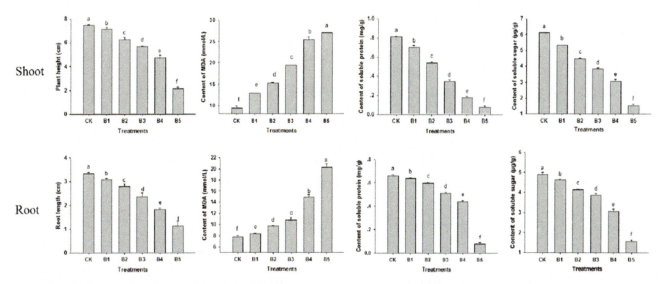

Figure 5. Effects of different enhanced UV-B radiation doses on 5-day-old wheat seedlings. CK, control group; B, treatment groups with graded doses of UV-B radiation (B1, 2.5 KJ/m^2/d; B2, 5 KJ/m^2/d; B3, 7.5 KJ/m^2/d; B4, 10 KJ/m^2/d; B5, 12.5 KJ/m^2/d). Data are means±SD (n = 3). Means with the same letter are not significantly different at Tukey's test (p≤0.05).

integrated into the plant tissues. Roots and leaves were separated, oven dried (70°C, 24 h) and weighed. Dried tissues were digested in 4:1 concentrated HNO$_3$:30% H$_2$O$_2$ for at least 2 h on a hotplate at 60°C. Samples were transferred to polypropylene tubes and centrifuged at 1000 g for 10 min. Supernatants were recovered and brought to 10 mL using deionized water. Cd analysis was performed using an X-Series ICP-MS instrument with an ICP-MS elements solution set used as standards.

Antioxidant Assays

Roots and shoots were separately homogenized, centrifuged and extracts assayed for catalase (CAT), guaiacol peroxidase (GPOX), superoxide dismutase (SOD), ascorbate peroxidase (APOX), dehydroascorbate reductase (DHAR) and glutathione reductase (GR) activities as previously described [31–35].

Measurement of ROS Production

Determination of H$_2$O$_2$ content in plant extracts. Frozen plant tissues (0.1 g) were homogenized in a 1:9 (w/v) phosphate buffer (50 mM, pH 6.0) at 4°C. The content of H$_2$O$_2$ was analyzed with a hydrogen peroxide assay kit (Beyotime, China) according to the manufacturer instruction. Briefly, test tubes containing 50 μL test solutions were placed at room temperature for 30 min and measured immediately with a spectrometer at a wavelength of 560 nm. Absorbance values were calibrated to a standard curve generated with known concentrations of H$_2$O$_2$ [36]. O$_2^-$ levels were monitored by staining for 20 min in a solution of 2 mM NBT in 20 mM phosphate buffer (pH 6.1). The reaction was stopped by transferring the seedlings into distilled water. O$_2^-$ content was quantified using the method of Ramel et al. [37]. The NBT-stained plantlets were ground in liquid nitrogen; the obtained powder was solubilized in 2 M KOH-dimethyl sulfoxide (1:1.16, v/v) and then centrifuged for 10 min at 12000 g. The A630 was immediately measured and compared with a standard curve obtained from known amounts of NBT in the KOH-dimethyl sulfoxide mixture [38].

Confocal Fluorescence Imaging Analysis

Cellular fluorescence was monitored using a FV-1000 Confocal system (Olympus, Co.) with a 1.4 NA, 60×oil immersion objective lens. Cell observations were performed on at least three replicate samples. Quantum dots were excited at 488 nm. Nuclei were stained with 4′,6-diamidino-2-phenylindole (DAPI) (Sigma, USA) and excited at 405 nm.

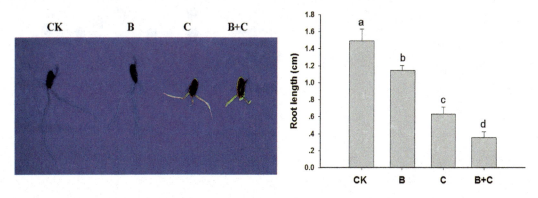

Figure 6. Two-day old seedlings visualized with UV light. Control, CK; UV-B treatment alone, B; CdTe-QDs treatment alone, C; combined CdTe-QDs and UV-B treatment, C+B.

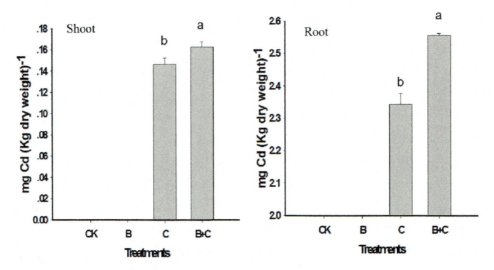

Figure 7. Cd concentration in tissues of 5-day-old wheat seedlings under different treatments. Control, CK; UV-B treatment alone, B; CdTe-QDs treatment alone, C; combined CdTe-QDs and UV-B treatment, C+B.

DNA laddering

Genomic DNA was extracted using a standard CTAB protocol [39]. DNA concentration was determined by spectrophotometry. DNA (5 μg) was analyzed using 1.5% agarose gel electrophoresis in the presence of ethidium bromide (5 μg/mL) and gels were visualized on a UV transilluminator.

Statistical Analysis

Data results are expressed as means ± standard deviations (SD). Statistical significance was assessed using one-way analysis of variance (ANOVA) tests using General Linear Model followed by Tukey test was performed using the SPSS 21.0 and Sigma-plot 10.0.

Results and Discussion

QDs characteristics

CdTe-QDs were synthesized and characterized using TEM. CdTe-QDs had an average diameter of 2.3±0.2 nm (Figure 1). X-ray diffraction (XRD) spectra scanned over the 2 theta (θ) range of 10–80° showed a cubic XRD structure of CdTe-QDs with diffractive peaks of 28°, 46°, and 57°, indicating well-crystallized QDs (Figure 2). The QDs exhibited narrow fluorescence emission spectra (λ max = 531 nm). Emission spectra collected over a period of 7 days are shown in Figure 3. QDs emission intensity decreased daily, with a total decrease of approximately 6.5% over 7 days (normalized intensity change from 561.8488 to 525.1871). These results indicated that almost 93.5% of QDs persisted during the experimental exposure period.

The effect of CdTe-QDs and UV-B irradiation on the growth of wheat seedlings

Wheat seedlings were treated with single agents of either CdTe-QDs or UV-B irradiation. Treatments of seedlings with five different concentrations of CdTe-QDs resulted in reductions in shoot height and root length, increased lipid oxidation as measured by the levels of the oxidation product MDA, as well as reductions in soluble sugar and soluble protein concentrations, in a dose dependent manner when compared with the control (CK) group (Figure 4). Of five CdTe-QDs concentrations tested,

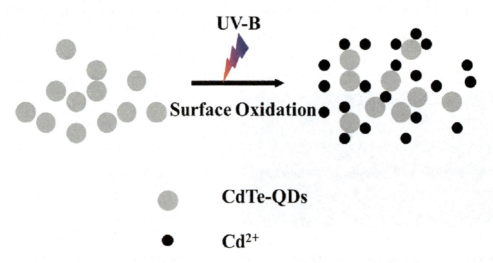

Figure 8. Schematic showing Cd^{2+} release from QDs as a result of UV-B oxidation of CdTe-QDs surfaces [41,42].

Table 2. Effects of QDs and UV-B radiation on growth of 5-day-old wheat seedlings.

Group	Treatments	Plant height (mm)	Root length (mm)	Fresh weight (g)	Dry weight (g)
CK	Control	75.63±1.379a	26.87±0.493a	0.1983±0.003a	0.0307±0.002a
B	UV-B	45.53±1.193c	16.26±0.404b	0.1217±0.011c	0.0143±0.003c
C	CdTe-QDs	51.23±1.101b	12.13±0.493c	0.1393±0.007b	0.0187±0.003b
B+C	UV-B+CdTe-QDs	31.47±1.026d	7.96±0.776d	0.0980±0.003d	0.0080±0.001d

Data are means±SD (n = 3). Means with the same letter are not significantly different at Tukey's test (p≤0.05).

the concentration of 200 mg/L (C4) was selected for further evaluations when taking into account of all parameters assessed (almost 75% shoot/root length reduction and 15 times MDA increase performed in the C5 treatment) (Figure 4). Treatments of seedlings with graded doses of UV-B irradiation led to similar growth inhibition as assessed by the above parameters (Figure 5). The UV-B dose of 10.0 KJ/m^2/d was selected for subsequent experiments since the dose higher than 10.0 KJ/m^2/d strongly inhibited wheat growth (Figure 5). This dose of UV-B irradiation should decrease the density of O_3 by 20% [40].

CdTe-QD accumulation in plant tissues

Wheat seedlings were randomly assigned to four treatment groups: control (CK), UV-B at 10 KJ/m^2/d (B), CdTe-QDs at 200 mg/L (C), and UV-B (10 KJ/m^2/d) plus CdTe-QDs (200 mg/L) (B+C). The uptake of CdTe-QDs was evident in two-day-old treated seedlings in the group treated by CdTe-QDs alone (C) and that treated by UV-B (10 KJ/m^2/d) plus CdTe-QDs (200 mg/L) (B+C) (Figure 6). Root length was reduced in all three treatment groups compared to the control group (Figure 6). CdTe-QDs fluorescence was observed in roots of seedlings treated with CdTe-QDs alone (C) and in seedlings received combined CdTe-QDs and UV-B (B+C), indicating CdTe-QDs nanoparticles uptake by roots.

Treatment of seedlings with CdTe-QDs resulted in a higher Cd accumulation in roots (2.344 mg/Kg DW) than in shoots (0.1461 mg/Kg DW) (Figure 7). This is likely due to the direct contact exposure of roots to the CdTe-QDs suspension. There was also a marked increase in Cd concentration in both shoots and roots of seedlings treated with CdTe-QDs in combination with UV-B irradiation (Figure 7). This increase in the levels of Cd^{2+} in the presence of UV-B radiation was reported previously as a consequence of QDs surface oxidation and Cd^{2+} release (Figure 8) [41,42]. Our results suggest a potential additive effect of CdTe-QDs and UV-B on plants.

Plant growth and chlorophyll content

The growth and chlorophyll contents of wheat seedlings exposed to different treatments were determined (Tables 2 and 3). UV-B radiation treatment resulted in a significantly reduction in plant height with an average height 30.1 mm shorter than that of controls (Table 2). Similarly, chlorophyll content, both chlorophyll a and b, were significantly lower than in controls (Table 3). The phytotoxic effects of CdTe-QDs treatment on plant height and chlorophyll content were less severe than those of UV-B radiation. However, root length was more severely affected in the CdTe-QDs group compared to the UV-B treated group (Table 2). Average root length in CdTe-QDs-treated plants was 14.74 mm shorter than in untreated controls. Total biomass was similar between the UV-B and QDs treated groups, but was significantly reduced compared to control untreated seedlings. The combined treatment group showed a significant reduction in plant height, root length, and total biomass when compared to the control group and the single treatment groups (Table 2). The enhanced toxicity in the combined treatment group may have been due to the release of free Cd^{2+} from CdTe-QDs in the presence of UV-B radiation.

Antioxidant defense in wheat seedlings

The cytotoxicity of QDs and UV-B radiaton have shown to be associated with the production of ROS [6,43,44]. H_2O_2 and O_2^- are the most common ROS produced during normal cellular metabolic processes. Their imbalance can be highly cytotoxic [35,45]. To determine the involvement of H_2O_2 and O_2^- during QDs and UV-B exposure, 5-day-old seedlings were examined for the presence of ROS following treatments with CdTe-QDs, UV-B, and combined CdTe-QDs and UV-B. The results showed that there was a marked increase in the concentrations of H_2O_2 in roots treated with CdTe-QDs, either alone or in combination with UV-B, compared to the UV-B treated and untreated groups. Furthermore, there was 11.5% increase in the levels of H_2O_2, from 215.37 nmol/g FW in the CdTe-QD treated group to 247.89 nmol/g FW in the combined CdTe-QD and UV-B treated

Table 3. Chlorophyll content in tissues of 5-day-old wheat seedlings.

Group	Treatments	Chlorophyll a (mg/g FW)	Chlorophyll b (mg/g FW)	Total chlorophyll (mg/g FW)	Chlorophyll a/b ratio
CK	Control	0.5943±0.0068a	0.2723±0.0042a	0.8667±0.0059a	2.1828±0.0510a
B	UV-B	0.4030±0.0076c	0.1970±0.0056c	0.6000±0.0026c	2.0474±0.0949b
C	CdTe-QDs	0.4990±0.0061b	0.2473±0.0057b	0.7463±0.0012b	2.0186±0.0714b
B+C	UV-B+CdTe-QDs	0.3443±0.0047d	0.1763±0.0084d	0.5207±0.0038d	1.9564±0.1165b

Data are means±SD (n = 3). Means with the same letter are not significantly different at Tukey's test (p≤0.05).

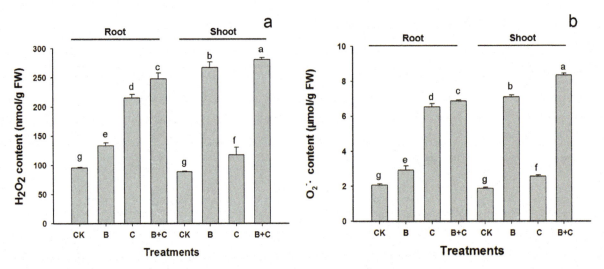

Figure 9. Contents of H_2O_2 and O_2^- in the root and shoot of 5 day old seedlings following different treatments. Data are means±SD (n = 3). Means with the same letter are not significantly different at Tukey's test (p≤0.05).

group (Figure 9). Similar results were observed for the O_2^- level. These results are consistent with the greater toxicity from higher levels of Cd following UV-B irradiation predicted for roots. We noted that such additive effect by UV-B was moderate in shoots where the production of H_2O_2 and O_2^- is found to be primarily associated with UV-B radiation. The relatively moderate effect in the Cd-associated ROS production in shoots is likely due to the low levels of Cd accumulation in shoots (Figure 7).

Plants use a highly complex antioxidant defense system to protect against oxidative stress that includes antioxidant enzymes such as SOD, CAT, GPOX, APOX, DHAR, and GR (Figure 10)

[35,46]. The O_2^- generated from mitochondria, chloroplasts, endoplasmic reticulum, and the cell wall is reduced to H_2O_2 by SOD. H_2O is then formed from H_2O_2 through the activities of CAT, and APOX. DHAR and glutathione reductase (GR) participate in the transformation of glutathion (GSH) to oxidized form of glutathione (GSSG) and generation of nicotinamide adenine dinucleotide phosphate (NADPH). GSH can bind to free Cd^{2+}, forming $Cd(GSH)_2$ and leading to the reduction of the Cd toxicity. In addition, phytochelatins (PCs) may bind Cd to form PC-Cd-S, which can then be stored in the vacuole [47]. Finally,

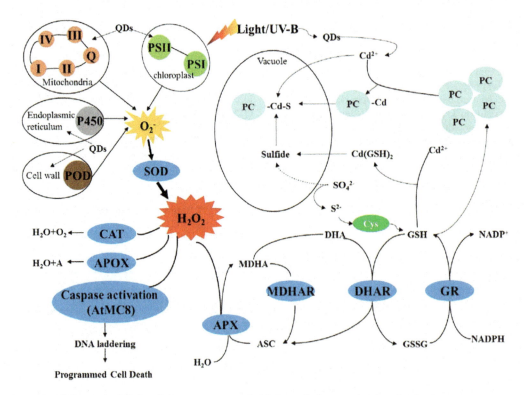

Figure 10. Schematic of the antioxidative defense system and Cd degradation mechanism in plants.

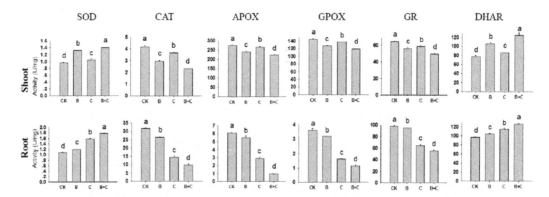

Figure 11. Antioxidant enzyme activities in shoots and roots of 5-day-old wheat seedlings. Data are means±SD (n = 3). Means with the same letter are not significantly different at Tukey's test (p≤0.05).

H_2O_2 activation of caspase can lead to programmed cell death [44,48].

Antioxidative defense enzymes activities were further assessed in the control, UV-B-only treated, CdTe-QDs treated, and UV-B plus CdTe-QDs treated seedlings (Figure 11). The inhibitory effect of CdTe-QDs upon antioxidant enzymes activities was milder than that of UV-B radiation treatment in shoots. Photosynthesis, which is susceptible to changes in light, mainly occurs in leaves [49]. Under ambient UV-B, the UV resistance locus 8 (UVR8) protein mediates antioxidant enzyme activities and regulates plant growth. However, it is currently unknown whether UV-B irradiation used in this study stimulates antioxidant enzyme activities in the same pathway.

In shoots, SOD and DHAR activities significantly increased in seedlings exposed to UV-B radiation when compared to controls. However, the other enzymes were significantly inhibited in the UV-B treated group compared to the control group. There were also significant difference in enzyme activities between the CdTe-QDs treated group and the control group, but the effects were not as marked as with the UV-B treated group (Figure 11 upper part). We inferred that CdTe-QDs affected metabolism in shoots through the release and transport of Cd^{2+} ions from QDs in root cells.

The cytotoxicity of Cd^{2+} has been known to be associated with oxidation stress in mammalian cells. We have demonstrated the additive effect of UV-B radiation on the Cd^{2+} toxicity in roots, manifested by the decreased levels of antioxidant enzymes such as CAT, APOX, GPOX and GR (Figure 11), and increased DNA fragmentation (Figure 12). The more pronounced effects in roots is presumably due to the release of additional Cd^{2+} as a result of surface oxidation of QDs under UV-B radiation [41,42]. We inferred that cytoplasmic diffusion of free Cd^{2+} occurred more rapidly than the diffusion of NPs. The greater root toxicity observed with the combined treatment compared to the single CdTe-QDs treatment may be the consequence of the increased accumulation of intracellular Cd^{2+}.

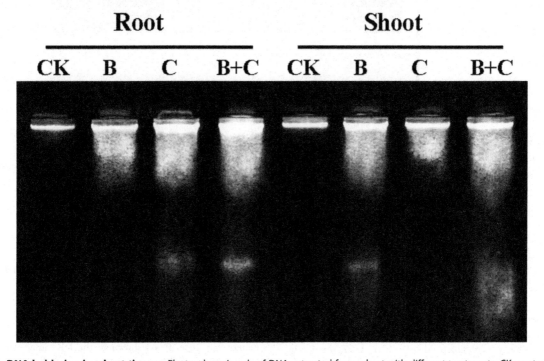

Figure 12. DNA laddering in wheat tissues. Electrophoresis gels of DNA extracted from wheat with different treatments. CK: control group; B: enhanced UV-B radiation; C: CdTe-QDs treatment; B+C: combined UV-B and CdTe-QDs treatment.

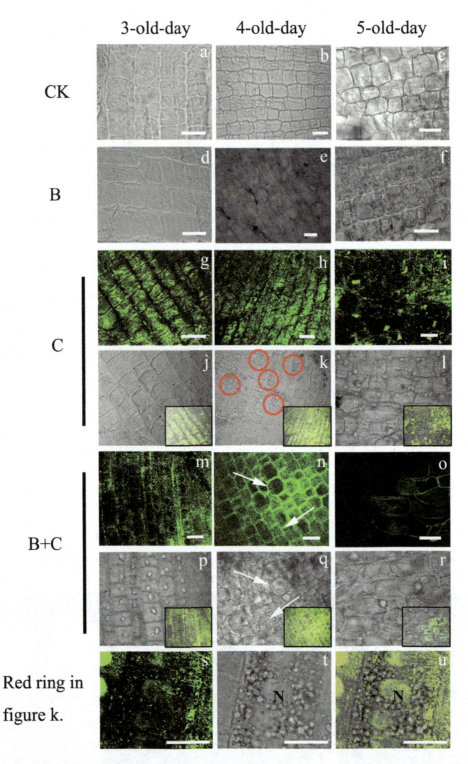

Figure 13. Confocal imaging of CdTe-QDs distribution in wheat root cells. CdTe-QDs are indicated by fluorescence imaging (g, h, i, m, n, o, s), DIC images demonstrate cell integrity (a, b, c, d, e, f, j, k, l, p, q, r, t). Regions highlighted in red in panel e are shown in panels s, t, and u. Pictures of the bottom right corner in figure j, k, l, p, q, r is the merge figures of g and j, h and k, i and l, m and p, n and q, o and r separately. Scale bars = 20 μm.

Distribution of CdTe-QDs in root cells

It has been demonstrated that CdSe-QDs, through the apoplastic pathway with the aid of silwet L-77, could be transferred into roots and were stable [50]. We therefore examined root cells of wheat seedling for the presence of CdSe-QDs using confocal microscopy (Figure 13). No fluorescence signal was detected in the untreated control (a, b, c) and in the UV-B treated cells (d, e, f). As shown in the DIC images, cells in the control group exhibited a clear outline of cell wall and regular shape ove three day period. In contrast, cells in the UV-B treated

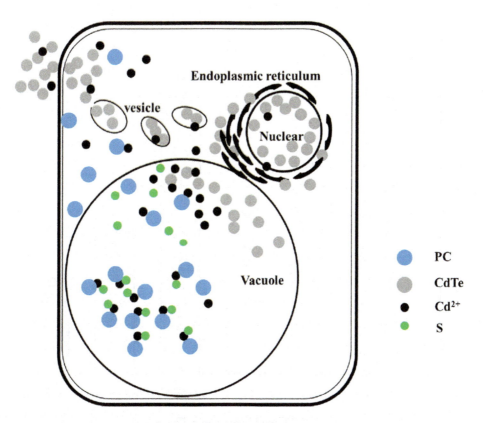

Figure 14. Schematic of a putative mechanism through which CdTe-QDs are processed by plant cells.

group showed the presence of intracellular vesicles on the fifth day and apparent abnormal rectangular shapes (f).

The presence of intracellular CdTe-QDs (g) was clearly visible after 3 days of CdTe-QDs treatment (g, j). Cell morphology appeared normal, with smooth surface and intact cell walls. After 4 days of treatment (h, k), vacuolation of cytoplasm appeared in some cells as shown ringed in red (k) and at higher magnification (s, t, u). Many small vesicles appeared around the nucleus (t), and CdTe-QDs were located inside the nucleus (u). This indicated the CdTe-QDs may enter the nucleus through the nuclear pore. CdTe-QDs were not uniformly distributed, but were found preferentially in and around the nucleus (u). A putative vesicle transport mechanism is shown in Figure 14. We propose that following the uptake of QDs by plant cells, PCs bind to Cd and form stable metal chelate complexes that are stored in the vacuole. Unbound excess QDs could spread into the nucleus leading to DNA damage. We inferred that NPs could produce a nanostructure that lead to an increase in the concentration of Cd around the nucleus, resulting in an increased cytotoxicity [12]. After 5 days of treatment (i, l), cell walls appeared looser and cells more variable in size (l), and the CdTe-QDs fluorescence intensity was reduced (i). The morphological characters resemble the features of programmed cell death.

In the combined UV-B and CdTe-QDs treated group, the situation is similar to the CdTe-QDs treated group. Cells exhibited normal morphology (p) on the third day and filled with CdTe-QDs (m). After 4 day treatment, cells are varied in size (n, q, white arrows). While following 5 day treatment, cells lost their square shape (r) and the fluorescence of CdTe-QDs was reduced dramatically (o).

Fifty cells were subsequently selected and the change in the fluorescence intensity over the treatment period was measured (Figure 15). CdTe-QD-derived fluorescence decreased by ~62.5% from the third to the fifth days of CdTe-QDs treatment and the decrease in intensity up to ~74.0% was observed in the combined treatment group. The results showed the UV-B radiation accelerated the CdTe-QDs-derived fluorescence decay, that is, ~11.5% fluorescence intensity decreased following the addition of UV-B radiation compared to single CdTe-QDs treatment. This was an order of magnitude higher than the inherent decrease in QDs emission intensity over 7 days (6.5%; Figure 3). The result indicated that CdTe-QDs were degraded by plant cells.

We detected the presence of QDs in shoots of seedlings but no fluorescence signal was observed in shoots. This suggested two possibilities. First, QDs may not have been transported to the top of the seedlings because QDs were only taken up by root epidermal cells and were not taken up by vascular tissues. Second, QDs that were taken up by root cells may have been degraded by PCs and stored in vacuoles, substantially decreasing the number of QDs were not available for transport into the shoot. Root cell took up the QDs and degraded them into Cd^{2+} partly. Cd^{2+} would bind to PCs or GSH, this is the cytotoxicity. While the other QDs changed ROS level and activated caspase, this would result in programmed cell death.

Programmed cell death in seedling cells

Apoptotic bodies visualized by DAPI staining were found in root and stem cells of all three treatment groups while absence in the control group (Figure 16), suggesting an induction of programmed cell death following the treatments.

DNA laddering or fragmentation is a feature of apoptosis [51]. Programmed cell death was investigated by using DNA ladder analysis (Figure 12). DNA fragmentation visualized as DNA

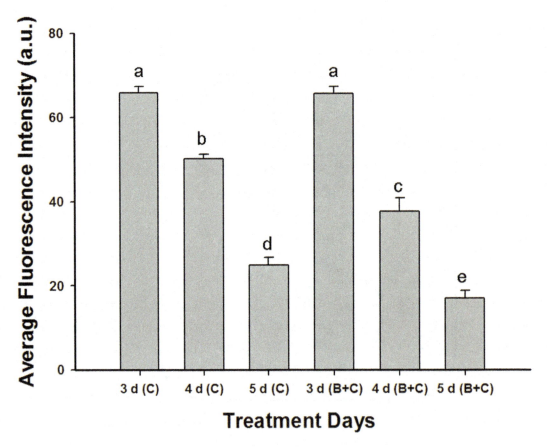

Figure 15. Average fluorescence intensity of QDs in 50 cells after different treatment durations. C, CdTe-QDs treatment alone; B+C, combined enhanced UV-B and CdTe-QDs treatment. Values are means±SD (n = 3). Means with the same letter are not significantly different at Tukey's test (p≤0.05).

laddering was evident in root cells of treatment groups involving CdTe-QDs. This may be due to nucleic acid damage caused by CdTe-QDs presence in the nuclei. Free Cd^{2+} would lead to further DNA damage [52]. As oxidation of aromatic DNA bases is the main source of DNA damage, an increase in intracellular ROS levels induced by CdTe-QDs would further induce DNA damage, leading to enhanced cytotoxicity. At the cellular level, Cd^{2+} alone could inhibit the biosynthesis of DNA, RNA and protein, and induce DNA strand breakage and lipid peroxidation [52]. In the combined treatment, Cd^{2+} release would be enhanced by UV-B radiation, which would further enhance the cytotoxicity.

DNA fragmentation in shoots was detected in the treatment groups involcing UV-B radiation, with the combined treatments producing the most DNA laddering. UV-B radiation causes DNA damage [53] through various mechanisms including formation of cyclobutyl pyrimidine dimer (CPD) adducts, (6-4) photoproducts

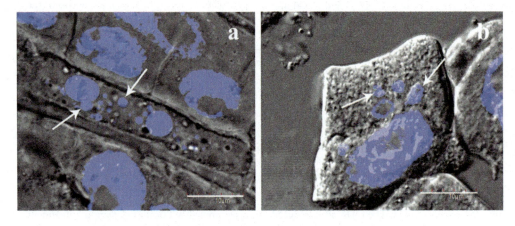

Figure 16. Cells undergoing programmed cell death. DAPI-stained DNA is shown in blue. Apoptotic bodies are indicated with white arrows. Shoot cells (a) and root cells (b) are shown. Scale bars = 10 μm.

((6-4) PPs), inter/intra cross links (ICLs), 8-oxoguanine, and DNA double-strand breaks (DSBs) [48]. We inferred that the damage caused by enhanced UV-B exposure in shoots masked the Cd^{2+} damage effects.

In summary, QDs are widely used and are becoming increasingly dispersed in the environment. Our study revealed the cytotoxicity of CdTe-QDs and UV-B radiation on wheat seedlings. Our results demonstrated that CdTe-QDs nanoparticles and UV-B radiation affected the antioxidant defense system and programmed cell death in the roots and shoots of wheat seedlings. At the doses used (200 mg CdTe-QDs/L and 10.0 $KJ/m^2/d$ enhanced UV-B), treatments induced negative effects on antioxidant enzyme activities and resulted in the formation of apoptotic bodies and DNA fragmentation. Combined treatments with both CdTe-QDs and enhanced UV-B exhibited the added deleterious effects. It is currently impossible to distinguish between Cd released from industrial waste and those released from QDs. The precise concentrations of Cd emissions from QDs are thus unknown. Therefore, in vitro studies such as ours are necessary for generating mechanistic insights into the specific effect of CdTe-QDs on agricultural plants.

Acknowledgments

We thank Dr Huiling Xu (Peter MacCallum Cancer Centre, Australia) for critical reading and editing the manuscript.

Author Contributions

Conceived and designed the experiments: RH. Performed the experiments: YG. Analyzed the data: HC. Contributed reagents/materials/analysis tools: YG. Contributed to the writing of the manuscript: HC.

References

1. Jones R (2009) Feynman's unfinished business. Nature nanotechnology 4: 785–785.
2. Djikanovic D, Kalauzi A, Jeremic M, Xu J, Micic M, et al. (2012) Interaction of the CdSe quantum dots with plant cell walls. Colloids Surf B Biointerfaces 91: 41–47.
3. Yang A, Zheng Y, Long C, Chen H, Liu B, et al. (2014) Fluorescent immunosorbent assay for the detection of alpha lactalbumin in dairy products with monoclonal antibody bioconjugated with CdSe/ZnS quantum dots. Food Chem 150: 73–79.
4. Sozer N, Kokini JL (2014) Use of quantum nanodot crystals as imaging probes for cereal proteins. Food Research International 57: 142–151.
5. Valizadeh A, Mikaeili H, Samiei M, Farkhani S, Zarghami N, et al. (2012) Quantum dots: synthesis, bioapplications, and toxicity. Nanoscale Research Letters 7: 1–14.
6. Rico CM, Hong J, Morales MI, Zhao LJ, Barrios AC, et al. (2013) Effect of Cerium Oxide Nanoparticles on Rice: A Study Involving the Antioxidant Defense System and In Vivo Fluorescence Imaging. Environmental Science & Technology 47: 5635–5642.
7. Miralles P, Church TL, Harris AT (2012) Toxicity, uptake, and translocation of engineered nanomaterials in vascular plants. Environmental science & technology 46: 9224–9239.
8. Nair R, Poulose AC, Nagaoka Y, Yoshida Y, Maekawa T, et al. (2011) Uptake of FITC labeled silica nanoparticles and quantum dots by rice seedlings: effects on seed germination and their potential as biolabels for plants. J Fluoresc 21: 2057–2068.
9. Nguyen KC, Willmore WG, Tayabali AF (2013) Cadmium telluride quantum dots cause oxidative stress leading to extrinsic and intrinsic apoptosis in hepatocellular carcinoma HepG2 cells. Toxicology 306: 114–123.
10. Liu Y, Wang P, Wang Y, Zhu Z, Lao F, et al. (2013) The influence on cell cycle and cell division by various cadmium-containing quantum dots. Small 9: 2440–2451.
11. Chen N, He Y, Su Y, Li X, Huang Q, et al. (2012) The cytotoxicity of cadmium-based quantum dots. Biomaterials 33: 1238–1244.
12. Su Y, Hu M, Fan C, He Y, Li Q, et al. (2010) The cytotoxicity of CdTe quantum dots and the relative contributions from released cadmium ions and nanoparticle properties. Biomaterials 31: 4829–4834.
13. Cho SJ, Maysinger D, Jain M, Röder B, Hackbarth S, et al. (2007) Long-term exposure to CdTe quantum dots causes functional impairments in live cells. Langmuir 23: 1974–1980.
14. Li X, Chen N, Su Y, He Y, Fan C, et al. (2013) Cytotoxicity of cadmium-based quantum dots. Chinese Science Bulletin (Chinese Version) 58: 1393.
15. Yu G, Tan Y, He X, Qin Y, Liang J (2014) CLAVATA3 Dodecapeptide Modified CdTe Nanoparticles: A Biocompatible Quantum Dot Probe for In Vivo Labeling of Plant Stem Cells. PloS one 9: e89241.
16. Gobe G, Crane D (2010) Mitochondria, reactive oxygen species and cadmium toxicity in the kidney. Toxicology letters 198: 49–55.
17. Cuypers A, Plusquin M, Remans T, Jozefczak M, Keunen E, et al. (2010) Cadmium stress: an oxidative challenge. Biometals 23: 927–940.
18. Lovrić J, Bazzi HS, Cuie Y, Fortin GR, Winnik FM, et al. (2005) Differences in subcellular distribution and toxicity of green and red emitting CdTe quantum dots. Journal of Molecular Medicine 83: 377–385.
19. Forster P, Thompson D, Baldwin M, Chipperfield M, Dameris M, et al. (2011) Scientific Assessment of Ozone Depletion: 2010. Global Ozone Research and Monitoring Project-Report 52: 516.
20. Taalas P, Amanatidis GT, Heikkilä A (2000) European conference on atmospheric UV radiation: overview. Journal of Geophysical Research: Atmospheres (1984–2012) 105: 4777–4785.
21. Choudhary KK, Agrawal SB (2014) Ultraviolet-B induced changes in morphological, physiological and biochemical parameters of two cultivars of pea (Pisum sativum L.). Ecotoxicol Environ Saf 100: 178–187.
22. Han R WX, Yue M (2002) Influence of He-Ne laser irradiation on the excision repair of cyclobutyl pyrimidine dimers in the wheat DNA. Chinese Science Bulletin 47: 818–821.
23. Hideg E, Jansen MA, Strid A (2013) UV-B exposure, ROS, and stress: inseparable companions or loosely linked associates? Trends Plant Sci 18: 107–115.
24. Wang G, Deng S, Li C, Liu Y, Chen L, et al. (2012) Damage to DNA caused by UV-B radiation in the desert cyanobacterium Scytonema javanicum and the effects of exogenous chemicals on the process. Chemosphere 88: 413–417.
25. Chen HZ ZJ, Du MT, Han R (2011) Influence of Enhanced UV-B Radiation on F-actin in Wheat Division Cells. Plant Diversity And Resources 33: 306–310.
26. Jenkins GI (2009) Signal Transduction in Responses to UV-B Radiation. Annu Rev Plant Biol: 407–431.
27. Gaponik N, Talapin DV, Rogach AL, Hoppe K, Shevchenko EV, et al. (2002) Thiol-capping of CdTe nanocrystals: an alternative to organometallic synthetic routes. The Journal of Physical Chemistry B 106: 7177–7185.
28. Schlemmer MR, Francis DD, Shanahan J, Schepers JS (2005) Remotely measuring chlorophyll content in corn leaves with differing nitrogen levels and relative water content. Agronomy Journal 97: 106–112.
29. Zhao S, Huang Q, Yang P, Zhang J, Jia H, et al. (2012) Effects of Ion Beams Pretreatment on Damage of UV-B Radiation on Seedlings of Winter Wheat (Triticum aestivum L.). Appl Biochem Biotechnol 168: 2123–2135.
30. Navarro DA, Bisson MA, Aga DS (2012) Investigating uptake of water-dispersible CdSe/ZnS quantum dot nanoparticles by Arabidopsis thaliana plants. J Hazard Mater 211–212: 427–435.
31. Lee YP, Kim SH, Bang JW, Lee HS, Kwak SS, et al. (2007) Enhanced tolerance to oxidative stress in transgenic tobacco plants expressing three antioxidant enzymes in chloroplasts. Plant Cell Rep 26: 591–598.
32. Verma S, Dubey RS (2003) Lead toxicity induces lipid peroxidation and alters the activities of antioxidant enzymes in growing rice plants. Plant Science 164: 645–655.
33. Shah K, Kumar RG, Verma S, Dubey R (2001) Effect of cadmium on lipid peroxidation, superoxide anion generation and activities of antioxidant enzymes in growing rice seedlings. Plant Science 161: 1135–1144.
34. Rao MV, Paliyath G, Ormrod DP (1996) Ultraviolet-B-and ozone-induced biochemical changes in antioxidant enzymes of Arabidopsis thaliana. Plant physiology 110: 125–136.
35. Hossain MA, Silva JATd, Fujita M (2011) Glyoxalase System and Reactive Oxygen Species Detoxification System in Plant Abiotic Stress Response and Tolerance: An Intimate Relationship.
36. Wang J, Wang Q, Li J, Shen Q, Wang F, et al. (2012) Cadmium induces hydrogen peroxide production and initiates hydrogen peroxide-dependent apoptosis in the gill of freshwater crab, Sinopotamon henanense. Comp Biochem Physiol C Toxicol Pharmacol 156: 195–201.
37. Ramel F, Sulmon C, Bogard M, Couée I, Gouesbet G (2009) Differential patterns of reactive oxygen species and antioxidative mechanisms during atrazine injury and sucrose-induced tolerance in Arabidopsis thaliana plantlets. BMC Plant Biology 9: 28.
38. Xu J, Yin H, Li Y, Liu X (2010) Nitric oxide is associated with long-term zinc tolerance in Solanum nigrum. Plant Physiol 154: 1319–1334.
39. Rogers SO, Bendich AJ (1985) Extraction of DNA from milligram amounts of fresh, herbarium and mummified plant tissues. Plant molecular biology 5: 69–76.
40. Zhi Qi MY, Rong Han, Xun-Ling Wang (2002) The damage repair role of He-Ne laser on plants exposed to different intensities of ultraviolet-B radiation. Photochemistry and Photobiology 75: 680–686.
41. Derfus AM, Chan WC, Bhatia SN (2004) Probing the cytotoxicity of semiconductor quantum dots. Nano letters 4: 11–18.

42. Kirchner C, Liedl T, Kudera S, Pellegrino T, Muñoz Javier A, et al. (2005) Cytotoxicity of colloidal CdSe and CdSe/ZnS nanoparticles. Nano Letters 5: 331–338.
43. Hideg É, Jansen MA, Strid Å (2013) UV-B exposure, ROS, and stress: inseparable companions or loosely linked associates? Trends in plant science 18: 107–115.
44. Huang W, Yang X, Yao S, LwinOo T, He H, et al. (2014) Reactive oxygen species burst induced by aluminum stress triggers mitochondria-dependent programmed cell death in peanut root tip cells. Plant Physiol Biochem 82C: 76–84.
45. Couee I, Sulmon C, Gouesbet G, El Amrani A (2006) Involvement of soluble sugars in reactive oxygen species balance and responses to oxidative stress in plants. J Exp Bot 57: 449–459.
46. Silva ECd, Albuquerque MBd, Neto ADdA, Junior CDdS (2013) Drought and Its Consequences to Plants – From Individual to Ecosystem.
47. Heiss S, Wachter A, Bogs J, Cobbett C, Rausch T (2003) Phytochelatin synthase (PCS) protein is induced in Brassica juncea leaves after prolonged Cd exposure. Journal of Experimental Botany 54: 1833–1839.
48. Nawkar GM, Maibam P, Park JH, Sahi VP, Lee SY, et al. (2013) UV-Induced Cell Death in Plants. Int J Mol Sci 14: 1608–1628.
49. Shen X, Zhou Y, Duan L, Li Z, Eneji AE, et al. (2010) Silicon effects on photosynthesis and antioxidant parameters of soybean seedlings under drought and ultraviolet-B radiation. J Plant Physiol 167: 1248–1252.
50. Hu Y, Li J, Ma L, Peng Q, Feng W, et al. (2010) High efficiency transport of quantum dots into plant roots with the aid of silwet L-77. Plant Physiol Biochem 48: 703–709.
51. Farage-Barhom S, Burd S, Sonego L, Mett A, Belausov E, et al. (2011) Localization of the Arabidopsis senescence- and cell death-associated BFN1 nuclease: from the ER to fragmented nuclei. Mol Plant 4: 1062–1073.
52. Fernández EL, Gustafson A-L, Andersson M, Hellman B, Dencker L (2003) Cadmium-induced changes in apoptotic gene expression levels and DNA damage in mouse embryos are blocked by zinc. Toxicological sciences 76: 162–170.
53. Rousseaux MC, Ballare CL, Giordano CV, Scopel AL, Zima AM, et al. (1999) Ozone depletion and UVB radiation: Impact on plant DNA damage in southern South America. Proceedings of the National Academy of Sciences of the United States of America 96: 15310–15315.

Novel Positively Charged Nanoparticle Labeling for *In Vivo* Imaging of Adipose Tissue-Derived Stem Cells

Hiroshi Yukawa[1]*, Shingo Nakagawa[2], Yasuma Yoshizumi[2], Masaki Watanabe[3], Hiroaki Saito[4], Yoshitaka Miyamoto[5], Hirofumi Noguchi[6], Koichi Oishi[7], Kenji Ono[7], Makoto Sawada[7], Ichiro Kato[4], Daisuke Onoshima[8], Momoko Obayashi[1], Yumi Hayashi[2], Noritada Kaji[1,3], Tetsuya Ishikawa[2], Shuji Hayashi[5], Yoshinobu Baba[1,3,9]

1 Research Center for Innovative Nanobiodevices, Nagoya University, Furo-cho, Chikusa-ku, Nagoya 464-8603, Japan, 2 Department of Medical Technology, Nagoya University, Graduate School of Medicine, Daikominami, Higashi-ku, Nagoya 461-8673, Japan, 3 Department of Applied Chemistry, Graduate School of Engineering, Nagoya University, Furo-cho, Chikusa-ku, Nagoya 464-8603, Japan, 4 Nagoya Research Laboratory, MEITO Sangyo Co., Ltd., Kiyosu 452-0067, Japan, 5 Department of Advanced Medicine in Biotechnology and Robotics, Graduate School of Medicine, Nagoya University, Higashi-ku, Nagoya 461-0047, Japan, 6 Department of Regenerative Medicine, Graduate School of Medicine, University of the Ryukyus, 207 Uehara, Nishihara, Okinawa 903-0215, Japan, 7 Research Institute of Environmental Medicine, Stress Adaption and Protection, Nagoya University, Furo-cho, Chikusa-ku, Nagoya, 464-8601, Japan, 8 Institute of Innovative for Future Society, Nagoya University, Furo-cho, Chikusa-ku, Nagoya 464-8603, Japan, 9 Health Research Institute, National Institute of Advanced Industrial Science and Technology (AIST), Hayashi-cho 2217-14, Takamatsu 761-0395, Japan

Abstract

Stem cell transplantation has been expected to have various applications for regenerative medicine. However, in order to detect and trace the transplanted stem cells in the body, non-invasive and widely clinically available cell imaging technologies are required. In this paper, we focused on magnetic resonance (MR) imaging technology, and investigated whether the trimethylamino dextran-coated magnetic iron oxide nanoparticle -03 (TMADM-03), which was newly developed by our group, could be used for labeling adipose tissue-derived stem cells (ASCs) as a contrast agent. No cytotoxicity was observed in ASCs transduced with less than 100 µg-Fe/mL of TMADM-03 after a one hour transduction time. The transduction efficiency of TMADM-03 into ASCs was about four-fold more efficient than that of the alkali-treated dextran-coated magnetic iron oxide nanoparticle (ATDM), which is a major component of commercially available contrast agents such as ferucarbotran (Resovist), and the level of labeling was maintained for at least two weeks. In addition, the differentiation ability of ASCs labeled with TMADM-03 and their ability to produce cytokines such as hepatocyte growth factor (HGF), vascular endothelial growth factor (VEGF) and prostaglandin E2 (PGE2), were confirmed to be maintained. The ASCs labeled with TMADM-03 were transplanted into the left kidney capsule of a mouse. The labeled ASCs could be imaged with good contrast using a 1T MR imaging system. These data suggest that TMADM-03 can therefore be utilized as a contrast agent for the MR imaging of stem cells.

Editor: Xing-Ming Shi, Georgia Regents University, United States of America

Funding: This research was supported by the Cabinet Office, Government of Japan and the Japan Society for the Promotion of Science (JSPS) through the Funding Program for World- Leading Innovative R& D on Science and Technology (FIRST Program) and partially supported by the Japan Science and Technology Agency (JST) through its "Research Center Network for Realization of Regenerative Medicine. The funders had no role in study design, data collection and analysis, decision to publish, or preparation of the manuscript.

Competing Interests: The authors have read the journal's policy and have the following conflicts: Hiroaki Saito and Ichiro Kato have ownership of stocks and paid employment at Meito Sangyo, Inc. The following authors have no competing interests: Hiroshi Yukawa, Watanabe Masaki, Yoshitaka Miyamoto, Noritada Kaji, Hirofumi Noguchi, Koichi Oishi, Kenji Ono, Makoto Sawada, Daisuke Onoshima, Yumi Hayashi, Tetsuya Ishikawa, Shuji Hayashi, Yoshinobu Baba. MEITO Sangyo Co., Ltd. provided the nanoparticles used in this study (Trimethylamino dextran-coated, magnetic iron oxide nanoparticles (TMADM-03)).

* Email: hiroshiy@med.nagoya-u.ac.jp

Introduction

Cell transplantation, which is a simple, rapid and minimally-invasive method relative to whole organ transplantation, has been demonstrated to be effective for treating various diseases such as diabetes, central nervous system (CNS) disorders and cancers including hematological diseases [1]. In particular, stem cell transplantation has been expected to have applications for regenerative medicine. Tsuji et al. showed that the transplantation of induced pluripotent stem (iPS) cells -derived neurospheres was effective for treating spinal cord injury [2]. Liu et al. showed that the transplantation of a combination of mesenchymal stromal cells and haploidentical hematopoietic stem cells facilitated platelet recovery without increasing the recurrence of leukemia [3]. However, the clinical application of stem cell transplantation for many internal organs has been restricted due to the lack of sufficient technology to trace such transplanted stem cells to confirm their correct implantation and to evaluate their growth and migration *in vivo* [4].

In order to reveal the location and accumulation of transplanted stem cells in various tissues and organs deep in the body, a non-invasive and widely clinically available cell imaging technology is needed [5,6]. We herein focus on magnetic resonance (MR) imaging as a method for tracing the transplanted stem cells, because it is a non-invasive, irradiation-free and clinically used method offering good tissue contrast [7]. The MR imaging of stem cells is currently an emerging strategy for tracing transplanted stem cells. To increase the contrast of issues in typical imaging studies, MR contrast agents such as gadolinium (Gd) and superparamagnetic iron oxide (SPIO) nanoparticles are generally used [8,9]. These agents cause hydrogen relaxivity changes and induce contrast modifications [8]. In particular, SPIO nanoparticles are known to generate a strong transverse relaxation time T2-negative contrast in MR images and to decrease the signal intensity [10]. In addition, T2-weighted agents including SPIO nanoparticles are preferentially used for cellular MR imaging since they are more biocompatible and more highly magnetic than T1-weighted agents, resulting in higher contrast modification on MR imaging with a lower concentration than T1-weighted agents [8].

Various SPIO nanoparticles have been developed as contrast agents, including ferucarbotran (Resovist), ferumoxide (Feridex, Endorem) and ferumoxtran-10 (Combidex, Sinerem) [11,12]. Ferucarbotran, an anionic SPIO nanoparticle with a carboxydextran coating has been successfully applied in the clinical setting as a liver contrast agent [13]. It was recently reported that ferucarbotran could more efficiency magnetically label stem cells than ferumoxide and ferumoxtran without including cytotoxicity [4,14]. In this study, we also demonstrate that stem cells can be labeled with ATDM which is a major component of ferucarbotran.

A more common method of labeling cells utilizes cationic transfection reagents to induce the formation of complexes with negatively charged SPIO nanoparticles, because positive charges have been generally considered to be effective for accelerating the intracellular incorporation of such particles [15-18]. Several groups have shown that protamine, which is a low molecular weight polycationic peptide approved by the U.S. FDA as an antidote for heparin anticoagulation, enhanced the uptake of ATDM into stem cells [19]. However, they could not form stable complexes with SPIO nanoparticles, and therefore, it is difficult to clarify the influence of these agents on stem cells [20].

In order to overcome these problems, we have developed five novel contrast agents to use for MR imaging; trimethylamino dextran-coated magnetic iron oxide nanoparticles with different positive charges [21,22]. TMADM-03 has proven to be stably dispersed in the culture medium including fetal bovine serum, and is efficient for labeling mature cells without exerting cytotoxic effect. In fact, Min6 cells, which are a β-cell line, could be efficiently labeled with TMADM-03 without signs of cytotoxicity [22,23]. However, the applicability of TMADM-03 for stem cells remains to be elucidated.

In our research group, adipose tissue-derived stem cells (ASCs) have been the major focus as the stem cell source for regenerative medicine, including stem cell transplantation [24]. ASCs can be easily obtained in abundance by minimally invasive harvest procedures, such as lipoaspiration under local anesthesia, and have the ability to differentiate into not only mesenchymal cells, but also epithelial and endothelial cells [25,26]. Moreover, ASCs have already been used for some clinical treatments [27]. ASCs thus are expected to provide a useful and effective source of the stem cells for regenerative medicine, including stem cell transplantation.

In this study, we investigated whether TMADM-03 could efficiently label ASCs without adverse effects, and determined whether the labeled ASCs could be observed *in vitro* and *in vivo* using MR imaging.

Materials and Methods

Materials

ATDM, which is a major component of ferucarbotran (Resovist), and TMADM-03 were provided by Meito Sangyo Co., Ltd. (Nagoya, Japan). The Cell Counting Kit-8 (CCK-8) was purchased from Dojindo Laboratories (Kumamoto, Japan). Iron standard solution (Fe 1000) and LabAssay-triglyceride were purchased from Wako Pure Chemical Industries, Ltd. (Osaka, Japan). Microhomogenizers for 1.5 mL microtubes ((3810)226AG) were purchased from Eppendorf Japan (Tokyo, Japan). Inductively coupled plasma - atomic emission spectrometry (ICP-AES) was employed to measure the iron concentrations. The Adipo-Inducer Reagent and Osteoblast-Inducer Reagent were purchased from Takara Bio. Inc. (Shiga, Japan). The Quantikine Mouse HGF Immunoassay and Quantikine Mouse VEGF Immunoassay were purchased from R&D systems (Minneapolis, USA). The mouse PGE2 ELISA kit was purchased from Cusabio Biotech Co., Ltd. (Wuhan, China). MACS LS column was purchased from Miltenyi Biotech (Tokyo, Japan).

Animals

C57BL/6 mice were purchased from SLC Japan. The mice were housed in a controlled environment (12 h light/dark cycles at 21°C) with free access to water and an alfalfa-free diet before sacrifice. All conditions and handing of animals in this study were conducted under protocols (024–002 and 025–018) approved by the Nagoya University Committee on Animal Use and Care.

Isolation and culture of ASCs

The isolation and culture of ASCs were reported previously [26]. Briefly, ASCs were collected from seven to fourteen-month-old female C57BL/6 mice. The adipose tissues in the inguinal groove were isolated and cut finely, then digested with type II collagenase (Collagenase Type II, Koken Co., Ltd., Tokyo, Japan) at 37°C in a shaking water bath for 90 min. Adipose tissue cells were when suspended in culture medium (Dulbecco's modified Eagle's medium (DMEM)/F12 containing 20% fetal bovine serum (FBS: Trace Scientific Ltd., Melbourne, Australia) and 100 U/mL penicillin/streptomycin). The cells were centrifuged at 1,200 rpm for five minutes at room temperature to obtain a pellet containing the ASCs. The cells were washed three times by suspension and centrifugation in the culture medium. The primary cells were then cultured for four to five days until they reached confluence and were defined as passage "0". The cells used in all of the experiments were between passages two and five.

Cytotoxicity of ATDM and TMADM-03 to ASCs

ASCs (1×10^4) were seeded in a 96-well plate (BD Biosciences) with 100 μL of culture medium for four hours at 37°C, which was then replaced with 100 μL of transduction medium (DMEM/F12 containing 2% FBS and 100 U/mL penicillin/streptomycin). ATDM (5 mg-Fe/mL) and TMADM-03 (5 mg-Fe/mL) were prepared at various concentrations (0, 5, 10, 50 and 100 μg-Fe/mL) with transduction medium, and were added into each well. After a one or 24 h incubation, the cells were counted using the CCK-8. The CCK-8 reagent (10 μL) was added to each well and the reaction was allowed to proceed for up to four hours. The absorbance of each sample at 450 nm was measured against a background control using a microplate reader.

Proliferation of ASCs labeled with TMADM-03

ASCs (2×10^3) were seeded in each well of a 96-well plate with 100 μL of culture medium and were incubated with various concentrations of TMADM-03. After one hour, the medium was changed to new incubation medium after the cells were washed with PBS three times to eliminate the remaining TMADM-03 in the culture medium. The cells were incubated for two or seven days, and then viable cells were counted using the CCK-8 in the same way as described above.

Electron microscopy analysis

Electron microscopy was used to visualize the presence of TMADM-03 inside the ASCs. ASCs labeled with TMADM-03 were fixed with 2% paraformaldehyde and 2% glutaraldehyde in 0.1 M phosphate buffer (pH 7.4) at 4°C for 24 h, followed by incubation in 2% osmium tetroxide at 4°C for 90 min. The cells were dehydrated in increasing concentrations of ethanol, immersed in propylenoxide and then embedded in Quetol 812 (Nissin EM, Tokyo). Ultrathin sections (70 nm) were stained using Reynold's lead citrate and examined using a JEM-1200EX transmission electron microscope (TEM) (JOEL, Ltd., Tokyo) at an accelerating voltage of 80 kV. These studies were done in cooperation with the Tokai Electron Microscopy Analysis Co., Ltd. (Aichi, Japan).

Quantitative determination of Fe in ASCs labeled with TMADM-03

ASCs (1×10^6) were incubated with ATDM or TMADM-03 at various concentrations (10, 30 and 50 μg-Fe/mL) in transduction medium for one hour. The amount of Fe was measured by phenanthroline spectrophotometric method and ICP-AES method. Briefly, in the ICP-AES method, the ASCs labeled with ATDM or TMADM-03 were washed with PBS three times and were collected by trypsinization. Concentrated nitric acid solution (2 mL) was added to the collected cells, and thermolysis of the solution was conducted at 200°C for four to five hours. After the volatilization of the solution, distilled water was added to the pellets derived from the labeled cells until they weigh 5 g. Next, the Fe concentration of the pellets was measured using the ICP-AES at the analytical wavelength of 259.74 nm. Iron standard solution (Fe 1000) (Wako) was serially diluted, and then used as a standard solution of Fe for comparison purposes.

The labeling efficiency of TMADM-03 for ASCs

The labeled ASCs with TMADM-03 were separated from unlabeled ASCs using MACS LS column in MACS technology according to the manufacture's procedure [28,29]. In brief, ASCs (3×10^5) were labeled with TMADM-03 (0, 10 and 30 μg-Fe/mL) in a one hour incubation, then the ASCs were washed with PBS three times and were collected by the centrifugation at 1200 rpm for 3 min. The ASCs were suspended with transduction medium (2 mL) and the cell suspension was filled into the prerinsed MACS LS column in the magnetic field of the MACS magnet. The ASCs labeled with TMADM-03 were bound to the column, whereas non-labeled ASCs passed through the column. The column was removed and the ASCs labeled with TMADM-03 were released from magnetic field. The column was washed three times with transduction medium (3 mL). The collected cells were counted, and the collected rate was calculated as the labeling efficiency of TMADM-03 for ASCs.

Analysis of the mechanism of TMADM-03 uptake

ASCs (5×10^5) were seeded in each well of a 6-well plate with 2 mL of culture medium and incubated for 24 h at 37°C. The cells were then treated with endocytosis inhibitors, 10 mM sodium azide and 2-deoxy-D-glucose, 5 mM amiloride, 5 μg filipin III, or 12.5 μg chlorpromazine (CPZ) at 37°C for one hour (15 min for amiloride), and then were treated with TMADM-03 (30 μg-Fe/mL) and incubated for one hour at 37°C. In addition, the treatment of incubation at 4°C for one hour was conducted to inhibit endocytosis. Then, the cells were collected and the Fe (II) concentration was measured as described above.

Adipogenic differentiation

The Adipo-Inducer Reagent was used for the adipogenic differentiation of ASCs. Their differentiation was conducted in accordance with the accompanying product manual. Briefly, the differentiation solution was prepared by adding insulin solution (1 mL), dexamethasone solution (0.5 mL) and 3-isobutyl-1-methylxanthine solution (0.1 mL) into the culture medium (100 mL). The incubation solution was prepared by adding insulin solution (1 mL) into the culture medium (100 mL). ASCs with or without the TMADM-03 label were incubated with the differentiation medium for two days. Thereafter, the medium was exchanged for the incubation medium, then cells were incubated for another five to ten days.

The adipogenic differentiation was confirmed by Oil Red O staining as an indicator of intracellular lipid accumulation. Briefly, the cells were fixed in a 10% solution of formaldehyde in PBS for at least 10 min at room temperature, and then were washed with 60% isopropanol. Next, the cells were stained with 2% (w/v) Oil Red O reagent for 10 min at room temperature, followed by repeated washing with distilled water and destaining in 100% isopropanol for one minute.

Osteogenic differentiation

The Osteoblast-Inducer Reagent was used for the osteogenic differentiation of ASCs as specified by the manufacture's product manual. Briefly, the differentiation solution was prepared by adding ascorbic acid (1 mL), hydrocortisone (0.2 mL) and β-glycerophosphate (1 mL) into the culture medium (100 mL). ASCs with or without the TMADM-03 label were incubated with the differentiation medium for 14 to 21 days. The medium was changed to fresh differentiation medium every seven days.

The osteogenic differentiation was confirmed by staining for alkaline phosphatase activity. The cells were then washed twice with PBS and fixed in 10% formalin for 15 min at room temperature. They were then washed and incubated with deionized water for 15 min, and were subsequently stained with a solution containing naphthol AS MX-PO$_4$ (Sigma, N-5000), N, N-dimethylformamide (Wako Pure Chemical Industries Ltd.), Red Violet LB salt (Sigma, F-1625) and Tris-HCl buffer (pH 8.3) for 45 min.

Triglyceride measurement

ASCs (2×10^5) were seeded in each well of a 12-well plate with 2 mL of culture medium and were transduced with TMADM-03 (30 μg-Fe/mL). After the process of adipogenic differentiation, the cells were treated with trypsin and collected into microtubes. PBS (100 μL) was added into the tubes, and then the cells were shredded with microhomogenizers. The amount of triglyceride in the microtubes was measured using the LabAssay Triglyceride Kit according to the manufacture's protocol. Briefly, the color-producing reagent was diluted with buffer solution and the coloring reagent was prepared. The coloring reagent was then added into the samples and standard solutions, and then incubated for five minutes at 37°C. The absorbance at 600 nm was measured by a BioPhotometer (Eppendorf, Tokyo, Japan) and the amount of triglyceride was calculated.

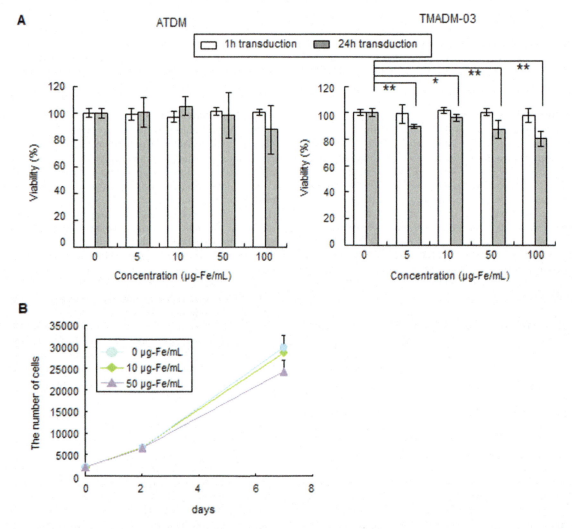

Figure 1. The viability and proliferation rate of ASCs labeled with ATDM or TMADM-03. A: The viability of ASCs labeled with ATDM or TMADM-03 (0, 5, 10, 50, 100 μg-Fe/cell) after a 1 h (white bars) or 24 h (gray bars) transduction at 37°C. There were significant differences in the viability of ASCs labeled with TMADM-03 after the 24 h transduction. B: The proliferation rate of ASCs labeled with TMADM-03 (0, 10, 50 μg-Fe/mL) at 0, 2 and 7 days after 1 h transduction. No significant differences were observed at any of the concentrations of TMADM-03. These data are shown as the means ± standard deviation of triplicate values. *$P<0.05$. **$P<0.01$.

Quantitative estimation of alkaline phosphatase expression

ASCs (1×10^5) were seeded in each well of a 24-well plate with 1 mL of culture medium, and were transduced with TMADM-03 (30 μg-Fe/mL). After the process of osteogenic differentiation, the alkaline phosphatase expression was evaluated by measuring the alkaline phosphatase staining area.

Enzyme-linked immunosorbent assays

ASCs (1×10^5) were seeded into each well of a 24-well plate, and were transduced with TMADM-03 (30 μg-Fe/mL) for one hour. Then, the cells were washed with culture medium, and incubated in fresh culture medium for 24 or 72 h at 37°C. The culture supernatants were collected, and then the levels of mouse HGF, VEGF and PGE2 produced by the ASCs labeled with TMADM-03 and non-labeled ASCs (Normal) in the medium were measured using specific ELISA kits according to the manufacturer's protocols.

ASCs transplantation

ASCs were labeled with TMADM-03 (30 μg-Fe/mL) for 1 h at 37°C. At the end of the uptake experiments, the ASCs were washed three times in the transduction medium, and were collected in microtubes. The ASCs (1×10^6) were transplanted into the renal subcapsular space of the right kidney of a mouse. Moreover, the ASCs (2×10^6) labeled with TMADM-03 (30 μg-Fe/mL) as the same condition were subcutaneously transplanted on the back of the mouse for *in vivo* imaging.

MR imaging

The mice were lightly anesthetized using isoflurane (3% induction and 1.5% maintenance) prior to imaging. MR imaging data were collected on a 1T MRI (MRTechnology, Tsukuba, Japan) according to the manufacture's procedure. In brief, the imaging parameters were as follows: T2 sequences with a TR/TE of 3000/69 ms, field of view (FOV): 30 and two averages were taken for a total acquisition time of about 14 min. T1 sequences were composed of a TR/TE of 500/9 ms, FOV: 30 and four

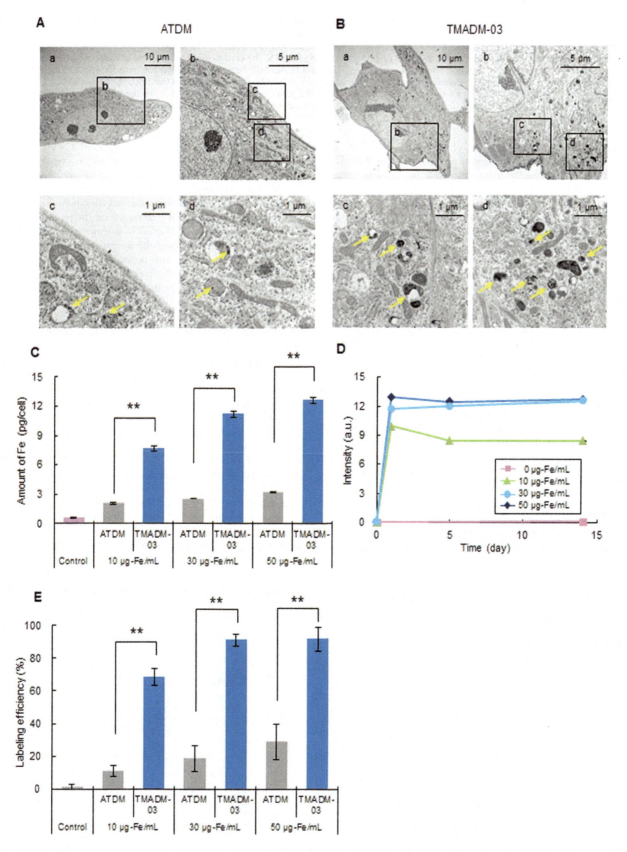

Figure 2. Confirmation of the uptake of ATDM and TMADM-03 by ASCs. A: The images obtained by transmission electron microscopy of ASCs labeled with ATDM (30 μg-Fe/mL) for 1 h at 37°C (a–d). A picture of the cells labeled with ATDM is shown (a). The surface of the cells labeled with ATDM is shown (b). The aggregates of the ATDM internalized by ASCs are shown by yellow arrows in (c) and (d). B: The images obtained by transmission electron microscopy of ASCs labeled with TMADM-03 (30 μg-Fe/mL) for 1 h at 37°C (a–d). A picture of the cells labeled with TMADM-03

is shown (a). The surface of the cells labeled with TMADM-03 is shown (b). The aggregates of the TMADM-03 internalized into ASCs are shown by yellow arrows in (c) and (d). The amount of TMADM-03 internalized in the cytoplasm of ASCs was found to be much higher than that of ATDM. C: The results of the quantitative determinations of the ATDM and TMADM-03 (10, 30, and 50 μg-Fe/mL) internalized into ASCs after a 1 h transduction by measuring the concentration of Fe derived from ATDM or TMADM-03 using ICP-AES. The control (Cont.) shows the amount of Fe normally in ASCs, without labeling by nanoparticles. Significant differences between ATDM and TMADM-03 were confirmed after the transduction at all concentrations. These data are shown as the means ± standard deviation of triplicate values. **$P<0.01$. D: The changes in the amount of TMADM-03 (0, 10, 30 and 50 μg-Fe/mL) internalized by ASCs after a 1 h transduction for two weeks. The data are shown as the means ± standard deviation of triplicate values. E: The labeling efficiency of TMADM-03 (0, 10, 30 and 50 μg-Fe/mL) for ASCs after a 1 h transduction using MACS Technology.

averages for a total acquisition time of about five minutes. All T1 and T2-weighted image data sets were visually evaluated to identify the location of the transplanted cells within each animal.

Prussian blue (PB) staining

The existence of iron particle (TMADM-03) within tissues was confirmed by the PB staining which is a traditional method for detecting the iron (ferric form) according to the manufacture's procedure [30,31]. In brief, the hydrochloric acid and potassium ferrocyanide were mixed and prepared immediately before use. The slides were immersed in this solution for 20 min, and then washed in distilled water three times. Next, the slides were treated with counterstain solution with for 5 minutes, and the slides were rinsed twice in distilled water. Then, the slides were dehydrated through 95% to 100% alcohol, and cleared in xylene two times for 3 minutes each. The slides were covered with resinous mounting medium.

Statistical analysis

Numerical values are presented as the means ± SD. Each experiment was repeated three times. The statistical significance was evaluated using unpaired Student's t-tests for comparisons between two groups; p-values <0.05 were considered to be statistically significant. All statistical analyses were performed using the SPSS software package.

Results

Cytotoxicity of ATDM and TMADM-03 to ASCs

ATDM and TMADM-03 were transduced into ASCs at various concentrations in transduction medium for one or 24 h incubations. Cytotoxicity was observed in the ASCs transduced for 24 h at all concentrations of TMADM-03, however, the degree of cytotoxicity was slight, and more than about 80% of the cells were still alive after the treatment. In addition, no cytotoxicity was observed after a one hour incubation at all concentrations of TMADM-03. On the other hand, no cytotoxicity of ATDM was observed under all of these experimental conditions (Fig. 1A).

Next, the influence of the compounds on the proliferation rate was examined for the non-cytotoxic conditions with TMADM-03. The cells were confirmed to exhibit a logarithmic growth rate that was nearly equal to that of normal, un-treated, ASCs. No significant differences were observed under these conditions (Fig. 1B). These data suggest that TMADM-03 could be used to label cells for one hour at a 100 μg-Fe/mL concentration.

Observation of ATDM and TMADM-03 internalization inside ASCs

To detect the internalization of ATDM and the TMADM-03 internalization by ASCs, the cells were transduced with 30 μg-Fe/mL of ATDM or TMADM-03 by a one hour incubation. The SPIO nanoparticles could be observed in ASCs transduced with both ATDM and TMADM-03 using TEM, and these nanoparticles were found in the cell cytoplasm and lysosomes. However, the degree of TMADM-03 incorporation was remarkably higher than that of ATDM (Figs. 2A, B). In addition, as shown in Fig. 2B-b, the surface of ASCs was found to be covered with TMADM-03. These data suggest that both ATDM and TMADM-03 could be transduced into ASCs within one hour of incubation, but the efficiency was markedly higher for TMADM-03.

Comparison of the uptake of ATDM and TMADM-03 by ASCs

To measure the uptake of ATDM and TMADM-03 by ASCs, the amount of Fe derived from ATDM and TMADM-03 in ASCs

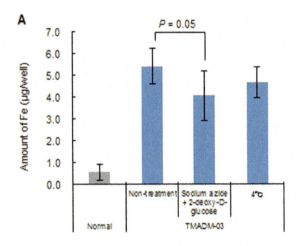
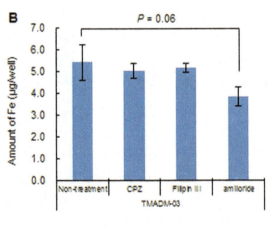

Figure 3. The mechanism of uptake of TMADM-03 by ASCs. A: The effect of endocytosis inhibitors on TMADM-03 internalization in ASCs. Cells were treated with sodium azide and 2-deoxy-D-glucose, or incubated at 4°C. B: The effect of pinocytosis inhibitors on TMADM-03 internalization in ASCs. Cells were treated with chlorpromazine (CPZ), Filipin III, or amiloride. The data are shown as the means ± standard deviation of triplicate values.

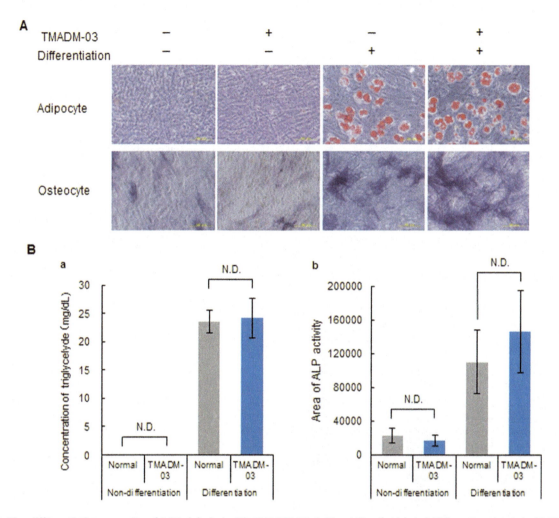

Figure 4. The differentiation capacity of ASCs labeled with TMADM-03. A: The ability of unlabeled ASCs or those labeled with TMADM-03 (30 μg-Fe/mL) to differentiate into adipocytes and osteocytes. The extent of adipogenic differentiation was assessed by Oil Red O staining. Red spherical bodies in the upper figures show lipid droplets produced by the differentiated ASCs (upper). The extent of osteogenic differentiation was assessed by ALP staining. Purple sites in the lower figures show the ALP produced by the differentiated ASCs (lower). B: The degree of differentiation into adipocytes by the concentration (mg/mL) of triglyceride present in the cells (a). The degree of differentiation into osteocytes by the ALP staining area (b). The data are shown as the means ± standard deviation of triplicate values.

was measured using ICP-AES. The amount of Fe was increased in a concentration-dependent manner for both types of nanoparticles. However, the amount of Fe in cells incubated with TMADM-03 was significantly higher (about four-fold) in comparison to that of ATDM at all concentrations (Fig. 2C). The amount of TMADM-03 was confirmed to remain approximately equal for at least 14 days in 30 and 50 μg-Fe/mL labeling conditions (Fig. 2D). In addition, the labeling efficiency was measured by MACS technology, and the efficiency of TMADM-03 was much higher than that of ATDM at all concentrations. Especially, the labeling efficiency of TMADM-03 in 30 and 50 μg-Fe/mL showed more than 90% (Fig. 2E). These data suggest that ASCs could be efficiently labeled with TMADM-03 at the concentration of 30 μg-Fe/mL and maintained the labeling state for at least 14 days.

Mechanism of TMADM-03 uptake by ASCs

To verify the mechanism of uptake of TMADM-03 in ASCs, the cells were treated with endocytosis inhibitors such as sodium azide and 2-deoxy-D-glucose (endocytosis inhibitors), amiloride (an inhibitor of the Na^+/H^+ exchanger required for macropinocytosis), filipin III (an inhibitor of caveolae formation) or chlorpromazine (CPZ: an inhibitor of AP-2-mediated clathrin-coated pit formation) at 37°C for one hour (15 min for amiloride). In addition, treatment by incubation at 4°C for one hour was also employed to inhibit endocytosis. The transduction of TMADM-03 was inhibited by the incubation at 4°C and the treatments with sodium azide and 2-deoxy-D-glucose, or amiloride (Figs. 3A, B). These data suggest that the uptake of TMADM-03 into ASCs was mainly dependent on the endocytosis, particularly macropinocytosis.

Differentiation of ASCs labeled with TMADM-03

To exam the influence of TMADM-03 on the differentiation capacity of ASCs, normal (non-labeled) and labeled ASCs were differentiated into adipocytes or osteoblasts, and then the degree of differentiation in the non-labeled and labeled ASCs was quantitatively compared. The differentiation of ASCs after treatment with TMADM-03 into either adipocytes or osteocytes was observed. There were also no significant differences between the

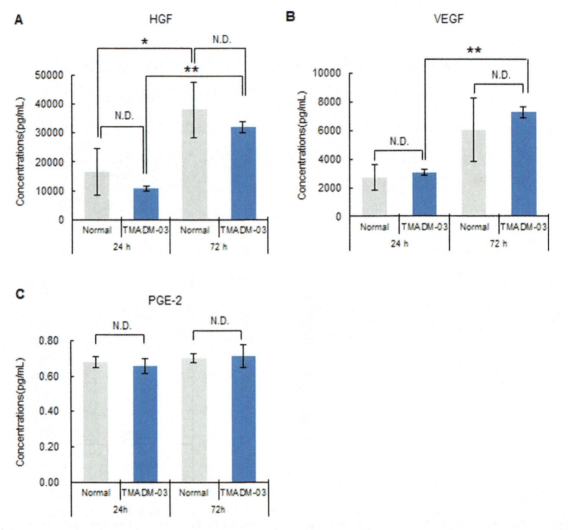

Figure 5. The levels of cytokines produced by ASCs labeled with TMADM-03. A: The concentration of HGF produced by non-labeled (normal) ASCs (1×10^5) or ASCs labeled with TMADM-03 incubated for 24 and 72 h in the culture medium. B: The concentration of VEGF produced by non-labeled (normal) ASCs (1×10^5) or ASCs labeled with TMADM-03 incubated for 24 and 72 h in the culture medium. C: The concentration of PGE2 produced by non-labeled (normal) ASCs (1×10^5) or ASCs labeled with TMADM-03 incubated for 24 and 72 h in the culture medium. The data are shown as the means ± standard deviation of triplicate. *$P<0.05$, **$P<0.01$.

non-labeled and labeled ASCs in terms of the concentration of triglycerides, indicating the degree of adipogenic differentiation (Figs. 4A, B–a). Moreover, similar expression of ALP indicating the degree of osteogenic differentiation was confirmed in the cells incubated with and without the TMADM-03 (Figs. 4A, B–b). These data suggest that TMADM-03 does not affect the differentiation of ASCs.

Cytokine production from ASCs labeled with TMADM-03

To confirm the production of HGF, VEGF and PGE2 from non-labeled ASCs or ASCs labeled with TMADM-03, the levels of these cytokines in the culture medium from ASCs cultured for 24 or 72 h were measured using specific ELISA kits. The production of these cytokines could be confirmed in both non-labeled and labeled ASCs, and no significant differences were observed in the production of any of these cytokines (Fig. 5). These data raised the possibility that the ability of ASCs to produce cytokines could be maintained after labeling with TMADM-03.

In vitro MRI of ASCs labeled with TMADM-03

To examine whether the cells labeled with 10, 30 and 50 μg-Fe/mL of TMADM-03 could be detected by MR imaging, the labeled cells (1×10^6) were collected in PBS and spun down, then the cell pellet was prepared for the MR analysis in microtubes. The labeled cell pellet could be detected at a lower intensity on both T1 and T2-weighted images in comparison to the unlabeled cell pellet (Fig. 6A). These results suggested that the cells labeled with more than 30 μg-Fe/mL of TMADM-03 could be detected with sufficient contrast for cell visualization by MR imaging.

MR imaging of ASCs labeled with TMADM-03 in mice

To assess whether images of transplanted ASCs labeled with TMADM-03 could be obtained in mice, the ASCs (1×10^6) labeled with 30 μg-Fe/mL of TMADM-03 after a one hour incubation were transplanted into the left kidney capsule of a mouse. The MR imaging data of both cross-section figures from the back and head three hour after transplantation showed remarkable decreases in signal intensity on T1 and T2-weighted images at the implanted

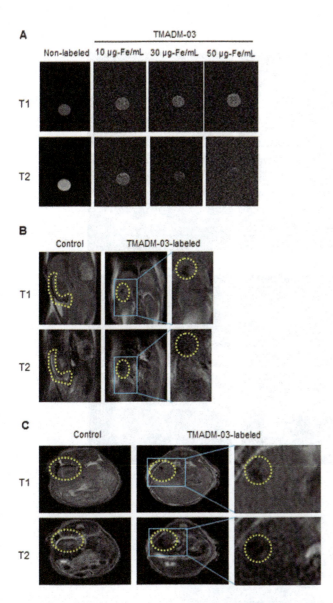

Figure 6. MR imaging of ASCs labeled with TMADM-03 in the kidney capsule. A: *In vitro* MR imaging of unlabeled and labeled ASCs (1×10^6). T1- (upper) and T2- (lower) weighted images were obtained for unlabeled ASCs and for ASCs labeled with TMADM-03 (10, 30 and 50 μg-Fe/mL). B: *In vivo* MR imaging of unlabelled ASCs (1×10^6) or the same number of ASCs labeled with TMADM-03 (30 μg-Fe/mL) in a cross-section figure from the back of the mouse. T1- (upper) and T2- (lower) weighted images were obtained for unlabeled ASCs, and for ASCs labeled with TMADM-03 3 hours after transduction. Yellow dotted circles show the transplanted ASCs. C: *In vivo* MR imaging of unlabeled ASCs (1×10^6) or the same number of ASCs labeled with TMADM-03 (30 μg-Fe/mL) in a cross-section figure from the head of the mouse. T1- (upper) and T2- (lower) weighted images were obtained for unlabeled ASCs and for ASCs labeled with TMADM-03. The yellow dotted circles show the transplanted ASCs. These images were obtained using a 1T MRI instrument (MR Technology).

site in the left kidney of a mouse that was transplanted with ASCs labeled with TMADM-03. On the other hand, in a mouse transplanted with unlabeled ASCs, no decrease in the signal intensity on T2 was observed in the MR imaging results (Figs. 6B C).

In addition, to investigate whether the labeled ASCs could be detected for 14 days, the ASCs (2×10^6) labeled with 30 μg-Fe/mL of TMADM-03 were transplanted under the skin of the back of a mouse at two sites (yellow dotted circles). The ASCs labeled with 30 μg-Fe/mL of TMADM-03 could be traced for at least 14 days after transplantation (Fig. 7A). In addition, to reveal whether the labeled ASCs were alive and did not affect the surrounding tissues or cells, the transplantation sites were treated with PB staining. The blue staining showing the existence of TMADM-03 was confirmed in transplantation sites, and there were no obvious abnormalities such as inflammation in the surrounding tissues or cells (Fig. 7B). These data suggest that the positively charged TMADM-03 was useful as a MR imaging contrast agent for assessing the disposition of transplanted ASCs.

Discussion

Various SPIO nanoparticles have been developed as contrast agents for MR imaging such as ferucarbotran (Resovist), ferristene (Abdoscan), ferumoxsil (GastroMARK, Lumirenr), ferumoxide (Feridex, Endorem), ferumoxtran-10 (Combidex, Sinerem) and feruglose (Crasican) etc. [11]. Numerous studies have recently revealed these agents to be useful for stem cell labeling for *in vivo* MR imaging [32–37]. Among these agents, there have been many studies on ferucarbotran (Resovist, Clivist), which is well known liver contrast agent currently used in the clinical setting [10,38,39]. Crabbe et al. revealed that Resovist was useful for labeling mouse mesenchymal stem cells, and that it was superior to Endoderm and Sinerem [4]. However, almost all of these agents have a negative charge coating site on the surface of the SPIO [40]. The surfaces of various cells, including stem cells, normally have many sugar chains whose termini are sialic acid, and these cells therefore have a negative charge on their surface, thus preventing the effective transduction of these cells with the SPIO [41]. We have previously succeeded in performing efficient quantum dots (QDs) labeling for ASCs through an endocytosis pathway using octa-arginine peptides with a positive charge known as cell penetrating peptides (CPPs) [42]. Various CPPs have been identified including the third helix of the homeodomain of antennapedia [43,44], VP22 herpesvirus protein [45] and the HIV-Tat protein [46]. Most of these peptides have a positive charge derived from amino acids such as arginine and lysine. In this study, we demonstrated that TMADM-03, which has a positive charge, can label ASCs more efficiently than ATDM which is a major component of ferucarbotran that has a negative charge.

We have already reported that the zeta voltages of ATDM and TMADM-03 were -15 mV and +2.0 mV, respectively [23]. When ASCs were transduced with TMADM-03 during a one hour incubation, the surface of ASCs was observed to be covered with TMADM-03 by a TEM analysis. The successful uptake of TMADM-03 by the ASCs was therefore thought to have occurred. The same phenomenon was not found in the case of ATDM. ATDM was thought to incidentally come into contacted with the surface of ASCs, and to subsequently be incorporated into the ASCs. As a result, about a four-fold higher uptake of TMADM-03 in comparison to ATDM was observed by ICP-AES in the present day. According to previous reports, positively charged substrates, such as protamine, can effectively increase the efficiency of transduction of magnetic nanoparticles into cells. Huang et al. reported that an approximately two-fold higher uptake of ATDM was observed when it was complexed with protamine in comparison to the uptake of ATDM alone [39]. In addition, Balakumaran reported that labeling by ferumoxide complexed with protamine did not affect the stemness of bone marrow

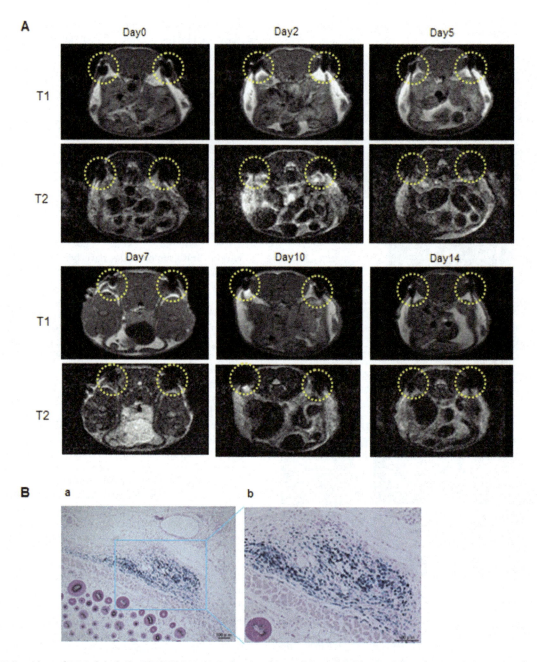

Figure 7. MR imaging of ASCs labeled with TMADM-03 under the skin and Prussian blue staining. A: *In vivo* MR imaging of ASCs (2×10^6) labeled with TMADM-03 (30 μg-Fe/mL) under the skin in a cross-section figure from the head of the mouse for 14 days. The two yellow dotted circles show the transplanted ASCs labeled with 30 μg-Fe/mL of TMADM-03. These images were obtained using a 1T MRI instrument (MR Technology). B: Prussian blue staining of the transplanted ASCs labeled with TMADM-03.

mesenchymal stem cells [34]. However, the efficiency of uptake of ATDM complexed with protamine is assumed to be lower than that of TMADM-03, and the influence of the released protamine on other types of stem cells remains unclear.

Slight cytotoxicity was observed in ASCs transduced with TMADM-03 during a 24 h incubation. However, no cytotoxicity was observed after one hour of incubation at a concentration of up to 100 μg/mL of TMADM-03, and the ASCs labeled with TMADM-03 under these non-cytotoxic conditions exhibited growth equivalent to that of normal ASCs, and could be successfully detected by MRI. The capacity of these cells to differentiate in adipocytes and osteocytes was not affected, and the ability of labeled ASCs to produce cytokines such as HGF, VEGF and PGE2, which are thought to be important for regenerative effects, was maintained after the labeling with TMADM-03. Moreover, the transduction of TMADM-03 into ASCs was inhibited by sodium azide and 2-deoxy-D-glucose (endocytosis inhibitors), and amiloride (a macropinocytosis inhibitor). Although the uptake mechanism of TMADM-03 had previously been unknown, our data indicate that the uptake pathway of TMADM-03 is thought to be mainly dependent on the endocytosis, partially macropinocytosis. These data suggest that TMADM-03 can be a safe and efficient MR contrast agent that can be used to label stem cells for clinical applications.

Using a 1T MR imaging system for small animals, we demonstrated that the ASCs labeled with TMADM-03 could be detected both *in vitro* and *in vivo*. As shown in Fig. 6A, the MR images of the pellet of ASCs labeled with TMADM-03 in a microtube had low signal, and a negative contrast effect could be confirmed. When ASCs labeled with TMADM-03 were transplanted under the skin and the left kidney capsule of a mouse, a negative effect on T2-weighted contrast images could be detected when TMADM-03 was used (Figs. 6B, 6C, 7A). Furthermore, the inflammatory state such as induced by the cell death could not be observed in the surrounding area of the transplantation of ASCs labeled with TMADM-03. These data suggest that TMADM-03 can be used as a contrast agent both *in vitro* and *in vivo* for the MR imaging of stem cells, and raise the possibility that TMADM-03 can provide insights into the location and accumulation of transplanted stem cells in tissues or organs deep in the body.

In conclusion, we investigated whether TMADM-03, which was previously developed by our group, could be used to label ASCs as a MR imaging contrast agent. No cytotoxicity was observed in the ASCs transduced with a concentration of up to 100 μg-Fe/mL of TMADM-03 for a one hour transduction time. The transduction efficiency of TMADM-03 into ASCs was about four-fold higher than that of ATDM, which is a major component of ferucarbotran (Resovist), a clinically-used contrast agent. Of note, the labeling level was maintained for at least two weeks. ASCs labeled with TMADM-03 were confirmed to be able to differentiate into both adipocytes and osteocytes to the same extent as non-labeled ASCs. In addition, the ability of ASCs labeled with TMADM-03 to product cytokines (HGF, VEGF and PGE2) was maintained. The ASCs labeled with TMADM-03 could be imaged with good contrast using a 1T MR imaging system when the labeled ASCs were transplanted into the left kidney capsule of a mouse. Together, these data suggest that TMADM-03 can be utilized as a MR imaging contrast agent for tracking transplanted stem cells.

Acknowledgments

This research is supported by the Japan Science and Technology Agency (JST) through its "Research Center Network for Realization of Regenerative Medicine." We appreciate the help of Naoko Kawakita (Nagoya University) for the treatment of ASCs and the cell labeling. We would also like to thank Tokai Electron Microscopy, Inc. for the technical assistance in the transmission electron microscope observation.

Author Contributions

Conceived and designed the experiments: HY. Performed the experiments: HY SN YY MW HS K. Oishi K. Ono MO YH. Analyzed the data: HY SN YY MW K. Ono DO. Contributed reagents/materials/analysis tools: HS YM HN MS IK NK TI SH YB. Wrote the paper: HY.

References

1. Bhirde A, Xie J, Swierczewska M, Chen X (2011) Nanoparticles for cell labeling. Nanoscale 3: 142–153.
2. Tsuji O, Miura K, Okada Y, Fujiyoshi K, Mukaino M, et al. (2010) Therapeutic potential of appropriately evaluated safe-induced pluripotent stem cells for spinal cord injury. Proc Natl Acad Sci USA 107: 12704–12709.
3. Liu K, Chen Y, Zeng Y, Xu L, Liu D, et al. (2011) Coinfusion of mesenchymal stromal cells facilitates platelet recovery without increasing leukemia recurrence in haploidentical hematopoietic stem cell transplantation: a randomized, controlled clinical study. Stem Cells Dev 20: 1679–1685.
4. Crabbe A, Vandeputte C, Dresselaers T, Sacido AA, Verdugo JM, et al. (2010) Effects of MRI contrast agents on the stem cell phenotype. Cell Transplant 19: 919–936.
5. Son KR, Chung SY, Kim HC, Kim HS, Choi SH, et al. (2010) MRI of magnetically labeled mesenchymal stem cells in hepatic failure model. World J Gastroenterol 16: 5611–5615.
6. Kim HM, Lee H, Hong KS, Cho MY, Sung MH, et al. (2011) Synthesis and high performance of magnetofluorescent polyelectrolyte nanocomposites as MR/near-infrared multimodal cellular imaging nanoprobes. ACS Nano 5: 8230–8240.
7. Tseng CL, Shih IL, Stobinski L, Lin FH (2010) Gadolinium hexanedione nanoparticles for stem cell labeling and tracking via magnetic resonance imaging. Biomaterials 31: 5427–5435.
8. Lalande C, Miraux S, Derkaoui SM, Mornet S, Bareille R, et al. (2011) Magnetic resonance imaging tracking of human adipose derived stromal cells within three-dimensional scaffolds for bone tissue engineering. Eur Cell Mater 21: 341–354.
9. Kim T, Momin E, Choi J, Yuan K, Zaidi H, et al. (2011) Mesoporous silica-coated hollow manganese oxide nanoparticles as positive T1 contrast agents for labeling and MRI tracking of adipose-derived mesenchymal stem cells. J Am Chem Soc 133: 2955–2961.
10. Chen R, Yu H, Jia ZY, Yao QL, Teng GJ (2011) Efficient nano iron particle-labeling and noninvasive MR imaging of mouse bone marrow-derived endothelial progenitor cells. Int J Nanomedicine 6: 511–519.
11. Rosen JE, Chan L, Shieh DB, Gu FX (2010) Iron oxide nanoparticles for targeted cancer imaging and diagnostics. Nanomedicine 8: 275–290.
12. Patel D, Kell A, Simard B, Xiang B, Lin HY, et al. (2011) The cell labeling efficacy, cytotoxicity and relaxivity of copper-activated MRI/PET imaging contrast agents. Biomaterials 32: 1167–1176.
13. Bae JE, Huh MI, Ryu BK, Do JY, Jin SU, et al. (2011) The effect of static magnetic fields on the aggregation and cytotoxicity of magnetic nanoparticles. Biomaterials 32: 9401–9414.
14. Mailänder V, Lorenz MR, Holzapfel V, Musyanovych A, Fuchs K, et al. (2008) Carboxylated superparamagnetic iron oxide particles label cells intracellularly without transfection agents. Mol Imaging Biol 10: 138–146.
15. Bulte JW, Kraitchman DL (2004) Iron oxide MR contrast agents for molecular and cellular imaging. NMR Biomed 17: 484–499.
16. Thorek DL, Tsourkas A (2008) Size, Charge and concentration dependent uptake of iron oxide particles by non-phagocytic cells. Biomaterials 29: 3583–3590.
17. Liu G, Tian J, Liu C, Ai H, Gu Z, et al. (2009) Cell labeling efficiency of layer-by-layer self-assembly modified silica nanoparticles. J Mat Res 24: 1317–1321.
18. Sponarová D, Horák D, Trchová M, Jendelová P, Herynek V, et al. (2011) The use of oligoperoxide-coated magnetic nanoparticles to label stem cells. J Biomed Nanotechnol 7: 384–394.
19. Bull BS, Huse WM, Brauer FS, Korpman RA (1975) Heparin therapy during extracorporeal circulation. II. the use of a dose-response curve to individualize heparin and protamine dosage. J Thorac Cardiovasc Surg 69: 685–689.
20. Arbab AS, Yocum GT, Wilson LB, Parwana A, Jordan EK, et al. (2004) Comparison of transfection agents in forming complexes with ferumoxides, cell labeling efficiency, and cellular viability. Mol Imaging 3: 24–32.
21. Oishi K, Noguchi H, Saito H, Yukawa H, Miyamoto Y, et al. (2010) Cell labeling with a novel contrast agent of magnetic resonance imaging. Cell Transplant 19: 887–892.
22. Oishi K, Noguchi H, Saito H, Yukawa H, Miyamoto Y, et al. (2012) Novel positive-charged nanoparticles for efficient magnetic resonance imaging of islet transplantation. Cell Medicine 3: 43–49.
23. Oishi K, Miyamoto Y, Saito H, Murase K, Ono K, et al. (2013) In vivo imaging of transplanted islets labeled with a novel cationic nanoparticle. PLoS One 8: e57046.
24. Yukawa H, Noguchi H, Oishi K, Takagi S, Hamaguchi M, et al. (2009) Cell transplantation of adipose tissue-derived stem cells in combination with heparin attenuated acute liver failure in mice. Cell Transplant 18: 601–609.
25. Oishi K, Noguchi H, Yukawa H, Miyazaki T, Kato R, et al. (2008) Cryopreservation of mouse adipose tissue-derived stem/progenitor cells. Cell Transplant 17: 35–41.
26. Yukawa H, Noguchi H, Oishi K, Miyazaki T, Kitagawa Y, et al. (2008) Recombinant sendai virus-mediated gene transfer to adipose tissue-derived stem cells (ASCs). Cell Transplant 17: 43–50.
27. Traktuev DO, Merfeld-Clauss S, Li J, Kolonin M, Arap W, et al. (2008) A population of multipotent CD34-positive adipose stromal cells share pericyte and mesenchymal surface markers, reside in a periendothelial location, and stabilize endothelial networks. Circ Res 102: 77–85.
28. Pierzchalski A, Mittag A, Bocsi J, Tarnok A (2013) An innovative cascade system for simultaneous separation of multiple cell types. PLoS One 8: e74745.
29. Kazemi T, Asgarian-Omran H, Hojjat-Farsangi M, Shabani M, Memarian A, et al. (2008) Fc receptor-like 1–5 molecules are similarly expressed in progressive and indolent clinical subtypes of B-cell chronic lymphocytic leukemia. Int J Cancer 123: 2113–2119.
30. Zhang B, Yang B, Zhai C, Jiang B, Wu Y (2013) The role of exendin-4-conjugated superparamagnetic iron oxide nanoparticles in beta-cell-targeted MRI. Biomaterials 34: 5843–5852.
31. Tai JH, Foster P, Rosales A, Feng B, Hasilo C, et al. (2006) Imaging islets labeled with magnetic nanoparticles at 1.5 Tesla. Diabetes 55: 2931–2938.

32. van Buul GM, Kotek G, Wielopolski PA, Farrell E, Bos PK, et al. (2011) Clinically translatable cell tracking and quantification by MRI in cartilage repair using superparamagnetic iron oxides. PLoS One 6: e17001.
33. Kim JI, Chun C, Kim B, Hong JM, Cho JK, et al. (2012) Thermosensitive/magnetic poly(organophosphazene) hydrogel as a long-term magnetic resonance contrast platform. Biomaterials 33: 218–224.
34. Balakumaran A, Pawelczyk E, Ren J, Sworder B, Chaudhry A, et al. (2010) Superparamagnetic iron oxide nanoparticles labeling of bone marrow stromal (mesenchymal) cells does not affect their "stemness". PLoS One 5: e11462.
35. Nohroudi K, Arnhold S, Berhorn T, Addicks K, Hoehn M, et al. (2010) In vivo MRI stem cell tracking requires balancing of detection limit and cell viability. Cell Transplant. 19: 431–441.
36. Hu SL, Zhang JQ, Hu X, Hu R, Luo HS, et al. (2009) In vitro labeling of human umbilical cord mesenchymal stem cells with superparamagnetic iron oxide nanoparticles. J Cell Biochem 108: 529–535.
37. Kim TH, Kim JK, Shim W, Kim SY, Park TJ, et al. (2010) Tracking of transplanted mesenchymal stem cells labeled with fluorescent magnetic nanoparticle in liver cirrhosis rat model with 3-T MRI. Magn Reson Imaging 28: 1004–1013.
38. Huang DM, Hsiao JK, Chen YC, Chien LY, Yao M, et al. (2009) The promotion of human mesenchymal stem cell proliferation by superparamagnetic iron oxide nanoparticles. Biomaterials 30: 3645–3651.
39. Chien LY, Hsiao JK, Hsu SC, Yao M, Lu CW, et al. (2011) In vivo magnetic resonance imaging of cell tropism, trafficking mechanism, and therapeutic impact of human mesenchymal stem cells in a murine glioma model. Biomaterials 32: 3275–3284.
40. Xiao L, Li J, Brougham DF, Fox EK, Feliu N, et al. (2011) Water-soluble superparamagnetic magnetite nanoparticles with biocompatible coating for enhanced magnetic resonance imaging. ACS Nano 5: 6315–6324.
41. Hart C, Chase LG, Hajivandi M, Agnew B (2011) Metabolic labeling and click chemistry detection of glycoprotein markers of mesenchymal stem cell differentiation. Methods Mol Biol 698: 459–484.
42. Yukawa H, Kagami Y, Watanabe M, Oishi K, Miyamoto Y, et al. (2010) Quantum dots labeling using octa-arginine peptides for imaging of adipose tissue-derived stem cells. Biomaterials 31: 4094–4103.
43. Derossi D, Calvet S, Trembleau A, Brunissen A, Chassaing G, et al. (1996) Cell internalization of the third helix of the antennapedia homeodomain is receptor-independent. J Biol Chem 271: 18188–18193.
44. Noguchi H, Kaneto H, Weir GC, Bonner-Weir S (2003) PDX-1 protein containing its own antennapedia-like protein transduction domain can transduce pancreatic duct and islet cells. Diabetes 52: 1732–1737.
45. Phelan A, Elliott G, O'Hare P (1998) Intercellular delivery of functional p53 by the herpesvirus protein VP22. Nat Biotechnol 16: 440–443.
46. Schwarze SR, Ho A, Vocero-Akbani A, Dowdy SF (1999) In vivo protein transduction: delivery of a biologically active protein into the mouse. Science 285: 1569–1572.

3-O-Galloylated Procyanidins from *Rumex acetosa* L. Inhibit the Attachment of Influenza A Virus

Andrea Derksen[1], Andreas Hensel[1], Wali Hafezi[2], Fabian Herrmann[1], Thomas J. Schmidt[1], Christina Ehrhardt[3], Stephan Ludwig[3], Joachim Kühn[2]*

[1] Institute of Pharmaceutical Biology and Phytochemistry, University of Münster, Münster, Germany, [2] Institute of Medical Microbiology - Clinical Virology, University Hospital Münster, Münster, Germany, [3] Institute of Molecular Virology, University of Münster, Münster, Germany

Abstract

Infections by influenza A viruses (IAV) are a major health burden to mankind. The current antiviral arsenal against IAV is limited and novel drugs are urgently required. Medicinal plants are known as an abundant source for bioactive compounds, including antiviral agents. The aim of the present study was to characterize the anti-IAV potential of a proanthocyanidin-enriched extract derived from the aerial parts of *Rumex acetosa* (RA), and to identify active compounds of RA, their mode of action, and structural features conferring anti-IAV activity. In a modified MTT (MTT_{IAV}) assay, RA was shown to inhibit growth of the IAV strain PR8 (H1N1) and a clinical isolate of IAV(H1N1)pdm09 with a half-maximal inhibitory concentration (IC_{50}) of 2.5 µg/mL and 2.2 µg/mL, and a selectivity index (SI) (half-maximal cytotoxic concentration (CC_{50})/IC_{50})) of 32 and 36, respectively. At RA concentrations>1 µg/mL plaque formation of IAV(H1N1)pdm09 was abrogated. RA was also active against an oseltamivir-resistant isolate of IAV(H1N1)pdm09. TNF-α and EGF-induced signal transduction in A549 cells was not affected by RA. The dimeric proanthocyanidin epicatechin-3-O-gallate-(4β→8)-epicatechin-3'-O-gallate (procyanidin B2-di-gallate) was identified as the main active principle of RA (IC_{50} approx. 15 µM, SI≥13). RA and procyanidin B2-di-gallate blocked attachment of IAV and interfered with viral penetration at higher concentrations. Galloylation of the procyanidin core structure was shown to be a prerequisite for anti-IAV activity; *o*-trihydroxylation in the B-ring increased the anti-IAV activity. *In silico* docking studies indicated that procyanidin B2-di-gallate is able to interact with the receptor binding site of IAV(H1N1)pdm09 hemagglutinin (HA). In conclusion, the proanthocyanidin-enriched extract RA and its main active constituent procyanidin B2-di-gallate protect cells from IAV infection by inhibiting viral entry into the host cell. RA and procyanidin B2-di-gallate appear to be a promising expansion of the currently available anti-influenza agents.

Editor: Cheryl A. Stoddart, University of California, San Francisco, United States of America

Funding: The authors acknowledge support by Deutsche Forschungsgemeinschaft and Open Access Publication Fund of University of Muenster. The funders had no role in study design, data collection and analysis, decision to publish, or preparation of the manuscript.

Competing Interests: The authors have declared that no competing interests exist.

* Email: kuehnj@uni-muenster.de

Introduction

Influenza A and B viruses (IAV, IBV) circulating in the human population are responsible for seasonal epidemics of varying extent. At present, the global annual disease burden of seasonal influenza is estimated to be 1 billion infections, 3 to 5 million of severe infections, and 300 000 to 500 000 fatalities. Without doubt, vaccination remains the most important strategy for prophylaxis and control of seasonal influenza [1]. Although predominantly associated with mild symptoms of upper respiratory tract infection, the first pandemic of the 21st century caused by IAV(H1N1)pdm09 impressively demonstrated the global health risks associated with IAV. Ongoing zoonotic infections with avian IAV(H5N1) and (H7N9) in the human population underscore the permanent threat of pandemic outbreaks, of which the "Spanish flu" pandemic of 1918–19 with an estimated number of 50 million deaths world-wide has been the most devastating [2].

Two classes of antiviral drugs have been licensed for the treatment and prophylaxis of influenza [3]. Matrix protein inhibitors, such as amantadine and rimantadine, inhibit viral uncoating. They are ineffective against IBV and are currently not recommended for the treatment of IAV infections due to high levels of resistance [4]. Neuraminidase inhibitors (NAI), such as oseltamivir and zanamivir, inhibit the release of virus progeny from infected cells and viral spread, are effective against IAV and IBV and have been licensed for first-line therapy of influenza. Although the vast majority of currently circulating IAV(H3N2) and (H1N1)pdm09 is sensitive to oseltamivir, the wide-spread use of oseltamivir has led to a high level of IAV(H1N1) resistance in 2008–9 [3,5]. In IAV(H1N1)pdm09 resistance against oseltamivir is almost exclusively caused by a single amino acid exchange (H275Y) in the neuraminidase [6]. Recently, two novel NAIs have been approved for the treatment of influenza, peramivir and laninamivir octanoate, the latter being effective also against oseltamivir-resistant influenza virus strains [3,7]. Since monotherapy with each of the NAIs currently licensed may eventually lead to the selection of resistant virus, drug combinations directed against different molecular targets of influenza virus may be a promising strategy to delay the development of resistance and to achieve synergistic effects. Thus, novel viral targets, antiviral agents and therapeutic strategies such as inhibitors of the viral RNA polymerase complex and broadly neutralizing antibodies should be developed and utilized for the treatment and prophylaxis of influenza [8,9].

Medicinal plant extracts with anti-IAV activity have been described in many publications [10–12]. Although in most plant-derived preparations active compounds and structure-activity relationships remain to be elucidated, polyphenols have been frequently identified to be the antiviral principle in plant extracts [13]. In particular, the broad antiviral and antimicrobial activity of green tea and its components has received much attention [14,15]. In green tea and a number of other polyphenol-rich plant extracts, catechins and proanthocyanidins, a subgroup of polyphenols derived from oligomerized flavan-3-ols, were found to exert antiviral effects against influenza viruses and other enveloped and non-enveloped viruses [16–20]. Recently, we have shown inhibition of viral attachment of herpes simplex virus type-1 by proanthocyanidin-enriched extracts from *Rumex acetosa* L. (Polygonaceae) and *Myrothamnus flabellifolia* Welw. [21,22]. Extracts from *R. acetosa* are a component of modern phytotherapeutical preparations with nationally registered drug status in Europe, and are used in the treatment of acute and chronic respiratory viral infections [23].

Aim of the present study was to investigate the anti-IAV activity of the *R. acetosa* extract (RA) *in vitro*, to identify relevant compounds and structural requirements for anti-IAV activity and to characterize their mode of action. Our results show that RA strongly inhibits growth of IAV by blocking viral entry. The dimeric, digalloylated procyanidin epicatechin-3-O-gallate-(4β→8)-epicatechin-3′-O-gallate (*syn.* procyanidin B2-di-gallate) was identified as main active principle in RA. Galloylation of the procyanidin backbone was found to be a prerequisite for anti-IAV activity.

Materials and Methods

Plant material, extract and isolated compounds of *Rumex acetosa*

Starting materials and preparation of the *Rumex acetosa* L. extract RA have been described recently [21]. Isolation and analytical characterization of proanthocyanidins from RA have been reported by Bicker et al. (2009) [24]. Structural features, sources and purity of flavan-3-ols, oligomeric proanthocyanidins, hydrolyzable tannins, depsides and building blocks of tannins used for antiviral bioassays used in this study are given in Figure 1 and Table 1. Sodium heparin (100,000 IU/g) was purchased from Roth (Karlsruhe, Germany).

Cells and viruses

MDCK II cells (canine kidney cells) were propagated in minimal essential medium (MEM; Biochrom, Berlin, Germany) supplemented with 5% fetal calf serum (FCS; Biochrom), 2 mM L-glutamine (Sigma-Aldrich), non-essential amino acids (1×) and 100 μg/mL penicillin/streptomycin (Biochrom). A549 cells (human lung epithelial cells) were grown in DMEM (PAA Laboratories, Pasching, Austria), supplemented with 10% FCS and 100 μg/mL penicillin/streptomycin. Cytotoxicity, antiviral and penetration assays (see below) were performed using serum-free media.

The influenza A virus laboratory strain A/Puerto Rico/8/34 (PR8), and three clinical isolates of IAV(H1N1)pdm09, i.e., A/Nordrhein-Westfalen/172/09 (NRW172), A/Nordrhein-Westfalen/173/09 (NRW173) [25] and isolate 1/09 (I1) obtained at the Institute of Medical Microbiology – Clinical Virology, University Hospital Münster, were propagated in embryonated chicken eggs. Viral stocks were prepared as described elsewhere [26].

The number of infectious particles in viral stocks was assessed by plaque titration. MDCK II cells were infected with serial dilutions of IAV in PBS containing 0.21% bovine albumin (MP Biochemicals, Eschwege, Germany), 100 U/mL penicillin (Biochrom), 100 μg/mL streptomycin (Biochrom), 230 μmol/L $MgCl_2$ (Roth) and 514 μmol/L $CaCl_2$ (Roth) for 30 min. at 37°C (500 μL/well). After discarding the inoculum, cells were washed with PBS and covered with 2 mL of overlay medium (MEM [Gibco, Life Technologies, Darmstadt, Germany] containing 100 U/mL penicillin, 100 μg/mL streptomycin, 0.21% $NaHCO_3$ [Gibco], 0.01% DEAE-dextran hydrochloride [Sigma-Aldrich], 0.21% bovine albumin, 232 μmol/L $MgCl_2$, 518 μmol/L $CaCl_2$, 0.00061 ‰ trypsin/829 nmol/L EDTA [Biochrom] and 0.62% Avicel type RC-591 NF [FMC BioPolymer, Philadelphia, PA, USA]). After 48 h of incubation at 37°C, overlay medium was discarded, cells were washed with PBS, fixed with 3.7% formaldehyde for 10 min. and stained with 0.1% crystal violet for 15 min. Subsequently, virus plaques were counted and the infectious titer (pfu/mL) was calculated.

Cytotoxicity assay, antiviral assays

Cytotoxicity assay. The effect of RA and its components on the proliferation of MDCK II cells was determined in 96-well plates (TPP, Trasadingen, Switzerland) using the MTT assay [27] essentially as described by Gescher et al. (2011) [21] with the exception that samples were incubated at 37°C for 1 h prior to addition to cells and remained on the cells for 48 h. The cytotoxic concentration of RA or its components which reduced the cells' viability by 50% (IC_{50}) was determined from dose-response curves. The untreated control was arbitrarily set as 100%.

MTT_{IAV} assay. The inhibitory effects of RA and other test compounds on the cytopathic effect induced by IAV replication was determined in a MDCK II cell-based assay measuring cell viability by MTT stain (MTT_{IAV} assay) [28]. An inoculum of 1×10^4 pfu IAV/well (corresponding to a multi plicity of infection of 0.1) was used to infect 96-well plates. All incubation steps were performed with serum-free MEM. In the elementary assay, IAV was pre-incubated with test compounds for 1 h at 37°C and subsequently MDCK II cells were incubated with this RA/IAV mixture for 48 h. In modified assays, either the test compound/IAV mixture was removed from the cells after 60 min., or cells were pre-incubated with test compounds alone for 1 h prior to infection with IAV, or test compounds were added to the cells following a 1 h infection period with IAV.

The antiviral activity was calculated according to the following formula [29]:

$$antiviral\ activity\ (\%) = \frac{(OD_T)_{IAV} - (OD_C)_{IAV}}{(OD_C)_{mock} - (OD_C)_{IAV}} \times 100$$

$(OD_T)_{IAV}$ represents the optical density of cells, which were infected by IAV (index: IAV) and treated with RA. $(OD_C)_{IAV}$ corresponds to the optical density measured for the untreated IAV-infected cells and $(OD_C)_{mock}$ is the optical density of untreated, mock-infected cells. The antiviral dose of RA which protected the cells by 50% was defined as the 50% inhibitory concentration (IC_{50}).

Plaque reduction assay. IAV was incubated with antiviral compounds for 1 h at 37°C, both diluted in PBS containing 100 U/mL penicillin, 100 μg/mL streptomycin, 230 μmol/L

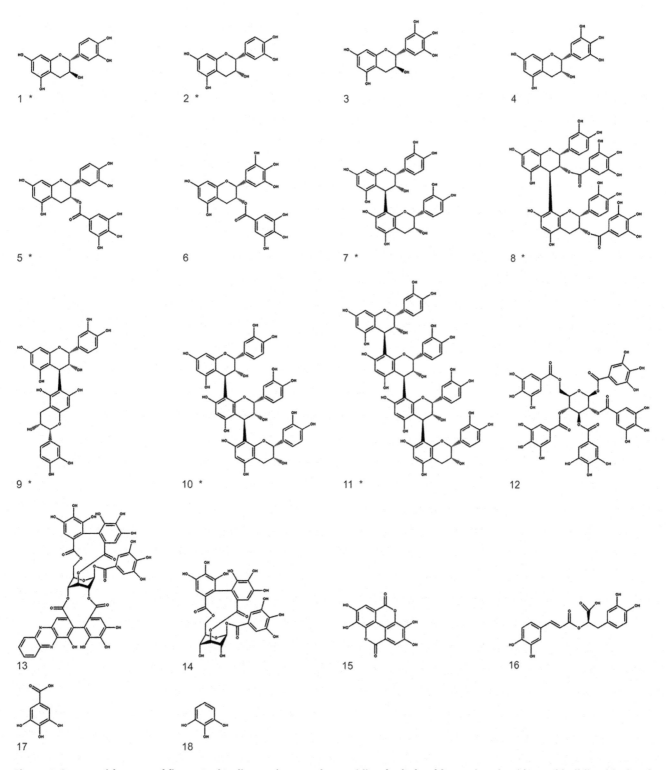

Figure 1. Structural features of flavan-3-ols, oligomeric proanthocyanidins, hydrolyzable tannins, depsides and building blocks of tannins tested for antiviral activity; compounds isolated from *Rumex acetosa* extract RA are marked by asterisk.

$MgCl_2$ and 514 µmol/L $CaCl_2$. MDCK II cells, cultivated in 12-well culture plates (Greiner Bio-One, Frickenhausen, Germany), were washed with PBS and infected with 300 µL/well IAV/RA-suspension (100 pfu/well). After 30 min. of incubation, the inoculum was removed, 1 mL of overlay-medium without bovine albumin was added and the plates were cultivated for 72 h at 37°C. Subsequently, cells were stained as described above, virus plaques were counted and antiviral activity was calculated by the following formula [21]:

Table 1. Flavan-3-ols, oligomeric proanthocyanidins, hydrolyzable tannins, depsides and building blocks of tannins tested for antiviral activity.

no.	compound	source	purity[1]	reference
1	(+)-catechin monohydrate	Sigma-Aldrich, Steinheim, Germany	≥98%	
2	(−)-epicatechin	Sigma-Aldrich, Steinheim, Germany	≥90%	
3	gallocatechin	IPBP[2], Münster, Germany	99%	[51]
4	epigallocatechin	IPBP, Münster, Germany	≥80%	[51]
5	epicatechin-3-O-gallate	IPBP, Münster, Germany	≥95%	[24]
6	epigallocatechin-3-O-gallate	Chengdu Biopurify Phytochemicals Ltd, Chengdu, China	≥95%	
7	epicatechin-(4β→8)-epicatechin (*procyanidin B2*)	IPBP, Münster, Germany	97%	[24]
8	epicatechin-3-O-gallate-(4β→8)-epicatechin-3'-O-gallate (*procyanidin B2-di-gallate*)	IPBP, Münster, Germany	91%	[24]
9	epicatechin-(4β→6)-epicatechin (*procyanidin B5*)	IPBP, Münster, Germany	99%	[24]
10	epicatechin-(4β→8)-epicatechin-(4β→8)-epicatechin (*procyanidin C1*)	IPBP, Münster, Germany	97%	[24]
11	epicatechin-(4β→8)-epicatechin-(4β→8)-epicatechin-(4β→8)-epicatechin (*procyanidin D1*)	IPBP, Münster, Germany	100%	[24]
12	1,2,3,4,6-penta-O-galloyl-β-D-glucose (PGG)	IPBP, Münster, Germany	≥95%	[37]
13	geraniin	IPBP, Münster, Germany	≥95%	[38]
14	corilagin	IPBP, Münster, Germany	≥95%	[38]
15	ellagic acid	Roth, Karlsruhe, Germany	≥95%	
16	rosmarinic acid	Sigma-Aldrich, Steinheim, Germany	97%	
17	gallic acid monohydrate	Roth, Karlsruhe, Germany	≥97%	
18	pyrogallol	Merck, Darmstadt, Germany	≥95%	

[1]purity was determined by quantitative HPLC (area %),
[2]IPBP: Institute of Pharmaceutical Biology and Phytochemistry.

$$\text{antiviral activity (\%)} = 1 - \frac{\text{plaque number}_{(assay)}}{\text{plaque number}_{(control)}} \times 100$$

Penetration assay. The effect of extract RA and antiviral compounds on viral penetration was determined by a modified plaque reduction assay. In contrast to the basic assay, cells were treated with RA after virus attachment to the cell surface. Penetration of IAV during the attachment and treatment phase was prevented by strictly performing all steps at 4°C.

MDCK II cells, cultivated to 95% confluence in 12-well culture plates, were pre-cooled to 4°C for 15 min. and washed with PBS. 600 pfu IAV, diluted in PBS (400 μL/well) containing 100 U/mL penicillin, 100 μg/mL streptomycin, 230 μmol/L $MgCl_2$ and 514 μmol/L $CaCl_2$, were allowed to attach to the cells. After 20 min. the inoculum was removed, cells were washed with PBS, PBS containing a 2-fold serial dilution of RA was added and cells were incubated for another 30 min. at 4°C. Before shifting culture plates to 37°C for initiation of viral penetration, cells were washed with PBS and covered with serum-free cultivation medium (see above). Following 30 min. incubation at 37°C, medium was removed and cells were treated with low pH citrate buffer (135 mM NaCl, 10 mM KCl, 40 mM citric acid, pH 3.0) for 15 s to stop penetration and inactivate attached, non-penetrated virions. Low pH buffer was removed by washing twice with PBS, and overlay medium was added. Further cultivation and quantitation of plaques was performed as described above. Mock-treatment of attached virus and inactivation of attached mock-treated virus by low pH citrate buffer immediately prior to the 37°C shift served as controls.

Hemagglutination inhibition test (HIT)

Twofold serial dilutions (25 μL) of test compounds in PBS and 4 hemagglutinating units (HU) of IAV (25 μl) were mixed carefully in 96-well plates with U-shaped bottom (Thermo Fisher Scientific Nunc, Schwerte, Germany). Plates were shaken for 5 min. and incubated for 25 min. at room temperature (RT). 50 μL of a 1.5% suspension of newborn chicken erythrocytes (RBC) in PBS (Labor Dr. Merk & Kollegen, Ochsenhausen, Germany) were added, and plates shaken again. Assays were read following a 2 h incubation period at RT, and the minimum inhibitory concentration (MIC), defined as the highest test compound dilution showing complete inhibition of the agglutination of erythrocytes, was determined. In every assay, a test compound control (compound plus RBC without addition of IAV), and erythrocyte controls (A: IAV plus RBC, without addition of test compound; B: RBC, without addition of test compound or IAV) were included. Test results were accepted if the back titration of IAV revealed 4 HU and the controls yielded correct results.

Immunoblotting

The effect of RA or test compounds on IAV envelope proteins was analyzed using recombinant purified HA (20 or 50 μg/mL) of influenza virus A/California/07/2009 (H1N1) (Sino Biological, Beijing, China). SDS-PAGE and blotting was performed essentially as described earlier [21]. To detect IAV HA, membranes were incubated with Anti-IAV H1N1 (Swine Flu 2009) HA antibody (dilution 1: 1000; Sino Biological) or QIAexpress

Penta-His Antibody (dilution 1: 500; Qiagen, Hilden, Germany) overnight.

Signal transduction assay

90–100% confluent A549 cells in 6-well culture plates were washed with PBS and pretreated with 100 μg/mL RA for 1 h at 37°C, or left untreated. Subsequently, cells were stimulated with EGF (30 ng/mL, 10 min.; R&D Systems, Minneapolis, MN, USA) or TNF-α (20 ng/mL, 30 min.; Sigma-Aldrich) in the presence of RA, or left untreated. Cells were washed with PBS twice and lysed with radioimmunoprecipitation assay buffer (25 mM Tris-HCl [pH 8; Roth], 137 mM NaCl [Merck], 10% glycerol [MP Biomedicals, Illkirch, France], 0.1% SDS [Roth], 0.5% DOC [Roth], 1% octylphenoxypolyethoxyethanol [IGEPAL; Sigma-Aldrich], 2 mM EDTA [pH 8; Roth], 50 mM sodium glycerophosphate [Merck Millipore, Billerica, MA, USA], 20 mM TSPP [Roth], plus 1 tablet cOmplete mini [Roche Diagnostics, Mannheim, Germany] per 10 mL buffer) for 45–60 min. at 4°C. Lysates were cleared by centrifugation, and protein content was quantified by the Bradford method. Briefly, 1 mL of 1: 5 diluted protein assay dye reagent concentrate (Bio-Rad Laboratories, Hercules, CA, USA) was added to 5 μL supernatant, absorption at 600 nm was determined and protein contents were adjusted to identical levels. Protein expression was analyzed by SDS-PAGE and immunoblot as described above. For protein detection Anti-ERK1/2 (pT202/pY204) antibody (dilution 1: 1000; BD, Franklin Lakes, NJ, USA) or Phospho-NF-κB p65 (Ser536)(93H1) antibody (dilution 1: 1000; Cell Signaling Technology, Danvers, MA, USA) was employed. Loading controls were performed with Anti-α-Tubulin (Clone DM 1A, dilution 1: 500; Sigma-Aldrich) or Anti-β-Actin (Clone AC-15, dilution 1: 1000; Sigma-Aldrich).

Statistical analysis

Data represent the means ±SD of at least three independent experiments. Statistical significance was evaluated by a two-tailed one sample t-test. A P value of <0.05 indicated a statistically significant difference.

In silico protein-ligand docking

For *in silico* analyses the HA of influenza virus A/California/04/2009 (H1N1) [30] (protein data base ID 3LZG) was used. HA of A/California/04/2009 (H1N1) is closely related to HA of the vaccine strain A/California/07/2009 (H1N1) and HAs of IAV(H1N1)pdm09 strains circulating in the post-pandemic era in Europe and Asia [31,32]. Epicatechin (**2**), epigallocatechin-3-O-gallate (EGCG) (**6**), procyanidin B2 (**7**) and procyanidin B2-di-gallate (**8**) were docked to the HA of influenza virus *in silico* by the software Molecular Operating Environment (MOE) version 2011.10 (Chemical Computing Group, Montreal, Canada). After identifying potential binding sites at HA with the MOE module "Site Finder", the test compounds were docked into the 30 cavities with the best PLB (propensity for ligand binding) score using the MMFF94× force field as implemented in MOE. The flexible docking method (induced fit, i.e. both the ligand and the protein binding site were treated as flexible) was applied. The best score of each cavity-compound pair was compared to the best score of the remaining 29 cavities for each of the four compounds. The docking pose represents the best geometry (lowest score) of all investigated orientations of all compounds with respect to all cavities taken into account.

Results and Discussion

Rumex acetosa extract RA specifically inhibits IAV-infection in cell culture

Extract RA and its constituents were screened for anti-IAV-activity by single cycle, MDCK II cell-based MTT_{IAV} assay. Depending on the IAV isolate, the screening window coefficient Z′ of the MTT_{IAV} assay ranged from approx. 0.6 to 0.63, indicating that this assay is well suited to detect inhibitors of IAV entry and replication [28,33]. Extract RA exhibited 100% antiviral activity against IAV PR8 at concentrations>5 μg/mL with an IC_{50} of 2.5 μg/mL. At extract concentrations≥25 μg/mL a dose-dependent, increasing reduction of cell vitality was observed. The CC_{50} of extract RA was determined to be approximately 80 μg/mL which corresponds to a selectivity index (SI = CC_{50}/IC_{50}) of 32 (Figure 2A). Almost identical data were found for the clinical isolate I1 of IAV(H1N1)pdm09 with an IC_{50} of 2.2 μg/mL, and a SI of 36 (Figure 2B). The results obtained by MTT_{IAV} assay were corroborated by plaque reduction assay. At a concentration of 100 ng/mL extract RA reduced plaque formation of IAV(H1N1)pdm09 I1 in a highly significant manner by 67%, at 1 μg/mL by 100% (Figure 3).

The antiviral effect of extract RA was tested in two additional clinical isolates of IAV(H1N1)pdm09 obtained in consecutive samples of a patient with acute respiratory distress syndrome. The oseltamivir-sensitive isolate NRW172 was obtained early after hospitalization, the oseltamivir-resistant isolate NRW173 was isolated after completion of oseltamivir therapy. Extract RA inhibited growth of NRW172 and NRW173 with similar efficiency. The IC_{50} values determined for NRW172 (19 μg/mL) and NRW173 (37 μg/mL) in MTT_{IAV} assay were approximately 10-fold higher as observed in IAV PR8 and IAV I1 (Figure 2C, D). Previous work indicated that a high protein load of samples may reduce the antiviral activity of extract RA [22]. Since stocks of IAV NRW172 (6.6×10^6 pfu/mL) and NRW173 (8.3×10^6 pfu/mL) contained significantly lower virus titers than stocks of IAV PR8 (3.2×10^8 pfu/mL) and I1 (3.4×10^7 pfu/mL), inhibitory effects of residual allantoic fluid on the anti-IAV activity of extract RA were studied. Retesting IAV I1 diluted to 6.6×10^6 pfu/mL in allantoic fluid of a noninfected egg led to an approx. four-fold increase in the IC_{50} of extract RA (8.2 μg/mL) (Figure S1). Thus, inhibitory effects of residual allantoic fluid on the anti-IAV activity of extract RA appear to account for the differences in IC_{50} values observed in MTT_{IAV} assay. Accordingly, the consistently lower IC_{50} values observed in plaque reduction assay are most likely due to higher dilution of virus stocks during incubation with extract RA. Whether strain specific factors also determine the susceptibility of IAV to extract RA as observed for a polyphenolic extract of *Pelargonium sidoides* DC [34] remains to be clarified.

Structure-activity relationship: epicatechin-3-O-gallate-(4β→8)-epicatechin-3′-O-gallate (procyanidin B2-di-gallate) (8) is responsible for the antiviral activity of RA

The lead compounds in extract RA have been recently described to be flavan-3-ols and oligomeric proanthocyanidins [24]. To pinpoint the plant secondary products responsible for the antiviral effect of the extract, the dominant proanthocyanidins isolated from extract RA were tested for antiviral effects against IAV I1 and cytotoxicity (Table 2) (for numbering of compounds compare Table 1) at concentrations of 2, 20 and 200 μM, respectively, by MTT_{IAV} and cytotoxicity assay. Additionally

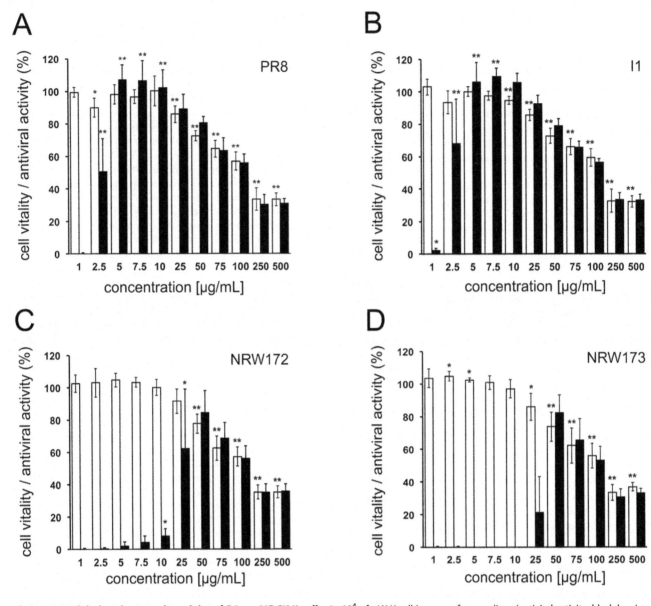

Figure 2. Antiviral and cytotoxic activity of RA on MDCK II cells. 1×10^4 pfu IAV/well in serum-free medium (antiviral activity, black bars) or serum-free medium (cytotoxic activity, white bars) were incubated with RA at different concentrations indicated for 1 h at 37°C. 48 h after adding the reaction mixtures to 96-well plates, the antiviral activity and cell vitality were determined by MTT_{IAV} assay and cytotoxicity assay, respectively. The following IAV laboratory strains and isolates were used: (A) laboratory strain PR8 [A/Puerto Rico/8/34], (B) clinical isolate I1 [A(H1N1)pdm09], (C) clinical isolate NRW172 [A(H1N1)pdm09], (D) clinical isolate NRW173 [A(H1N1)pdm09]. Values represent mean ±SD of ≥3 independent experiments. * $p<0.05$, ** $p<0.01$ (two-tailed, unpaired Student's t-test). Statistical significance of antiviral activity was calculated for nontoxic concentrations only (A: 1 to 10 μg/mL, B: 1 to 7.5 μg/mL, C: 1 to 25 μg/mL, D: 1 to 10 μg/mL).

EGCG (**6**), a known inhibitor of IAV replication from extracts of green tea which is not present in extract RA [17,24] was included (Table 2).

The monomeric flavan-3-ols catechin (**1**) and epicatechin (**2**) did not show antiviral activity. Trihydroxylation of the B-ring in gallocatechin (**3**) and epigallocatechin (**4**) led to a slightly increased cytotoxicity. Esterification with gallic acid also increased cytotoxicity. Epicatechin-3-O-gallate (**5**) did not show antiviral activity, while EGCG (**6**) exhibited strong activity at concentrations of about 20 μM (estimated SI≥17). These results indicated that an o-trihydroxylation in the B-ring and galloylation at position O-3 is responsible for the antiviral effects of flavan-3-ols detected by MTT_{IAV} assay.

Strong antiviral activity was determined for the oligomeric proanthocyanidins in the cases where the epicatechin building blocks are galloylated. While the dimeric epicatechin-(4β→8)-epicatechin (procyanidin B2) (**7**) was inactive, the corresponding di-galloylated procyanidin epicatechin-3-O-gallate-(4β→8)-epicatechin-3'-O-gallate (procyanidin B2-di-gallate) (**8**) exhibited a prominent antiviral activity (IC_{50} of approx. 15 μM) with an SI of about ≥13. It should be noted that the increasing cytotoxicity of active compounds such as procyanidin B2-digallate (**8**) and EGCG (**6**) at high concentrations reduces the extent of cytoprotection against influenza virus detectable by MTT_{IAV} assay. Using the formula given in Materials and Methods to calculate the results of

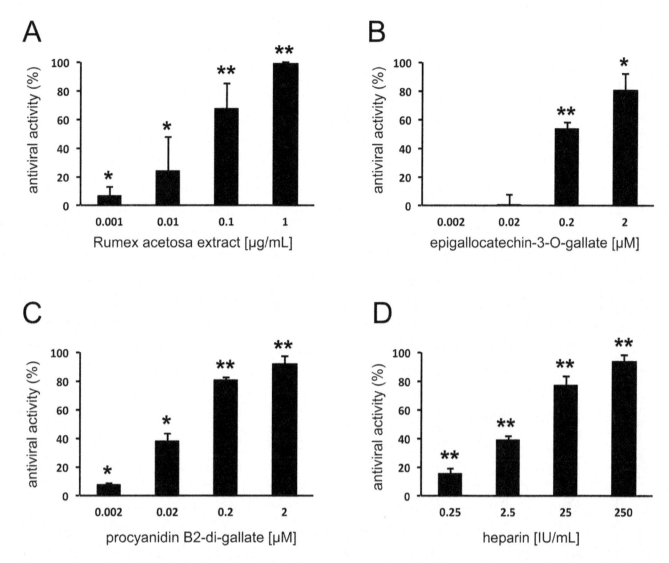

Figure 3. Reduction of IAV plaque formation by the *Rumex acetosa* extract RA (A), epigallocatechin-3-O-gallate (6) (B) and procyanidin B2-digallate (8) (C). IAV and test compounds were co-incubated for 1 h at 37°C prior to the addition to MDCK II cells. Heparin served as positive control (D). Values (% of plaque reduction) ±SD relate to the respective mock-treated controls (= 100%). * $p<0.05$, ** $p<0.01$ (two-tailed, unpaired Student's t-test).

MTT_{IAV} assay, this seemingly reduces the antiviral activity of active compounds at cytotoxic concentrations (200 µM) (Table 2).

Other non-galloylated di- and oligomeric procyanidins from RA with different structural features were inactive. Compared to the epicatechin-(4β→8)-epicatechin (procyanidin B2) (**7**), dimeric epicatechin procyanidins with 4β→6-interflavan linkage such as epicatechin-(4β→6)-epicatechin (procyanidin B5) (**9**) did not show an altered antiviral profile. However, the 4β→6-linked compound (**9**) exerted higher cytotoxicity compared to (**7**) indicating that changes in the planarity of the molecules may significantly influence the effects on cell physiology. The trimeric and tetrameric procyanidins epicatechin-(4β→8)-epicatechin-(4β→8)-epicatechin (procyanidin C1) (**10**) and epicatechin-(4β→8)-epicatechin-(4β→8)-epicatechin-(4β→8)-epicatechin (procyanidin D1) (**11**), respectively, offered no relevant antiviral activity but showed weak cytotoxic effects.

Thus, within the complex mixture of extract RA dominated by flavan-3-ols and proanthocyanidins with different degrees of polymerization and galloylation, the antiviral activity is mostly mediated by galloylated oligomers. The dimeric compound procyanidin B2-di-gallate (**8**) was assessed as the main principle of antiviral activity in extract RA. The content of procyanidin B2-di-gallate (**8**) in extract RA was determined by UHPLC to be 0.96%. The strong antiviral effect of procyanidin B2-di-gallate (**8**) was confirmed by plaque reduction assay (Figure 3). Purified galloylated higher oligomers present in extract RA were not available for antiviral testing, however, most likely are also active against influenza virus. Generally, a higher number of pyrogalloyl moieties, an increased degree of polymerization and a 4β→8 interflavan linkage amplify the anti-IAV activity of polyphenols from extract RA. These findings are in accordance with the results published by De Bruyne et al. (1999) [35] describing similar structural requirements of polyphenols active against HSV and HIV. In addition, trihydroxylation of the B-ring of non-galloylated oligomeric proanthocyanidins has been reported to mediate anti-influenza virus activity [34].

An insignificant anti-influenza activity of the monomeric flavan-3-ols catechin (**1**) and epicatechin (**2**) has been reported earlier

Table 2. Anti-IAV activity and effect on cell vitality of flavan-3-ols and oligomeric proanthocyanidins from *Rumex acetosa* extract RA and structurally related polyphenolic compounds.

no.	compound	cell vitality[1]			CC_{50} (µM)	anti-IAV activity[2]			IC_{50} (µM)
		2 µM	20 µM	200 µM		2 µM	20 µM	200 µM	
1	catechin monohydrate	105±3	102±5	119±9	>200	0±0	0±0	0±0	>200
2	epicatechin	101±2	104±4	124±20	>200	0±0	0±0	1±1	>200
3	gallocatechin	106±5	108±1	75±17	>200	0±0	0±0	66±5	≤156
4	epigallocatechin	101±4	106±1	86±17	>200	0±0	0±0	26±22	>200
5	epicatechin-3-O-gallate	107±3	106±4	41±2	175	0±0	1±0	38±2	≤258
6	epigallocatechin-3-O-gallate	103±4	92±7	62±9	>200	1±1	87±25	60±7	≤12
7	procyanidin B2	107±6	108±9	117±8	>200	0±0	0±0	1±1	>200
8	procyanidin B2-di-gallate	106±5	90±3	48±4	191	1±1	71±35	46±4	≤15
9	procyanidin B5	100±3	84±4	57±4	>200	0±0	0±0	63±4	≤163
10	procyanidin C1	104±2	99±4	122±6	>200	0±0	0±0	87±5	123
11	procyanidin D1	101±6	86±8	54±9	>200	0±0	1±0	44±7	≤225
12	PGG	91±7	57±14	37±3	83	3±3	46±9	35±1	≤22
13	geraniin	99±1	107±2	35±3	162	0±0	1±1	25±0	≤388
14	corilagin	101±1	103±1	8±1	120	0±-1	1±0	3±2	uncalc.[3]
15	ellagic acid	106±1	110±3	108±2	>200	0±1	1±1	4±1	>200
16	rosmarinic acid	102±1	103±1	102±1	>200	0±0	0±0	1±1	>200
17	gallic acid monohydrate	106±5	107±8	49±18	197	0±1	-1±0	14±11	>200
18	pyrogallol	98±4	96±1	43±1	176	0±0	7±3	42±1	≤241

[1] cytotoxicity was determined by cytotoxicity assay,
[2] antiviral effects against the IAV(H1N1)pdm09 isolate I1 were determined by MTT_{IAV} assay.
[3] uncalculable due to strong cytotoxicity.

[16,19]. Interestingly, Song et al. (2005) [19] showed that ECG (**5**) a main constituent from green tea strongly inhibited anti-IAV and IBV in cell culture whereas EGC (**4**) exhibited little antiviral activity. Yang et al. (2014) [16] found that procyanidin B2 (**7**) significantly inhibited growth of IAV. This is in contrast to our findings where ECG (**5**) and procyanidin B2 (**7**) were screened negative for anti-IAV activity at noncytotoxic concentrations. Most likely, this reflects differences in the test format used, e.g. MTT$_{IAV}$ assay *vs.* plaque reduction assay and cytopathic effect inhibition assay, respectively. In particular, the assays used by Song et al. (2005) [19] and Yang et al. (2014) [16] imply multi-cycle replication of IAV and thus should also detect inhibitory effects of compounds on late steps of the viral replication cycle, such as assembly, maturation and release as reviewed by Beyleveld et al. (2013) [28]. Accordingly, Song et al. (2005) [19] detected a direct inhibition of the viral neuraminidase activity by ECG (**5**), however, not by EGC (**4**).

A prominent virucidal activity of EGCG (**6**) from green tea has been first reported by Nakayama et al. (1993) [17]. As reported for ECG (**5**), EGCG (**6**) also directly inhibits the viral neuraminidase. In addition to anti-influenza activity, EGCG offers broad anti-infective properties against various viral, bacterial and fungal pathogens as reviewed by Steinmann et al. (2012) [15].

After oral application, proanthocyanidins exhibit a very limited bioavailability as reviewed by Zumdick et al. (2012) [36]. Thus, the oral application of active compounds such as procyanidin B2-di-gallate (**8**) for the systemic treatment of influenza virus infection appears to be inappropriate. As an alternative, the local application of procyanidins in the upper respiratory tract, either by lozenges, chewing gums etc. or by inhaling devices allows the active compounds to directly contact the virus and should be preferred.

Because proanthocyanidins are known to have tannin-like effects it might be assumed that these polyphenols from extract RA nonspecifically inactivate essential viral structural proteins. Therefore we included other polyphenols not being part of extracts from *R. acetosa*, but with known strong astringent activity (Table 1). Pentagalloyl-glucose (PGG) (**12**), a well characterized hydrolyzable tannin [37], showed moderate antiviral activity, however, significant cell toxicity in the MTT$_{IAV}$ assay (Table 2). Also the ellagitannins geraniin (**13**), corilagin (**14**) [38] and ellagic acid (**15**) were inactive at the highest concentration tested (200 µM) (Table 2). When added at concentrations in the millimolar range, ellagic acid (**15**) has been reported to exhibit broad anti-influenza activity *in vitro* and *in vivo* [39]. The depside rosmarinic acid (**16**), known as tannin-like compound, was also inactive. Keeping in mind that also oligomeric procyanidins such as procyanidin B2, C1 or D1 (**7, 10, 11**) are known to interact strongly with proteins in a tannin-like manner, nonspecific denaturing effects do not appear to account for most of the antiviral activity observed for procyanidin B2-di-gallate (**8**). Otherwise, a more potent activity of the hydrolyzable tannins geraniin (**13**) and corilagin (**14**) should have been observed. An exception appears to be PGG (**12**), which exhibited moderate anti-IAV activity in MTT$_{IAV}$ assay with an IC$_{50}$ of 22 µM. This might be due to its flexible structure. In contrast to geraniin (**13**), PGG (**12**) owns the capacity to rotate its galloyl moieties relatively to the glucose. As a result PGG (**12**) may be able to bind more strongly to proteins. In accordance with our results, PGG (**12**) has been recently reported to possess anti-IAV activity at micromolar concentrations and to inhibit viral entry, budding and release [40].

Since only the galloylated compounds (**6**) and (**8**) exhibited prominent antiviral activity, we tested the effect of free gallic acid (**17**) and pyrogallol (**18**), mimicking a trihydroxylated phenyl system. Both compounds, however, showed only moderate antiviral activity yet relevant cytotoxicity at a concentration of 200 µM. Theissen et al. (2014) [41] recently reported that gallic acid (**17**) inhibits reporter gene expression of the recombinant IAV laboratory strain A/Puerto Rico/8/34-NS116-GFP in a multi-cycle assay with an EC$_{50}$ of approx. 50 µM and a SI of approx. 15. Similar to our findings, however, preincubation of IAV(H1N1)pdm09 particles for 2 h with 50 µg/mL (corresponding to 265 µM) gallic acid (**17**) had only little effect on virus replication in A549 cells. Furthermore, gallic acid (**17**) poorly inhibited IAV neuraminidase with an IC$_{50}$ of >500 µM. Thus, the inhibitory mechanism of gallic acid (**17**) on IAV replication remains to be clarified.

Extract RA affects viral attachment

To identify steps in the viral life cycle that were affected by extract RA, virus and cells were treated with extract RA at different times pre and post infection. If pre-treated IAV was added to cells for 1 h, viral replication was inhibited completely at concentrations of extract RA>10 µg/mL. In contrast, if cells were infected with IAV and extract RA was added after 1 h, no antiviral effect was observed at ≤10 µg/mL, indicating that extract RA does not operate in the post-entry phase (data not shown).

To determine whether extract RA interacts with target molecules of the host cells or of the virus, MDCK II cells were incubated with extract RA for 1 h and subsequently infected with IAV. At concentrations of ≤10 µg/mL this preincubation of the host cells did not result in any antiviral effects (data not shown). This suggests that the anti-IAV activity of extract RA is caused by direct interaction with IAV particles and inhibition of viral entry as shown for a number of polyphenol and tannin-rich plant extracts in earlier reports [17–19,39,41–44].

To reconnoiter the effect of extract RA to inhibit penetration of IAV particles already attached to the cell surface we used a penetration assay. Cells were infected at 4°C, unbound viral particles were removed by washing, extract RA was added at 4°C for 30 min., and penetration was allowed to occur by a temperature shift to 37°C (30 min.) followed by washing with pH 3.0 citrate buffer to inactivate non-penetrated virus. As shown in Figure 4, extract RA also blocks viral penetration. However, in comparison to incubation of IAV with extract RA prior to entry, significantly higher concentrations of extract RA were needed to achieve comparable antiviral effects. Washing of cells with pH 3.0 citrate buffer at 4°C immediately after the adsorption period and prior to shifting the temperature to 37°C completely abrogated plaque formation. These observations suggested that RA affects virus entry primarily by inhibiting viral attachment. Similar results were also obtained with EGCG (**6**) and procyanidin B2-di-gallate (**8**) (Figure 4). As discussed above, the relatively high protein load due to the presence of cells and culture media components may increase the concentration of RA and its active constituents needed to inhibit penetration of IAV already attached to the cell surface. When added after the infection of MDCK cells, high concentrations of green tea extract and EGC (**4**) have been reported to affect the early phase of influenza virus infection, possibly by interference of the polyphenolic compounds with the acidification of endosomes [18].

RA and galloylated oligomeric procyanidins interact with IAV hemagglutinin

Data presented above suggested that extract RA, EGCG (**6**) and procyanidin B2-di gallate (**8**) may interfere with the sialic acid receptor binding function of the viral HA. Therefore, effects on

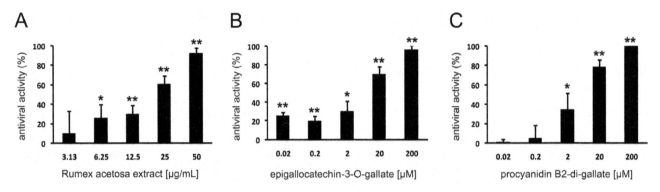

Figure 4. Effect of *Rumex acetosa* extract RA (A), epigallocatechin-3-O-gallate (6) (B) and procyanidin B2-digallate (8) (C) on the penetration of IAV. Effects on the penetration of IAV were determined by a modified plaque reduction assay. Test compounds were added for 30 min. after attachment of IAV to MDCK II cells at 4°C. Values (% of plaque reduction) ±SD relate to the respective mock-treated controls (=100%) and represent ≥3 independent experiments. * p<0.05, ** p<0.01 (two-tailed, unpaired Student's t-test).

HA-mediated attachment of IAV to the cell surface were further investigated in a hemagglutination inhibition assay. Using four hemagglutinating units of IAV(H1N1)pdm09 I1 in allantoic fluid (5.5×10^7 pfu/mL) to agglutinate chicken erythrocytes, pretreatment of the IAV suspension with extract RA inhibited erythrocyte agglutination at a minimum inhibitory concentration of 156 µg/mL (Table 3). At higher concentrations, hemagglutination reappeared due to direct agglutination of erythrocytes by extract RA. By serial dilution of extract RA in PBS the minimal concentration needed to agglutinate erythrocytes in the absence of IAV was determined to be 156 µg/mL. Thus, treatment of IAV with extract RA appears to directly interfere with the cell surface receptor-binding function of IAV HA. Procyanidin B2-di-gallate (**8**) did not inhibit IAV-mediated hemagglutination, however, was able to directly agglutinate erythrocytes at a concentration ≥ 39 µM. In accordance to Theissen et al. (2014) [41] EGCG (**6**) showed no inhibitory effect on IAV-mediated hemagglutination, however, directly agglutinated erythrocytes (Table 3). None of the test compounds induced hemolysis (data not shown). Strong, IAV-strain specific differences in the concentrations of EGCG (**6**) needed to inhibit hemagglutination have been reported earlier [19], and may account for the failure to detect inhibitory effects of procyanidin B2-di-gallate (**8**) and EGCG (**6**) on IAV(H1N1)pdm09 induced hemagglutination.

In addition, the physical interaction of extract RA and its active compounds with recombinant, soluble HA was studied by SDS-PAGE and immunoblotting. Incubation of HA with high concentrations of extract RA, i.e. 2.5 to 10 mg/mL, for 1 h led to the almost complete disappearance of the 75 – 85 kDa HA-specific band in SDS-PAGE (Figure 5) and abrogated reactivity of HA with an HA-specific monoclonal antibody in immunoblotting (data not shown). Extract RA-treated HA appeared to be retained in the gel pockets, most likely due to the formation of large, electrophoretically immobile complexes. At lower concentrations, i.e. 1 to 0.1 mg/mL, extract RA had no effect on the electrophoretic mobility and immunoreactivity of HA, respectively. Taking into consideration that the IAV-specific IC_{50} value of extract RA in MTT and plaque reduction assay is approximately 100 to 1,000-fold lower, this finding supports the conclusion that most of the anti-IAV activity of extract RA is not due to non-specific tannin-like effects on viral proteins.

Incubation of HA with high concentrations of procyanidin B2-di-gallate (**8**) (1.13 mM) and EGCG (**6**) (2.18 mM) led to a time dependent slight reduction of the monomeric HA band and the appearance of HA aggregates being visible in Coomassie-stained gels as a broad 75 to >200 kDa "smear" (Figure 6A, C). After incubation of HA with EGCG (**6**) for 4 h to 24 h a faint band corresponding to HA dimers became visible (Figure 6A). Higher oligomers of HA could not be detected. As compared to mock treated HA, incubation with the galloylated oligomeric proanthocyanidins (**6**) and (**8**) only led to a moderate decrease in the intensity of the band corresponding to monomeric HA in Coomassie-stained gels (Figure 6A, C). Both compounds, however, reduced the strength of the HA monomer-specific signal in immunoblot (Figure 6B, D). The decrease in immunoreactivity of HA appeared to be more pronounced for (**6**).

Thus, (**6**) and (**8**) exhibit tannin-like astringent effects on HA when applied for prolonged times at high concentrations, i.e., at concentrations approx. 100 to 10,000-fold higher than the respective IC_{50} values in MTT_{IAV} assay and plaque reduction

Table 3. Effect of *Rumex acetosa* extract RA and single compounds on IAV-mediated hemagglutination.

compound[1]	MIC	direct agglutination	highest concentration tested
Rumex acetosa extract	156 µg/mL	156 µg/mL	10 mg/mL
epigallocatechin-3-O-gallate (**6**)	n.d.[2]	156 µM	5 mM
procyanidin B2-di-gallate (**8**)	n.d.	39 µM	5 mM

[1]compounds are numbered as given in Table 1,
[2]n.d.: not detectable.

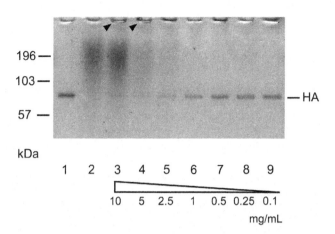

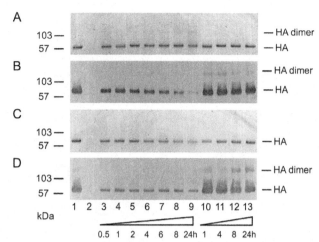

Figure 5. Effect of RA on the electrophoretic mobility of recombinant soluble HA. Mock-treated HA (lane 1), RA (10 mg/mL) (lane 2), and HA treated with RA (0.1 to 10 mg/mL) as indicated for 1 h (lanes 3 to 9) were loaded onto 10% bis-tris SDS-PAGE gels and analyzed by Coomassie-staining. The positions of molecular weight marker (mwm) and HA are indicated. HA conglomerates in the gel pockets are marked by arrowhead.

Figure 6. Effect of EGCG (6) (A, B) and procyanidin B2-di-gallate (8) (C, D) on electrophoretic mobility and detection of HA by immunoblotting. Recombinant soluble HA was either mock-treated (lanes 1), incubated with EGCG (6) (2.18 mM) or procyanidin B2-di-gallate (8) (1.13 mM) dissolved in PBS for the times indicated (lanes 3 to 9) or incubated with PBS only (lanes 10 to 13); EGCG (6) (2.18 mM) and procyanidin B2-di-gallate (8) (1.13 mM) incubated in the absence of HA served as control (lanes 2). Figure 6A, C: Coomassie-stained SDS-PAGE. Figure 6B, D: Detection of HA by immunoblot using a penta-His-specific monoclonal antibody. The expected position of monomeric (approx. 75 kDa) and dimeric HA (approx. 150 kDa) is indicated. Required parameters are missing or incorrect.

assay, respectively. The observed "smear" in SDS-PAGE and immunoblots may stem from HA literally coated with various amounts of (**6**) and (**8**). This may also account for the reduced reactivity of the His-tag-specific monoclonal antibody used to detect recombinant soluble HA. Similar effects were observed with an HA-specific monoclonal antibody (data not shown). The effects of high concentrations of extract RA and its active compounds on HA are in good accordance with the model suggested by Haslam (1996) [45] by describing the aggregation of proteins by polyphenols, and confirms earlier findings in HSV-1 [21]. On the other hand, antiviral effects of (**6**) and (**8**) are detectable at much lower concentrations. Therefore, similar to what was observed for RA, tannin-like astringent effects are unlikely to mediate most of the antiviral activity of these compounds.

Procyanidin B2-di-gallate (8) is predicted *in silico* to interact with the sialic acid binding site of viral hemagglutinin

To visualize the binding of components from RA to the viral surface proteins, four selected compounds were docked to HA of influenza virus A/California/04/2009 (H1N1) [30] *in silico* by means of the software package MOE. Exemplary for the docking results of all investigated cavities of HA, the score of the docking at the sialic acid binding site [46] was -6.29 for procyanidin B2-di-gallate (**8**), -5.55 for procyanidin B2 (**7**), -5.89 for EGCG (**6**), and -5.28 for epicatechin (**2**), with (**8**) showing the best score. The data demonstrated a better score of galloylated compounds in comparison to the respective ungalloylated molecules. Additionally, inspection of the best docking pose revealed the binding of (**8**) (Figure 7) with both galloyl moieties and the B-ring of the second epicatechin gallate unit deep inside the sialic acid binding pocket, suggesting a notably stronger anchorage of galloylated molecules in contrast to ungalloylated compounds and offering a straightforward explanation for the strong activity of this digalloylated dimer. Aside from this, the investigated dimers (**7**) and (**8**) yielded a better docking score than the monomeric (**6**) and (**2**). These results further corroborate the observation depicted in the functional bioassays: An increase in the degree of polymerization and galloylation enhances the binding of proanthocyanidins to HA. As discussed already above, these results are in contrast to a model favoring the unspecific "coating" of HA by polyphenols. The strong anchoring of the galloylated compounds (**6**) and (**8**) in the sialic acid binding pocket of HA disclosed by *in silico* visualization may block the receptor binding site of HA and consequently specifically inhibit the viral adsorption process.

EGCG (**6**) blocks binding of HIV gp120 to its cellular receptor CD4, and it has been suggested that there is an appropriate binding site of EGCG (**6**) in the region of CD4 interacting with gp120. The galloyl ring D of EGCG (**6**) appears to stack against aromatic and basic amino acid side chains within the gp120 binding site of CD4, e.g., Phe 43, Arg 59, Trp62 of CD4, thereby abrogating interaction of gp120 with CD4 [47]. Notably, crystal structure analyses revealed that a subgroup of neutralizing antibodies interferes with receptor binding of HA by targeting the highly conserved Tyr98 and Trp153 at the hydrophobic cavity base of the sialic acid binding site with an aromatic side chain [48,49]. It is therefore worth mentioning that in our docking model, the galloyl moiety of the second epicatechin gallate unit of procyanidin B2-di-gallate (**8**) is close to the aromatic side chain of Trp153 in the sialic acid binding pocket of HA, where it might interact in terms of a T-shaped π-π interaction. Furthermore, the B-ring of the second subunit is in a position where its phenolic oxygens might form hydrogen bonds with the hydroxyl proton of Tyr98 (both distances O...H<3 Å; see Figure 7B).

RA does not interfere with cellular responses to TNF-α and EGF

While the extract RA showed little cytotoxic effect over a wide range of concentrations it might still elicit or interfere with intracellular responses in treated cells. Thus, the effect of the addition of high concentrations of RA (100 μg/mL) close to the calculated CC_{50} for 1 h at 37°C on TNF-α and EGF induced signal transduction was studied. As shown in Figure 8A stimula-

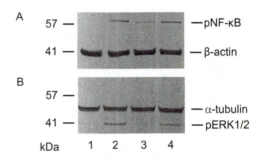

Figure 8. Influence of extract RA on TNF-α (A) and EGF (B) induced signal transduction in A549 cells. Lanes 1 and 2 represent cells preincubated for 1 h with medium, lanes 3 and 4 with RA (100 μg/mL). (**A**) Stimulation of cells with TNF-α (20 ng/mL, 30 min.) (lane 2, 4), and detection of phosphorylated NF-κB; loading control β-actin; (**B**) stimulation of cells with EGF (30 ng/mL, 10 min.) (lane 2, 4), and detection of phosphorylated ERK1/2; loading control α-tubulin.

tion of A549 cells by TNF-α led to similar increases in phosphorylated NF-κB (pNF-κB) in RA-treated or mock-treated cells, respectively. In the absence of TNF-α, neither RA nor mock-treatment led to a significant induction of pNF-κB. Potential effects of RA on Raf/MEK/ERK-signaling were investigated by stimulation of A549 cells by EGF (Figure 8B). While non-EGF-stimulated cells did not express pERK1/2, regardless if pretreated with RA or not (lanes 1 and 3), EGF treatment activated its expression (lane 2). Pretreatment of the cells with RA, followed by stimulation with EGF did not result in a significant decrease in pERK1/2 expression. It was thus concluded that even high concentrations of RA close to the CC_{50} are unlikely to significantly elicit or interfere with TNF-α and EGF-induced signal transduction. This is in accordance to recent results showing that cells are inert to LADANIA067, a polyphenol-rich extract of *Ribes nigrum folium* inhibiting entry of IAV [50].

Conclusions

The proanthocyanidin-enriched extract RA and its main active constituent epicatechin-3-O-gallate-(4β→8)-epicatechin-3′-O-gallate (procyanidin B2-di-gallate) protect cells from IAV infection by blocking IAV adsorption and interfering with penetration at higher concentrations. Anti-IAV-activity is dependent on galloylation of the procyanidin backbone. At effective concentrations, cells are unaffected by RA and procyanidin B2-di-gallat. Regarding the need for new and abundantly available anti-influenza therapeutics, RA and procyanidin B2-di-gallate appear to be a promising expansion of the currently available anti-influenza agents.

Supporting Information

Figure S1 Inhibitory effect of residual allantoic fluid on the antiviral activity of RA. To demonstrate that titres of viral stocks prepared from allantoic fluid of infected eggs have an impact on the outcome of the MTT_{IAV} assay, stocks of isolate I1 (H1N1)pdm09 were approx. 50-fold prediluted in allantoic fluid (from 3.2×10^8 pfu/mL to 6.6×10^6 pfu/mL). Subsequently, virus was diluted to 1×10^4 pfu IAV/well in serum-free medium and the antiviral activity and cell vitality were determined by MTT_{IAV} assay and cytotoxicity assay, respectively (compare Figure 2). Values represent mean ±SD of ≥3 independent experiments, * $p<0.05$, ** $p<0.01$ (two-tailed, unpaired Student's t-test). Statistical significance of antiviral activity was calculated for nontoxic concentrations only (1 to 5 μg/mL).

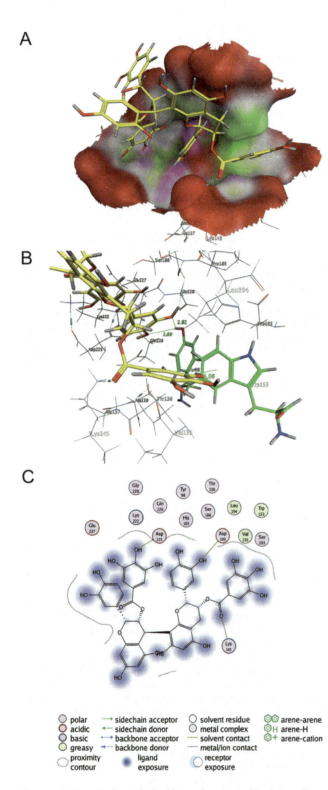

Figure 7. Protein-ligand docking of epicatechin-3-O-gallate-(4β→8)-epicatechin-3′-O-gallate (8) into the sialic acid binding cavity of hemagglutinin. (A) 3D model; protein: green: hydrophobic, purple: polar, red: exposed; ligand: yellow: carbon, light grey: hydrogen, red: oxygen, blue: nitrogen; (B) Interactions of Tyr98 and Trp153; (C) 2D.

Acknowledgments

The expert technical assistance of Maria Hovens and Marie-Luise Romberg is highly acknowledged.

Author Contributions

Conceived and designed the experiments: AD AH WH TJS CE SL JK. Performed the experiments: AD FH TJS. Analyzed the data: AD AH WH FH TJS CE SL JK. Contributed reagents/materials/analysis tools: WH TJS CE SL JK. Wrote the paper: AD AH WH FH TSH CE SL JK.

References

1. Lambert LC, Fauci AS (2010) Influenza vaccines for the future. N Engl J Med 363: 2036–2044.
2. Taubenberger JK, Morens DM (2006) 1918 Influenza: the mother of all pandemics. Emerg Infect Dis 12: 15–22.
3. Kamali A, Holodniy M (2013) Influenza treatment and prophylaxis with neuraminidase inhibitors: a review. Infect Drug Resist 6: 187–198.
4. Fiore AE, Fry A, Shay D, Gubareva L, Bresee JS, et al. (2011) Antiviral agents for the treatment and chemoprophylaxis of influenza --- recommendations of the Advisory Committee on Immunization Practices (ACIP). MMWR Recomm Rep 60: 1–24.
5. Thorlund K, Awad T, Boivin G, Thabane L (2011) Systematic review of influenza resistance to the neuraminidase inhibitors. BMC Infect Dis 11: 134.
6. Dixit R, Khandaker G, Ilgoutz S, Rashid H, Booy R (2013) Emergence of oseltamivir resistance: control and management of influenza before, during and after the pandemic. Infect Disord Drug Targets 13: 34–45.
7. De Clercq E (2013) Antivirals: past, present and future. Biochem Pharmacol 85: 727–744.
8. De Clercq E (2013) A Cutting-Edge View on the Current State of Antiviral Drug Development. Med Res Rev 33: 1249–1277.
9. Laursen NS, Wilson IA (2013) Broadly neutralizing antibodies against influenza viruses. Antiviral Res 98: 476–483.
10. Wang X, Jia W, Zhao A, Wang X (2006) Anti-influenza agents from plants and traditional Chinese medicine. Phytother Res 20: 335–341.
11. Ge H, Wang YF, Xu J, Gu Q, Liu HB, et al. (2010) Anti-influenza agents from Traditional Chinese Medicine. Nat Prod Rep 27: 1758–1780.
12. Jassim SA, Naji MA (2003) Novel antiviral agents: a medicinal plant perspective. J Appl Microbiol 95: 412–427.
13. Daglia M (2012) Polyphenols as antimicrobial agents. Curr Opin Biotechnol 23: 174–181.
14. Song JM, Seong BL (2007) Tea catechins as a potential alternative anti-infectious agent. Expert Rev Anti Infect Ther 5: 497–506.
15. Steinmann J, Buer J, Pietschmann T, Steinmann E (2013) Anti-infective properties of epigallocatechin-3-gallate (EGCG), a component of green tea. Br J Pharmacol 168: 1059–1073.
16. Yang ZF, Bai LP, Huang WB, Li XZ, Zhao SS, et al. (2014) Comparison of in vitro antiviral activity of tea polyphenols against influenza A and B viruses and structure-activity relationship analysis. Fitoterapia 93: 47–53.
17. Nakayama M, Suzuki K, Toda M, Okubo S, Hara Y, et al. (1993) Inhibition of the infectivity of influenza virus by tea polyphenols. Antiviral Res 21: 289–299.
18. Imanishi N, Tuji Y, Katada Y, Maruhashi M, Konosu S, et al. (2002) Additional inhibitory effect of tea extract on the growth of influenza A and B viruses in MDCK cells. Microbiol Immunol 46: 491–494.
19. Song JM, Lee KH, Seong BL (2005) Antiviral effect of catechins in green tea on influenza virus. Antiviral Res 68: 66–74.
20. Ubillas R, Jolad SD, Bruening RC, Kernan MR, King SR, et al. (1994) SP-303, an antiviral oligomeric proanthocyanidin from the latex of Croton lechleri (Sangre de Drago). Phytomedicine 1: 77–106.
21. Gescher K, Hensel A, Hafezi W, Derksen A, Kuhn J (2011) Oligomeric proanthocyanidins from Rumex acetosa L. inhibit the attachment of herpes simplex virus type-1. Antiviral Res 89: 9–18.
22. Gescher K, Kuhn J, Lorentzen E, Hafezi W, Derksen A, et al. (2011) Proanthocyanidin-enriched extract from Myrothamnus flabellifolia Welw. exerts antiviral activity against herpes simplex virus type 1 by inhibition of viral adsorption and penetration. J Ethnopharmacol 134: 468–474.
23. Glatthaar-Saalmuller B, Rauchhaus U, Rode S, Haunschild J, Saalmuller A (2011) Antiviral activity in vitro of two preparations of the herbal medicinal product Sinupret(R) against viruses causing respiratory infections. Phytomedicine 19: 1–7.
24. Bicker J, Petereit F, Hensel A (2009) Proanthocyanidins and a phloroglucinol derivative from Rumex acetosa L. Fitoterapia 80: 483–495.
25. Pabst D, Kuehn J, Schuler-Luettmann S, Wiebe K, Lebiedz P (2011) Acute Respiratory Distress Syndrome as a presenting manifestation in young patients infected with H1N1 influenza virus. Eur J Intern Med 22: e119–124.
26. Hrincius ER, Wixler V, Wolff T, Wagner R, Ludwig S, et al. (2010) CRK adaptor protein expression is required for efficient replication of avian influenza A viruses and controls JNK-mediated apoptotic responses. Cell Microbiol 12: 831–843.
27. Mosmann T (1983) Rapid colorimetric assay for cellular growth and survival: application to proliferation and cytotoxicity assays. J Immunol Methods 65: 55–63.
28. Beyleveld G, White KM, Ayllon J, Shaw ML (2013) New-generation screening assays for the detection of anti-influenza compounds targeting viral and host functions. Antiviral Res 100: 120–132.
29. Pauwels R, Balzarini J, Baba M, Snoeck R, Schols D, et al. (1988) Rapid and automated tetrazolium-based colorimetric assay for the detection of anti-HIV compounds. J Virol Methods 20: 309–321.
30. Xu R, Ekiert DC, Krause JC, Hai R, Crowe JE Jr, et al. (2010) Structural basis of preexisting immunity to the 2009 H1N1 pandemic influenza virus. Science 328: 357–360.
31. Pariani E, Amendola A, Ranghiero A, Anselmi G, Zanetti A (2013) Surveillance of influenza viruses in the post-pandemic era (2010-2012) in Northern Italy. Hum Vaccin Immunother 9.
32. Khandaker I, Suzuki A, Kamigaki T, Tohma K, Odagiri T, et al. (2013) Molecular evolution of the hemagglutinin and neuraminidase genes of pandemic (H1N1) 2009 influenza viruses in Sendai, Japan, during 2009–2011. Virus Genes.
33. Zhang JH, Chung TD, Oldenburg KR (1999) A Simple Statistical Parameter for Use in Evaluation and Validation of High Throughput Screening Assays. J Biomol Screen 4: 67–73.
34. Theisen LL, Muller CP (2012) EPs(R) 7630 (Umckaloabo(R)), an extract from Pelargonium sidoides roots, exerts anti-influenza virus activity in vitro and in vivo. Antiviral Res 94: 147–156.
35. De Bruyne T, Pieters L, Witvrouw M, De Clercq E, Vanden Berghe D, et al. (1999) Biological evaluation of proanthocyanidin dimers and related polyphenols. J Nat Prod 62: 954–958.
36. Zumdick S, Deters A, Hensel A (2012) In vitro intestinal transport of oligomeric procyanidins (DP 2 to 4) across monolayers of Caco-2 cells. Fitoterapia 83: 1210–1217.
37. Wang R, Lechtenberg M, Sendker J, Petereit F, Deters A, et al. (2013) Wound-healing plants from TCM: in vitro investigations on selected TCM plants and their influence on human dermal fibroblasts and keratinocytes. Fitoterapia 84: 308–317.
38. Agyare C, Lechtenberg M, Deters A, Petereit F, Hensel A (2011) Ellagitannins from Phyllanthus muellerianus (Kuntze) Exell.: Geraniin and furosin stimulate cellular activity, differentiation and collagen synthesis of human skin keratinocytes and dermal fibroblasts. Phytomedicine 18: 617–624.
39. Park S, Kim JI, Lee I, Lee S, Hwang MW, et al. (2013) Aronia melanocarpa and its components demonstrate antiviral activity against influenza viruses. Biochem Biophys Res Commun 440: 14–19.
40. Liu G, Xiong S, Xiang YF, Guo CW, Ge F, et al. (2011) Antiviral activity and possible mechanisms of action of pentagalloylglucose (PGG) against influenza A virus. Arch Virol 156: 1359–1369.
41. Theisen LL, Erdelmeier CA, Spoden GA, Boukhallouk F, Sausy A, et al. (2014) Tannins from Hamamelis virginiana Bark Extract: Characterization and Improvement of the Antiviral Efficacy against Influenza A Virus and Human Papillomavirus. PLoS One 9: e88062.
42. Ehrhardt C, Hrincius ER, Korte V, Mazur I, Droebner K, et al. (2007) A polyphenol rich plant extract, CYSTUS052, exerts anti influenza virus activity in cell culture without toxic side effects or the tendency to induce viral resistance. Antiviral Res 76: 38–47.
43. Droebner K, Ehrhardt C, Poetter A, Ludwig S, Planz O (2007) CYSTUS052, a polyphenol-rich plant extract, exerts anti-influenza virus activity in mice. Antiviral Res 76: 1–10.
44. Haidari M, Ali M, Ward Casscells S 3rd, Madjid M (2009) Pomegranate (Punica granatum) purified polyphenol extract inhibits influenza virus and has a synergistic effect with oseltamivir. Phytomedicine 16: 1127–1136.
45. Haslam E (1996) Natural polyphenols (vegetable tannins) as drugs: possible modes of action. J Nat Prod 59: 205–215.
46. Sauter NK, Hanson JE, Glick GD, Brown JH, Crowther RL, et al. (1992) Binding of influenza virus hemagglutinin to analogs of its cell-surface receptor, sialic acid: analysis by proton nuclear magnetic resonance spectroscopy and X-ray crystallography. Biochemistry 31: 9609–9621.
47. Williamson MP, McCormick TG, Nance CL, Shearer WT (2006) Epigallocatechin gallate, the main polyphenol in green tea, binds to the T-cell receptor, CD4: Potential for HIV-1 therapy. J Allergy Clin Immunol 118: 1369–1374.
48. Xu R, Krause JC, McBride R, Paulson JC, Crowe JE Jr, et al. (2013) A recurring motif for antibody recognition of the receptor-binding site of influenza hemagglutinin. Nat Struct Mol Biol 20: 363–370.
49. Ekiert DC, Kashyap AK, Steel J, Rubrum A, Bhabha G, et al. (2012) Cross-neutralization of influenza A viruses mediated by a single antibody loop. Nature 489: 526–532.
50. Ehrhardt C, Dudek SE, Holzberg M, Urban S, Hrincius ER, et al. (2013) A plant extract of Ribes nigrum folium possesses anti-influenza virus activity in vitro and in vivo by preventing virus entry to host cells. PLoS One 8: e63657.
51. Danne A, Petereit F, Nahrstedt A (1994) Flavan-3-ols, prodelphinidins and further polyphenols from Cistus salvifolius. Phytochemistry 37: 533–538.

Lichen Secondary Metabolites in *Flavocetraria cucullata* Exhibit Anti-Cancer Effects on Human Cancer Cells through the Induction of Apoptosis and Suppression of Tumorigenic Potentials

Thanh Thi Nguyen[1,2], Somy Yoon[3], Yi Yang[1], Ho-Bin Lee[4], Soonok Oh[1], Min-Hye Jeong[1], Jong-Jin Kim[4], Sung-Tae Yee[4], Florin Crişan[5], Cheol Moon[4], Kwang Youl Lee[6], Kyung Keun Kim[3], Jae-Seoun Hur[1]*, Hangun Kim[4]*

[1] Korean Lichen Research Institute, Sunchon National University, Sunchon, Republic of Korea, [2] Faculty of Natural Science and Technology, Tay Nguyen University, Buon Ma Thuot, Vietnam, [3] Medical Research Center for Gene Regulation, Chonnam National University Medical School, Gwangju, Republic of Korea, [4] College of Pharmacy and Research Institute of Life and Pharmaceutical Sciences, Sunchon National University, Sunchon, Republic of Korea, [5] Department of Taxonomy and Ecology, Faculty of Biology and Geology, Babes-Bolyai University, Cluj-Napoca, Romania, [6] College of Pharmacy, Chonnam National University, Gwangju, Korea

Abstract

Lichens are symbiotic organisms which produce distinct secondary metabolic products. In the present study, we tested the cytotoxic activity of 17 lichen species against several human cancer cells and further investigated the molecular mechanisms underlying their anti-cancer activity. We found that among 17 lichens species, *F. cucullata* exhibited the most potent cytotoxicity in several human cancer cells. High performance liquid chromatography analysis revealed that the acetone extract of *F. cucullata* contains usnic acid, salazinic acid, Squamatic acid, Baeomycesic acid, d-protolichesterinic acid, and lichesterinic acid as subcomponents. MTT assay showed that cancer cell lines were more vulnerable to the cytotoxic effects of the extract than non-cancer cell lines. Furthermore, among the identified subcomponents, usnic acid treatment had a similar cytotoxic effect on cancer cell lines but with lower potency than the extract. At a lethal dose, treatment with the extract or with usnic acid greatly increased the apoptotic cell population and specifically activated the apoptotic signaling pathway; however, using sub-lethal doses, extract and usnic acid treatment decreased cancer cell motility and inhibited *in vitro* and *in vivo* tumorigenic potentials. In these cells, we observed significantly reduced levels of epithelial-mesenchymal transition (EMT) markers and phosphor-Akt, while phosphor-c-Jun and phosphor-ERK1/2 levels were only marginally affected. Overall, the anti-cancer activity of the extract is more potent than that of usnic acid alone. Taken together, *F. cucullata* and its subcomponent, usnic acid together with additional component, exert anti-cancer effects on human cancer cells through the induction of apoptosis and the inhibition of EMT.

Editor: Chengfeng Yang, Michigan State University, United States of America

Funding: This study was supported by the Basic Science Research Program through the National Research Foundation of Korea (NRF-2013R1A1A2004677, NRF-2013R1A2A2A07067609) and by the Korea National Research Resource Center Program (NRF-2012M3A9B8021726). This study also received support from a research grant funded by the Sunchon Research Center for Natural Medicine. The funders had no role in study design, data collection and analysis, decision to publish, or preparation of the manuscript.

Competing Interests: The authors have declared that no competing interests exist.

* Email: jshur1@sunchon.ac.kr (JSH); hangunkim@sunchon.ac.kr (HK)

Introduction

Cancer is a major cause of death worldwide. As a group, cancers account for approximately 13% of all deaths each year with the most common being lung cancer (1.37 million deaths), stomach cancer (736,000 deaths), liver cancer (695,000 deaths), colorectal cancer (608,000 deaths), and breast cancer (458,000 deaths) [1]. Invasive cancer is the leading cause of death in the developed world and the second leading cause of death in the developing world [2], so for these reasons, various cancer therapies have been developed, including a wide range of anti-cancer agents with known cytotoxic effects on cancer cells.

Lichens are symbiotic organisms, usually composed of a fungal partner (mycobiont) and one or more photosynthetic partners (photobiont), which is most often either a green alga or a cyanobacterium [3]. Although the dual nature of most lichens is now widely recognized, it is less commonly known that some lichens are symbioses involving three (tripartite lichens) or more partners. In general, lichens exist as discrete thalli and are implicitly treated as individuals in many studies, even though they may be a symbiotic entity involving species from three kingdoms. From a genetic and evolutionary perspective, lichens cannot be regarded as individuals but rather as composites, and this has major implications for many areas of investigation such as development and reproduction.

Many lichen secondary products are unpalatable and may serve as defensive compounds against herbivores as well as decomposers. For this reason, these secondary products are frequently used by the pharmaceutical industry as antibacterial and antiviral compounds [4,5]. In addition, lichens and their secondary metabolites have long been studied for anti-cancer therapy [6–15]. In the present study, we tested the cytotoxic activity of 17 lichen species collected from the Romanian Carpathian mountains against several human cancer cells and further investigated the molecular mechanisms underlying their anti-cancer activity to identify potential compounds for novel anti-cancer agents.

Materials and Methods

Preparation of lichen extracts

Thalli of *F. cucullata* were collected from Romania in 2011 during the field trip in the National Park Călimani and the Natural Park Bucegi organized by Dr. Crișan at Babeș-Bolyai University, Cluj-Napoca, Romania. The permit to collect lichen specimens from those locations was issued by the Administration of the National Park Călimani and the Administration of the Natural Park Bucegi, with the approval of the Commission for Protection of Natural Monuments (Romanian Academy). The field studies did not involve any endangered or protected species. The duplicates were deposited into the Korean Lichen Research Institute (KoLRI), Sunchon National University, Korea. Finely dried ground thalli of the lichen (150 g) were extracted using acetone in a Soxhlet extractor. The extracts were filtered and then concentrated under reduced pressure in a rotary evaporator. The dry extracts were stored at $-25°C$ until further use. The extracts were dissolved in dimethylsulfoxide (DMSO) for all experiments.

High performance liquid chromatography (HPLC) analysis of lichen materials

Dry lichen extracts were redissolved in 2 mL of acetone and then subjected to HPLC (SHIMADZU, LC-20A). HPLC analyses were carried out on YMC-Pack ODS-A (150×3.9 mm I.D.) reversed-phase column fully endcapped C18 material (particle size, 5 μm; pore size, 12 nm). Elution was performed at a flow rate of 1 mL/min under the following conditions: column temp, 40°C; solvent system, methanol: water: phosphoric acid (80:20:1, v/v/v) before subsequent injection. The analysis was monitored by a photodiode array detector (SPD-M20A) with a range of 190–800 nm during the entire HPLC run. Observed peaks were scanned between 190 and 400 nm. The sample injection volume was 10 μL. The standards used were obtained from the following sources: salazinic acid ($t_R = 2.27 \pm 0.2$ min) isolated from lichen *Lobaria pulmonaria*, usnic acid ($t_R = 11.3 \pm 0.3$ min) from *Usnea longissima* and protolichesterinic acid ($t_R = 22.3 \pm 0.2$ min) and lichesterinic acid ($t_R = 26.5 \pm 0.2$ min) from lichen *Cetraria islandica*.

Cell culture

The human cancer cell lines HT29 (colon cancer), AGS (gastric cancer), A549 (lung cancer), and CWR22Rv-1 (prostate cancer) were maintained in Roswell Park Memorial Institute (RPMI) 1640 medium (Gen Depot, USA) supplemented with 10% fetal bovine serum (FBS) (Gen Depot, USA) and 1% penicillin and streptomycin (RPMI complete medium) (Gen Depot, USA). HaCaT (human keratinocyte), NIH 3T3 (mouse embryonic fibroblast cells), HEK293T (human embryonic kidney) cells, RIE (rat intestinal epithelial) cells, and Madin-Darby canine kidney (MDCK) cells were maintained in Dulbecco's Modified Eagle Medium (DMEM) (Gen Depot, USA) supplemented with 10% FBS and 1% penicillin and streptomycin. Cells were cultured in 5% CO_2 in a humidified atmosphere at 37°C. Cell lines were purchased from the Korean Cell Line Bank (http://cellbank.snu.ac.kr), Korea.

MTT assay

Lichen extracts were dissolved in DMSO (Sigma-Aldrich, St. Louis, USA) and serially diluted with DMEM or RPMI 1640 to obtain concentrations of 6.125, 12.5, 25, 50, 100 μg/mL. Cells (2×10^4 cells/well) were seeded on a 96-well plate, grown overnight, and then treated with the acetone extract or main compounds of *F. cucullata* at concentrations of 100 μg/mL or μM to 10 μg/mL or μM for 48 hr. Once treatment was completed, cultures were supplemented with MTT. After incubation with MTT at 37°C, cells were lysed with lysis buffer containing 50% DMSO and 20% SDS, and absorbance was measured at 570 nm using a microplate reader (VERSAmax, Molecular Devices, Minnesota, USA). The percentage of viable cells was calculated using the following formula: percentage cell viability = (optical density (OD) of the experiment samples/OD of the control)×100. IC_{50} values were calculated using the Statistical Package for Social Science (SPSS) software.

Fluorescence microscopy of apoptotic morphology

Cells were cultured on chamber slides at a density of 4×10^5 cells/well and allowed to attach overnight, followed by treatment with the *F. cucullata* acetone extract or usnic acid for 24 hr or 48 hr. Cells were washed with phosphate-buffered saline (PBS) and incubated with Annexin V FITC labeling solution for 15 min. Then, cells were washed twice in PBS and analyzed using a Nikon Eclipse 400 (Nikon Instech Co., Ltd., Kawasaki, Japan) fluorescent microscope.

Cells were cultured as described above. After 24 hr or 48 hr treatment with the *F. cucullata* acetone extract or usnic acid, cells were washed with PBS three times and fixed in 4% paraformaldehyde at room temperature, then incubated in 0.1% Triton x-100 (Sigma-Aldrich, St. Louis, USA) for 30 min. Subsequently, the samples were stained with Hoechst 33257 (Sigma-Aldrich, St. Louis, USA) at room temperature after washing three times in fixative solution in PBS. The cells were washed twice in PBS and mounted onto a glass slide. The slides were analyzed using a Nikon Eclipse 400 (Nikon Instech Co., Ltd., Kawasaki, Japan) fluorescent microscope and evaluated as the percentage of cells with condensed or fragmented nuclei from a total number of 300 cells.

Flow cytometry assay for cell cycle

After 24 hr of incubation, untreated and acetone extract- or usnic acid-treated MDCK, HEK293T, HT29, AGS, A549, and CWR22Rv-1 cells were trypsinized. Then, an RNase inhibitor was added and incubated for 15 min at room temperature. Finally, the samples were centrifuged to remove the supernatant, and pellet cells were diluted in 100 μL of propidium iodide (Sigma-Aldrich, St. Louis, USA) and incubated for another 30 min at 4°C. Flow cytometry was performed with a FACS Caliber (BD Biosciences, San Diego, USA).

Wound-healing assay

AGS and A549 cells were plated at a density of 2.5×10^5 cells/well on 6-well tissue culture plates (Corning, New York, USA) and grown overnight to confluence. Monolayer cells were scratched with a pipette tip to create a wound. The cells were then washed

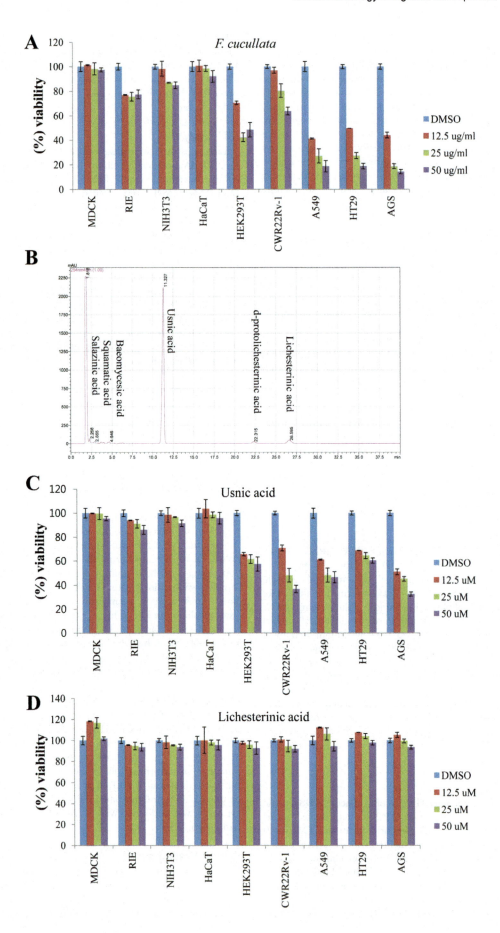

Figure 1. Cytotoxic effects of the acetone extract of *F. cucullata* and its main component, usnic acid, on human cancer cells. (A) Percent viability of cells treated with the acetone extract of *F. cucullata*. Cells were treated with the *F. cucullata* extract in a concentration ranging from 10–50 µg/mL for 48 hr, and cell viability was measured by an MTT assay. (B) High performance liquid chromatography chromatograms of the *F. cucullata* extract. The identity of each subcomponent is noted on the corresponding peak. (C–D) The percent viability of cells treated with either usnic acid (C) or lichesterinic acid (D). Cells were treated with the indicated subcomponent of *F. cucullata* in a concentration ranging from 12.5–50 µM for 48 hr, and cell viability was measured by an MTT assay. Data represent means ± S.E.M. (standard error of the mean), n = 3.

twice with serum-free RPMI 1640 to remove floating cells and incubated in medium with 5 µg/mL of the *F. cucullata* extract or 10 µM usnic acid. Photographs of cells were taken at 0, 24, 48, and 72 hr after wounding to measure the width of the wound. The distance migrated by the cells was calculated as the difference between the edges of the wound at time point 1 and at time point 2. For each cell line, an average of eight wound assays was taken to determine the average rate of migration at a given concentration of acetone extract or usnic acid. Experiments were repeated at least three times.

Invasion assay

Tumor cell invasion was analyzed using a transwell chamber (Corning Coster, Corning, NY, USA) assay with a topchamber of 8 µm pore-size polycarbonate membrane coated with 1% gelatin. AGS and A549 cells were plated at 2.5×10^5 cells/well in culture medium containing 0.2% bovine serum albumin (BSA) in the upper compartment of the chamber. The lower compartment was filled with culture medium containing 0.2% BSA and 1 µg/mL fibronectin as a chemo-attractant. Cells were cultured in the absence or presence of 5 µg/mL acetone extract or 10 µM usnic acid for 24 hr. The upper chambers were fixed and stained with Diff Quick kit (Sysmex, Kobe, Japan). The invaded cells were analyzed under a light microscope in five randomly selected fields. Each experiment was performed in triplicate. The results are expressed as the mean number of cells migrating per high-power field.

Clonogenic assay

A549 and AGS cells were washed, trypsinized, and resuspended in RPMI 1640. Cells (500 cells/well) were seeded on 6-well plates in 2.5 mL RPMI 1640 medium per well and were incubated for attachment. Subsequent to 48 hr treatment, media containing the acetone extract or usnic acid was replaced with fresh medium for 12 days. Colonies were fixed in 4% paraformaldehyde, stained with 0.5% crystal violet, and counted under a stereomicroscope. The plating efficiency (PE) of untreated cells and the survival fraction (SF) of treated cells were then determined (n = 3) [16].

Soft agar colony-formation assay

AGS (1×10^4) and A549 (1×10^4) cells were suspended in 1.5 mL of soft agar (0.35% agarose in RPMI complete medium), plated onto 1.5 mL of solidified agar (0.6% agarose in RPMI complete medium) in 6-well plates and cultured for 3 weeks. Cells were fed two times per week with cell culture media containing the acetone extract (1 µg/mL or 5 µg/mL), usnic acid (5 µM or 10 µM), lichesterinic acid (10 µM), or DMSO (0.01%). Pixel intensity of colony area was measured by the IMT iSolution software (IMT i-Solution Inc., Northampton, NJ, USA) in randomly selected microscope fields in each plate. To measure the percent area of colony, pixel amount of colony area were normalized to pixel×pixel square. Data represent the mean of three experiments.

Detection of proteins in cell lysates

Cells treated with various concentrations of the acetone extract or subcomponents for 48 hr were harvested and analyzed by western blot as previously described [17]. The antibodies used were purchased from Cell signaling Technology (PARP, caspase-3, Bax, Bcl_xL, α-tubulin), and BD Biosciences (E-cadherin). All results are representative from at least three independent experiments. To analyze the level of phosphoproteins, bead-based multiplex assay (Bio-Plex phosphoprotein assay, Bio-Rad, Hercules, CA, USA) was performed according to the manufacturer's instructions [18,19]. Briefly, this assay measured multiple phosphoprotein signals from a single lysate [20].

qRT-PCR analysis

Total RNA (1 µg) from each group of treated cells was converted to cDNA using a M-MLV reverse Transcriptase kit (Invitrogen, Carlsbad, CA, USA) and SYBR green (Enzynomics, Seoul, Korea). The primers used for real-time PCR were E-cadherin (forward) 5′-cagaaagttttccaccaaag-3′ and (reverse) 5′-aaatgtgagcaattctgctt-3′; N-cadherin (forward) 5′-ctcctatgagtggaa-caggaacg-3′ and (reverse) 5′-ttggatcaatgtcataatcaagtgctgta-3′; Snail (forward) 5′-gaggcggtggcagactag-3′ and (reverse) 5′-gaca-catcggtcagaccag-3′; Twist (forward) 5′-cgggagtccgcagtctta-3′ and (reverse) 5′-tgaatcttgctcagcttgtc-3′; GAPDH (forward) 5′-atcac-catcttccaggagcga-3′ and (reverse) 5′-agttgtcatggatgaccttggc-3′. qRT-PCR reaction and analysis were performed using CFX (Bio-Rad, Hercules, CA, USA).

In vivo tumorigenicity assay

The experimental protocol was approved by the Chonnam National University Medical School Research Institutional Animal Care & Use Committee. Maintenance of animals and all in vivo experiments were performed according to the Guiding Principles in the Care and Use of Animals (DHEW publication, NIH 80-23). A549 cells were prepared in RPMI 1640 medium (1×10^6 cells/mouse) and suspended cells were pretreated with one-tenth of lethal concentration of *F. cucullata* acetone extract, usnic acid, lichesterinic acid, or DMSO (Vehicle) just before injection. Cells were injected subcutaneously into the flank region of Balb/c nude mouse and tumor was measured after two weeks.

Statistical analysis

All experiments were assayed in triplicates (n = 3). Data were expressed as means ± standard deviation. All statistical analyses were performed using the SPSS version 17. Treatment effects were determined using one-way ANOVA post-hoc analysis. A p-value < 0.05 was considered significant unless indicated otherwise.

Results

Flavocetraria cucullata acetone extract has potent cytotoxic effects on cancer cells

To identify the cytotoxic substance from Romanian lichens, we measured the IC_{50} values of acetone extracts from 17 lichen species on HT29 (colorectal cancer cells) and AGS (gastric cancer cells) cells. Among the lichen species, *F. cucullata* exerted the most potent cytotoxic effects on both HT29 (IC_{50} = 10.9 µg/mL) and AGS (IC_{50} = 11.6 µg/mL) compared to other lichen species (IC_{50} values ranged around 25–100 µg/mL, Table S1 in File S1). To

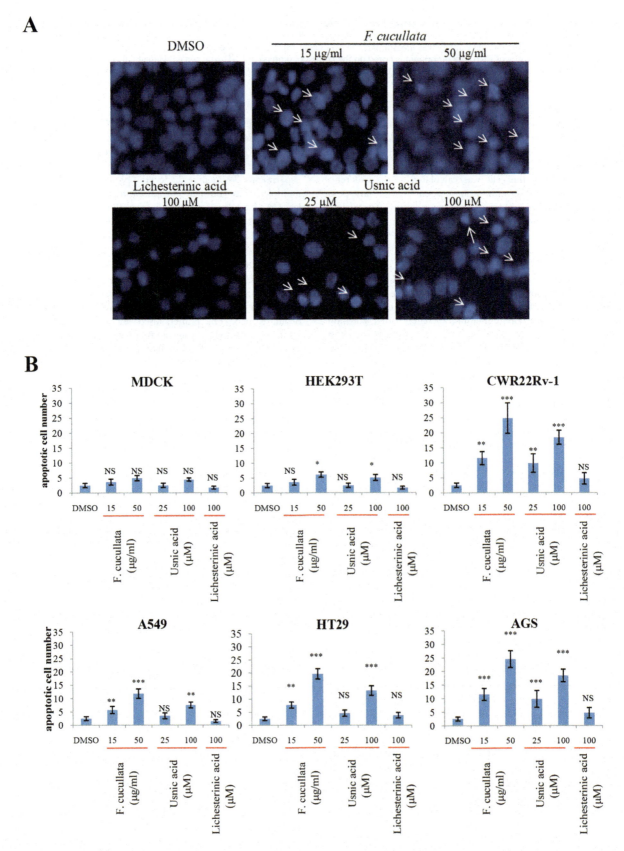

Figure 2. Induction of nuclear condensation of human cancer cells by the acetone extract of *F. cucullata* and its main component, usnic acid in lethal concentrations. (A) Hoechst 33258 staining of AGS (human gastric cancer cell line) cells treated with the *F. cucullata* extract or its subcomponents, usnic acid and lichesterinic acid. Arrows indicate cells showing condensed or fragmented nuclear morphology. Representative images are shown from three independent experiments. (B) Quantificational analysis of condensed or fragmented nuclear morphology in various

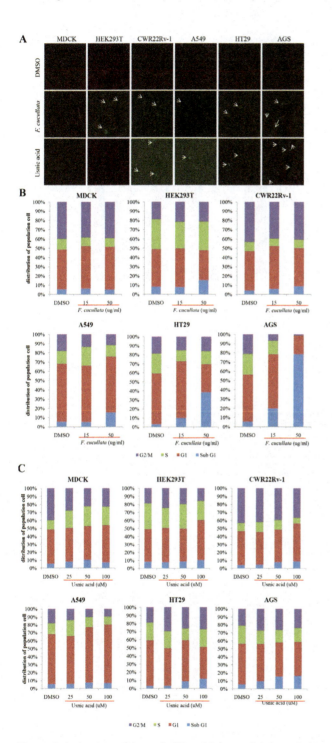

Figure 3. Induction of Annexin V positivity and accumulation of sub G1 population on human cancer cells by the acetone extract of *F. cucullata* and usnic acid in lethal concentrations. (A) FITC-Annexin V staining of cells treated with the *F. cucullata* extract or usnic acid. Arrows indicate cells showing FITC positivity. (B–C) Flow cytometric analysis of cell-cycle distributions after *F. cucullata* extract (B) or usnic acid (C) treatment and graphical representation of the results. Representative images or results are shown from three independent experiments.

cells treated with *F. cucullata* extract or its subcomponents. Data represent mean ± S.E.M. (standard error of the mean), n = 3. **$p<0.01$; ***$p<0.001$; NS, no significant difference compared to the dimethylsulfoxide-treated group.

verify whether the cytotoxicity of the *F. cucullata* extract was specific to cancer cells, we conducted further tests on additional cancer cells including A549 (lung cancer cells) and CWR22Rv-1 (prostate cancer cells) cells and on non-cancer cells including MDCK (Madin-Darby canine kidney) and RIE (rat intestinal epithelial cell), NIH 3T3 (mouse embryonic fibroblast), HaCaT (human keratinocyte) cells. The results showed that the *F. cucullata* acetone extract specifically affected the viability of cancer cells while non-cancer cells were not severely damaged (Fig. 1A).

To identify the subcomponents of *F. cucullata*, HPLC was performed on the acetone extract of *F. cucullata*; the resulting chromatograms and mass spectrometric analyses of each peak are presented in Figure 1B and Table S2 in File S1. As shown in Figure 1B, salazinic acid (Tr = 2.268 min), squamatic acid (Tr = 2.855), baeomycesic acid (Tr = 4.646), usnic acid (Tr = 11.327), d-protolichesterinic acid (Tr = 22.315), and lichesterinic acid (Tr = 26.595) were detected in the acetone extract of *F. cucullata*. Among the subcomponents, usnic acid had the highest peak (% intensity = 91.49±0.0025), while d-protolichesterinic acid and lichesterinic acid showed lower peaks (% intensity = 2.27±0.1, 2.22±0.1, respectively) (Table S2 in File S1). After identifying the lichen subcomponents, two main metabolites, usnic acid (Sigma-Aldrich, St. Louis, USA) and lichesterinic acid (isolated from *F. cucullata* extract which share their chemical structure with d-protolichesterinic acid except one unsaturated carbon bond) were used for further experiments. To determine which subcomponent was responsible for the cytotoxicity of lichen, we measured the cytotoxicity of usnic acid and lichesterinic acid and found that usnic acid showed similar cytotoxic effects in non-cancer and cancer cells while lichesterinic acid exhibited no apparent cytotoxic effect on any of the tested cells (Fig. 1C and 1D). In Table S3 in File S1, the IC_{50} values of acetone extract, usnic acid, and lichesterinic acid in various cells are presented. Interestingly, given the molecular weight (MW = 344) and % intensity of usnic acid in the acetone extract of *F. cucullata*, IC_{50} values of usnic acid in HEK293T, HT29, and A549 cells were likely higher than those of calculated usnic acid concentration in the extract. These results suggest that unidentified subcomponents of the *F. cucullata* extract likely potentiate the cytotoxicity of usnic acid. However, it is worth noting that IC_{50} values of usnic acid, especially in non-cancer cells such as MDCK, RIE, NIH 3T3, and HaCaT cells, were much lower than those of usnic acid concentration in the *F. cucullata* extract, suggesting that there may be a resistant mechanism underlying the cytotoxicity of usnic acid in cells or that other subcomponent(s) can lessen the cytotoxicity of usnic acid to the cells. Taken together, these results suggest that the acetone extract of *F. cucullata* has selective cytotoxicity to cancer cells and that usnic acid may act as a major effector of these effects.

Lethal concentrations of *Flavocetraria cucullata* and usnic acid induce apoptosis of cancer cells

To determine whether the cytotoxicity of *F. cucullata* and usnic acid was due to the induction of apoptosis, cells treated with a lethal concentration of *F. cucullata* (50 μg/mL) or usnic acid (100 μM) were stained with Hoechst 33258 and their nuclear morphology was observed. As shown in Figure 2A, condensed nuclear morphology was seen in AGS cells treated with either *F. cucullata* extract or usnic acid. In Figure 2B, quantifications of cell numbers in various cell lines are shown. Interestingly, induction of

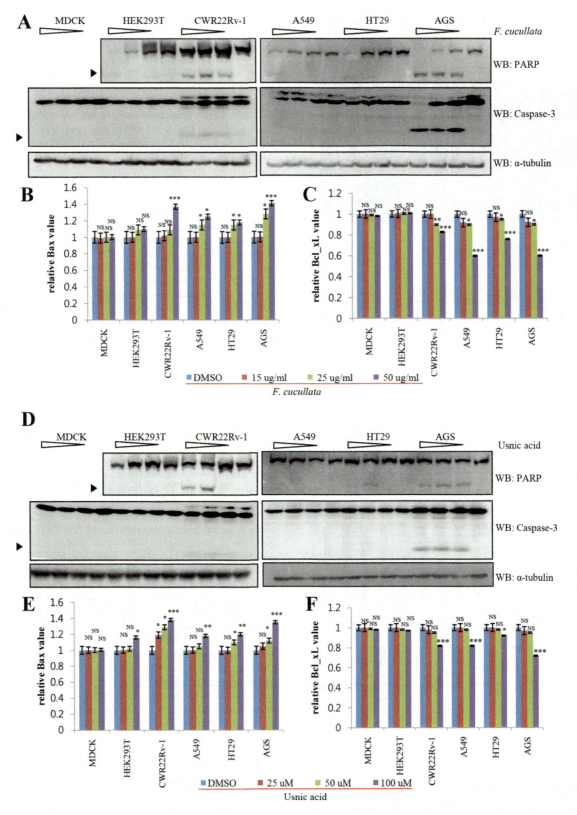

Figure 4. Activation of apoptosis pathway on human cancer cells by the acetone extract of *F. cucullata* and usnic acid in lethal concentrations. (A and D) Western blot analysis of poly (ADP-ribose) polymerase (PARP) and caspase-3 in cells treated with the *F. cucullata* (A) or usnic acid (D). Arrowheads indicate cleaved fragments of each protein. (B–C and E–F) Quantificational analysis of Bax (B and E) and Bcl-xL (C and F) protein expression levels in cells treated with the *F. cucullata* or usnic acid, respectively. Data represent mean ± S.E.M. (standard error of the mean). *$p<0.05$; **$p<0.01$; ***$p<0.001$; NS, no significant difference compared to the dimethylsulfoxide-treated group.

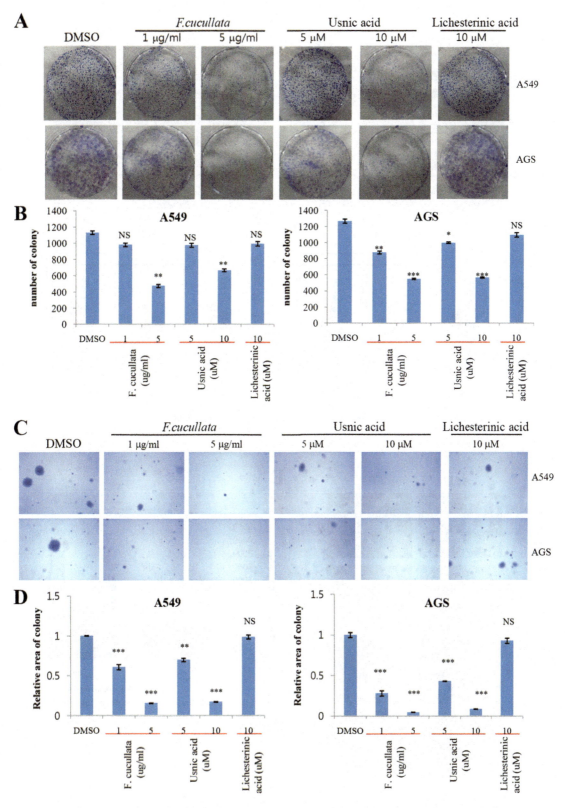

Figure 5. **Inhibition of anchorage-independent growth of A549 and AGS cancer cells by the acetone extract of *F. cucullata* and usnic acid in sub-lethal concentrations.** (A–B) Clonogenic assay of A549 and AGS cells treated with the *F. cucullata* extract, usnic acid, or lichesterinic acid (A) and quantificational analysis of colony number in each group (B). (C–D) Soft agar colony-formation assay of A549 and AGS cells treated with *F. cucullata* extract, usnic acid, or lichesterinic acid (C) and quantificational analysis of percent colony area in each group (D). Representative images are shown from three independent experiments. Data represent mean ± S.E.M. (standard error of the mean), n = 3. *p<0.05; **p<0.01; ***p<0.001; NS, no significant difference compared to the dimethylsulfoxide-treated group.

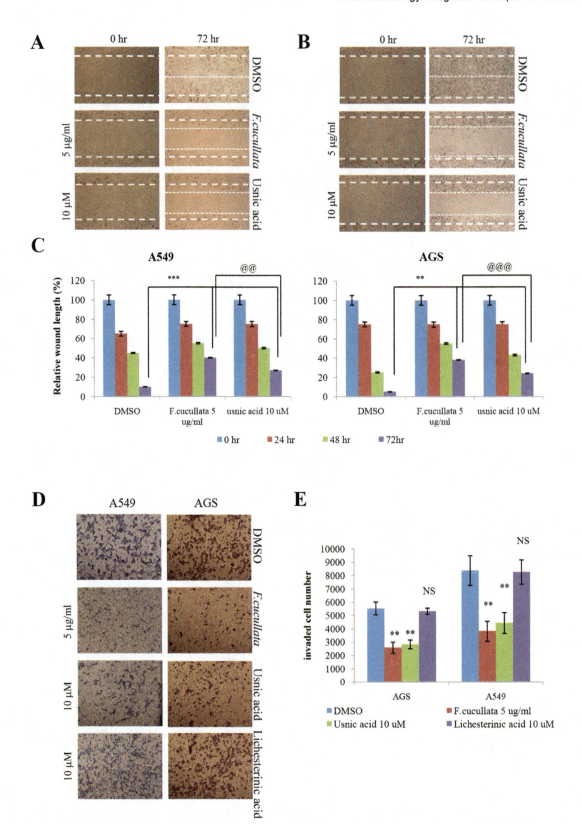

Figure 6. Inhibition of the motility of A549 and AGS cancer cells by the acetone extract of *F. cucullata* and usnic acid in sub-lethal concentrations. (A–C) Migration assay of A549 (A) and AGS (B) cells treated with the *F. cucullata* extract or usnic acid, and quantificational analysis of wound length in each group (C). (D–E) Invasion assay of A549 and AGS cells treated with the *F. cucullata* extract, usnic acid, or lichesterinic acid (D), and quantificational analysis of invaded cell numbers in each group (E). Representative images are shown from three independent experiments. Data represent mean ± S.E.M. (standard error of the mean), n = 3. **$p<0.01$; ***$p<0.001$; NS, no significant difference when compared to the dimethylsulfoxide-treated group in each cell lines. @@$p<0.01$; @@@$p<0.001$ when compared to the indicated group.

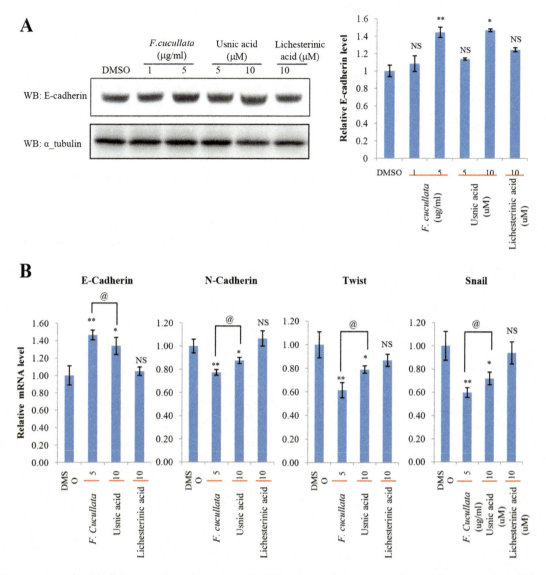

Figure 7. Suppression of epithelial-mesenchymal transition (EMT) by the acetone extract of *F. cucullata* and usnic acid in sub-lethal concentrations. (A) E-cadherin level in A549 cells treated with the *F. cucullata* extract, usnic acid, or lichesterinic acid for 48 hr, and quantificational analysis of E-cadherin band in each group. Values were obtained by measuring the intensity of E-cadherin band normalized to α-tubulin. (B) Quantitative analysis of the mRNA level of EMT markers in A549 cells treated with the *F. cucullata* extract, usnic acid, or lichesterinic acid for 48 hr. Data represent mean ± S.E.M. (standard error of the mean), n = 3. *p<0.05; **p<0.01; NS, no significant difference when compared to the dimethylsulfoxide-treated group; @p<0.05 when compared to the indicated group.

nuclear condensation was significantly increased in treated cancer cells but was not seen in the non-cancer cell line MDCK, suggesting that *F. cucullata* and usnic acid are selectively cytotoxic to cancer cells through the induction of apoptosis.

To confirm this, we stained the cells with FITC-Annexin V to detect exposure of phosphatidylserine on the outer plasma membrane, which is a characteristic finding in cells undergoing apoptosis. As shown in Figure 3A, cancer cells treated with either *F. cucullata* extract or usnic acid showed FITC positivity. To determine the percentage of apoptotic cells, flow cytometric analysis of cells stained with propidium iodide was performed. As shown in Figures 3B and 3C, the population of cells in the sub G1 phase increased following 24 hr treatment in cancer cells. This quantification analysis revealed that the induction of apoptosis by the *F. cucullata* extract was dose-dependent except in MDCK cells, with significant increases seen in AGS, HT29, and A549 cells (Fig. 3B). However, as shown in Figure 3C, the effectiveness of usnic acid in increasing the number of apoptotic cells was significantly lower than that of the *F. cucullata* extract. These findings again suggest that unidentified subcomponent(s) of *F. cucullata* may potentiate the effects of usnic acid although usnic acid plays a major role in inducing apoptosis in various cancer cells.

To further confirm changes in the level of apoptotic proteins, we performed western blot analysis for poly (ADP-ribose) polymerase (PARP), caspase-3, Bax, and Bcl-xL. As shown in Figures 4A and 4D, extract and usnic acid treatment increased the levels of cleaved PARP and cleaved caspase-3 in CWR22Rv-1, AGS, HT29, and A549 cells. In addition, the level of the pro-apoptotic protein, Bax, was significantly increased in these treated cells, but

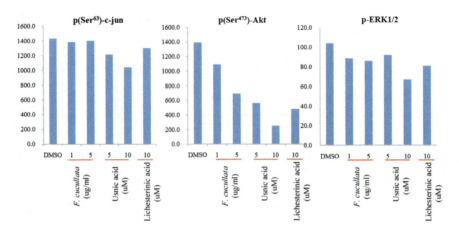

Figure 8. Reduction of phosphor-Akt level by the acetone extract of *F. cucullata* and usnic acid in sub-lethal concentrations. Phosphoprotein analysis for p(Ser^{63})-c-jun, p(Ser^{473})-Akt, and p-(Thr^{202}/Tyr^{204}, Thr^{185}/Tyr^{187})-ERK1/2 in A549 cells treated with the *F. cucullata* extract, usnic acid, or lichesterinic acid.

not in MDCK and HEK293T cells (Figs. 4B and 4E). By contrast, the level of the anti-apoptotic protein, Bcl-xL, was significantly decreased only in treated cancer cells (Figs. 4C and 4F). Consistently, *F. cucullata* was more effective in inducing apoptosis than usnic acid and was more effective in cancer cells than non-cancer cell. Taken together, the results demonstrate that lethal concentrations of the acetone extract of *F. cucullata* and the subcomponent of usnic acid induce apoptosis of cancer cells.

Sub-lethal concentrations of *Flavocetraria cucullata* and usnic acid inhibit tumorigenicity and motility of cancer cells

To further explore the anti-cancer activity of the *F. cucullata* extract and usnic acid, we used one-tenth of the lethal concentrations of these compounds which did not showing the cytotoxicity (sub-lethal concentration) and tested the *in vitro* tumorigenicity and motility of A549 and AGS cells. A clonogenic assay of these cells at sub-lethal concentrations of the extract

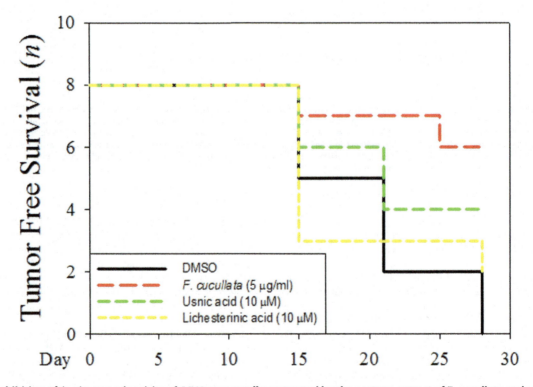

Figure 9. Inhibition of *in vivo* tumorigenicity of A549 cancer cells pretreated by the acetone extract of F. cucullata and usnic acid in sub-lethal concentrations. A549 cells were pretreated with indicated concentration of *F. cucullata*, usnic acid, or lichesterinic acid before subcutaneous injection into Balb/c nude mouse (n = 8) and tumor free survival number in each group during 4 weeks were measured.

(5 μg/mL) or usnic acid (10 μM) showed a significant decrease in the number of colonies, indicating that cell proliferation was inhibited at these concentrations (Figs. 5A and 5B). Interestingly, treatment by 10 μg/mL extract or 15 μM usnic acid completely inhibited the formation of colonies in both cell types (data not shown). By contrast, lichesterinic acid showed no inhibitory effect on cell proliferation. A soft agar colony-formation assay was performed to test whether sub-lethal concentrations of *F. cucullata* and usnic acid inhibited anchorage-independent growth of A549 and AGS cells. As shown in Figures 5C and 5D, colony formation of A549 and AGS cells on soft agar was significantly decreased by treatment with the *F. cucullata* extract or usnic acid in a dose-dependent manner, while lichesterinic acid did not affect anchorage-independent growth. These results demonstrate that both the *F. cucullata* extract and usnic acid have anti-tumorigenic activity at sub-lethal concentrations. A wound-healing assay and invasion assay were further performed to test whether *F. cucullata* and usnic acid affect migration and invasion, respectively, of cancer cells at sub-lethal concentrations. In Figures 6A–C, *F. cucullata* extract and usnic acid treatment significantly inhibited the migration of A549 and AGS cells. As shown in Figures 6D–E, the *F. cucullata* extract and usnic acid also inhibited the invasion of A549 and AGS cells, while no such inhibition of invasion was detected in lichesterinic acid-treated cancer cells. The results clearly show that *F. cucullata* and usnic acid inhibit cancer cell motility and decrease tumorigenicity of cancer cells at sub-lethal concentrations.

As *F. cucullata* and usnic acid were found to significantly decrease cancer cell motility and tumorigenicity, we then investigated whether epithelial-mesenchymal transition (EMT) plays a role in mediating these effects. The expression level of E-cadherin was analyzed in A549 cells treated with a sub-lethal concentration of *F. cucullata*, usnic acid, or lichesterinic acid. The data showed that the acetone extract of *F. cucullata* and usnic acid significantly increased the protein level of E-cadherin (Fig. 7A). Consistently, the expression level of E-cadherin mRNA was also increased in these cells, while mRNA levels of N-cadherin, Twist, and Snail were decreased in these cells. These findings indicate that *F. cucullata* and usnic acid can inhibit EMT (Fig. 7B). Lichesterinic acid treatment induced no significant changes in the levels of these EMT markers. In addition, changes in the phosphorylation levels of c-jun, Akt, and ERK1/2 were analyzed in A549 cells treated with a sub-lethal concentration of *F. cucullata*, usnic acid, or lichesterinic acid. As shown in Figure 8, the level of p-(Ser^{473})-Akt was dramatically decreased by both *F. cucullata* and usnic acid treatment in a dose-dependent manner while the levels of p-(Ser^{63})-c-jun and p-(Thr^{202}/Tyr^{204}, Thr^{185}/Tyr^{187})-ERK1/2 were only marginally affected by usnic acid. These results suggest that sub-lethal concentrations *F. cucullata* extract and usnic acid can exert anti-cancer effects possibly through inhibiting EMT and Akt signaling.

To further support the anti-cancer effects of *F. cucullata* extract and usnic acid at sub-lethal concentration, we performed the *in vivo* tumorigenicity assay. As shown in Figure 9 and Figure S1 in File S1, tumor free survival number in *F. cucullata* pretreated group is highest (tumor free in six out of eight mouse) among DMSO (zero out of eight), usnic acid (four out of eight), or lichesterinic acid (two out of eight) pretreated group. Interestingly, when comparing the *F. cucullata* and usnic acid pretreated group, it is worth noting that tumor free survival number was less in the usnic acid treated group than that of the *F. cucullata* treated group. Taken together, these results demonstrate that *F. cucullata* extract and usnic acid have *in vitro* and *in vivo* anti-cancer effects at sub-lethal concentration.

Discussion

Lichen species living at high elevation are occasionally exposed to strong sunlight, including UV radiation, and to severe fluctuations in temperature during their growing seasons. Severe environmental stresses can stimulate the production of chemical protectants for lichens to cope with stress-induced damage, e.g., many lichen pigments are well known to protect lichen thalli from strong UV radiation [5]. Furthermore, several antioxidant compounds have been extracted from lichens growing in harsh environmental conditions [21]. In this study, we investigated the anti-cancer activity of Romanian Carpathian lichens against several cancer cell lines. Among the 17 lichens species tested in this study, *F. cucullata* exhibited the most potent cytotoxicity against HT29 and AGS cancer cell lines. To the best of our knowledge, this is the first report at the molecular level on the anti-cancer activity of lethal and sub-lethal doses of *F. cucullata* and usnic acid against several cancer cell lines. We found the following: 1) the acetone extract of *F. cucullata* and its subcomponent, usnic acid, exert selective cytotoxicity on cancer cells through inducing apoptosis at lethal concentrations; 2) the extract of *F. cucullata* and usnic acid inhibit tumorigenesis and motility of cancer cells at sub-lethal concentrations; 3) the extract of *F. cucullata* and usnic acid suppress EMT and inhibit Akt phosphorylation; and 4) the anti-cancer activity of the extract is more potent than that of usnic acid alone.

Lichen is easily recognized on moss or soil due to its yellow color and curled thalli, and the yellowish thalli indicate that lichen contains usnic acid. HPLC analysis of the acetone extract of thalli confirmed usnic acid as the major compound of the extract, which has been shown to possess many biological activities [5]. Salazinic acid, squamatic acid, baeomycesic acid, d-protolichesterinic acid, and lichesterinic acid have also been detected as additional compounds in thalli. Usnic acid has been previously shown to induce apoptosis of various cancer cell lines, such as human ovarian carcinoma A2780, human colon adenocarcinoma HT29, human breast adenocarcinoma MCF-7, human cervix adenocarcinoma HeLa, human promyelocytic leukemia, human T-cells lymphocyte leukemia, Jurkat, and human breast adenocarcinoma SK-BR-3 cells, at lethal doses through a caspase-dependent pathway by activating caspase-3 [5–10,22,23]. More specifically, Singh et al. [24] reported that usnic acid inhibits the growth of A549 human lung carcinoma cells and induces cell-cycle arrest and apoptosis. In addition, recent reports showed that the anti-cancer activity of lethal doses of protolichesterinic acid in several cancer cell lines acts via induction of apoptosis through inhibition of the expression of protein Hsp70 in prostate cancer cell lines and activation of caspase-3 in HeLa cell lines [10,11]. Salazinic acid was also reported to have cytotoxic effects on several cancer cell lines, such as FemX (human melanoma) and LS174 (human colon carcinoma) cells [25]. In this study, the acetone extract of lichen thalli and usnic acid at lethal doses showed selective cytotoxicity to several cancer cell lines by inducing apoptosis; however, the acetone extract showed more potent cytotoxic effects on the tested cancer cell lines than usnic acid alone. This finding suggests that additional compounds of the lichen such as protolichesterinic and salazinic acid may contribute to the cytotoxic effects of the acetone extract.

There are many examples of compounds derived from natural products possessing inhibitory activity on invasion and metastasis [26–28]. However, nothing is known from lichen species. Instead, strong wound closure effect was observed in HaCaT cells (human keratinocyte) in the presence of sub-lethal doses of usnic acid and gyrophoric acid suggesting its possible role in tissue regeneration

[29]. Sub-lethal doses of the acetone extract of *F. cucullata* and usnic acid inhibited tumorigenesis and motility of cancer cell lines. Investigation of the expression of intracellular signaling markers involved in the metastatic pathway showed that the extract suppressed the expression of EMT markers and inhibited phosphorylation of Akt. Similar to our findings of the synergistic effects with several compounds (e.g., salazinic acid) of the extract on apoptosis at lethal doses, the acetone extract also exerted more potent inhibition of markers of the metastatic pathway compared to usnic acid alone. Recently, Song et al. reported that usnic acid at sub-lethal doses suppressed the angiogenic potential in a mouse xenograft tumor model and significantly inhibited endothelial cell proliferation, migration and tube formation by inhibiting pAKT and pERK1/2 levels in endothelial cells [30]. Consistently, our results showed that usnic acid also decreased pAKT and pERK1/2 level in A549 cells (Fig. 8). However, the potent effects of the acetone extract of *F. cucullata* was not observed in decreasing pAKT level suggesting that inhibition of EMT is more prominent by the acetone extract of *F. cucullata* and act a crucial role in the inhibition of tumorigenesis and motility of cancer cells.

In this study, our present results suggest that usnic acid plays a major role in the regulation of apoptosis, tumorigenesis, and motility of cancer cells, while additional subcomponents such as salazinic acid synergistically exert anti-cancer activity against the cancer cells alongside usnic acid. In this regards, our findings add novel insight into an anti-cancer activity of lichen species. First, as the acetone extract of lichen thalli and usnic acid showed either selective cytotoxicity or inhibitory activity on tumorigenesis and motility of cancer cells at lethal or sub-lethal doses, respectively, selective cytotoxicity to cancer cells might be obtained via dose-adjustment of the acetone extract of lichen thalli and suggest that this novel anti-cancer chemotherapeutic agent can be used as a selective and effective agent against various cancers. Second, as the acetone extract of lichen thalli showed more potent cytotoxic effects on the tested cancer cells than usnic acid alone, whole acetone extract of lichen thalli may be more effective as a new therapeutic agent than usnic acid alone in treating cancer patients. Therefore, these findings support a rationale for combined using of additional compounds of the lichen as well as usnic acid to improve responses to anti-cancer therapy in patients resistant to routine cancer chemotherapy. Further study is required to reveal additional molecular mechanisms underlying the anti-cancer activity of the lichen species and their secondary metabolites.

Supporting Information

File S1 Includes Figure S1, Tables S1–S3. **Figure S1.** In vivo tumorigenicity assay using A549 cells pretreated with DMSO, acetone extract of *F. cucullata*, usnic acid, or lichesterinic acid. A549 cells were pretreated with DMSO, *F. cucullata* (5 μg/mL), Usnic acid (10 μM) or Lichesterinic acid (10 μM) before injection. Pictures were taken after 28 days of subcutaneous cell injections. **Table S1.** IC_{50} values of the acetone extract from thalli of the Romania lichens. **Table S2.** Mass spectrometry of the *Flavocetraria cucullata* acetone extract. **Table S3.** IC_{50} values of the acetone extract of *F. cucullata* and usnic acid, lichesterinic acid, on various cancer cells.

Author Contributions

Conceived and designed the experiments: JSH HK. Performed the experiments: TTN SY YY HBL. Analyzed the data: TTN CM KYL KKK HK. Contributed reagents/materials/analysis tools: SO MHJ JJK STY FC. Contributed to the writing of the manuscript: TTN JSH HK.

References

1. WHO (2013) World Health Statistics 2013.
2. Siegel R, Naishadham D, Jemal A (2013) Cancer statistics, 2013. CA Cancer J Clin 63: 11–30.
3. Nash TH (2008) Lichen biology. Cambridge; New York: Cambridge University Press. ix, 486 p.
4. Fashelt D (1994) Secondary biochemistry of lichens. Symbiosis 16: 117–165.
5. Shrestha G, St. Clair LL (2013) Lichens: a promising source of antibiotic and anticancer drugs. Phytochem Rev 12: 229–244.
6. Kupchan SM, Kopperman HL (1975) l-usnic acid: tumor inhibitor isolated from lichens. Experientia 31: 625.
7. Takai M, Uehara Y, Beisler JA (1979) Usnic acid derivatives as potential antineoplastic agents. J Med Chem 22: 1380–1384.
8. Cardarelli M, Serino G, Campanella L, Ercole P, De Cicco Nardone F, et al. (1997) Antimitotic effects of usnic acid on different biological systems. Cell Mol Life Sci 53: 667–672.
9. Kumar KC, Muller K (1999) Lichen metabolites. 1. Inhibitory action against leukotriene B4 biosynthesis by a non-redox mechanism. J Nat Prod 62: 817–820.
10. Haraldsdottir S, Guolaugsdottir E, Ingolfsdottir K, Ogmundsdottir HM (2004) Anti-proliferative effects of lichen-derived lipoxygenase inhibitors on twelve human cancer cell lines of different tissue origin in vitro. Planta Med 70: 1098–1100.
11. Russo A, Caggia S, Piovano M, Garbarino J, Cardile V (2012) Effect of vicanicin and protolichesterinic acid on human prostate cancer cells: role of Hsp70 protein. Chem Biol Interact 195: 1–10.
12. Ren MR, Hur JS, Kim JY, Park KW, Park SC, et al. (2009) Anti-proliferative effects of Lethariella zahlbruckneri extracts in human HT-29 human colon cancer cell lines. Food Chem Toxicol 47: 2157–2162.
13. Molnar K, Farkas E (2010) Current results on biological activities of lichen secondary metabolites: a review. Z Naturforsch C 65: 157–173.
14. Shukla V, Joshi GP, Rawat MSM (2010) Lichens as a potential natural source of bioactive compounds: a review. Phytochem Rev 9: 303–314.
15. Zambare VP, Christopher LP (2012) Biopharmaceutical potential of lichens. Pharm Biol 50: 778–798.
16. Franken NA, Rodermond HM, Stap J, Haveman J, van Bree C (2006) Clonogenic assay of cells in vitro. Nat Protoc 1: 2315–2319.
17. Kim H, Ki H, Park HS, Kim K (2005) Presenilin-1 D257A and D385A mutants fail to cleave Notch in their endoproteolyzed forms, but only presenilin-1 D385A mutant can restore its gamma-secretase activity with the compensatory overexpression of normal C-terminal fragment. J Biol Chem 280: 22462–22472.
18. Chang L, Karin M (2001) Mammalian MAP kinase signalling cascades. Nature 410: 37–40.
19. Fulton RJ, McDade RL, Smith PL, Kienker IJ, Kettman JR, Jr. (1997) Advanced multiplexed analysis with the FlowMetrix system. Clin Chem 43: 1749–1756.
20. Gingrich JC, Davis DR, Nguyen Q (2000) Multiplex detection and quantitation of proteins on western blots using fluorescent probes. Biotechniques 29: 636–642.
21. Backor M, Pawlik-Skowronska B, Tomko J, Budova J, Sanita di Toppi L (2006) Response to copper stress in aposymbiotically grown lichen mycobiont Cladonia cristatella: uptake, viability, ergosterol and production of non-protein thiols. Mycol Res 110: 994–999.
22. Mayer M, O'Neill MA, Murray KE, Santos-Magalhaes NS, Carneiro-Leao AM, et al. (2005) Usnic acid: a non-genotoxic compound with anti-cancer properties. Anticancer Drugs 16: 805–809.
23. Backorova M, Jendzelovsky R, Kello M, Backor M, Mikes J, et al. (2012) Lichen secondary metabolites are responsible for induction of apoptosis in HT-29 and A2780 human cancer cell lines. Toxicol In Vitro 26: 462–468.
24. Singh N, Nambiar D, Kale RK, Singh RP (2013) Usnic acid inhibits growth and induces cell cycle arrest and apoptosis in human lung carcinoma A549 cells. Nutr Cancer 65 Suppl 1: 36–43.
25. Manojlovic N, Rankovic B, Kosanic M, Vasiljevic P, Stanojkovic T (2012) Chemical composition of three Parmelia lichens and antioxidant, antimicrobial and cytotoxic activities of some their major metabolites. Phytomedicine 19: 1166–1172.
26. Pavese JM, Farmer RL, Bergan RC (2010) Inhibition of cancer cell invasion and metastasis by genistein. Cancer Metastasis Rev 29: 465–482.
27. Lecomte N, Njardarson JT, Nagorny P, Yang G, Downey R, et al. (2011) Emergence of potent inhibitors of metastasis in lung cancer via syntheses based on migrastatin. Proc Natl Acad Sci U S A 108: 15074–15078.
28. Wang J, Tan XF, Nguyen VS, Yang P, Zhou J, et al. (2014) A quantitative chemical proteomics approach to profile the specific cellular targets of

andrographolide, a promising anticancer agent that suppresses tumor metastasis. Mol Cell Proteomics 13: 876–886.
29. Burlando B, Ranzato E, Volante A, Appendino G, Pollastro F, et al. (2009) Antiproliferative effects on tumour cells and promotion of keratinocyte wound healing by different lichen compounds. Planta Med 75: 607–613.
30. Song Y, Dai F, Zhai D, Dong Y, Zhang J, et al. (2012) Usnic acid inhibits breast tumor angiogenesis and growth by suppressing VEGFR2-mediated AKT and ERK1/2 signaling pathways. Angiogenesis 15: 421–432.

Fasting Enhances TRAIL-Mediated Liver Natural Killer Cell Activity via HSP70 Upregulation

Vu T. A. Dang[1], Kazuaki Tanabe[1]*, Yuka Tanaka[1], Noriaki Tokumoto[2], Toshihiro Misumi[1], Yoshihiro Saeki[1], Nobuaki Fujikuni[1], Hideki Ohdan[1]

1 Department of Gastroenterological and Transplant Surgery, Applied Life Sciences, Institute of Biomedical and Health Sciences, Hiroshima University, Hiroshima, Japan,
2 Department of Surgery, Hiroshima City Hospital, Hiroshima, Japan

Abstract

Acute starvation, which is frequently observed in clinical practice, sometimes augments the cytolytic activity of natural killer cells against neoplastic cells. In this study, we investigated the molecular mechanisms underlying the enhancement of natural killer cell function by fasting in mice. The total number of liver resident natural killer cells in a unit weight of liver tissue obtained from C57BL/6J mice did not change after a 3-day fast, while the proportions of tumor necrosis factor–related apoptosis-inducing ligand (TRAIL)$^+$ and CD69$^+$ natural killer cells were significantly elevated (n = 7, p <0.01), as determined by flow cytometric analysis. Furthermore, we found that TRAIL$^-$ natural killer cells that were adoptively transferred into Rag-2$^{-/-}$ γ chain$^{-/-}$ mice could convert into TRAIL$^+$ natural killer cells in fasted mice at a higher proportion than in fed mice. Liver natural killer cells also showed high TRAIL-mediated antitumor function in response to 3-day fasting. Since these fasted mice highly expressed heat shock protein 70 (n = 7, p <0.05) in liver tissues, as determined by western blot, the role of this protein in natural killer cell activation was investigated. Treatment of liver lymphocytes with 50 μg/mL of recombinant heat shock protein 70 led to the upregulation of both TRAIL and CD69 in liver natural killer cells (n = 6, p < 0.05). In addition, HSP70 neutralization by intraperitoneally injecting an anti-heat shock protein 70 monoclonal antibody into mice prior to fasting led to the downregulation of TRAIL expression (n = 6, p <0.05). These findings indicate that acute fasting enhances TRAIL-mediated liver natural killer cell activity against neoplastic cells through upregulation of heat shock protein 70.

Editor: Jianhua Yu, The Ohio State University, United States of America

Funding: This work was supported by Grants-in-Aid for Scientific Research C (25461949 and 25462023) from the Japan Society for the Promotion of Science and Research on Hepatitis, and BSE grant from the Japanese Ministry of Health, Labor, and Welfare. The funders had no role in study design, data collection and analysis, decision to publish, or preparation of the manuscript.

Competing Interests: The authors have declared that no competing interests exist.

* Email: ktanabe2@hiroshima-u.ac.jp

Introduction

Natural killer (NK) cells, the front-line defense for the immune system, do not require priming to exert their effector function on neoplastic cells, modified cells, and invading infectious microbes [1–3]. Although it has been demonstrated that acute starvation, which is frequently observed in clinical practice, sometimes augments the cytolytic activity of NK cells against neoplastic cells [4], the molecular mechanisms underlying this phenomenon remain unclear. In addition, few studies have addressed the question of whether such augmentation of NK cell activity by nutritional alteration is of practical benefit.

It has been shown that many transformed cells, including virus-infected and tumor cells, can be attacked by tumor necrosis factor–related apoptosis-inducing ligand (TRAIL)-expressing NK cells [5–8]. A variety of mechanisms are involved in the control of neoplastic cells by NK cells. One is the direct release of cytolytic granules containing perforin, granzymes, and granulysin via the granule exocytosis pathway [1,2]. Another mechanism is mediated by death-inducing ligands such as Fas ligand (FasL) and TRAIL [2,6,8].

TRAIL, an Apo2 ligand, is a type II transmembrane protein belonging to the TNF family. There are 5 TRAIL receptors: two can induce apoptotic signals and the others act as decoy receptors [6,9,10]. The ligation of TRAIL on NK cells with its two apoptotic receptors, TRAIL receptor 1 (death receptor 4) and TRAIL receptor 2 (death receptor 5), on target cells is an important mechanism of target cell lysis via the extrinsic pathway of apoptosis (as opposed to the mitochondrial pathway of apoptosis) [6,7,9].

Heat shock proteins (HSPs) are overproduced in many stressful conditions, including fasting. They are also involved in immune cell activation [11–15]. In particular, extracellular HSP70 is involved in immune stimulation [11,14,16,17]. HSP70 is expressed on the surface of some tumor cells and acts as a recognition structure for NK cells, promoting NK cell cytotoxicity [18–20]. Furthermore, in some stressful situations, HSP70 is actively released in the extracellular space as a soluble protein or bound to exosomes to activate antigen-presenting cells [21] or NK cells [18,22]. It has also been shown that recombinant HSP70 can stimulate the proliferation and antitumor function of NK cells [19].

Based on these studies, we hypothesized that acute starvation may lead to the enhancement of NK cell activity against neoplastic cells by inducing the expression of HSP70. In this study, we show that both the proportion of TRAIL$^+$ NK cells and the expression of HSP70 were significantly elevated in the liver of fasted mice. Moreover, treatment of liver NK cells with recombinant HSP70 upregulated both TRAIL and CD69 expression, and neutralization of HSP70 in fasted mice by intraperitoneal injection of an anti-HSP70 monoclonal antibody downregulated TRAIL expression. Thus, our findings indicate that acute fasting enhances TRAIL-mediated liver NK cell activity against neoplastic cells through upregulating HSP70.

Materials and Methods

Ethics statements

This study was performed in strict accordance with the Guide for the Care and Use of Laboratory Animals and the local committee for animal experiments. The experimental protocol was approved by the Ethics Review Committee for Animal Experimentation of the Graduate School of Biomedical Sciences, Hiroshima University (Permit Number: A13-112). Surgery was performed under diethyl ether anesthesia, and all efforts were made to minimize the suffering of the mice.

Mice and fasting protocol

C57BL/6J (B6) female mice aged 8–10 weeks were purchased from CLEA Japan, Inc. (Osaka, Japan). B6-based Rag-2$^{-/-}$ γ chain$^{-/-}$ mice aged 8–12 weeks were purchased from Taconic Farms (Hudson, NY, USA). The mice were housed in the animal facility of Hiroshima University, Japan, in a pathogen-free, microisolated environment. Prior to the start of the fasting experiments, mice were allowed *ad libitum* access to food. During the fasting experiments, the mice in the control group were allowed *ad libitum* access to food and fasted mice were deprived of food for 1 or 3 days. All mice were allowed free access to water. Mouse body weight was checked every day until the day of sacrifice. Liver weight was determined on the day of sacrifice.

Lymphocyte isolation

After mice were anesthetized by diethyl ether, peripheral blood from the orbital sinus was collected into heparinized tubes. The peripheral blood cells (PBCs) were collected by centrifugation and red blood cells were removed using ammonium chloride potassium (ACK) lysing buffer. Liver lymphocytes were prepared according to a previously described method [23]. In brief, after injection of 1 mL phosphate-buffered saline (PBS) supplemented with 10% heparin via the portal vein, the liver was dissected out and perfused with 50 mL PBS supplemented with 0.1% ethylenediamine tetraacetic acid. Blood cells were harvested from the liver perfusate by centrifugation and erythrocytes were then removed using the ACK lysing buffer. Splenic lymphocytes were prepared as a single cell suspension by gently crushing the spleens in PBS and the erythrocytes were removed by treatment with the ACK buffer. The bone marrow cells were harvested by flushing the femurs and tibias with PBS, lymphocytes were then harvested after centrifuging and lysing red blood cells with ACK buffer. All lymphocytes were stored in RPMI medium for culture, ^{51}Cr-release assay or in fluorescence-activated cell sorting (FACS) buffer to determine their phenotype by flow cytometry.

Flow cytometric analysis

The lymphocytes were first incubated with an anti-CD16/32 (2.4G2) antibody to block nonspecific Fc-γ receptor binding and then stained with the following monoclonal antibodies (mAbs): fluorescein isothiocyanate (FITC) or BD Horizon BV421-conjugated anti-mouse NK1.1 (PK136), allophycocyanin (APC) or APC-Cy7-conjugated anti-mouse TCR-β chain (H57-597), FITC-conjugated anti-mouse CD49b (DX5) or rat IgM, k isotype control (R4-22), Alexa Fluor 647-conjugated anti-mouse CD49a (Ha31/8) or IgG2, λ1 isotype control (Ha4/8), phycoerythrin (PE)-conjugated anti-mouse CD253 (TRAIL; N2B2), CD69 (H1.2F3), CD122 (TM-Beta1), CD25 (3C7), CD314 (NKG2D; CX5), CD335 (NKp46; 29A1.4), CD178 (Fas Ligand; MFL3), or PE-conjugated mouse immunoglobulin G (IgG) 2a,k as the isotype-matched control antibody. Liver lymphocytes were also stained simultaneously with PE-Cy7 anti-mouse CD69 (H1.2F3) or PE-Cy7 Hamster IgG1, λ1 isotype control to analyze the relation between TRAIL and CD69 under fasting conditions. The apoptosis-related markers on Hepa1-6 cells were also analyzed using PE-conjugated anti-mouse CD95 (Fas/APO-1; Jo2), anti-mouse CD262 (DR5; MD5-1), anti-mouse decoy TRAIL-receptor 1 (mDcR1-3) and 2 (mDcR2-1), or PE-conjugated IgG2, λ1 isotype control antibody. All antibodies were purchased from BD Biosciences, except for CD253 (TRAIL) and CD262 (DR5) (eBioscience) and anti-mouse decoy TRAIL-receptor 1 and 2 antibodies (BioLegend). Dead cells were excluded by light scatter and propidium iodide or 7-AAD staining. Depending on the number of dyes to be detected, flow cytometric analyses were performed using the FACSCalibur (BD Biosciences), BD FACS-Canto II flow cytometer (BD Biosciences), or the BD LSRFortessa X-20 (BD Biosciences). Data were analyzed using FlowJo 7.6.5 software (TreeStar, San Carlos, CA, USA).

Isolation of NK cells and adoptive transfer assay

Liver leukocytes were obtained from wild type B6 mice. Liver NK cells were then negatively separated by using a mouse NK cell isolation kit II (Miltenyi Biotec, Auburn, CA, USA). TRAIL$^-$ NK cells were further sorted magnetically using biotin-conjugated anti-mouse CD253 (TRAIL; N2B2; eBioscience) and streptavidin microbeads (Miltenyi Biotec) in the negative fraction. The purity of isolated TRAIL$^-$ NK cells was assessed by flow cytometry. The liver TRAIL$^-$ NK cells were intravenously injected into Rag-2$^{-/-}$ γ chain$^{-/-}$ mice (0.5×10^6 cells/mouse). The transferred mice were then divided into two groups. The fasted mice received only water and fed mice received both food and water for 3 days. The lymphocytes from the liver, spleen, and bone marrow of transferred or non-transferred (control) mice were harvested after the fasting period, and NK cell phenotyping was performed.

Cytotoxicity assay

Mouse lymphoma cells (YAC-1) and mouse hepatoma cells (Hepa1-6), both purchased from the RIKEN Cell Bank (Tsukuba, Japan), were used as the target cells. The effector cells were fresh liver lymphocytes obtained from fed (control) mice and mice that had been fasted for 3 days. The YAC-1 and Hepa1-6 cells were labeled with Na$_2$[^{51}Cr]O$_4$ and then incubated with the effector cells in round-bottomed 96-well plates for 4 hours. The culture medium was RPMI 1640 (Gibco BRL, Grand Island, NY, USA) supplemented with 10% heat-inactivated fetal bovine serum (Sanko Chemical Co. Ltd., Tokyo, Japan), 100 IU/mL penicillin, 100 μg/mL streptomycin (Gibco BRL), 1 mM sodium pyruvate, and 1 mM nonessential amino acids (NEAA; Gibco, Grand Island, NY, USA). For the control, target cells were incubated either in culture medium to determine spontaneous release or in a

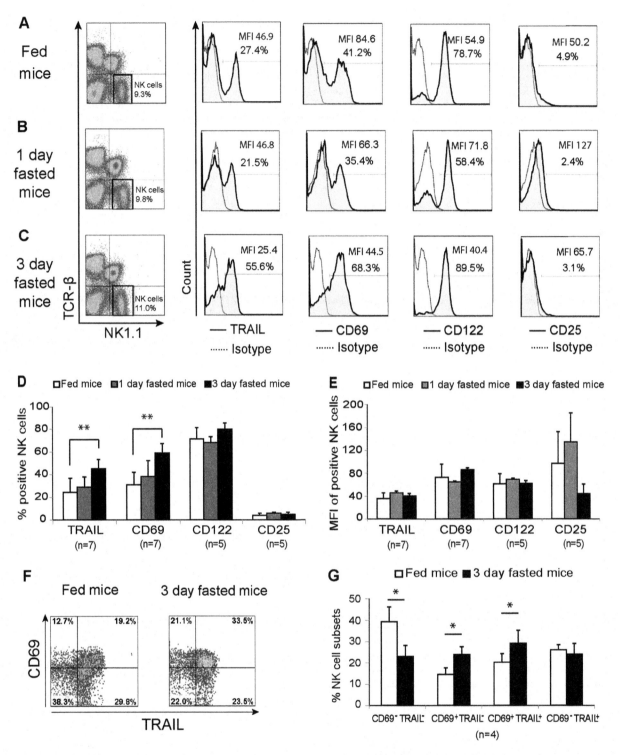

Figure 1. **Phenotype of liver natural killer cells under starvation.** Isolated liver lymphocytes from 3 mouse groups were stained with monoclonal antibodies against the cell surface markers TRAIL, CD69, CD122, and CD25 prior to analysis by flow cytometry. Representative natural killer (NK) cell phenotype analyses from (A) fed, (B) 1-day-fasted and (C) 3-day-fasted mice are presented in dot plots and histograms. TCRβ$^-$ NK1.1$^+$ cells were gated as NK cells. The dotted lines represent the negative control. The distribution of TRAIL, CD69, CD122, and CD25 expression in NK cells is indicated by the solid lines (shaded areas) and the percentage and mean fluorescence intensity (MFI) of positive cells are provided. (D) The percentages or (E) MFI of liver NK cells that are positive for TRAIL, CD69, CD122, and CD25 are shown in bar graphs as mean plus standard deviation. (F) Dot plots of representative data and (G) bar graph present the mean plus standard deviation of proportion of NK cell subsets regarding to TRAIL and CD69 expression in fed and fasted mice; *p <0.05, **p <0.01 as analyzed by the independent samples T test.

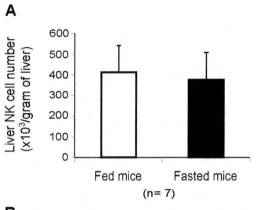
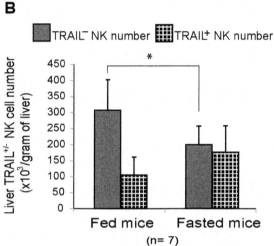
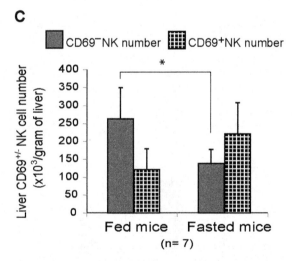

Figure 2. Distribution of TRAIL and CD69 expression in liver natural killer cells in response to starvation. Liver lymphocytes from fed mice and 3-day-fasted mice were stained with monoclonal antibodies and counted using flow cytometry. Numbers of (A) TCRβ⁻ NK1.1⁺ natural killer (NK) cells, (B) TRAIL$^{+/-}$ NK cells, and (C) CD69$^{+/-}$ NK cells per gram of liver tissue are presented in bar graphs as mean plus standard deviation (n = 7); *$p < 0.05$ as analyzed by the independent samples T test.

mixture of 2% Nonidet P-40 to define the maximum ^{51}Cr release. For the blocking assay, the effector cells were pre-incubated for 1 hour at 37°C with 50 nM concanamycin A (CMA; Sigma-Aldrich, Saint Louis, MO, USA), and/or 10 μg/mL anti-mouse CD253 (TRAIL; N2B2; eBioscience), and/or 10 μg/mL anti-mouse CD178 (FasL; MFL3; BD Biosciences), or the isotype-matched controls. Cell-free supernatants were carefully harvested and the radioactivity from the ^{51}Cr that had been released into the supernatants was measured using a gamma counter (Aloka ARC-380). The cytotoxicity percentage, as indicated by ^{51}Cr release, was calculated using the following equation: percent cytotoxicity = [(cpm of experimental release − cpm of spontaneous release)] / [(cpm of maximum release − cpm of spontaneous release)] × 100.

Western blotting

Western blotting was performed to detect HSP70, HSP27, and β-actin expression in liver tissues. For each sample, 5 mg of fresh or frozen liver tissue from either fed mice or mice that had been fasted for 3 days was homogenized in 1 mL NP-40 lysis buffer (containing 1 μL leupeptin, 1 μL aprotinin, and 10 μL 100 mM phenylmethylsulfonyl fluoride). The lysates were centrifuged at 15,000 g for 15 minutes at 4°C. The supernatant was then harvested, and its protein concentration was determined using a spectrophotometer (NanoDrop 2000c). The sample was then mixed with 3× SDS solution (containing 960 μL 3× Laemmli buffer and 60 μL 2-mercaptoethanol per milliliter) and boiled at 100°C for 10 minutes. For each sample, 5 mg of fresh or frozen liver tissue from either fed mice or mice that had been fasted for 3 days was homogenized in 1 mL NP-40 lysis buffer (containing 1 μL leupeptin, 1 μL aprotinin, and 10 μL 100 mM phenyl-methylsulfonyl fluoride). The lysates were centrifuged at 15,000 g for 15 minutes at 4°C. The supernatant was then harvested, and its protein concentration was determined using a spectrophotometer (NanoDrop 2000c). The sample was then mixed with 3× SDS solution (containing 960 μL 3× Laemmli buffer and 60 μL 2-mercaptoethanol per milliliter) and boiled at 100°C for 10 minutes. For each sample, 10 μg protein was resolved by electrophoresis on 10% polyacrylamide gels with 0.1% SDS and transferred to nitrocellulose transfer membranes (Schleicher & Schuell, Keene, NH, USA), which were then incubated with an anti-HSP70 mAb (C92F3A-5; SMC-100A, StressMarq Biosciences Inc., Victoria, BC, Canada), an anti-HSP27 mAb (G3.1; ADI-SPA-800, Enzo Life Sciences), or an anti-β-actin mAb (6D1, MBL). Blots were then incubated with a peroxidase-labeled goat anti-mouse immunoglobulin antibody (NA 931; Amersham International, Buckinghamshire, UK) and developed using X-ray film and an enhanced chemiluminescence detection reagent (Amersham Pharmacia Biotech). The band density on the X-ray film was quantified using ImageJ software (NIH, Bethesda, MD, USA).

Treatment of liver lymphocytes with recombinant HSP70

Liver lymphocytes (2 million/well) isolated from fed B6 mice were cultured with recombinant mouse HSP70-A1 (ADI-SPP-502, Enzo Life Sciences) at different concentrations (0 μg/mL as the control or 0.5, 5, and 50 μg/mL) with or without 20 ng/mL recombinant mouse interleukin (IL)-2 (eBioscience) in RPMI 1640 supplemented with 10% fetal bovine serum, 100 IU/mL penicillin, 100 μg/mL streptomycin (Gibco BRL, Carlsbad, CA, USA), 1 mM sodium pyruvate, and 1 mM NEAA (Gibco BRL). After 2, 3, or 5 days of culture, the lymphocytes were harvested and the NK cell phenotype was analyzed by flow cytometry.

HSP70 inhibition by anti-HSP70 antibody *in vivo*

Eight-week-old B6 female mice were intraperitoneally injected with 200 μL PBS containing 100 μg of either mouse anti-HSP70 mAb (clone C92F3A-5; without sodium azide; StressMarq

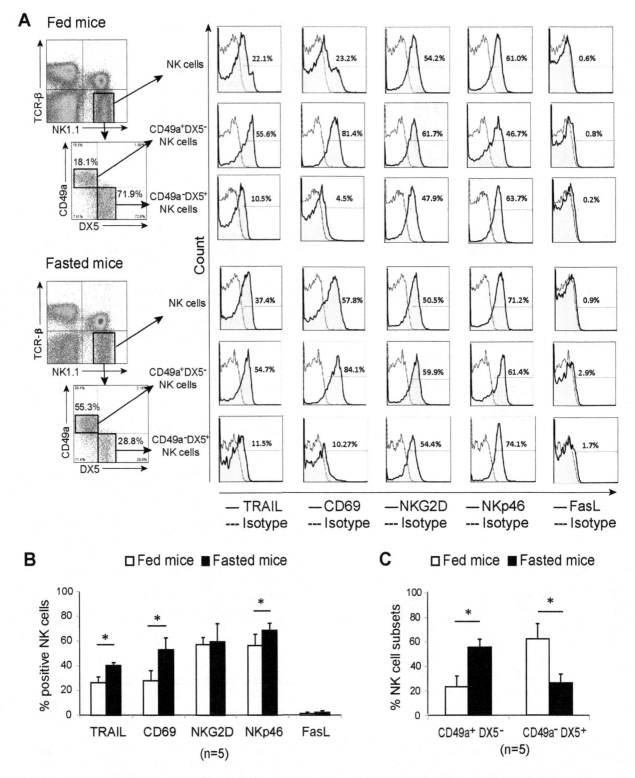

Figure 3. Analysis of functional markers in liver natural killer cells and their CD49a$^+$ DX5$^-$ and CD49a$^-$ DX5$^+$ subgroups. Liver lymphocytes from fed and 3-day-fasted mice were simultaneously stained with monoclonal antibodies against DX5, CD49a, TRAIL, CD69, NKG2D, NKp46, and FasL. (A) Representative dot plots of gated TCRβ$^-$ NK1.1$^+$ natural killer (NK) cells and its two subsets, CD49a$^+$ DX5$^-$ and CD49a$^-$ DX5$^+$ NK cells, in fed and fasted mice are presented. Histograms show the expression of TRAIL, CD69, NKG2D, NKp46, and FasL (solid lines) on whole NK cells and their subsets with the percentage of NK cells that are positive for those markers, dotted lines present negative control. (B) Bar graph shows the mean percentage plus standard deviation of NK cells that are positive for TRAIL, CD69, NKG2D, NKp46, or FasL. (C) The proportion of NK cell subsets, CD49a$^+$ DX5$^-$ and CD49a$^-$ DX5$^+$ NK cells, in fed and fasted mice are shown as mean ratio plus standard deviation; *p <0.05 as analyzed by the independent samples T test.

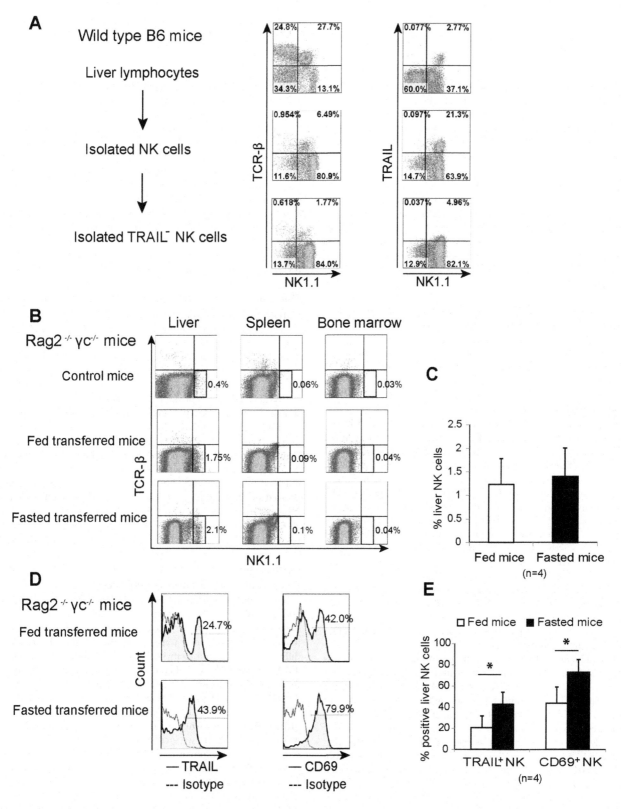

Figure 4. Adoptive transfer assay for TRAIL and CD69 expression on liver natural killer cells in response to starvation. (A) Isolated TRAIL⁻ natural killer (NK) cells were separated from liver lymphocytes of wild type B6 mice. Proportion of lymphocytes expressing TCRβ, NK1.1, and TRAIL in whole liver lymphocytes, isolated NK cells, and isolated TRAIL⁻ NK cells are presented in dot plots. The isolated TRAIL⁻ NK cells were adoptively transferred into Rag-2$^{-/-}$ γ chain$^{-/-}$ mice (0.5×10^6 cells/mouse), which were then fed or fasted for 3 days before determining their NK phenotype. (B) Dot plots show the gated TCRβ⁻ NK1.1⁺ NK cells and their percentage in the liver, spleen, and bone marrow of non-transferred (control), fed-transferred, and fasted-transferred mice. (C) Bar graph presents the mean percentage plus standard deviation of NK cells in the liver of fed and fasted-transferred mice. (D) Expression of TRAIL and CD69 (solid lines) on the liver NK cells of representative fed- and fasted-transferred mice

with their percentages of positive cells are presented in histograms; dotted lines showed the negative control. (E) The proportion of liver TRAIL$^+$ and CD69$^+$ NK cells in fed and fasted-transferred mice are shown in bar graph as mean plus standard deviation; *p <0.05 as analyzed by the independent samples T test.

Biosciences Inc.) or a mouse IgG isotype-matched control antibody (Jackson ImmunoResearch Laboratories Inc.) just before fasting (6 mice per group). Mouse body weight was measured every day. After fasting for 3 days, the mice were sacrificed, and their liver lymphocytes were harvested to determine TRAIL and CD69 expression on NK cells by flow cytometry.

Statistical analysis

Data are presented as mean plus standard deviation or standard error of the mean. The statistical differences between 2 groups were analyzed using an independent samples T test (2-tailed) in SPSS Statistics version 16.0 (IBM, Rockford, IL, USA); p-values of 0.05 or less were considered to indicate significance.

Results

The proportion of TRAIL$^+$ and CD69$^+$ NK cells increased in mouse livers in response to starvation

The phenotypic characteristics of NK cells in mice that had been fasted for 1–3 days were examined by flow cytometry. Liver lymphocytes from both fed and fasted mice were harvested and stained with various antibodies to identify the membrane markers TRAIL, CD69, CD122 (IL-2 receptor β chain), and CD25 (IL-2 receptor α chain).

Electronically gated TCRβ$^-$ NK1.1$^+$ NK cells and NK cell markers from a representative fed, 1-day-fasted, or 3-day-fasted mouse are shown in Figure 1 A–C. Notably, compared to fed mice, 3-day-fasted mice showed significantly higher proportions of TRAIL and CD69 in liver NK cells (Figure 1D). Mean fluorescence intensity (MFI) of TRAIL or CD69 positive NK cells showed no significant differences among the groups (Figure 1E). Next, the distribution analysis of CD69 and TRAIL expression revealed that the proportion of CD69$^+$TRAIL$^+$ double positive NK cells significantly increased in fasted mice, while CD69$^-$TRAIL$^-$ NK cells significantly decreased. The proportion of CD69$^+$ TRAIL$^-$ cells also increased (Figure 1F, G). There was no difference in CD122 and CD25 expression in liver NK cells among the groups (Figure 1D, E) as well as in splenic NK cells (data not shown). The proportion of NK cells in the liver mononuclear cell fractions from 3-day-fasted mice did not differ from that from fed mice (Figure S1A).

The influence of fasting on the absolute number of NK cells was also examined. The total number of liver resident NK cells in a unit weight of liver tissue did not differ between fasted and fed mice, indicating that, under fasting conditions, the number of TRAIL$^-$ NK cells decreased, while that of TRAIL$^+$ NK cells increased (Figure 2A, B).

Analysis of other functional markers of NK cells indicated that whole liver NK cells from 3-day fasted mice highly expressed not only TRAIL and CD69 but also NKp46 when compared with fed mice. There was no significant difference in NKG2D or FasL expression (Figure 3A, B). Additionally, changes in CD49a and DX5 phenotype characteristics in NK cells were examined based on a report that recently demonstrated that liver-resident CD3$^-$ NK1.1$^+$ NK subsets are characterized according to the differential expression of CD49a and DX5 [24]. While proportions of CD49a$^-$ DX5$^+$ NK cells significantly decreased in fasted mice, the proportion of CD49a$^+$ DX5$^-$ NK cells, which highly expressed TRAIL and CD69, significantly increased (Figure 3A,

C). Taken together, our results indicate that, under 3-day fasting, TRAIL and CD69 are highly expressed in mouse liver-resident CD49a$^+$ DX5$^-$ NK cells.

The phenotypic characteristics of NK cells in the spleen, bone marrow, and peripheral blood were also examined under starvation (Figure S1A-G). The proportion of NK cells did not differ in the spleen as well as in the liver, while it increased in the bone marrow and decreased in peripheral blood under fasting conditions (Figure S1A). Splenic NK cells from fasted mice showed a trend similar to that of liver NK cells in terms of CD69 expression, but NK cells in other organs did not show a similar trend. Unlike the findings for the liver, the spleens from both fed and fasted mice presented a very low CD49a$^+$ DX5$^-$ NK cell fraction (data not shown).

TRAIL upregulation on liver NK cells in adoptive transferred fasted mice

We next examined the mechanism of TRAIL upregulation in fasted mice. To clarify whether TRAIL$^-$ NK cells convert into TRAIL$^+$ NK cells in fasting mice, we transferred TRAIL$^-$ NK cells that were isolated from liver lymphocytes obtained from wild type B6 mice into Rag-2$^{-/-}$ γ chain$^{-/-}$ B6 mice. The NK cell purity and TRAIL expression rate on the isolated NK cells are shown in Figure 4A. It is noteworthy that these mice present macrophages, but not NK cells or other lymphocytes. The absence of NK cells in Rag-2$^{-/-}$ γ chain$^{-/-}$ mice was analyzed in Figure 4B (control mice). Three days after injection, the injected NK cells homed to the liver, but not to the spleen or the bone marrow (Figure 4B, C). Furthermore, fasted transferred mice showed significantly high expression of TRAIL and CD69 in liver NK cells in comparison with fed transferred mice (Figure 4D, E). These results indicate that TRAIL upregulation is induced in liver-resident NK cells by converting TRAIL$^-$ cells into TRAIL$^+$ cells.

Cytotoxicity of liver lymphocytes against TRAIL-sensitive cancer cells increased in fasted mice

The cytotoxic potential of NK cells against the cell lines YAC-1 and Hepa1-6, which differ in their sensitivity to TRAIL, was determined using the ^{51}Cr release assay. Liver lymphocytes from fed and 3-day-fasted mice were used as the effectors. There was no difference in the cytotoxicity of the two lymphocyte groups against TRAIL-resistant YAC-1 (Figure 5A). However, liver lymphocytes from fasted mice showed significantly higher cytotoxicity against TRAIL-sensitive Hepa1-6 than liver lymphocytes from fed mice at effector: target ratios of 40:1, 20:1, and 10:1 (Figure 5B). To further investigate whether the upregulated cytotoxicity was mediated via TRAIL, we incubated liver lymphocytes from fasted mice with perforin inhibitor (CMA), anti-TRAIL mAb, anti-FasL mAb, or their combination at an effector: target ratio of 40:1. Hepa1-6 receptor expression was also examined. Hepa1-6 cells highly expressed both Fas and death receptor 5 (TRAIL receptor 2) (Figure 5C). Lymphocytes treated with CMA, anti-TRAIL mAb, or their combination presented a significantly reduced cytotoxicity in comparison with the untreated group (Figure 5D). In contrast, the group treated with anti-FasL showed no significant difference. These results indicate that liver NK cells from fasted mice presented an increased perforin- and TRAIL-mediated antitumor activity.

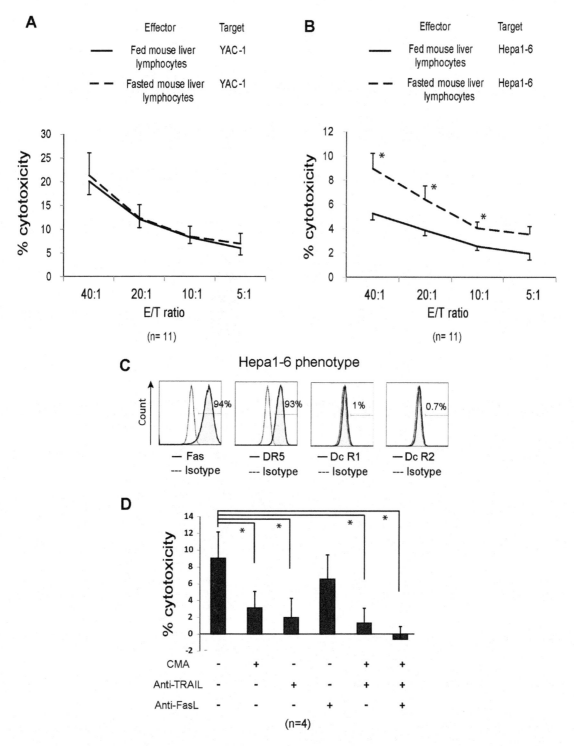

Figure 5. Assay analyzing cytotoxic effects of liver lymphocytes obtained from fasted mice on tumor cells. (A) The cytotoxic activity of freshly isolated liver lymphocytes from fed mice (solid lines) and 3-day-fasted mice (dashed lines) against TRAIL-resistant YAC-1 and (B) TRAIL-sensitive Hepa1-6 cells was analyzed using the ^{51}Cr-release assay. The effector to target (E/T) ratios were 40:1, 20:1, 10:1, and 5:1. The cytotoxicity percentage was calculated as the percentage of specific ^{51}Cr release, as described in the materials and methods section. Data are presented as mean ± standard error of the mean from triplicate samples of 11 repeated assays, each including 1 fed and 1 fasted mouse. (C) Histograms show the phenotype of Hepa1-6 cells that was analyzed using antibodies against mouse Fas, death receptor 5 (DR5), and decoy TRAIL receptor 1 and 2 (DcR1 and DcR2) in solid lines. Negative controls, which were stained with isotype-math antibodies, are indicated using dotted lines. The proportion of Hepa1-6 cells positive for those markers is provided. (D) Liver lymphocytes that were obtained from 3-day-fasted mice were incubated with CMA, anti-TRAIL mAb, anti-FasL mAb, or their combination before incubation with ^{51}Cr-labeled-Hepa1-6 for 4 hours, at a lymphocyte: Hepa1-6 ratio of 40:1. Bar graph shows the mean cytotoxicity percentage plus standard deviation for each group. Statistical analysis was performed for each ratio using the independent samples T test; *$p < 0.05$.

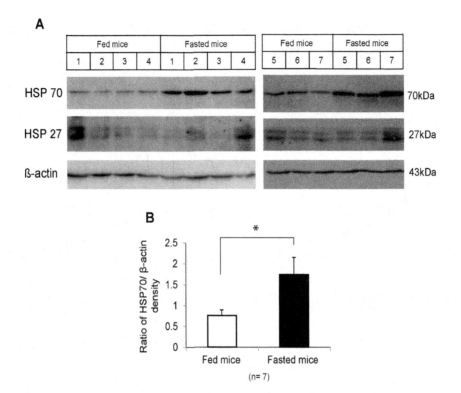

Figure 6. Western blot analysis of heat shock protein expression in fasted mouse livers. (A) Heat shock protein (HSP)70, HSP27, and β-actin expression in the livers from fed mice (control) and 3-day-fasted mice (7 mice in each group) was determined by western blot. (B) The bar graph shows the average HSP70/β-actin densities plus standard error of the mean; densities were analyzed using ImageJ software. Statistical analyses were performed using the independent samples T test. *$p < 0.05$.

Overexpression of HSP70 was induced in livers from fasted mice

It has been demonstrated that HSP70 actively released in the extracellular space activates NK cells [18,22]. Hence, HSPs induced by acute starvation may play a role in TRAIL-mediated antitumor activity. We found that HSP70 expression was significantly higher in 3-day-fasted mouse liver than in fed mouse liver ($p < 0.05$), while HSP27 expression was not changed (Figure 6).

Treatment with recombinant HSP70 induced the proliferation and activation of liver NK cells

The contribution of HSP70 to NK cell activation was assessed *in vitro* by examining the phenotypic characteristics of mouse liver NK cells after culturing liver lymphocytes with IL-2 and different concentrations of recombinant HSP70 (0 μg/mL as the control, 0.5, 5, or 50 μg/mL) for 3 days. Treatment with ≥5 μg/mL HSP70 induced NK cell proliferation ($p < 0.05$; Figure 7B), whereas treatment with 50 μg/mL HSP70 led to an upregulation of TRAIL and CD69 expression in liver NK cells as compared to the control (Figure 7C, D).

Anti-HSP70 neutralizing antibody reduced TRAIL expression in liver NK cells in fasted mice

To further clarify the relationship between HSP70 and TRAIL-mediated NK cell function, an *in vivo* HSP70 neutralization assay was performed. Either an anti-HSP70 mAb or a mouse IgG isotype-matched control antibody was intraperitoneally injected (100 μg per mouse) into mice on day 0 before fasting. After the mice had been fasted for 3 days, their liver lymphocytes were harvested for NK cell phenotypic determination. The two groups of mice did not differ in terms of their body weight or liver lymphocyte yield (data not shown). TRAIL and CD69 expression in the TCRβ$^-$ NK1.1$^+$ NK cells was then assessed by flow cytometry (Figure 8A). Although there was no difference in NK cell frequency between the two groups (Figure 8B), TRAIL expression in liver NK cells from mice injected with the anti-HSP70 mAb was significantly lower than that in cells from the control group (Figure 8C). CD69 expression was also downregulated in cells from mice injected with the anti-HSP70 mAb, but no significance was observed ($p = 0.07$; Figure 8C). MFI of TRAIL or CD69 positive NK cells did not significantly differ between two groups of mice (Figure 8D).

Discussion

Acute starvation is well known to induce physiological changes in the body. Consistent with previous studies [4,25], our study showed a decrease in body weight and liver weight as well as in the number of lymphocytes from various organs in fasted mice as compared to fed mice (Figure S2A–H). Interestingly, we observed that, although the liver weight decreased proportionately with body weight (i.e., the liver:body weight ratio was unchanged), the lymphocyte number notably decreased under starvation.

We previously reported that liver NK cells constitute a unique NK population characterized by high TRAIL expression and high production of perforin, granzymes, and cytokines and have the capacity to kill various kinds of cancer cells, virus-infected cells, or other transformed cells [26,27]. The ligation of TRAIL with death receptor 4 or 5 on target cells induces NK cell activation [7]. On the other hand, CD69, which is a type II transmembrane

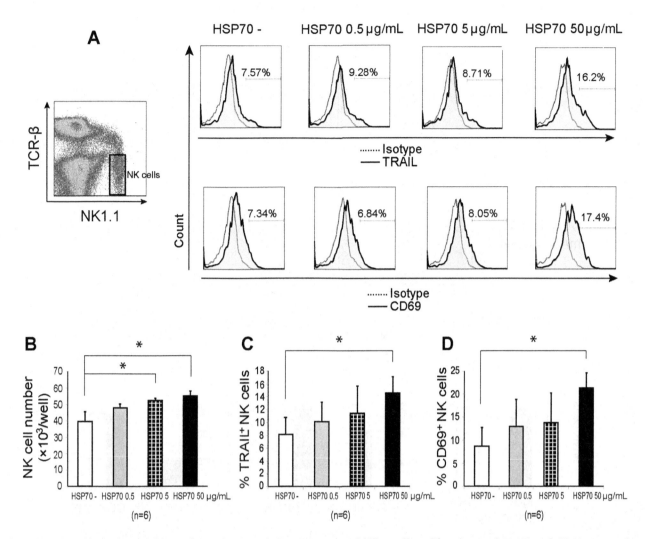

Figure 7. The effect of recombinant heat shock protein 70 on natural killer cell proliferation and TRAIL and CD69 expression. Isolated liver lymphocytes (2 million cells/well) were cultured with mouse recombinant heat shock protein (HSP) 70 at various concentrations: 0, 0.5, 5, or 50 μg/mL. After 3 days of culture, the lymphocytes were harvested for phenotypic determination. (A) Representative flow cytometric analysis of TRAIL and CD69 expression in TCRβ− NK1.1+ natural killer (NK) cells is shown. The dotted lines represent the expression distribution in the negative control cells and the solid lines (shaded areas) with numbers indicate the distribution of TRAIL+ and CD69+ NK cells. (B) TCRβ− NK1.1+ NK cell number per well, (C) TRAIL+ and (D) CD69+ NK cell percentages are shown in bar graphs as mean plus standard deviation (n=6). Data were statistically analyzed using the independent samples T test; *$p < 0.05$.

glycoprotein, is highly induced in many activated lymphocytes, in particular in NK cells [28]. This study represents the first report showing that the proportion of liver-resident NK cells expressing TRAIL and CD69 is significantly higher in fasted mice than in fed mice (Figures 1 and 3). The adoptive transfer assay indicated that TRAIL− NK cells could turn into TRAIL+ NK cells under fasting condition (Figure 4). Taken together with the fact that the total number of liver resident NK cells, including both TRAIL+ and TRAIL−, in a unit weight of liver tissue did not differ between fasted and fed mice (Figure 2), our results confirm that fasting leads to the activation of liver NK cells.

Liver NK cells from fasted mice have previously been demonstrated to have high antitumor activity [4]. However, the mechanism underlying this activity has been entirely unknown. Our study indicates that liver lymphocytes from fasted mice showed high cytotoxicity against TRAIL-sensitive Hepa1-6 cells and related to the TRAIL-mediated apoptotic pathway (Figure 5). Furthermore, these lymphocytes contained a higher proportion of TRAIL+ NK cells than those from fed mice (Figure 1D). In contrast, TRAIL expression in other kind of lymphocytes such as T cells and NKT cells was very low and did not differ between fed and fasted mice (data not shown). These observations suggest that the cytoxicity in liver NK cells from fasted mice is linked to the specific upregulation of TRAIL by acute starvation.

Our result may help understand the innate immune response in post-operative fasted and cachectic patients or patients with other conditions suffering from fasting. Besides many negative effects of starvation, such as fatigue and weight loss, fasting may still exert high level of antitumor effects via TRAIL-mediated NK cell activity. This might provide a new therapeutic approach to activate TRAIL-mediated NK cell activity in patients; further studies are needed in this regard.

Many factors contribute to the regulation of TRAIL expression in NK cells. Interferon gamma (IFN-γ) is one of the most important factor, which can both induce TRAIL expression in NK cells and mediate NK cell cytotoxic activity [8,29,30]. Other

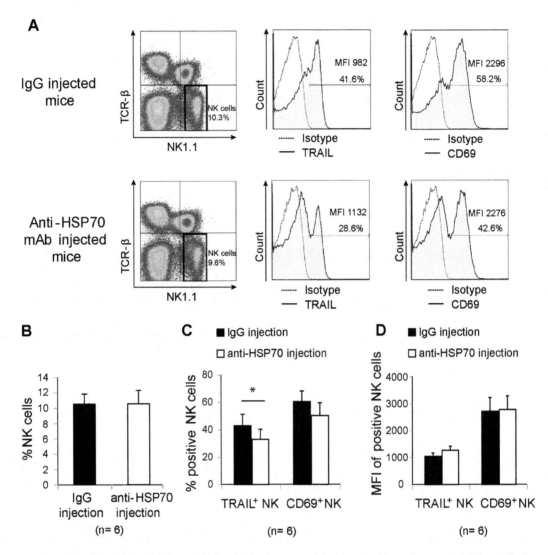

Figure 8. Neutralization effect of an anti-heat shock protein 70 monoclonal antibody on the natural killer cell phenotype. Mice received intraperitoneal injections of an anti-heat shock protein (HSP) 70 monoclonal antibody or isotype-matched mouse immunoglobulin G (6 mice per group) just before fasting. After a 3-day fast, liver lymphocytes were harvested for phenotyping by flow cytometry. (A) The distribution of TRAIL and CD69 expression on electronically gated TCRβ$^-$ NK1.1$^+$ natural killer (NK) cells is indicated with solid lines (shaded areas). The percentage and mean fluorescence intensity (MFI) of TRAIL$^+$ or CD69$^+$ NK cells are provided. The dotted lines represent the distribution in the negative control. (B) TCRβ$^-$ NK1.1$^+$, (C) TRAIL$^+$ and CD69$^+$ NK cell proportions, and (D) MFI from NK cells positive for those markers are shown in bar graphs as mean plus standard deviation (n = 6). The difference among the groups was analyzed using the independent samples T test; *p <0.05.

cytokines such as IL-2, IL-12, IL-15, IL-18, and IL-21 have been shown to be involved in the survival and antitumor activity of NK cells [31]. However, neither IFN-γ nor IL-12 is upregulated in 3-day-fasted mice [4], and neither IL-12 nor IL-18 induced TRAIL expression in liver NK cells [30].

It is well known that HSPs are strongly induced in various stressful situations to cope with stimuli. HSP60 and GRP78 were found to be induced in response to fasting [13,32]. In this study, we found that HSP70 was significantly overexpressed in the liver of fasted mice (Figure 6). HSP70 can actively translocate into the plasma membrane following some stresses and even be released into the extracellular space to stimulate immune cells [21,33].

Previous studies have shown that HSP70 is linked to NK cell cytotoxicity. Membrane-bound HSP70 on tumor cells has been identified as a recognition structure for NK cells that promotes NK cell cytotoxicity [18–20,34], and an *in vitro* study has shown that culturing NK cells with HSP70 leads to an increase in their cytotoxicity [19,20]. In addition, adoptive infusion of HSP70/IL-2 pre-stimulated NK cells induced shrinking of tumor masses in tumor-bearing mice and improved survival [18–20,35]. Despite such striking facts, it is still not fully understood which molecules are responsible for NK cell immunostimulatory response to HSP70.

In the present study, we cultured recombinant HSP70 with liver lymphocytes and found that NK cell proliferation increased with HSP70 stimulation (Figure 7B). Furthermore, both TRAIL and CD69 expression in liver NK cells from fed mice were upregulated in response to HSP70 in a dose-dependent manner (Figure 7C, D). This result suggests that HSP70 may play a role in the stimulation of TRAIL expression in NK cells during fasting. Thus, to determine the effect of HSP70 on TRAIL expression, HSP70 inhibition using an anti-HSP70 mAb was performed *in vivo*. As expected, TRAIL$^+$ NK cell proportion was significantly downregulated in the anti-HSP70 mAb–treated mice. To our knowledge, this is the first report to provide evidence that HSP70 can induce NK cell activation in fasted mice via TRAIL. Since TRAIL downregulation by HSP70 inhibition is not complete, there may be other factors that regulate TRAIL-mediated NK activity; further studies are needed in this regard.

In conclusion, our mouse-model study showed that starvation has a positive effect on innate immunity by activating liver NK cells through TRAIL upregulation. We also showed that the underlying mechanism is, at least in part, due to HSP70 overexpression in the liver. This insight into HSP70-mediated NK cell activation may lead to the development of new therapeutic approaches that use NK cells to target cancer or virus-infected cells.

Supporting Information

Figure S1 Additional phenotypic analysis of natural killer cells from the spleen, bone marrow, and blood under starvation. (A) The mean proportion plus standard deviation of gated TCRβ^- NK1.1$^+$ natural killer (NK) cells from the liver, spleen, bone marrow, and blood of fed and 3-day-fasted mice are shown in bar graphs. (B) Histograms show the representative expression of the indicated markers on NK cells (solid lines) with the percentages of positive NK cells from the spleen, (D) bone marrow, and (F) blood; dotted lines represent negative control. Bar graphs represent the mean percentage plus standard deviation of positive NK cells in (C) the spleen, (E) bone marrow, and (G) blood. Data were analyzed using the independent samples T test; *p <0.05.

Figure S2 Physiological characteristics of the fasted mice. (A) Mouse body weight was measured every day during the fasting period. (B, C) Liver weight and ratio of liver:body weight were determined on the day of sacrifice. Lymphocytes from (D, E) the liver, (F) spleen, (G) bone marrow, and (H) blood from fed and fasted mice were counted using a hemocytometer; average numbers plus standard deviation are shown. The difference between groups was analyzed using the independent samples T test; *p <0.05; **p <0.01.

Acknowledgments

We would like to thank Dr. Tomoyuki Abe, Naoki Tanimine, JinLian Piao, Yuka Igarashi, and Yuko Ishida for their advice, encouragement, and expert technical assistance. This work was carried out in part at the Research Facilities for Laboratory Animal Science, Natural Science Center for Basic Research and Development (N-BARD), Hiroshima University.

Author Contributions

Conceived and designed the experiments: KT YT HO NT VTAD. Performed the experiments: VTAD TM YS YT. Analyzed the data: VTAD TM NF YT YS. Contributed reagents/materials/analysis tools: TM NF YT. Wrote the paper: VTAD KT HO YT.

References

1. Langers I, Renoux VM, Thiry M, Delvenne P, Jacobs N (2012) Natural killer cells: role in local tumor growth and metastasis. Biologics 6: 73–82.
2. Smyth MJ, Cretney E, Kelly JM, Westwood JA, Street SE, et al. (2005) Activation of NK cell cytotoxicity. Mol Immunol 42: 501–510.
3. Kiessling R, Klein E, Pross H, Wigzell H (1975) "Natural" killer cells in the mouse. II. Cytotoxic cells with specificity for mouse Moloney leukemia cells. Characteristics of the killer cell. Eur J Immunol 5: 117–121.
4. Shen J, Ren H, Tomiyama-Miyaji C, Watanabe M, Kainuma E, et al. (2009) Resistance and augmentation of innate immunity in mice exposed to starvation. Cell Immunol 259: 66–73.
5. Wiley SR, Schooley K, Smolak PJ, Din WS, Huang CP, et al. (1995) Identification and characterization of a new member of the TNF family that induces apoptosis. Immunity 3: 673–682.
6. Almasan A, Ashkenazi A (2003) Apo2L/TRAIL: apoptosis signaling, biology, and potential for cancer therapy. Cytokine Growth Factor Rev 14: 337–348.
7. Falschlehner C, Schaefer U, Walczak H (2009) Following TRAIL's path in the immune system. Immunology 127: 145–154.
8. Takeda K, Hayakawa Y, Smyth MJ, Kayagaki N, Yamaguchi N, et al. (2001) Involvement of tumor necrosis factor-related apoptosis-inducing ligand in surveillance of tumor metastasis by liver natural killer cells. Nat Med 7: 94–100.
9. Maksimovic-Ivanic D, Stosic-Grujicic S, Nicoletti F, Mijatovic S (2012) Resistance to TRAIL and how to surmount it. Immunol Res 52: 157–168.
10. Srivastava RK (2001) TRAIL/Apo-2L: mechanisms and clinical applications in cancer. Neoplasia 3: 535–546.
11. Joly AL, Wettstein G, Mignot G, Ghiringhelli F, Garrido C (2010) Dual Role of Heat Shock Proteins as Regulators of Apoptosis and Innate Immunity. Journal of Innate Immunity 2: 238–247.
12. Schmid TE, Multhoff G (2012) Radiation-induced stress proteins - the role of heat shock proteins (HSP) in anti- tumor responses. Curr Med Chem 19: 1765–1770.
13. Nishihara M, Sumimoto R, Sakimoto H, Sanada O, Fukuda Y, et al. (1998) Examination of TNF-alpha and heat shock protein gene expression in ischemic injured livers from fasted and nonfasted rats. Transplant Proc 30: 3697–3699.
14. Schmitt E, Gehrmann M, Brunet M, Multhoff G, Garrido C (2007) Intracellular and extracellular functions of heat shock proteins: repercussions in cancer therapy. J Leukoc Biol 81: 15–27.
15. Pockley AG, Muthana M, Calderwood SK (2008) The dual immunoregulatory roles of stress proteins. Trends Biochem Sci 33: 71–79.
16. Giuliano JS Jr, Lahni PM, Wong HR, Wheeler DS (2011) Extracellular Heat Shock Proteins: Alarmins for the Host Immune System. The Open Inflammation Journal 4: 12.
17. Jolesch A, Elmer K, Bendz H, Issels RD, Noessner E (2012) Hsp70, a messenger from hyperthermia for the immune system. European Journal of Cell Biology 91: 48–52.
18. Elsner L, Muppala V, Gehrmann M, Lozano J, Malzahn D, et al. (2007) The heat shock protein HSP70 promotes mouse NK cell activity against tumors that express inducible NKG2D ligands. Journal of Immunology 179: 5523–5533.
19. Multhoff G, Mizzen L, Winchester CC, Milner CM, Wenk S, et al. (1999) Heat shock protein 70 (Hsp70) stimulates proliferation and cytolytic activity of natural killer cells. Exp Hematol 27: 1627–1636.
20. Multhoff G, Pfister K, Gehrmann M, Hantschel M, Gross C, et al. (2001) A 14-mer Hsp70 peptide stimulates natural killer (NK) cell activity. Cell Stress Chaperones 6: 337–344.
21. Vega VL, Rodriguez-Silva M, Frey T, Gehrmann M, Diaz JC, et al. (2008) Hsp70 translocates to the plasma membrane after stress and is released into the extracellular environment in a membrane-associated form that activates macrophages. Journal of Immunology 180: 4299–4307.
22. Lv LH, Wan YL, Lin Y, Zhang W, Yang M, et al. (2012) Anticancer Drugs Cause Release of Exosomes with Heat Shock Proteins from Human Hepatocellular Carcinoma Cells That Elicit Effective Natural Killer Cell Antitumor Responses in Vitro. Journal of Biological Chemistry 287: 15874–15885.
23. Bouwens L, Remels L, Baekeland M, Van Bossuyt H, Wisse E (1987) Large granular lymphocytes or "pit cells" from rat liver: isolation, ultrastructural characterization and natural killer activity. Eur J Immunol 17: 37–42.
24. Peng H, Jiang X, Chen Y, Sojka DK, Wei H, et al. (2013) Liver-resident NK cells confer adaptive immunity in skin-contact inflammation. J Clin Invest 123: 1444–1456.
25. Clinthorne JF, Beli E, Duriancik DM, Gardner EM (2013) NK cell maturation and function in C57BL/6 mice are altered by caloric restriction. J Immunol 190: 712–722.
26. Ochi M, Ohdan H, Mitsuta H, Onoe T, Tokita D, et al. (2004) Liver NK cells expressing TRAIL are toxic against self hepatocytes in mice. Hepatology 39: 1321–1331.
27. Ishiyama K, Ohdan H, Ohira M, Mitsuta H, Arihiro K, et al. (2006) Difference in cytotoxicity against hepatocellular carcinoma between liver and periphery natural killer cells in humans. Hepatology 43: 362–372.
28. Marzio R, Mauel J, Betz-Corradin S (1999) CD69 and regulation of the immune function. Immunopharmacol Immunotoxicol 21: 565–582.
29. Smyth MJ, Cretney E, Takeda K, Wiltrout RH, Sedger LM, et al. (2001) Tumor necrosis factor-related apoptosis-inducing ligand (TRAIL) contributes to interferon gamma-dependent natural killer cell protection from tumor metastasis. J Exp Med 193: 661–670.
30. Takeda K, Cretney E, Hayakawa Y, Ota T, Akiba H, et al. (2005) TRAIL identifies immature natural killer cells in newborn mice and adult mouse liver. Blood 105: 2082–2089.
31. Zwirner NW, Domaica CI (2010) Cytokine regulation of natural killer cell effector functions. Biofactors 36: 274–288.
32. Takahashi Y, Tamaki T, Tanaka M, Konoeda Y, Kawamura A, et al. (1998) Efficacy of heat-shock proteins induced by severe fasting to protect rat livers

preserved for 72 hours from cold ischemia/reperfusion injury. Transplant Proc 30: 3700–3702.

33. Juhasz K, Thuenauer R, Spachinger A, Duda E, Horvath I, et al. (2013) Lysosomal Rerouting of Hsp70 Trafficking as a Potential Immune Activating Tool for Targeting Melanoma. Current Pharmaceutical Design 19: 430–440.

34. Multhoff G, Botzler C, Jennen L, Schmidt J, Ellwart J, et al. (1997) Heat shock protein 72 on tumor cells: a recognition structure for natural killer cells. J Immunol 158: 4341–4350.

35. Stangl S, Wortmann A, Guertler U, Multhoff G (2006) Control of metastasized pancreatic carcinomas in SCID/beige mice with human IL-2/TKD-activated NK cells. J Immunol 176: 6270–6276.

Synergism between Basic Asp49 and Lys49 Phospholipase A₂ Myotoxins of Viperid Snake Venom *In Vitro* and *In Vivo*

Diana Mora-Obando[1], Julián Fernández[1], Cesare Montecucco[2], José María Gutiérrez[1], Bruno Lomonte[1]*

[1] Instituto Clodomiro Picado, Facultad de Microbiología, Universidad de Costa Rica, San José, Costa Rica, [2] Department of Biomedical Sciences, University of Padova, Padova, Italy

Abstract

Two subtypes of phospholipases A$_2$ (PLA$_2$s) with the ability to induce myonecrosis, 'Asp49' and 'Lys49' myotoxins, often coexist in viperid snake venoms. Since the latter lack catalytic activity, two different mechanisms are involved in their myotoxicity. A synergism between Asp49 and Lys49 myotoxins from *Bothrops asper* was previously observed *in vitro*, enhancing Ca^{2+} entry and cell death when acting together upon C2C12 myotubes. These observations are extended for the first time *in vivo*, by demonstrating a clear enhancement of myonecrosis by the combined action of these two toxins in mice. In addition, novel aspects of their synergism were revealed using myotubes. Proportions of Asp49 myotoxin as low as 0.1% of the Lys49 myotoxin are sufficient to enhance cytotoxicity of the latter, but not the opposite. Sublytic amounts of Asp49 myotoxin also enhanced cytotoxicity of a synthetic peptide encompassing the toxic region of Lys49 myotoxin. Asp49 myotoxin rendered myotubes more susceptible to osmotic lysis, whereas Lys49 myotoxin did not. In contrast to myotoxic Asp49 PLA$_2$, an acidic non-toxic PLA$_2$ from the same venom did not markedly synergize with Lys49 myotoxin, revealing a functional difference between basic and acidic PLA$_2$ enzymes. It is suggested that Asp49 myotoxins synergize with Lys49 myotoxins by virtue of their PLA$_2$ activity. In addition to the membrane-destabilizing effect of this activity, Asp49 myotoxins may generate anionic patches of hydrolytic reaction products, facilitating electrostatic interactions with Lys49 myotoxins. These data provide new evidence for the evolutionary adaptive value of the two subtypes of PLA$_2$ myotoxins acting synergistically in viperid venoms.

Editor: Chi Zhang, University of Texas Southwestern Medical Center, United States of America

Funding: Funding support by the Graduate Studies Program, Universidad de Costa Rica; International Centre for Genetic Engineering and Biotechnology, Italy (CRP/COS13-01); and Vicerrectoria de Investigacion, Universidad de Costa Rica (741-B4-100). The funders had no role in study design, data collection and analysis, decision to publish, or preparation of the manuscript.

* Email: bruno.lomonte@ucr.ac.cr

Introduction

Phospholipases A$_2$ (PLA$_2$s) are widespread enzymes in snake venoms, where they play major toxic roles in the immobilization and/or killing of prey [1,2]. Among their diverse activities, myotoxicity is a clinically relevant effect which may lead to severe tissue damage and associated sequelae in envenomings [3–5]. Two divergent ancestral PLA$_2$ genes representing the group I and group II scaffolds, respectively, were recruited and expressed in the venom gland secretions of Elapidae and Viperidae [6]. Through a process of accelerated evolution [7], these genes accumulated mutations that converted their corresponding non-toxic proteins into potent toxins, most notably displaying neurotoxicity and/or myotoxicity. The independent emergence of such toxic activities in these two lineages of advanced snakes illustrates a case of convergent evolution [8,9]. A growing body of knowledge has been gathered on the characterization of PLA$_2$ toxins, but the structural bases for their toxicity and precise modes of action remain only partially understood, thus leaving opened a number of challenging questions [10].

In the venoms of viperid snakes, two subtypes of myotoxic PLA$_2$s can be found, commonly referred to as 'Asp49' and 'Lys49' variants. The latter, first described in the venom of *Agkistrodon piscivorus piscivorus* [11] and then isolated from many viperid venoms [9], present the substitution of Asp49 by Lys49, a critical change in the catalytic center of the molecule which, together with key amino acid substitutions located in the calcium-binding loop, precludes catalysis [12–14]. Therefore, in sharp contrast with their Asp49 PLA$_2$ counterparts, the Lys49 myotoxins are enzymatically-inactive PLA$_2$ homologues, or 'PLA$_2$-like' proteins [13,15–18].

Notwithstanding their difference in catalytic activity, both Lys49 and Asp49 PLA$_2$ variants display myotoxicity *in vivo* [4,19–21]. The Asp49 PLA$_2$s depend on their enzymatic activity to induce skeletal muscle damage, since their catalytic inactivation by covalently modifying His48 with *p*-bromophenacyl bromide results in the loss of myotoxicity [22–24]. Furthermore, the toxic effects of

Asp49 PLA$_2$s on myogenic cells in culture can be mimicked by the products of their hydrolytic activity, i.e. fatty acids and lysophospholipids [25], and hydrolysis of muscle phospholipids of the external monolayer of the sarcolemma by these enzymes has been demonstrated in myotubes in culture as well as in injected mouse muscles [26]. On the other hand, the catalytic-independent mechanism by which Lys49 PLA$_2$ homologues induce myonecrosis, has been shown to depend on a cluster of amino acids at their C-terminal region which directly affect the integrity of the sarcolemma [9,18,27–32].

The venom of *Bothrops asper*, the snake species causing the majority of envenomings in Central America [33], contains multiple Asp49 and Lys49 myotoxin isoforms [34] as well as a non-myotoxic, acidic Asp49 PLA$_2$ [35]. In a previous study, a synergistic action between purified Asp49 and Lys49 myotoxins was observed *in vitro*, whereby these two proteins induced a more pronounced Ca^{2+} entry and cell death by acting together, rather than individually [25]. The present work extends these observations by exploring for the first time whether the same phenomenon occurs *in vivo*, and characterizes in further detail relevant features of this synergistic action using an *in vitro* model.

Materials and Methods

Isolation of phospholipases A$_2$ from *Bothrops asper* venom

Snake venom was collected from specimens kept at the Serpentarium of Instituto Clodomiro Picado, under authorization of the University of Costa Rica. Pooled venom of *Bothrops asper* from the Pacific versant of Costa Rica was fractionated as previously described, to obtain myotoxin II (Lys49; UniProt accession P24605; [36,37]), a mixture of myotoxins I/III (Asp49; P20474; [24,38]), and an acidic BaspPLA$_2$-II (non-myotoxic, Asp49; P86389; [35]). Fractionation steps included ion-exchange chromatography followed by semi-preparative reverse-phase HPLC on a C$_8$ support. Purity was assessed by nano-electrospray mass spectrometry in a QTrap-3200 instrument (ABSciex) operated in positive ion-enhanced multicharge mode, as described [24]. The lack of contaminating Asp49 PLA$_2$s in the Lys49 myotoxin II preparation was evaluated by assaying PLA$_2$ activity using the synthetic substrate 4-nitro-3-octanoyloxybenzoic acid [39]. Conversely, the lack of contaminating Lys49 myotoxins in the basic Asp49 PLA$_2$ myotoxin preparation was ascertained by automated N-terminal amino acid sequencing using a PPSQ-33A

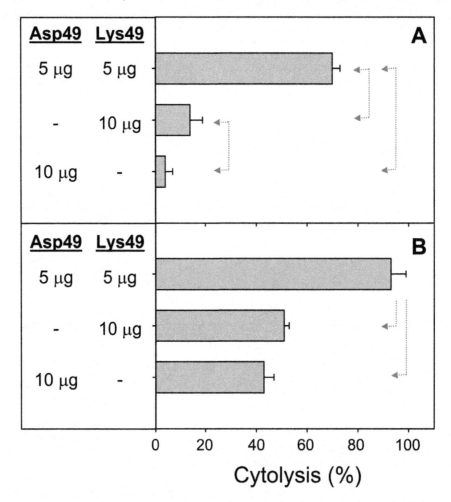

Figure 1. Cytotoxic activity of Asp49 and Lys49 myotoxins from *Bothrops asper*, alone or in combination, upon C2C12 myoblasts (A) or myotubes (B). The indicated amounts of toxins were added in a total volume of 150 µL. Cytolysis was determined by the release of lactate dehydrogenase to the medium 3 h after exposure of the cells to the toxins, as described in Materials and Methods. Reference values of 0 and 100% cytolysis were established using medium or 0.1% Triton X-100 in medium, respectively. Each bar represents mean ± SD of triplicate cell cultures. Statistically significant differences (p<0.05) between two groups are indicated by dotted arrow lines.

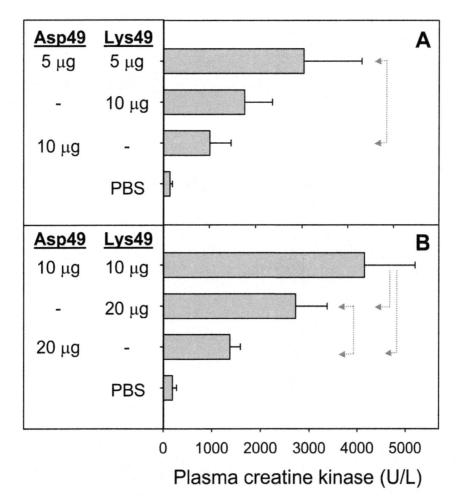

Figure 2. Myotoxic activity of Asp49 and Lys49 myotoxins from *Bothrops asper*, alone or in combination, injected by intramuscular route in CD-1 mice. Plasma creatine kinase activity was determined 3 h after injection of the indicated amounts of toxins. Control mice received only vehicle (PBS). Each bar represents mean ± SD of five animals. Statistically significant differences (p<0.05) between two groups are indicated by dotted arrow lines. Synergistic action is shown at a total dose of 10 μg in (A) or 20 μg in (B), respectively.

instrument (Shimadzu Biotech), to confirm the absence of a Leucine signal in the fifth cycle [24].

Asp49 PLA$_2$ myotoxin inactivation by *p*-bromophenacyl bromide

Three mg of the Asp49 myotoxin were dissolved in 1 mL of 0.1 M Tris, 0.7 mM EDTA, pH 8.0 buffer. Then, 125 μL of *p*-bromophenacyl bromide (*p*-BPB; 1.5 mg/mL in ethanol; Sigma Chemical Co.) were added and incubated at room temperature (20–25°C) for 24 h [22]. Excess *p*-BPB and salts were eliminated by RP-HPLC on a semi-preparative C$_8$ column, as described [24]. The protein was collected and finally dried by vacuum centrifugation at 45°C. Enzymatic inactivation was determined on the 4-nitro-3-octanoyloxybenzoic acid substrate in comparison to a control sample of the toxin which was processed identically but omitting the *p*-BPB reagent [24].

Synthetic peptide of *B. asper* myotoxin II

A synthetic peptide from the C-terminal region of *B. asper* myotoxin II, corresponding to the sequence 115–129 (KKYR-YYLKPLCKK; p$^{115-129}$), was obtained from a commercial provider (Peptide 2.0, Inc.). The peptide was synthesized with native endings by Fmoc chemistry, and its molecular mass was in agreement with the expected value. Its purity level was at least 95% by RP-HPLC analysis. This 13-mer peptide has been shown to reproduce, albeit with a lower potency, the cytolytic effect of myotoxin II *in vitro* [27,29].

Cytotoxic activity

Cytolysis was determined on the murine myogenic cell line C2C12 (ATCC-CRL1772) using a lactate dehydrogenase release assay, as previously described [40]. Cells were grown at subconfluent densities in 25 cm^2 bottles using Dulbecco's modified Eagle's medium supplemented with 10% fetal calf serum (DMEM, 10% FCS), and after detachment by trypsin, they were seeded in 96-well plates for cytotoxicity assays. These were performed either at the myoblast stage in near-confluent cell monolayers, or after their differentiation to fused myotubes in DMEM 1% FCS during 4–6 additional days. In brief, different amounts of toxins, alone or in combination, dissolved in 150 μL of assay medium (DMEM, 1% FCS) were added to the cells immediately after removal of their medium, and incubated for 3 h at 37°C. Then, an aliquot of cell supernatant (60 μL) was collected from each well and the lactacte dehydrogenase (LDH) activity was quantified by a UV kinetic assay (LDH-BR Cromatest, Linear Chemicals). Controls for 0 and 100% cytotoxicity consisted of assay medium, and 0.1%

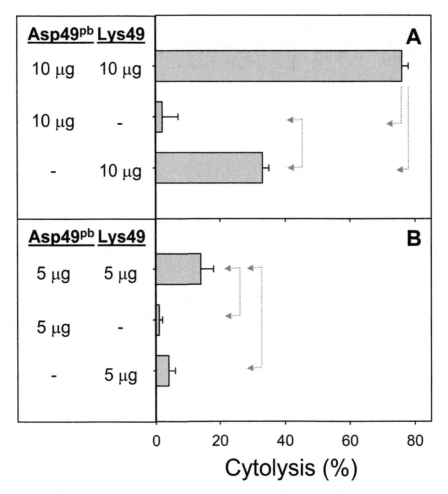

Figure 3. Cytotoxic activity of *p*-bromophenacyl bromide-modified Asp49 myotoxin (Asp49^{pb}) and Lys49 myotoxin, alone or in combination at 10 μg (A) or 5 μg (B), upon C2C12 myotubes. The indicated amounts of toxins were added in a total volume of 150 μL. Cytolysis was determined by the release of lactate dehydrogenase to the medium, 3 h after exposure of the cells to the toxins. Each bar represents mean ± SD of triplicate cell cultures. Statistically significant differences (p<0.05) between two groups are indicated by dotted arrow lines.

Triton X-100 diluted in assay medium, respectively. All samples were assayed in triplicate wells.

Myotoxic activity

Myotoxic activity was determined in CD-1 mice of 18 to 20 g of body weight, using five animals per group. These *in vivo* assays were kept to a minimum, and followed protocols authorized by the Institutional Committee for the Use and Care of Animals (CICUA; #132-13), University of Costa Rica. Mice were housed in cages for groups of 4–6, and provided food and water *ad libitum*. Different amounts of the toxins, alone or in combination, dissolved in 50 μL of phosphate-buffered saline (PBS; 0.12 M NaCl, 0.04 M sodium phosphate buffer, pH 7.2), were injected into the gastrocnemius muscle [36]. A control group of mice received an identical injection of PBS. After 3 h, blood was collected from the tip of the tail into a heparinized capillary and centrifuged. The plasma creatine kinase (CK) activity, expressed in U/L, was determined using a UV kinetic assay (CK-Nac, Biocon Diagnostik). Mice were sacrificed by CO_2 inhalation, at the end of the experiment.

Statistical analysis

ANOVA was used for the comparison of mean values from more than two groups, followed by Tukey-Kramer tests, with a statistical significance of $p<0.05$. Calculations were performed with the aid of the Instat (GraphPad) software.

Results

The cytolytic effect of Asp49 and Lys49 myotoxins, when added alone or in combination to cultures of the C2C12 cell line at the myoblast or myotube stages, is shown in Fig. 1. A higher effect of these toxins was observed in myotubes than in myoblasts, and this difference was more conspicuous in the case of the Asp49 myotoxin, which was extremely weak against myoblasts (Fig. 1A). In both stages of cell differentiation, the combination of the myotoxins induced a significantly higher cytotoxicity in comparison to the effect of either toxin alone (Fig. 1). The observed effect was clearly synergistic and not just additive. Following these *in vitro* findings, experiments were performed in mice to determine whether synergism also occurs in mature skeletal muscle, under conditions that mimic envenomings. Results revealed a clear enhancement of myotoxicity, as judged by the higher release of creatine kinase from damaged muscle to the

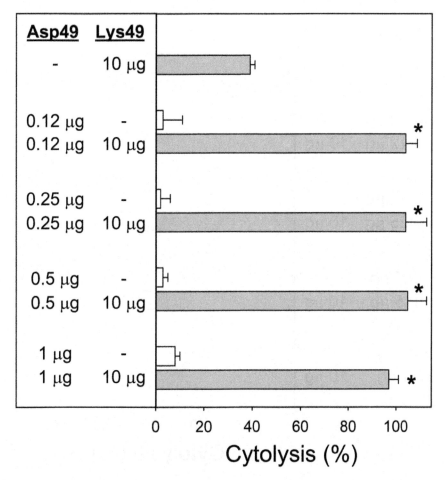

Figure 4. Cytotoxic activity of a fixed amount of Lys49 myotoxin, alone or in combination with low amounts of Asp49 myotoxin, upon C2C12 myotubes. The indicated amounts of toxins were added in a total volume of 150 μL. Cytolysis was determined by the release of lactate dehydrogenase to the medium, 3 h after exposure of the cells to the toxins. Each bar represents mean ± SD of triplicate cell cultures. All values from cultures where the Lys49 myotoxin was added together with Asp49 myotoxin were significantly different ($p<0.05$) from the value of cultures exposed only to Lys49 myotoxin (indicated by asterisks).

plasma, when the Asp49 and Lys49 toxins acted in combination (Fig. 2). When injected individually, the myotoxic effect of the Lys49 myotoxin was significantly higher than that of the Asp49 myotoxin at the dose of 20 μg (Fig. 2B), although at 10 μg (Fig. 2A) this same trend did not reach statistical significance.

The role of enzymatic activity of the Asp49 myotoxin in the synergistic effect was studied by using a p-BPB-treated enzyme. This protein incorporated a single molecule of the alkylating agent, as confirmed by mass spectrometry, and its catalytic activity was inactivated by 97% in comparison to the untreated enzyme [24]. As shown in Fig. 3, the cytolytic action of the p-BPB-treated Asp49 myotoxin alone was negligible, as expected. However, the combined action of this protein and the Lys49 myotoxin caused a significant enhancement of the cytotoxic effect (Fig. 3). Since the p-PBP-treated Asp49 protein had a residual enzymatic activity of 3%, further experiments were designed to determine whether the synergistic effect observed in Fig. 3 could be due to this low residual catalytic action or, alternatively, depended on a non-catalytic mechanism of the Asp49 myotoxin. Therefore, low amounts of native Asp49 myotoxin, within a range comparable to the proportion of enzymatically-active protein remaining in the p-PBP-treated toxin, were combined with a fixed amount of Lys49 myotoxin (Fig. 4). Results showed that Asp49 myotoxin amounts as low as 0.12 μg (representing 1.2% in proportion to the Lys49 myotoxin), efficiently enhanced the cytotoxicity of the final mixture. Importantly, these low amounts of Asp49 myotoxin were essentially non-toxic when added alone to the myotube cultures (Fig. 4). Further titration of the effect of Asp49 myotoxin in this assay showed that the minimal amount of enzyme capable of inducing synergism was 0.012 μg. The reverse combination, i.e. addition of low quantities of Lys49 myotoxin to a fixed amount of Asp49 myotoxin (Fig. 5) did not enhance toxicity, thus revealing the directionality of the synergistic mechanism.

Since results indicated that the Asp49 myotoxin, even in low amounts, enhanced the toxicity of the Lys49 myotoxin, an experiment was performed to determine whether this synergy was dependent on the time lapse when a low amount of the enzyme was in contact with myotubes, before the addition of the Lys49 myotoxin. The Asp49 enzyme was incubated with the cells for the time periods indicated in Fig. 6 (0, 15, 30, or 60 min) and, after five washings of the cell cultures, the Lys49 myotoxin was added. A significant enhancement in cytotoxicity was recorded at all time periods of cell exposure to the Asp49 myotoxin and, remarkably, even when the Asp49 enzyme was added and the cultures were immediately washed (Fig. 6).

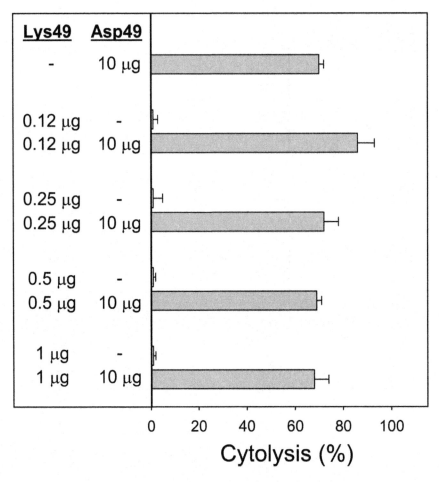

Figure 5. Cytotoxic activity of a fixed amount of Asp49 myotoxin, alone or in combination with low amounts of Lys49 myotoxin, upon C2C12 myotubes. The indicated amounts of toxins were added in a total volume of 150 μL. Cytolysis was determined by the release of lactate dehydrogenase to the medium, 3 h after exposure of the cells to the toxins. Each bar represents mean ± SD of triplicate cell cultures. None of the values from cultures where the Asp49 myotoxin was added together with Lys49 myotoxin were significantly different from the value of cultures exposed only to Asp49 myotoxin.

Since *B. asper* venom also contains non-myotoxic Asp49 PLA$_2$s whose role in venom's toxicity is uncertain [35], the effect of a non-myotoxic, acidic-type PLA$_2$ on the cytotoxic activity of Lys49 myotoxin was investigated in the same assay system, as shown in Fig. 7. As expected, the acidic Asp49 enzyme alone was not cytotoxic. The combination of this enzyme with the Lys49 myotoxin caused a significant, although only modest increase at 5 μg, but at 10 μg was unable to significantly enhance cytotoxicity of Lys49 myotoxin (Fig. 7).

The synergistic effect of a low amount of Asp49 myotoxin toward the cytolytic action of the synthetic peptide p$^{115-129}$ of the Lys49 myotoxin was evaluated. As presented in Fig. 8, the cytotoxicity induced by this short peptide was markedly enhanced by acting in combination with the Asp49 enzyme.

Finally, the cytotoxic action of Asp49 and Lys49 myotoxins was tested under conditions of osmotic imbalance of the cells. Culture medium was rendered hypotonic by the addition of varying proportions of purified water (8:2, 9:1, or 10:1 water:medium), and cytolysis was determined in the absence or presence of the toxins. As shown in Fig. 9A, myotubes exposed to a low amount of Asp49 myotoxin became significantly more susceptible to the deleterious action of the hypotonic media, at 8:2 and 9:1 water:medium proportions. At the 10:0 proportion (100% water), the high cytolysis in the control cells did not allow the assessment of the effect of myotoxin. In contrast, when the same experiment was performed with Lys49 myotoxin, it revealed that this protein does not alter the susceptibility of myotubes exposed to hypotonic conditions, since similar values of cytolysis were observed in the absence or in the presence of the toxin (Fig. 9B).

Discussion

The venoms of many viperid snake species contain variable combinations of PLA$_2$s, often including acidic and basic variants, and among the latter, Asp49 and Lys49 myotoxin subtypes [1,2,41]. Phylogenetic analyses indicate that the myotoxic Lys49 PLA$_2$ homologues diverged from ancestral, group II Asp49 PLA$_2$s before the separation of Viperinae and Crotalinae [42–46]. Intriguingly, however, a comprehensive examination of the bioactivities displayed by myotoxic Asp49 and Lys49 variants does not provide evident clues on the possible evolutionary advantages conferred by the emergence of the latter, since both types of myotoxins share similar toxicological profiles and often coexist in viperid venoms [41]. Nevertheless, the abundance and common occurrence of these coexisting myotoxins in many viperid species strongly suggest that they provided an important adaptive value in this family of snakes. Several speculative hypotheses have

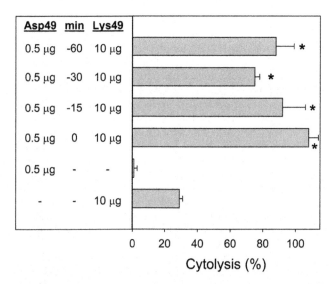

Figure 6. Cytotoxic activity of a fixed amount of Lys49 myotoxin, alone or in combination with a low amount of Asp49 myotoxin. In this experiment, Asp49 myotoxin was first incubated for variable periods of time with C2C12 myotubes, and then washed five times, before the addition of Lys49 myotoxin. The indicated amounts of toxins were added in a total volume of 150 μL. Cytolysis was determined by the release of lactate dehydrogenase to the medium 3 h after exposure of the cells to the toxins. Each bar represents mean ± SD of triplicate cell cultures. All values from cultures where the Lys49 myotoxin was added together with Asp49 myotoxin were significantly different (p<0.05) from the value of cultures exposed only to Lys49 myotoxin (indicated by asterisks).

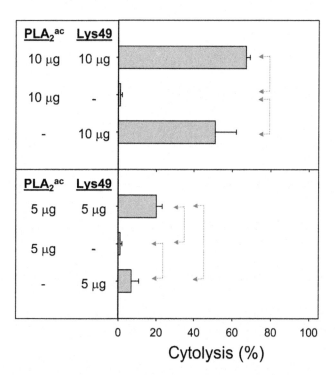

Figure 7. Cytotoxic activity of *Bothrops asper* acidic Asp49 phospholipase A_2 (PLA_2^{ac}) and Lys49 myotoxin, alone or in combination, upon C2C12 myotubes. The indicated amounts of toxins were added in a total volume of 150 μL. Cytolysis was determined by the release of lactate dehydrogenase to the medium, 3 h after exposure of the cells to the toxins. Each bar represents mean ± SD of triplicate cell cultures. Statistically significant differences (p<0.05) between two groups are indicated by dotted arrow lines.

been proposed to envisage their possible biological significance and adaptive value, one of them being synergism [41]. A synergistic action upon myogenic cells in culture was first described by Cintra-Francischinelli et al. [25] using the C2C12 cell line as a target for Asp49 and Lys49 myotoxins isolated from the venom of *B. asper*. The present study extends such observations by demonstrating the *in vivo* synergism between these two toxin subtypes in the induction of myonecrosis, and provides further insights into the mechanisms of this synergistic effect.

In agreement with previous studies [47], a higher susceptibility of myotubes over myoblasts to the cytotoxic action of the myotoxins was observed. Also, myoblasts were more resistant to the Asp49 than to the Lys49 myotoxin, as previously noted by Cintra-Francischinelli et al. [25]. In agreement with their study, a cytotoxic synergism between the two toxins was confirmed at both stages of cell differentiation, i.e. myoblasts and myotubes. In order to determine whether these *in vitro* observations would also apply to the biologically-relevant target of myotoxins, i.e. skeletal muscle, similar experiments were conducted in mice. Results demonstrate, for the first time *in vivo*, a clear enhancement of myotoxicity by the combined action of Asp49 and Lys49 myotoxins in comparison to the effect of either protein alone. Therefore, these *in vivo* results add new evidence for the adaptive value of the emergence of two subtypes of PLA_2 myotoxins in viperid venoms, conferring a selective advantage in the light of the high energetic costs of venom protein synthesis [48,49].

The *in vivo* synergism hereby shown helps to clarify previous observations in the study of viperid PLA_2 myotoxins, in which crude venoms have generally been found to induce stronger myonecrosis than their isolated myotoxins [50]. Although the contribution to muscle damage of other toxin types in crude venoms (for example hemorrhagic metalloproteinases that promote myonecrosis as a consequence of ischemia [51]) cannot be excluded, the combined action of Asp49 and Lys49 myotoxins in crude venoms may explain the higher magnitude of myonecrosis

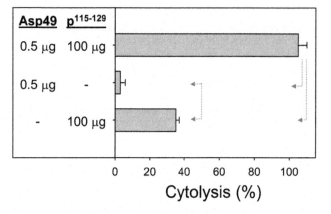

Figure 8. Cytotoxic activity of Asp49 myotoxin and the synthetic C-terminal peptide p115-129 of Lys49 myotoxin II from *Bothrops asper*, alone or in combination, upon C2C12 myotubes. The indicated amounts of toxin or synthetic peptide were added in a total volume of 150 μL. Cytolysis was determined by the release of lactate dehydrogenase to the medium, 3 h after exposure of the cells to the toxins. Each bar represents mean ± SD of triplicate cell cultures. Statistically significant differences (p<0.05) between two groups are indicated by dotted arrow lines.

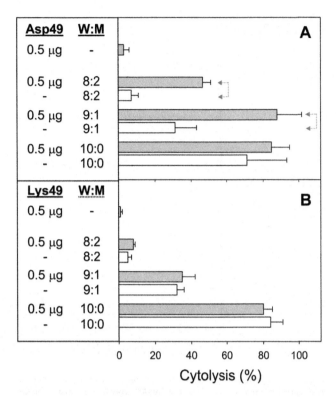

Figure 9. Cytotoxic activity of Asp49 and Lys49 myotoxins upon C2C12 myotubes under conditions of osmotic imbalance. Myotubes were grown and differentiated as described in Methods, and then the toxins (0.5 µg) were added to cultures using medium that contained the indicated proportion of water (gray bars). (**A**) Asp49 myotoxin, (**B**) Lys49 myotoxin. Control cultures exposed to the same medium conditions, in the absence of toxin, were tested in parallel (empty bars). Cytolysis was determined by the release of lactate dehydrogenase to the medium after 3 h. Each bar represents mean ± SD of triplicate cell cultures. Statistically significant differences (p<0.05) between two groups are indicated by dotted arrow lines.

observed in comparison to experiments analyzing isolated myotoxins. Also noteworthy, the extent of muscle damage induced by the Lys49 myotoxin was higher than that caused by the Asp49 myotoxin. This result is in agreement with the proposal that Lys49 PLA_2 homologues in viperids provided an adaptive value due to their increased myotoxic potency, as discussed by Kihara et al. [52]. From the biological standpoint, an enhanced capacity to induce acute muscle damage might contribute to a more efficient digestion of the abundant muscle mass characteristic of mammalian prey [41].

In order to determine whether the synergistic mechanism depends on the PLA_2 activity of Asp49 myotoxins, this enzyme was inactivated by p-BPB [22,24]. As expected, the modified enzyme essentially lost its cytotoxic effect upon myotubes, but surprisingly, still enhanced the cytotoxic action of the Lys49 myotoxin. This prompted us to evaluate the residual catalytic activity of the p-BPB-treated protein, which revealed a low, but detectable hydrolysis of the 4-nitro-3-octanoyloxybenzoic acid substrate, estimated at the level of 3% of the unmodified toxin. On this basis, it was hypothesized that such low residual catalytic activity could either be sufficient for the occurrence of synergism, or, alternatively, the synergistic action recorded for the p-BPB-modified enzyme would be caused by a catalytically-independent mechanism. To address this point, the synergism was subsequently tested with low amounts of the Asp49 PLA_2, mimicking the proportion of the corresponding residual enzymatic activity of the p-BPB-treated myotoxin. Results confirmed that these minute amounts of the Asp49 PLA_2, in sublytic concentrations per se, are able to enhance the cytolytic effect of the Lys49 myotoxin. Therefore, the mechanism of synergism can be attributed to the enzymatic action of the Asp49 PLA_2, rather than a catalytically-independent activity. A similar conclusion was reached by Cintra-Francischinelli et al. [25] by observing that, in the absence of external Ca^{2+}, the Asp49 myotoxin was unable to synergize with the Lys49 myotoxin due to the requirement of this ion for enzymatic activity. Moreover, the present observations underscore that even a very low enzymatic activity of Asp49 myotoxins is enough for the observed synergism. The directionality of this 'micro-synergism' was determined to be an enhancement of the Lys49 myotoxin toxicity by the Asp49 enzyme, and not the converse, since low quantities of the Lys49 myotoxin did not increase the toxic action of the Asp49 enzyme.

Using this experimental model of 'micro-synergism', additional aspects of the mechanisms involved were explored. Since the enhancing action of the Asp49 enzyme was found to depend on its catalytic activity, an experiment was designed to evaluate the effect of time by which cells were exposed to the enzyme, then washed, and finally exposed to the Lys49 myotoxin. The addition of a low amount of the Asp49 PLA_2, independently of the time of contact with the cells, and even when washing was performed immediately after toxin addition, led to a similar cytotoxic outcome. One possibility to explain these findings would be that the enzyme binds rapidly and tightly to the cell membrane interface, and is not removed by gentle washing, thus continuing its enzymatic phospholipid hydrolysis. The assessment of this hypothesis awaits experiments on the binding of myotoxins to myotubes.

Considering that the venom of B. asper contains, in addition to basic PLA_2s, an acidic Asp49 PLA_2 enzyme which is devoid of myotoxicity (BaspPLA$_2$-II [35]), it was of interest to evaluate whether this enzyme would be able to synergize with the basic Lys49 myotoxin. In agreement with its previous characterization, this acidic PLA_2 did not induce cytotoxicity per se. Interestingly, this acidic PLA_2 did not induce the marked synergistic effect observed with the basic Asp49 PLA_2. Only a minor increase in cytotoxicity was observed when using 5 µg of the enzyme, and twice this amount did not result in a statistically significant difference of toxicity in comparison to the Lys49 myotoxin alone. This result is noteworthy because the acidic enzyme displays a higher catalytic activity than the Asp49 myotoxin [35]. This suggests that the acidic enzyme might be unable to hydrolyze the membrane phospholipids of myotubes, which in turn would explain both its lack of toxicity and its inability to synergize effectively with Lys49 myotoxin in this model. This hypothesis awaits the study of phospholipid hydrolysis in the membranes of myotubes and muscle cells by using highly sensitive methodologies such as mass spectrometry [26]. Hence, the role of this non-cytotoxic acidic PLA_2 in the overall toxicity of the venom of B. asper, if any, remains uncertain.

A key question arising from the present and previous studies on the synergism between Asp49 PLA_2 and Lys49 myotoxins concerns how does the enzymatic activity of the former enhance the toxicity of the latter. To the best of our knowledge, the first evidence of a synergism between these two myotoxin subtypes was reported by Shen and Cho [53], who demonstrated that an Asp49 PLA_2 from A. p. piscivorus venom enhanced the liposome-permeabilizing effect of a Lys49 PLA_2 homologue isolated from the same source. These authors proposed that the Asp49 enzyme would generate anionic patches of hydrolytic reaction products on the surface of the liposomes, which in turn would facilitate the

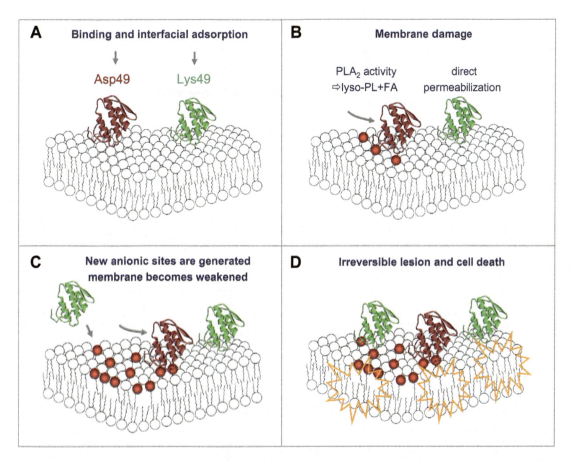

Figure 10. Cartoon representation of the hypothetical synergistic mechanism involved in the membrane-damaging activity of Asp49 and Lys49 myotoxins. Toxins bind to the muscle cell membrane (A), although acceptor moieties for this event are unknown. Each toxin type by its own has the ability to induce cytotoxicity *in vitro* or myonecrosis *in vivo* through membrane damage. Asp49 myotoxins destabilize the membrane by the enzymatic hydrolysis of phospholipids (PL) and consequent production of lyso-PL and fatty acids (FA), whereas Lys49 myotoxins exert a direct permeabilization mechanism via their C-terminal region (B). When acting in combination, FA produced by the Asp49 myotoxin generate new anionic sites (red spheres) that facilitate the binding of Lys49 myotoxin through electrostatic interactions (C). The membrane becomes more unstable due to PL hydrolysis *per se*, and to the accumulation of the reaction products (lysoPL and FA). As a result of these combined actions of Asp49 and Lys49 myotoxins, membrane damage is enhanced and the cell becomes irreversibly damaged (D). Note that the toxin cartoons are represented as monomers for simplicity, although these toxins actually occur as homodimers. Cartoons are not drawn to scale, and the orientation of the toxins interacting with the membrane is only for illustrative purposes.

electrostatic interaction with the Lys49 protein, and the consequent permeabilization of the vesicle by the non-enzymatic, bilayer penetrating mechanism of the latter [53]. A second, non-mutually exclusive explanation for the synergistic mechanism was proposed [25], whereby the products of phospholipid hydrolysis generated by the Asp49 myotoxin would enhance the toxicity of the Lys49 myotoxin by rendering the cell membrane more unstable, based on the observation that a mixture of lysophospholipids and fatty acids can mimic *per se* the membrane-damaging effects of Asp49 myotoxin.

In the present study, two further observations shed light into the possible mechanisms of the synergy here characterized. First, the bioactive C-terminal synthetic peptide of the Lys49 myotoxin, $p^{115-129}$, reproduced the synergy phenomenon observed with the parent protein, i.e. the concomitant addition of a low amount of Asp49 PLA$_2$ and peptide resulted in a significant enhancement of myotube cell lysis. Since this peptide is highly cationic [27], this finding (as well as results with the parent Lys49 myotoxin) would be compatible with the hypothesis that proposed the generation of new anionic sites by the Asp49 enzyme [53], thus facilitating the electrostatic interaction of the peptide or the toxin with the membrane [54,55], and ultimately its permeabilization [8,25,56]. However, the higher cytotoxic effect of the peptide when acting in synergy with the Asp49 myotoxin might as well be explained by the weakening of membrane stability caused by the catalytic action of the enzyme and by the generation of fatty acids and lysophospholipids. Thus, results of this experiment would be compatible with both mechanisms. The hypothesis of a general membrane-destabilizing effect caused by phospholipid hydrolysis and generation of products that alter its biophysical properties [25] is hereby experimentally supported. It was hypothesized that, if the myotube cell membrane becomes more unstable due to the enzymatic action of Asp49 PLA$_2$, it would be less capable of resisting a non-specific stress such as osmotic imbalance. Results confirmed this assumption, showing that myotubes were significantly more susceptible to the cytolysis induced by hypotonic media if they were exposed to minute amounts of Asp49 PLA$_2$ myotoxin. In contrast, myotubes exposed to equivalent amounts of Lys49 myotoxin were equally susceptible to lysis in such hypotonic media, as in the absence of toxin. Taken together, these experiments indicate that the enhancing mechanism for the toxicity of Lys49 myotoxins exerted by Asp49 PLA$_2$ myotoxin involves at least the weakening of cell membrane integrity by the latter. On the other hand, the possibility of the generation of new anionic sites by the accumulation of products of catalysis in the membrane remains to be tested, but clearly, both mechanisms would rely on the enzymatic activity of the Asp49 PLA$_2$ myotoxin (Fig. 10).

The synergistic mechanism hereby characterized contributes to rationalize the evolutionary advantage for the emergence of two different subtypes of PLA$_2$ myotoxins in the venom of many viperids, which are known to use two contrasting molecular mechanisms that lead to the same outcome: skeletal muscle necrosis. The synergy between Asp49 and Lys49 myotoxins represents at least one advantageous feature for the snakes, but additional mechanisms of adaptive value for these toxins may also exist [41], for example in their possible functional interactions with other snake venom components [57,58]. On a more general ground, our findings stress the need to study the action of snake venoms from a holistic perspective, i.e. by analyzing not only the action of purified toxins, but also the interaction of different components in the context of the complexity of snakebite envenoming.

Acknowledgments

The valuable contribution of Juan Manuel Ureña and Wan-Chih Tsai in various aspects of this work is gratefully acknowledged. This study was performed in partial fulfillment of the M.Sc degree of D. Mora-Obando at the University of Costa Rica.

Author Contributions

Conceived and designed the experiments: BL DMO. Performed the experiments: DMO. Analyzed the data: DMO JF CM JMG BL. Contributed reagents/materials/analysis tools: JF. Contributed to the writing of the manuscript: BL JMG CM.

References

1. Kini RM (1997) Venom Phospholipase A$_2$ Enzymes. Structure, Function, and Mechanisms. John Wiley & Sons, Chichester, 511.
2. Kini RM (2003) Excitement ahead: structure, function and mechanism of snake venom phospholipase A$_2$ enzymes. Toxicon 42: 827–840.
3. Harris JB, Cullen MJ (1990) Muscle necrosis caused by snake venoms and toxins. Electron Microsc Rev 3: 183–211.
4. Gutiérrez JM, Ownby CL (2003) Skeletal muscle degeneration induced by venom phospholipases A$_2$: insights into the mechanisms of local and systemic myotoxicity. Toxicon 42: 915–931.
5. Warrell DA (2010) Snakebite. Lancet 375, 77–88.
6. Fry BG, Wüster W (2004) Assembling an arsenal: origin and evolution of the snake venom proteome inferred from phylogenetic analysis of toxin sequences. Mol Biol Evol 21: 870–883.
7. Nakashima KI, Nobuhisa I, Deshimaru M, Nakai M, Ogawa T, et al. (1995) Accelerated evolution in the protein-coding regions is universal in crotalinae snake venom gland phospholipase A$_2$ isozyme genes. Proc Natl Acad Sci USA 92: 5605–5609.
8. Lomonte B, Gutiérrez JM (2011) Phospholipases A$_2$ from Viperidae snake venoms: how do they induce skeletal muscle damage? Acta Chim Slovenica 58: 647–659.
9. Lomonte B, Rangel J (2012) Snake venom Lys49 myotoxins: from phospholipases A$_2$ to non-enzymatic membrane disruptors. Toxicon 60: 520–530.
10. Gutiérrez JM, Lomonte B (2013) Phospholipases A$_2$: unveiling the secrets of a functionally versatile group of snake venom toxins. Toxicon 62: 27–39.
11. Maraganore JM, Merutka G, Cho W, Welches W, Kézdy FJ, et al. (1984) A new class of phospholipases A$_2$ with lysine in place of aspartate 49. J Biol Chem 259: 13839–13843.
12. Arni RK, Ward RJ (1996) Phospholipase A$_2$ - a structural review. Toxicon 34: 827–841.
13. Petan T, Križaj I, Pungerčar J (2007) Restoration of enzymatic activity in a Ser-49 phospholipase A$_2$ homologue decreases its Ca^{2+}-independent membrane-damaging activity and increases its toxicity. Biochemistry 46: 12795–12809.
14. Fernandes CAH, Marchi-Salvador DP, Salvador GM, Silva MCO, Costa TR, et al. (2010) Comparison between apo and complexed structures of bothropstoxin-I reveals the role of Lys122 and Ca2+-binding loop region for the catalytically inactive Lys49-PLA$_2$s. J Structural Biol 171: 31–43.
15. Scott DL, Achari A, Vidal JC, Sigler PB (1992) Crystallographic and biochemical studies of the (inactive) Lys-49 phospholipase A$_2$ from the venom of *Agkistrodon piscivorus piscivorus*. J Biol Chem 267: 22645–22657.
16. Ward RJ, Chioato L, de Oliveira AHC, Ruller R, Sá JM (2002) Active-site mutagenesis of a Lys49-phospholipase A$_2$: biological and membrane-disrupting activities in the absence of catalysis. Biochem J 362: 89–96.
17. Lomonte B, Angulo Y, Calderón L (2003) An overview of Lysine-49 phospholipase A$_2$ myotoxins from crotalid snake venoms and their structural determinants of myotoxic action. Toxicon 42: 885–901.
18. dos Santos JI, Fernandes CAH, Magro AJ, Fontes MRM (2009) The intriguing phospholipases A$_2$ homologues: relevant structural features on myotoxicity and catalytic inactivity. Prot Peptide Lett 16: 887–893.
19. Gutiérrez JM, Lomonte B (1995) Phospholipase A$_2$ myotoxins from *Bothrops* snake venoms. Toxicon 33: 1405–1424.
20. Gutiérrez JM, Lomonte B (1997) Phospholipase A$_2$ myotoxins from Bothrops snake venoms. In: Kini RM (Ed), Venom phospholipase A$_2$ enzymes: structure, function, and mechanism. John Wiley & Sons, England, 321–352.
21. Montecucco C, Gutiérrez JM, Lomonte B (2008) Cellular pathology induced by snake venom phospholipase A$_2$ myotoxins and neurotoxins: common aspects of their mechanisms of action. Cell Mol Life Sci 65: 2897–2912.
22. Díaz-Oreiro C, Gutiérrez JM (1997) Chemical modification of histidine and lysine residues of myotoxic phospholipases A$_2$ isolated from *Bothrops asper* and *Bothrops godmani* snake venoms: effects on enzymatic and pharmacological properties. Toxicon 35: 241–252.
23. Soares AM, Giglio JR (2003) Chemical modifications of phospholipases A$_2$ from snake venoms: effects on catalytic and pharmacological properties. Toxicon 42: 855–868.
24. Mora-Obando D, Díaz-Oreiro C, Angulo Y, Gutiérrez JM, Lomonte B (2014) Role of enzymatic activity in muscle damage and cytotoxicity induced by *Bothrops asper* Asp49 phospholipase A$_2$ myotoxins: are there additional effector mechanisms involved? Peer J (in press). dx.doi.org/10.7717/peerj.569.
25. Cintra-Francischinelli M, Pizzo P, Rodrigues-Simioni L, Ponce-Soto L, Rossetto O, et al. (2009) Calcium imaging of muscle cells treated with snake myotoxins reveals toxin synergism and presence of receptors. Cell Mol Life Sci 66: 1718–1728.
26. Fernández J, Caccin P, Koster G, Lomonte B, Gutiérrez JM, et al. (2013) Muscle phospholipid hydrolysis by *Bothrops asper* Asp49 and Lys49 phospholipase A$_2$ myotoxins - distinct mechanisms of action. FEBS J 280: 3878–3886.
27. Lomonte B, Moreno E, Tarkowski A, Hanson LÅ, Maccarana M (1994) Neutralizing interaction between heparins and myotoxin II, a Lys-49 phospholipase A$_2$ from *Bothrops asper* snake venom. Identification of a heparin-binding and cytolytic toxin region by the use of synthetic peptides and molecular modeling. J Biol Chem 269: 29867–29873.
28. Lomonte B, Angulo Y, Santamaría C (2003) Comparative study of synthetic peptides corresponding to region 115–129 in Lys49 myotoxic phospholipases A$_2$ from snake venoms. Toxicon 42: 307–312.
29. Núñez CE, Angulo Y, Lomonte B (2001) Identification of the myotoxic site of the Lys49 phospholipase A$_2$ from *Agkistrodon piscivorus piscivorus* snake venom: synthetic C-terminal peptides from Lys49, but not from Asp49 myotoxins, exert membrane-damaging activities. Toxicon 39: 1587–1594.
30. Chioato L, de Oliveira AHC, Ruller R, Sá JM, Ward RJ (2002) Distinct sites for myotoxic and membrane-damaging activities in the C-terminal region of a Lys49-phospholipase A$_2$. Biochem J 366: 971–976.
31. Chioato L, Ward RJ (2003) Mapping structural determinants of biological activities in snake venom phospholipases A$_2$ by sequence analysis and site directed mutagenesis. Toxicon 42, 869–883.
32. Cintra-Francischinelli M, Pizzo P, Angulo Y, Gutiérrez JM, Montecucco C, et al. (2010) The C-terminal region of a Lys49 myotoxin mediates Ca^{2+} influx in C2C12 myotubes. Toxicon 55: 590–596.
33. Gutiérrez JM (1995) Clinical toxicology of snakebite in Central America. In: Handbook of Clinical Toxicology of Animal Venoms and Poisons (Meier J, White J, eds), 645–665. CRC Press, Boca Ratón.
34. Angulo Y, Lomonte B (2009) Biochemistry and toxicology of toxins purified from the venom of the snake *Bothrops asper*. Toxicon 54: 949–957.
35. Fernández J, Gutiérrez JM, Angulo Y, Sanz L, Juárez P, et al. (2010) Isolation of an acidic phospholipase A$_2$ from the venom of the snake *Bothrops asper* of Costa Rica: Biochemical and toxicological characterization. Biochimie 92: 273–283.
36. Lomonte B, Gutiérrez JM (1989) A new muscle damaging toxin, myotoxin II, from the venom of the snake *Bothrops asper* (terciopelo). Toxicon 27: 725–733.
37. Francis B, Gutiérrez JM, Lomonte B, Kaiser II (1991) Myotoxin II from *Bothrops asper* (Terciopelo) venom is a lysine-49 phospholipase A$_2$. Archs Biochem Biophys 284: 352–359.
38. Kaiser II, Gutierrez JM, Plummer D, Aird SD, Odell GV (1990) The amino acid sequence of a myotoxic phospholipase from the venom of *Bothrops asper*. Archs Biochem Biophys 278: 319–325.
39. Holzer M, Mackessy SP (1996) An aqueous endpoint assay of snake venom phospholipase A$_2$. Toxicon 34: 1149–1155.
40. Lomonte B, Angulo Y, Rufini S, Cho W, Giglio JR, et al. (1999) Comparative study of the cytolytic activity of myotoxic phospholipases A$_2$ on mouse

endothelial (tEnd) and skeletal muscle (C2C12) cells *in vitro*. Toxicon 37: 145–158.

41. Lomonte B, Angulo Y, Sasa M, Gutiérrez JM (2009) The phospholipase A_2 homologues of snake venoms: biological activities and their possible adaptive roles. Prot Peptide Lett 16: 860–876.

42. Moura-da-Silva AM, Paine MJI, Diniz MRV, Theakston RDG, Crampton JM (1995) The molecular cloning of a phospholipase A_2 from *Bothrops jararacussu* snake venom: evolution of venom group II phospholipase A_2's may imply gene duplications. J Mol Evol 41: 174–179.

43. Tsai IH, Chen YH, Wang YM, Tu MC, Tu AT (2001) Purification, sequencing, and phylogenetic analyses of novel Lys-49 phospholipases A_2 from the venoms of rattlesnakes and other pit vipers. Archs Biochem Biophys 394: 236–244.

44. Angulo Y, Olamendi-Portugal T, Alape-Girón A, Possani LD, Lomonte B (2002) Structural characterization and phylogenetic relationships of myotoxin II from *Atropoides (Bothrops) nummifer* snake venom, a Lys49 phospholipase A_2 homologue. Int J Biochem Cell Biol 34: 1268–1278.

45. Lynch VJ (2007) Inventing an arsenal: adaptive evolution and neofunctionalization of snake venom phospholipase A_2 genes. BMC Evolut Biol 7: 2, doi:10.1186/1471-2148-7-2.

46. dos Santos JI, Cintra-Francischinelli M, Borges RJ, Fernandes CAH, Pizzo P, et al., (2010) Structural, functional, and bioinformatics studies reveal a new snake venom homologue phospholipase A_2 class. Proteins 79: 61–78.

47. Angulo Y, Lomonte B (2005) Differential susceptibility of C2C12 myoblasts and myotubes to group II phospholipase A_2 myotoxins from crotalid snake venoms. Cell Biochem Funct 23: 307–313.

48. McCue MD (2006) Cost of producing venom in three North American pitviper species. Copeia 2006: 818–825.

49. Morgenstern D, King GF (2013) The venom optimization hypothesis revisited. Toxicon 63: 120–128.

50. Gutiérrez JM, Ownby CL, Odell GV (1984) Isolation of a myotoxin from *Bothrops asper* venom: partial characterization and action on skeletal muscle. Toxicon 22: 115–128.

51. Gutiérrez JM, Romero M, Núñez J, Chaves F, Borkow G, et al., (1995) Skeletal muscle necrosis and regeneration after injection of BaH1, a hemorrhagic metalloproteinase isolated from the venom of the snake *Bothrops asper* (terciopelo). Exp Mol Pathol 62: 28–41.

52. Kihara H, Uchikawa R, Hattori S, Ohno M (1992) Myotoxicity and physiological effects of three *Trimeresurus flavoviridis* phospholipases A_2. Biochem Int 28: 895–903.

53. Shen Z, Cho W (1995) Membrane leakage induced by synergetic action of Lys-49 and Asp-49 *Agkistrodon piscivorus piscivorus* phospholipases A_2: implications in their pharmacological activities. Int J Biochem Cell Biol 27: 1009–1013.

54. Díaz C, Gutiérrez JM, Lomonte B, Gené JA (1991) The effect of myotoxins isolated from *Bothrops* snake venoms on multilamellar liposomes: relationship to phospholipase A_2, anticoagulant and myotoxic activities. Biochim Biophys Acta 1070: 455–460.

55. Rufini S, Cesaroni P, Desideri A, Farias R, Gubenšek F, et al., (1992) Calcium ion-independent membrane leakage induced by phospholipase-like myotoxins. Biochemistry 31: 12424–12430.

56. Cintra-Francischinelli M, Caccin P, Chiavegato A, Pizzo P, Carmignoto G, et al., (2010) *Bothrops* snake myotoxins induce a large efflux of ATP and potassium with spreading of cell damage and pain. Proc Natl Acad Sci USA 107: 14140–14145.

57. Bustillo S, Gay CC, García Denegri ME, Ponce-Soto LA, Bal de Kier Joffe E, et al., (2012) Synergism between baltergin metalloproteinase and Ba SPII RP4 PLA_2 from *Bothrops alternatus* venom on skeletal muscle (C2C12) cells. Toxicon 59, 338–343.

58. Caccin P, Pellegatti P, Fernández J, Vono M, Cintra-Francischinelli M, et al. (2013) Why myotoxin-containing snake venoms possess powerful nucleotidases? Biochem Biophys Res Comm 430, 1289–1293.

The Protective Effect of Esculentoside A on Experimental Acute Liver Injury in Mice

Fang Zhang[1,2,9], Xingtong Wang[1,9], Xiaochen Qiu[3,9], Junjie Wang[1], He Fang[1], Zhihong Wang[1], Yu Sun[1], Zhaofan Xia[1]*

1 Department of Burn Surgery, the Second Military Medical University affiliated Changhai Hospital, Shanghai, China, 2 Number 73901 Troop of PLA, Shanghai, China, 3 Department of General Surgery, 309th Hospital of PLA, Beijing, China

Abstract

Inflammatory response and oxidative stress are considered to play an important role in the development of acute liver injury induced by carbon tetrachloride (CCl_4) and galactosamine (GalN)/lipopolysaccharides (LPS). Esculentoside A (EsA), isolated from the Chinese herb phytolacca esculenta, has the effect of modulating immune response, cell proliferation and apoptosis as well as anti-inflammatory effects. The present study is to evaluate the protective effect of EsA on CCl_4 and GalN/LPS-induced acute liver injury. In vitro, CCK-8 assays showed that EsA had no cytotoxicity, while it significantly reduced levels of TNF-α and cell death rate challenged by CCl_4. Moreover, EsA treatment up-regulated PPAR-γ expression of LO2 cells and reduced levels of reactive oxygen species (ROS) challenged by CCl_4. In vivo, EsA prevented mice from CCl_4-induced liver histopathological damage. In addition, levels of AST and ALT were significantly decreased by EsA treatment. Furthermore, the mice treated with EsA had a lower level of TNF-α, Interleukin (IL)-1β and IL-6 in mRNA expression. EsA prevented MDA release and increased GSH-Px activity in liver tissues. Immunohistochemical staining showed that over-expression of F4/80 and CD11b were markedly inhibited by EsA. The western bolt results showed that EsA significantly inhibited CCl_4-induced phosphonated IkBalpha (P-IκB) and ERK. Furthermore, EsA treatment also alleviated GalN/LPS-induced acute liver injury on liver enzyme and histopathological damage. Unfortunately, our results exhibited that EsA had no effects on CCl_4-induced hepatocyte apoptosis which were showed by TUNEL staining and Bax, Caspase-3 and cleaved Caspase-3 expression. Our results proved that EsA treatment attenuated CCl_4 and GalN/LPS-induced acute liver injury in mice and its protective effects might be involved in inhibiting inflammatory response and oxidative stress, but not apoptosis with its underlying mechanism associated with PPAR-γ, NF-κB and ERK signal pathways.

Editor: Hervé Guillou, INRA, France

Funding: This work was financially supported by the key project of the National Natural Science Foundation of China (No. 81120108015), the National "973" key project of China (No. 2012CB518100) and the 1255 Foundation of Changhai Hospital (No. CH125510200). The funders had no role in study design, data collection and analysis, decision to publish, or preparation of the manuscript.

Competing Interests: The authors have declared that no competing interests exist.

* Email: xiazhaofan@163.com

9 These authors contributed equally to this work.

Introduction

Liver is one of the most important internal organs in human body with multiple of functions such as detoxification, protein synthesis, and production of biochemicals necessary for digestion etc [1]. In addition, liver is also the most vulnerable organ attacked by chemical toxic agents [2]. Acute liver injury is usually referred as the rapid development of hepatocellular dysfunction with a poor prognosis. It frequently results from the induction of drugs, virus infection, toxins or hepatic ischemic-reperfusion injury, et al [3,4]. CCl_4 is a well-known hepatotoxin widely used to induce acute and chronic toxic liver injury in a wide range of laboratory animals [1,5]. The toxicity of CCl_4 results from its reductive dehalogenation by cytochrome P450 into the highly reactive free radical trichloromethyl radical (•CCl_3). Free radicals probably activate Kupffer cells and mediate the hepatic inflammation process through producing TNF-α and other pro-inflammatory cytokines. In the presence of excess oxygen, •CCl_3 can transform into trichloromethylperoxy radical CCl_3OO•, another highly reactive species [2,3]. This molecule can also decrease polyunsaturated fatty acids and cause lipid peroxidation, which contributes to severe cellular damage [6,7]. Another classical animal model achieved by intraperitoneal injection of GalN/LPS has often been used for the study of acute liver injury. GalN acts as a sensitizing agent because it depletes hepatic stores of uridine triphosphate via the galactose pathway. Low doses of LPS cause modest inflammatory responses resulting in increased susceptibility to numerous hepatotoxic chemicals, combined with GalN. As a response, hepatocytes strive to clear LPS, which is followed by inflammatory response, oxidative stress and even hepatic necrosis [8].

EsA is a saponin isolated from the root of Phytolacca esculenta, which is identified as 3-O-[b-D-glucopyranosyl-(1,4)-b-D-xylopyranosyl] phytolaccagenin (Fig. 1.) [9]. EsA has the effect of modulating immune response, cellular proliferation and apoptosis as well as anti-inflammatory effects in acute and chronic experimental models [10,11]. Ju DW et al have demonstrated that EsA has the ability to inhibit pro-inflammatory cytokine production such as TNF-α, IL-1β, IL-2, IL-6 and prostaglandin E2 in several cell types [12,13]. EsA is also referred to reduce the radiation-induced cutaneous and fibrovascular toxicities both in vivo and vitro [14]. Furthermore, EsA can also suppress inflammatory responses in LPS-induced acute lung injury through inhibiting the over-activity of NF-κB and mitogen activated protein kinase (MAPK) signal pathways [15]. However, it remains unclear whether EsA has a protective effect on CCl_4 and GalN/LPS-induced acute liver injury, which might be associated with inhibiting inflammatory response and oxidative stress.

This is our first study to investigate the protective effect of EsA treatment on experimental acute liver injury. Therefore, we investigated the protective effect of EsA on experimental acute liver injury using both cell culture and animal experimental systems. In our study, we found that EsA treatment attenuated CCl_4 and GalN/LPS-induced acute liver injury and its protective effect might be involved in inhibiting inflammatory response and oxidative stress, the underlying mechanism was associated with PPAR-γ, ERK and NF-κB signal pathways.

Materials and Methods

Cell culture and experimental animals

The human normal hepatocyte cell lines LO2 were kindly provided by the Eastern Hepato-Biliary Hospital, Second Military Medical University (SMMU), Shanghai. The cell line was cultured in Dulbecco's Modified Eagles Medium (DMEM) and 10% FBS at 37°C under a humidified atmosphere of 5% CO_2.

Male C57Bl/6 mice (20–25g) were obtained from the Experimental Animal Center, SMMU, Shanghai. They were maintained under controlled conditions (23±3°C, 50±10% humidity and 12 h day/night rhythm) and fed standard laboratory chaw. All animal experiments were approved by Institutional Animal Care and Use Committee of SMMU in accordance with the Guide for Care and Use of Laboratory Animals published by U.S. National Institutes of Health (NIH) (publication No. 96-01).

Material and reagents

EsA was kindly provided by the Department of Phytochemistry, College of Pharmacy, SMMU, Shanghai. Cell culture reagents were purchased from Invitrogen (Carlsbad, CA, USA). The ELISA kits of TNF-α was obtained from R&D Systems (Minneapolis, MN, USA). CCl_4, GalN and LPS were purchased from Sigma (St. Louis, MO, USA). The rabbit monoclonal antibody Bax, Caspase-3, cleaved Caspase-3, ERK, P-ERK, IκB, P-IκB and GAPDH were purchased from Cell Signaling Technology Inc (Beverly, MA, USA). F4/80 and CD11b were purchased from Abcam (Cambridge, MA, USA). The rabbit monoclonal antibody PPAR-γ was purchased from Wanlei Biotechnology (Shenyang, China). The horseradish peroxidase econjugated goat anti-rabbit and goat anti-mouse antibodies were provided by Santa Cruz Biotechnology (Dallas, Texas, USA). CCK-8 assays were obtained from Dojindo Laboratories, Kumamoto, Japan. Trizol Reagent was purchased from Invitrogen (Carlsbad, CA, USA). MDA and GSH-px assays were obtained from Jiancheng Bioengineering Institute (Jiangsu, China). ROS assays were purchased from Beyotime institute of biotechnology (Jiangsu, China). All other chemicals used were of reagent grade.

Experiment protocol

In vitro, LO2 cells were seeded at 5×10^3 per well into 96 well microplate and incubated with DMEM and 10% FBS for 24 hours. The cell culture mediums were removed, different concentrations of EsA were added respectively (1.25 mg/L, 2.5 mg/L, 5 mg/L and 10 mg/L) and 70% CCl_4 injury liquid was added as reported (n = 5 in each group) [16]. Parts of the cells were incubated for 4 hours, then 20 ul of CCK-8 solution was added to each well and incubated for another 4 hours at 37°C [17]. Other parts of LO2 cells were incubated with CCl_4 and 5 mg/L EsA for 8 hours as above. Then the cell culture medium was sent for measurement of TNF-α. LO2 cells were observed for cell death rate using flow cytometry analysis. In order to evaluate the effect of EsA on the expression of PPAR-γ gene, LO2 cells were seeded at 5×10^6 per well into 6 well microplate and incubated with DMEM and 10% FBS for 24 hours. PPAR-γ siRNA was cultured with LO2 cells for 24 hours according to the

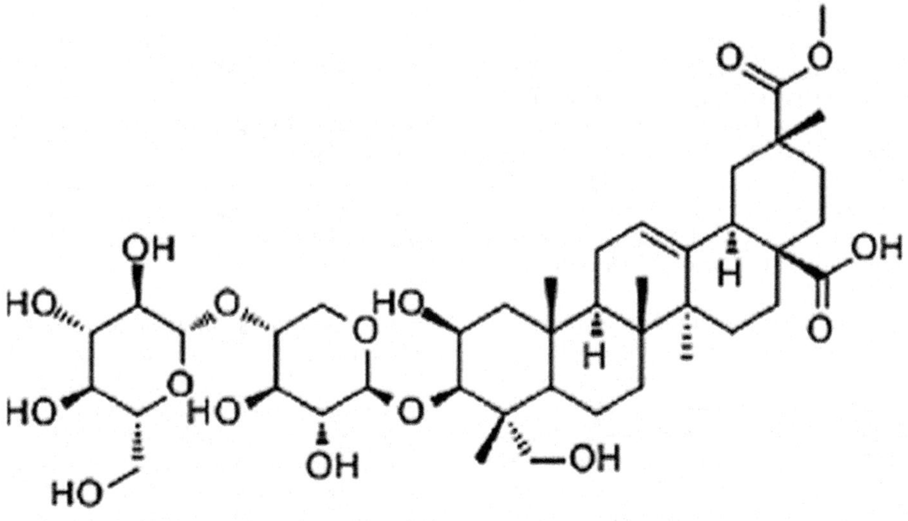

Figure 1. The molecular structure of Esculentoside A (EsA).

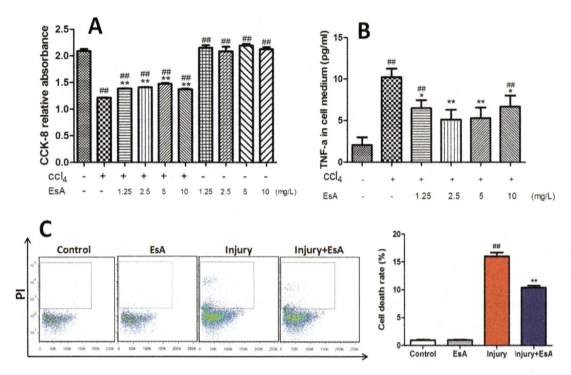

Figure 2. Measurement of EsA cytotoxicity and effects of EsA on CCl_4-induced LO_2 cell injury in vitro. The EsA cytotoxicity was measured using CCK-8 assays (A). Levels of TNF-α in LO2 culture mediums challenged by CCl_4 increased to approximately 4-fold and which was dramatically prevented by EsA treatment, and the concentration of 2.5 mg/L reduced the level of TNF-α most obviously (B). The cell death rate was observed by flow cytometric analysis (C). The values presented are the means ± standard error of the mean (n = 5). $^{\#\#}P<0.01$ versus the Control group. $^{*}P<0.05$, $^{**}P<0.01$ versus the Injury group.

instruction manuals (F, 5′-CUGGCCUCCUUGAUGAAUAUU-3′, R, 5′-UAUUCACAAGGAGGCCAGTT-3′ designed by Jima institute of biotechnology, Shanghai), then the cell culture mediums were removed, 2.5 mg/L EsA and 70% CCl_4 injury liquid were added as above. After 4 hours, ROS assays, real-time PCR and western blot were performed.

In vivo, CCl_4-induced acute liver injury was firstly performed to evaluate the effect of EsA treatment. Twenty-four mice were randomly divided into the following four groups (n = 6 in each group): (1) Control group, mice were injected i.p. with glycerol and distilled water (2:3 v/v, 5 ml/kg) and olive oil (5 ml/kg). (2) EsA group, EsA was dissolved in glycerol and distilled water (2:3 v/v) and given (i.p., 5 mg/kg) 30 minutes after administration of olive oil (i.p., 5 ml/kg). (3) Injury group, CCl_4 mixed with olive oil (1:9 v/v, 5 ml/kg) was injected i.p. for acute liver injury model, glycerol and distilled water (2:3 v/v) were given (i.p., 5 ml/kg) 30 minutes later. (4) Injury + EsA group, EsA was dissolved in glycerol and distilled water (2:3 v/v) and given (i.p., 5 mg/kg) 30 minutes after administration of CCl_4 and olive oil as the Injury group.

GalN/LPS-induced acute liver injury model was performed as described [18]. The grouping was as above (n = 6 in each group): (1) Control group, mice were injected i.p. with glycerol and distilled water (2:3 v/v, 5 ml/kg) and PBS water (5 ml/kg). (2) EsA group, EsA was dissolved in glycerol and distilled water as above and given (i.p., 5 mg/kg) 30 minutes after administration of PBS water (i.p., 5 ml/kg). (3) Injury group, GalN/LPS were dissolved in PBS water respectively and injected (i.p., GalN 800 mg/kg, LPS 5 ug/kg, PBS 5 ml/kg). After 30 minutes, glycerol and distilled water (i.p., 2:3 v/v, 5 ml/kg) were given. (4) Injury + EsA group, EsA was given 30 minutes after GalN/LPS administration. The mice were sacrificed by an overdose of pentobarbital sodium (i.p., 20 mg/body weight) with blood sample and liver tissues collection 12 hours after CCl_4 or GalN/LPS administration.

Cytotoxicity assays in vitro

The EsA cytotoxicity to LO2 cells was measured by CCK-8 assays after CCl_4 challenge. Cell viability was expressed as optical density (OD), which was proportional to the numbers of living cells. The absorbance of each well was measured by multiskan spectrum microplate reader (Biotek, USA) at 490 nm. The assays were performed as reported [19].

Measurement of pro-inflammatory cytokines in LO2 culture medium

In order to test the anti-inflammatory effect of EsA in vitro, TNF-α in LO2 culture mediums were measured with a commercial ELISA kit following the instructions of the manufacturer.

Flow cytometric analysis of cell death in vitro

To observe the effect of EsA on LO2 cell death rate induced by CCl_4, LO2 cells treated with CCl_4 were centrifuged at 1000 rpm for 10 minutes. The resulting pellet was suspended and adjusted to 1×10^6 cells/ml in 10 ul propidium iodide (PI) buffer solution and 2 ul PI staining was performed to observe dead cells. The cells were analyzed by flow cytometry using a FACScan (Mitenyi Biotech, Germany). The measurement of cell death rate was obtained following the instructions of the manufacturer (Baihao biology CO., LTD, Beijing).

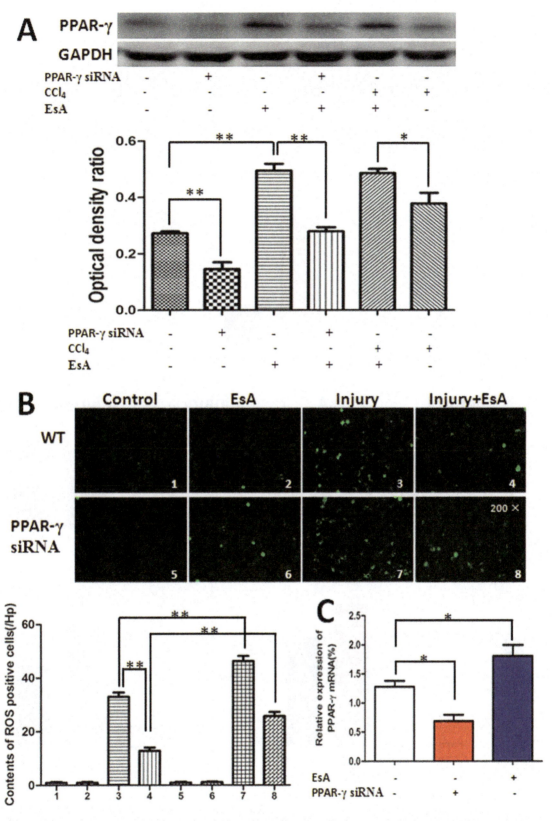

Figure 3. Effects of EsA on CCl_4-induced LO_2 cell injury and PPAR-γ expression. The treatment effects of EsA and protein expression of PPAR-γ were measured using western blot (A). Levels of ROS in LO2 cells challenged by CCl_4 were shown (B Magnification, 200×). The mRNA expression of PPAR-γ was measured using quantitative real-time PCR (C). The values presented are the means ± standard error of the mean (n = 5). *P<0.05, **P<0.01.

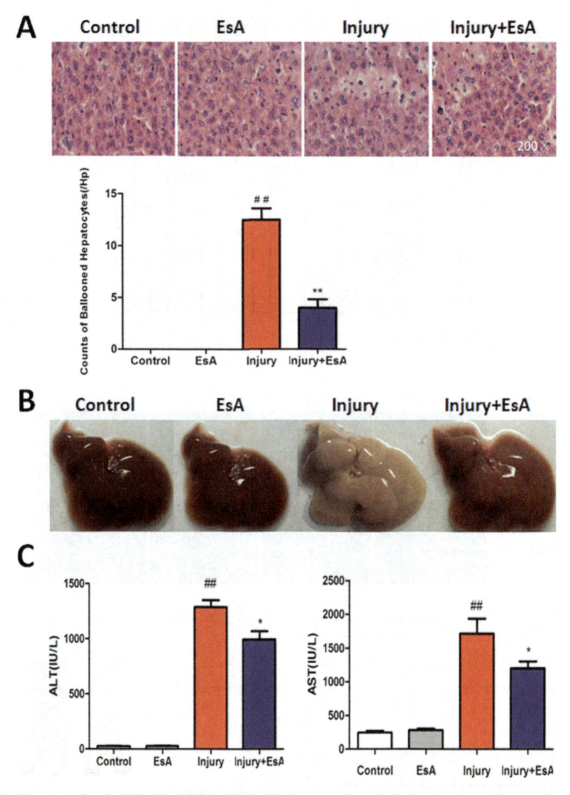

Figure 4. EsA protected against CCl$_4$-induced histopathological damage and hepatic dysfunction. Hematoxylin and eosin staining (A Magnification, 200×) showed that livers in Injury group exhibited more ballooned hepatocytes than those in Control group and EsA group, and symptoms of those histopathological damage were significantly alleviated by EsA treatment (n=6). Photographs of livers were taken 12 hours post-CCl$_4$ injection, livers in Injury group turned white (B). Levels of AST and ALT increased obviously after CCl$_4$ challenge. However, AST and ALT levels did not markedly increase in mice treated with EsA alone, and AST and ALT levels were significantly decreased with EsA treatment. (n=6 C). The values presented are the means ± standard error of the mean. ##$P<0.01$ versus the Control group. *$P<0.05$, **$P<0.01$ versus the Injury group.

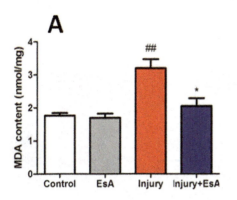
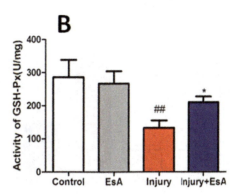

Figure 5. Effects of EsA on CCl$_4$-induced liver oxidative stress. EsA treatment significantly decreased levels of MDA (A) and increased the activity of GSH-Px (B) compared with the Injury group. The values presented are the means ± standard error of the mean (n = 6). ##P<0.01 versus the Control group. *P<0.05 versus the Injury group.

Measurement of serum liver enzymes

To assess EsA toxicity to livers and the effect of EsA treatment for CCl$_4$ and GalN/LPS-induced acute liver injury, serum enzymes (AST and ALT) were measured by an automatic blood biochemical analyzer (7600-120, Hitachi High-Technologies Corp., Tokyo, Japan) using commercial kits [20].

Hematoxylin and eosin staining (H&E)

For histological analysis, a portion of liver from the left lobe was fixed in 10% neutral-buffered formalin and embedded in paraffin. Sections of 5 µm thickness were affixed to slides, and stained with H&E. Finally, histopathological changes in the slices were observed with a light photomicroscope and were evaluated for pathological change using double blind method.

Immunohistochemistry for CD11b and F4/80

Immunohistochemistry was performed with CD11b and F4/80 antibody by the methods as described previously [21]. Briefly, sections of liver tissues were deparaffinized and incubated with anti-mice-CD11b and F4/80 antibody overnight at 4°C. The sections were washed and then incubated with anti-rabbit-IgG. Secondary labeling was achieved by biotinylated rabbit anti-rat antibody. Horseradish peroxidase-conjugated avidin and brown-colored diaminobenzidine were used to visualize the labeling. Finally, the slides were counterstained with hematoxylin.

Measurement of MDA levels and GSH-Px activity in vivo and ROS levels *in vitro*

MDA levels and GSH-Px activity in liver tissues were measured using commercial reagent kits (Jiancheng Bioengineering Institute, Jiangsu, China) according to the instruction manuals [22]. The measurement of ROS levels was performed as reported [23]. LO2 cells were stained with 2′,7′-dichlorofluorescein diacetate (DCFH-DA) for 30 minutes at 37°C in the dark, then the cells were washed three times with serum-free DMEM medium, the fluorescence intensity was detected with a multi-detection microplate reader with excitation at 488 nm and emission at 530 nm.

Quantitative real-time PCR (SYBR Green method)

Total RNA was extracted from liver tissues and LO2 cells using Trizol. Quantitative real-time PCR was carried out using SYBR Green PCR Master Mix in a total volume of 10 ul on Step One Plus Real-Time PCR System (Applied Biosystems) as follows: 95°C for 30s, 40 cycles of 95°C for 15s, 60°C for 30s and 72°C for 35s. GAPDH and 18S were used as the reference genes. The relative levels of gene expression were represented as $\Delta Ct = Ct$ gene $-$ Ct reference, and the fold change of gene expression was calculated using the $2^{-\Delta\Delta Ct}$ method [24].

Primer Sequences

- TNF-α (Mouse); F, 5′-TGTCTCAGCCTCTTCTCATT-3′, R, 5′-AGATGATCTGAGTGTGAGGG-3′
- IL-1β (Mouse); F 5′- GCAGGCAGTATCACTCATTG-3′, R, 5′-CACACCAGCAGGTTATCATC-3′
- IL-6 (Mouse); F, 5′-ATGAAGTTCCTCTCTGCAAGAGACT-3′, R, 5′-CACTAGGTTTGCCGAGTAGATCTC-3′
- GAPDH (Mouse); F, 5′-AGAACATCATCCCTGCATCC-3′, R, 5′- TCCACCACCCTGTTGCTGTA-3′
- PPAR-γ (Human); F, 5′-CAGGAAAGACAACAGACAAATCA-3′, R, 5′-GGGGTGATGTGTTTGAACTTG-3′
- 18S (Human); F, 5′-GGAAGGGCACCACCAGGAGT-3′, R, 5′-TGCAGCCCCGGACATCTAAG-3′

TUNEL stain

With the sections of liver tissues, terminal deoxynucleotidyl transferase dUTP nick end labeling (TUNEL) assay was performed using the In SituCell Death Detection Kit according to the manufacturer's instructions. TUNEL-positive cells were counted by randomly selecting high-power fields [5].

Western blot analysis

About 200 mg liver tissues or 5×10^6 LO2 cells were homogenized in 1 ml tissue protein extraction reagent. The homogenates were centrifuged at 12,000 rpm for 20 minutes at 4°C, and the supernatants were collected. Protein concentration of the supernatants was determined by BCA protein assay kit. Western blot analysis was performed with ERK, P-ERK, Bax, Caspase-3, cleaved Caspase-3, IκB, P-IκB, PPAR-γ and GAPDH monoclonal antibodies as previously described [25].

Statistical analysis

Statistical description was performed using SPSS 16.0 for windows (SPSS Inc., Chicago, USA). All data were expressed as

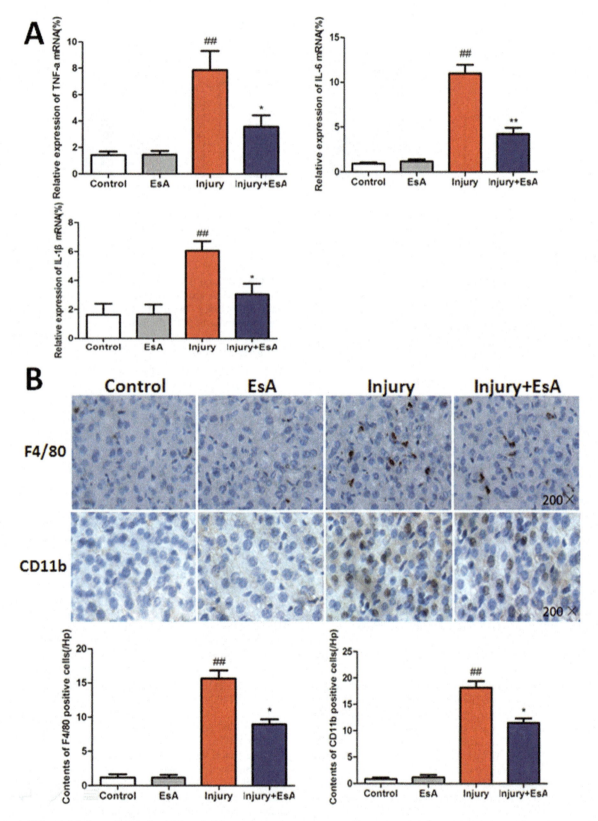

Figure 6. Effects of EsA on CCl$_4$-induced liver inflammation. mRNA expression of TNF-a, IL-1β and IL-6 (A) and Immunohistochemical staining of F4/80 and CD11b cells (B) accumulating in liver tissues were determined at 12 hours post CCl$_4$-induced acute liver injury (Magnification, 200×). The values presented are the means ± standard error of the mean (n=6). $^{\#\#}$P<0.01 versus the Control group. *P<0.05, **P<0.01 versus the Injury group.

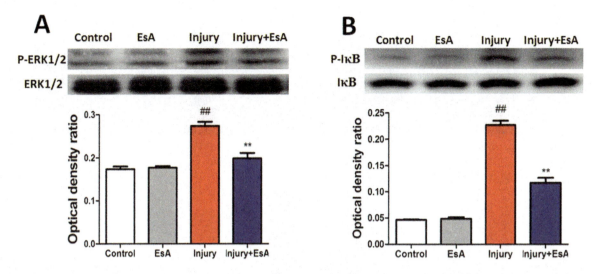

Figure 7. The underlying mechanism of EsA against CCl$_4$-induced acute liver injury in mice. The activity of ERK (A) and IκB (B) were determined by western blot. Relative protein levels were quantified by densitometry and expressed as optical density ratio. The values presented are the means ± standard error of the mean (n = 6). ## P<0.01 versus the Control group. **P<0.01 versus the Injury group.

means ± standard error of the mean (SEM). The statistical significance of differences between groups was analyzed using one-way analysis of variance and two-tailed Student t-test. p<0.05 was considered statistically significant.

Results

Measurement of EsA cytotoxicity and effects of EsA on CCl$_4$-induced LO2 cell injury

The effect of EsA cytotoxicity to LO2 was assessed by CCK-8 assays. Absorbance in LO2 was not reduced by different concentrations of EsA (1.25, 2.5, 5 and 10 mg/L) compared with that in Control group (p>0.05). Furthermore, absorbance of LO2 treated with CCl$_4$ and different concentrations of EsA was higher than that treated with CCl$_4$ alone (p<0.01, Fig. 2. A). These results demonstrated that there was no cytotoxicity for EsA to LO2 cell lines at the concentration of lower than 10 mg/L and the viability of LO2 challenged by CCl$_4$ might be effectively elevated by EsA treatment.

Levels of TNF-α in LO2 culture mediums challenged by CCl$_4$ increased approximately 4-fold. However, different concentrations of EsA (1.25, 2.5, 5 and 10 mg/L) dramatically prevented TNF-α over-production, and EsA treatment reduced levels of TNF-α most obviously at the concentration of 2.5 mg/L (p<0.01, Fig. 2. B). The effect of EsA on cell death rate induced by CCl$_4$ was observed by flow cytometric analysis. The cell death rate in Control group and EsA group were less than 1% respectively, the rate was more than 15% in the Injury group and which was significantly reduced by EsA treatment (p<0.01 Fig. 2. C).

As shown in Fig. 3., levels of cell ROS in the Control group and EsA group were both low, which were elevated rapidly after CCl$_4$ challenge, and EsA treatment decreased levels of ROS significantly. However, the treatment effect of EsA on CCl$_4$ injured cells was affected by PPAR-γ siRNA (p<0.01 Fig. 3. B). The western blot and real-time PCR results exhibited that PPAR-γ expression of LO2 cells were shut down significantly using siRNA technology, and expression of PPAR-γ was up-regulated obviously on cells treated with EsA (p<0.01 Fig. 3. A and p<0.05 Fig. 3. C). Moreover, western blot showed that EsA treatment could also up-regulate PPAR-γ expression of LO2 cells challenged by CCl$_4$ (p<0.05 Fig. 3. A).

EsA administration prevented CCl$_4$-induced liver histopathological damage and hepatic dysfunction

At 12 hours after CCl$_4$-induced liver injury, liver sections showed normal cell morphology, with well-preserved cytoplasm and a clear plump nucleus in the Control and EsA group. However, significant anomalies of liver cells were observed in CCl$_4$-injured mice, where many ballooned cells were exhibited, and symptoms of those histopathological damage were significantly alleviated by EsA treatment (p<0.01 Fig. 4. A). Furthermore, livers of the Injury group turned white at 12 hours after CCl$_4$ injection, suggesting that CCl$_4$ has induced severe liver cell injury. And livers treated with EsA seemed much better than those of the Injury group (Fig. 4. B).

To examine the effects of EsA on CCl$_4$-induced hepatic dysfunction and toxicity of EsA to livers in mice, serum enzymes of liver function were measured. In the Control group, the ALT and AST activities were 24.17±8.01 and 244.17±68.88 IU/L respectively, and there were no markedly increase with a single injection with EsA, whereas the injection of CCl$_4$ in mice led to a rapid increase of ALT and AST activities up to 1285.83±156.28 and 1798.33±440.18 IU/L respectively, with an obvious increases compared to those in the Control and EsA group (p<0.01). However, with the treatment of EsA, the serum activities were significantly decreased compared to the CCl$_4$-intoxicated mice (p<0.05 Fig. 4. C).

EsA treatment lessened oxidative stress in acute liver injury induced by CCl$_4$

In order to evaluate the effects of EsA treatment on oxidative stress induced by CCl$_4$ in liver, we monitored MDA and GSH-Px. As shown in Fig. 5., EsA treatment significantly decreased MDA, a lipid peroxidative product of cell membranes, as indicated by a significant increase in MDA content from 1.76±0.18 and 1.69±0.31 nmol/mg in the Control and EsA group to 3.20±0.66 nmol/mg in the Injury group (p<0.05 Fig. 5. A).

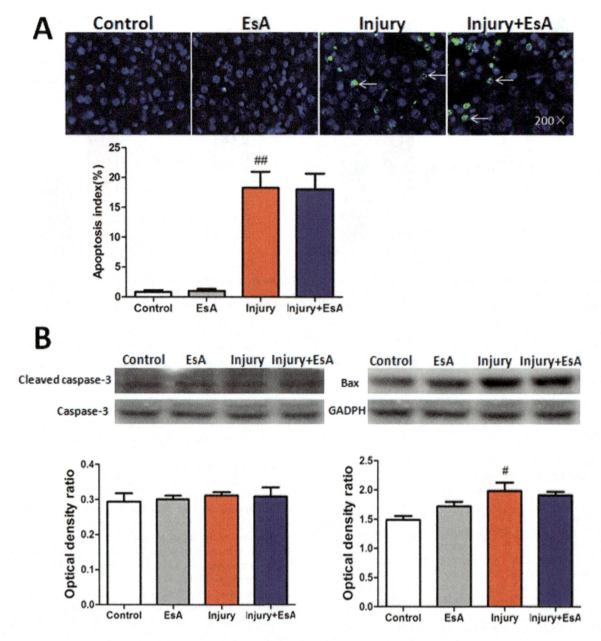

Figure 8. Effects of EsA on cell apoptosis at 12 hours post-CCl$_4$ injection. Liver tissues sections were stained with TUNEL method (Magnification, ×200). There were no obvious difference for rates of positive TUNEL stained cells between the Injury and Injury+EsA groups (A). The activity of Bax, Caspase-3 and cleaved Caspase-3 were determined by western blot. Relative protein levels were quantified by densitometry and expressed as optical density ratio (B). The values presented are the means ± standard error of the mean (n=6). $^{\#}P<0.05$, $^{\#\#}P<0.01$ versus the Control group.

Furthermore, treament with EsA also increased the activity of GSH-Px compared with the Injury group markedly (p<0.05 Fig. 5. B) [26].

Effects of EsA on pro-cytokine production and inflammatory cell infiltration following CCl$_4$ challenge

As Fig. 6. showed that mice treated with EsA exhibited a lower mRNA expression of TNF-α, IL-1β and IL-6 compared with those in the Injury group (p<0.05 and p<0.01, Fig. 6. A). To characterize the inflammatory infiltration, liver sections were subjected to F4/80 antibody staining to identify the presence and distribution of macrophages, and CD11b antibody to identify neutrophils [27,28]. Immunohistochemical staining showed that number of F4/80 and CD11b positive cells accumulating in liver sections was decreased by EsA treatment compared with that in Injury group (p<0.05, Fig. 6. B).

Effects of EsA on ERK/NF-κB pathways activation in acute liver injury induced by CCl$_4$

MAPK families play an important role in CCl$_4$-induced liver inflammatory response [29]. Herein, we tested the effects of EsA on ERK and NF-κB signal pathways in CCl$_4$-induced acute liver

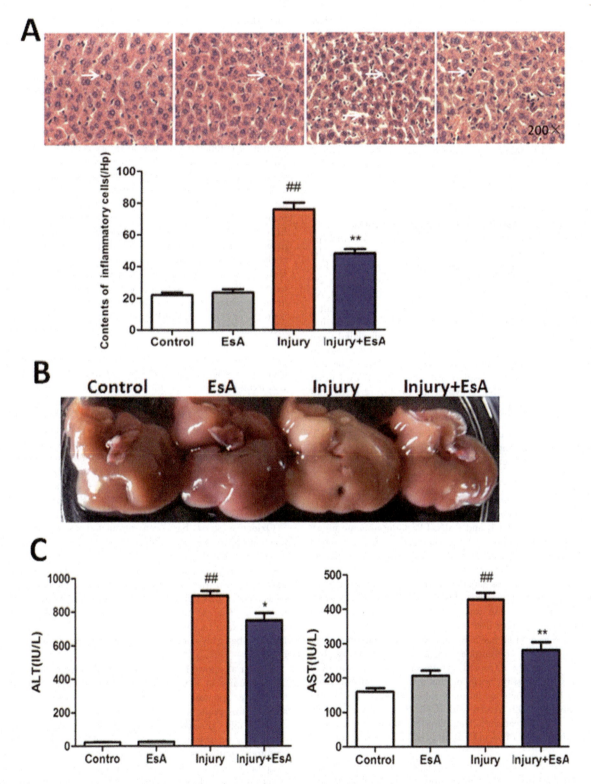

Figure 9. EsA protected against GalN/LPS-induced histopathological damage and hepatic dysfunction. Hematoxylin and eosin staining (A Magnification, 200×) showed that livers in Injury group exhibited more inflammatory cells than those in Control group and EsA group, which were significantly alleviated by treatment of EsA (n = 6). Liver photographs were taken 12 hours post-GalN/LPS administration, and livers in Injury group turned white (B). Levels of AST and ALT increased obviously after GalN/LPS challenge, and which were significantly decreased with EsA treatment (n = 6 C). The values presented are the means ± standard error of the mean. ##$P<0.01$ versus the Control group. *$P<0.05$, **$P<0.01$ versus the Injury group.

injury. With the treatment of EsA, protein expression of P-ERK was significantly lower than that in Injury group. Furthermore, we found that EsA treatment also decreased over-expression of P-IκB induced by CCl_4 compared with the Injury group (p<0.01, Fig. 7.).

EsA treatment had no obvious effects on hepatocyte apoptosis induced by CCl_4

As Fig. 8. showed that treatment with EsA had no obvious effects on TUNEL stain and protein expression of Bax, Caspase-3 and cleaved Caspase-3 compared with the Injury group (p>0.05, Fig. 8.).

EsA protected against GalN/LPS-induced liver histopathological damage and hepatic dysfunction

At 12 hours after GalN/LPS-induced liver injury, abnormal cell morphology and many inflammatory cells were observed in the Injury group compared with those in Control group and EsA group. However, symptoms of these histopathological damage were significantly alleviated by EsA treatment (p<0.01 Fig. 9. A). And livers of the Injury group turned white at 12 hours after GalN/LPS administration, suggesting severe liver cell injury has been induced by GalN/LPS, and EsA treatment alleviated these liver damage (Fig. 9. B). Serum enzymes were measured to evaluate effects of EsA treatment on GalN/LPS-induced hepatic dysfunction in mice. The injection of GalN/LPS led to a rapid increase of ALT and AST activities up to 897.5±71.75 and 427.5±50.07 IU/L respectively, with an obvious increases compared to those in the Control and EsA group (p<0.01). However, with the treatment of EsA, the serum activities of ALT and AST were significantly decreased compared to the mice in the Injury group (p<0.05 and p<0.01 Fig. 9. C).

Discussion

The present study demonstrated that treatment with EsA could protect the liver from CCl_4 and GalN/LPS-induced acute injury in both cell culture and animal experimental systems. We found that EsA treatment significantly reduced hepatic enzymes release, pro-inflammatory cytokine production, inflammatory cells infiltration and oxidative stress damage. Importantly, EsA was proved to have no cytotoxicity in vitro. This must be a preliminary study in demonstrating that EsA treatment can ameliorate CCl_4 and GalN/LPS-induced acute liver injury.

Wu et al. referred that haemolytic activity was the main toxicity of EsA and the high concentration might have cytotoxicity [16]. Therefore, we firstly measured cytotoxicity for EsA to LO2 in vitro by CCK-8 assays, we found that there was no cytotoxicity for EsA to LO2 at the concentration of lower than 10 mg/L and the viability of LO2 treated with CCl_4 might be effectively promoted by EsA treatment. Therefore, we started investigating the protective effect of EsA in CCl_4 and GalN/LPS-induced acute liver injury.

As the acute liver injury induced by CCl_4 and GalN/LPS was characterized with liver dysfunction and cell morphology deterioration, the liver histopathological changes and liver function were investigated. In our study, it was found that EsA treatment could significantly mitigate liver histopathological changes as evidenced by H&E staining. Meanwhile, high levels of ALT and AST challenged by CCl_4 and GalN/LPS, which are direct indicators of hepatic function and correlated with the severity of liver injury, were markedly prevented by treatment with EsA. Our results showed that EsA treatment could lessen hepatic dysfunction and cell morphology deterioration in acute liver injury induced by CCl_4 and GalN/LPS.

Inflammatory cell infiltration and inflammatory response were proved to be involved in the process of CCl_4-induced acute chemical liver injury [30]. In our study, F4/80 (marker for mature mouse macrophages) and CD11b antibodies (marker of neutrophil activation) were used to stain inflammatory cells in liver sections and we found that EsA treatment obviously reduced inflammatory infiltration compared with that in Injury group [27,28]. Previous studies have showed that EsA could decrease both extracellular and cellular TNF-α in a dose dependent manner at concentrations of higher than 1 μmol/L [31]. Similarly, levels of pro-inflammatory cytokines, which are direct indicators of inflammatory response, were also significantly reduced by EsA administration. In our study, EsA treatment also showed obvious effect of preventing the over-production of TNF-α in LO2 cell medium challenged by CCl_4. However, we found that levels of TNF-α were reduced not in a dose dependent manner, and the effect of EsA treatment was best at concentrations of 2.5 mg/L. To explore the underlying anti-inflammatory mechanism of EsA on CCl_4-induced acute liver injury, NF-κB and ERK signal pathways were investigated. Previous works have proved that NF-κB regulated the expression of multiple genes involved in the early inflammatory response, which played a central role in the pathology of acute liver injury and inflammation [32]. Zhong et al. exhibited that EsA-treatment decreased the NF-κB expression in LPS-induced acute lung injury in mice [15]. We found that the active NF-κB signal pathway challenged by CCl_4 was inhibited by EsA treatment, similarly with the ERK. We also found that EsA treatment could up-regulate PPAR-γ gene expression of LO2 cells, and the low expression of PPAR-γ affected the treatment effects of EsA. Thus, the beneficial effect of EsA may be partly due to attenuating inflammatory response in CCl_4 and GalN/LPS-induced acute liver injury via PPAR-γ, ERK and NF-κB signal pathways.

Oxidative stress has been postulated as major molecular mechanisms in acute liver injury induced by CCl_4 [33,34]. Yu et al. referred that the levels of MDA and GSH-Px were associated with CCl_4-induced liver oxidative stress injury [35]. Increased MDA, a lipid peroxidative product of cell membranes, was prevented by EsA treatment in our study [36]. Furthermore, EsA treatment led to an obvious increase in GSH-Px activity, compared with the Injury group. Overall, the protective effect of EsA may be partly due to attenuating oxidative stress in acute liver injury.

Xiao et al. showed that EsA has the positive curative effect on autoimmunity in a mouse model through the acceleration of thymocyte apoptosis [37]. Hu et al. demonstrated that EsA affected pro-apoptotic genes included Fas, p53, redox metabolism, calcium and glucocorticoid-associated apoptosis signals [11]. Therefore, we investigated the effect of EsA on mitochondrial apoptotic pathways including Bax, Caspase-3 and cleaved Caspase-3. But our works reflected that EsA treatment had no effect on CCl_4-induced hepatocyte apoptosis, which were proved by the TUNEL staining and apoptosis–associated protein expression.

In summary, treatment with EsA attenuated CCl_4 and GalN/LPS-induced acute liver injury in mice, and the protective mechanism might be involved in inhibiting inflammatory response and oxidative stress, but not apoptosis. Accordingly, EsA may have potential applications as a supportive treatment for acute liver injury due to its unique advantages.

Supporting Information

Figure S1 The primary data for EsA cytotoxicity and treatment effect of EsA in vitro.

Figure S2 The primary data for EsA treatment on CCl₄-induced LO2 cell injury and PPAR-γ expression.

Figure S3 The primary data for protection of EsA against CCl₄-induced histopathological damage and hepatic dysfunction.

Figure S4 The primary data for EsA treatment on CCl₄-induced liver oxidative stress in mice.

Figure S5 The primary data for EsA treatment on CCl₄-induced liver inflammation in mice.

Figure S6 The primary data for underlying mechanism of EsA against CCl₄-induced acute liver injury.

Figure S7 The primary data for effects of EsA on cell apoptosis after CCl₄ injection.

Figure S8 The primary data for protection of EsA against GalN/LPS-induced histopathological damage and hepatic dysfunction.

Acknowledgments

The authors are grateful for the excellent technical support from Yingying Liu and Li Wang (Burn institute of PLA).

Author Contributions

Conceived and designed the experiments: ZX. Performed the experiments: FZ XW XQ JW HF. Analyzed the data: FZ XW ZW YS. Contributed reagents/materials/analysis tools: FZ XW XQ JW ZW YS. Contributed to the writing of the manuscript: FZ XW XQ ZX.

References

1. Ma JQ, Ding J, Zhang L, Liu CM (2014) Hepatoprotective properties of sesamin against CCl₄ induced oxidative stress-mediated apoptosis in mice via JNK pathway. Food Chem Toxicol 64: 41–8.
2. Bhondave PD, Devarshi PP, Mahadik KR, Harsulkar AM (2014) 'Ashvagandharishta' prepared using yeast consortium from Woodfordia fruticosa flowers exhibit hepatoprotective effect on CCl₄ induced liver damage in Wistar rats. J Ethnopharmacol 151(1): 183–90.
3. Hydes T, Wright M, Jaynes E, Nash K (2014) Nitrofurantoin immune-mediated drug-induced liver injury: a serious complication of a commonly prescribed medication. BMJ Case Rep pii: bcr2013203136.
4. Patel RP, Lang JD, Smith AB, Crawford JH (2014) Redox therapeutics in hepatic ischemia reperfusion injury. World J Hepatol 6(1): 1–8.
5. Kaneko M, Nagamine T, Nakazato K, Mori M (2013) The anti-apoptotic effect of fucoxanthin on carbon tetrachloride-induced hepatotoxicity. J Toxicol Sci 38(1): 115–26.
6. R Domitrovic, H Jakovac, G Blagojevic (2011) Hepatoprotective activity of berberineis mediated by inhibition of TNF-alpha, COX-2, and iNOS expression in CCl(4)-intoxicated mice. Toxicology 280: 33–43.
7. Liu CM, Zheng GH, Ming QL, Chao C, Sun JM (2013) Sesamin protects mouse liver against nickel-induced oxidative DNA damage and apoptosis by the PI3K–Akt pathway. J Agric Food Chem 61(5): 1146–54.
8. Wang Y, Gao LN, Cui YL, Jiang HL (2014) Protective effect of danhong injection on acute hepatic failure induced by lipopolysaccharide and d-galactosamine in mice. Evid Based Complement Alternat Med. Epub: 153902.
9. Wu F, Yi Y, Sun P, Zhang D (2007) Synthesis, in vitro inhibitory activity towards COX-2 and haemolytic activity of derivatives of esculentoside A. Bioor Med Chem Lett 17: 6430.
10. Ma H, Zhang X, Zhang X, Yang D, Meng L, et al. (2013) The effect of esculentoside A on lupus nephritis-prone BXSB mice. Arch Med Sci 9(2): 354–60.
11. Hu Z, Qiu L, Xiao Z, Wang J, Yu Q, et al. (2010) Effects of esculentoside A on autoimmune syndrome induced by Campylobacter jejuni in mice and its modulation on T-lymphocyte proliferation and apoptosis. Int Immunopharmacol 10(1): 65–71.
12. Xiao ZY, Zheng QY, Jiang YY, Zhou B, Yin M, et al. (2004) Effects of esculentoside A on production of interleukin-1, 2, and prostaglandin E2. Acta Pharmacol Sin 25(6): 817–21.
13. Ju DW, Zheng QY, Cao X, Fang J, Wang HB (1998) Esculentoside A inhibits tumor necrosis factor, interleukin-1, and interleukin-6 production induced by lipopolysaccharide in mice. Pharmacology 56(4): 187–95.
14. Xiao Z, Su Y, Yang S, Yin L, Wang W, et al. (2006) Protective effect of esculentoside A on radiation-induced dermatitis and fibrosis. Int J Radiat Oncol Biol Phys 65(3): 882–9.
15. Zhong WT, Jiang LX, Wei JY, Qiao AN, Wei MM, et al. (2013) Protective effect of esculentoside A on lipopolysaccharide-induced acute lung injury in mice. J Surg Res 185(1): 364–72.
16. Wu HJ, Gong X, Yang YT, Wang YZ, Li X, et al. (2012) Improvement of carbon tetrachloride drug-induced liver injury model in vitro. Zhongguo Zhong Yao Za Zhi 37(23): 3633–6.
17. Fan Q, Lu M, Xia ZY, Bao L (2013) Mycobacterium tuberculosis MPT64 stimulates the activation of murine macrophage modulated by IFN-γ. Eur Rev Med Pharmacol Sci 17(24): 3296–305.
18. Sun H, Chen L, Zhou W, Hu L, Li L, et al. (2011) The protective role of hydrogen-rich saline in experimental liver injury in mice. J Hepatol 54(3): 471–80.
19. Zhou RM, Jing YY, Guo Y, Gao C, Zhang BY, et al. (2011) Molecular interaction of TPPP with PrP antagonized the CytoPrP-induced disruption of microtubule structures and cytotoxicity. PLoS One 6(8): e23079.
20. El-Naggar SA, Alm-Eldeen AA, Germoush MO, El-Boray KF (2014) Ameliorative effect of propolis against cyclophosphamide-induced toxicity in mice. Pharm Biol [Epub ahead of print].
21. Hagiwara S, Iwasaka H, Hasegawa A, Koga H, Noguchi T (2008) Effects of hyperglycemia and insulin therapy on high mobility group box 1 in endotoxin-induced acute lung injury in a rat model. Crit Care Med 36: 2407–13.
22. Yin G, Cao L, Xu P, Jeney G, Nakao M, et al. (2011) Hepatoprotective and antioxidant effects of Glycyrrhiza glabra extract against carbon tetrachloride (CCl(4))-induced hepatocyte damage in common carp (Cyprinus carpio). Fish Physiol Biochem 37(1): 209–16.
23. Tao L, Li X, Zhang L, Tian J, Li X, et al. (2011) Protective effect of tetrahydroxystilbene glucoside on 6-OHDA-induced apoptosis in PC12 cells through the ROS-NO pathway. PLoS One 6(10): e26055.
24. Man X, He J, Kong C, Zhu Y, Zhang Z (2014) Clinical significance and biological roles of CARMA3 in human bladder carcinoma. Tumour Biol [Epub ahead of print].
25. Li W, Qiu X, Wang J, Li H, Sun Y, et al. (2013) The therapeutic efficacy of glutamine for rats with smoking inhalation injury. Int Immunopharmacol 16(2): 248–53.
26. Cui Y, Han Y, Yang X, Sun Y, Zhao Y (2013) Protective effects of quercetin and quercetin-5′,8-disulfonate against carbon tetrachloride-caused oxidative liver injury in mice. Molecules 19(1): 291–305.
27. Sato A, Nakashima H, Nakashima M, Ikarashi M, Nishiyama K, et al. (2014) Involvement of the TNF and FasL produced by CD11b Kupffer cells/macrophages in CCl4-induced acute hepatic injury. PLoS One 25; 9(3): e92515.
28. Seki A, Sakai Y, Komura T, Nasti A, Yoshida K, et al. (2013) Adipose tissue-derived stem cells as a regenerative therapy for a mouse steatohepatitis-induced cirrhosis model. Hepatology 58(3): 1133–42.
29. He DK, Shao YR, Zhang L, Shen J, Zhong ZY, et al. (2014) Adenovirus-delivered angiopoietin-1 suppresses NF-κB and p38 MAPK and attenuates inflammatory responses in phosgene-induced acute lung injury. Inhal Toxicol 26(3): 185–92.
30. Mukhopadhyay P, Rajesh M, Cao Z, Horváth B, Park O, et al. (2013) Poly (ADP-ribose) polymerase-1 is a key mediator of liver inflammation and fibrosis. Hepatology doi:10.1002/hep.26763.
31. Jun F, Yue ZQ, Bin WH, Wen JD, Hua YY (1992) Effects of esculentoside A on turnour necrosis factor production by mice peritoneal macrophages. Mediators Inflamm 1(6): 375–7.
32. Liu SF, Malik AB (2006) NF-kappa B activation as a pathological mechanism of septic shock and inflammation. Am J Physiol Lung Cell Mol Physiol 290(4): L622–L645.

33. Sun F, Hamagawa E, Tsutsui C, Ono Y, Ogiri Y, et al. (2001) Evaluation of oxidative stress during apoptosis and necrosis caused by carbon tetrachloride in rat liver. Biochim Biophys Acta 1535(2): 186–91.
34. Weber LW, Boll M, Stampfl A (2003) Hepatotoxicity and mechanism of action of haloalkanes: carbon tetrachloride as a toxicological model. Crit Rev Toxicol 33(2): 105–36.
35. Yu H, Zheng L, Yin L, Xu L, Qi Y, et al. (2014) Protective effects of the total saponins from Dioscorea nipponica Makino against carbon tetrachloride-induced liver injury in mice through suppression of apoptosis and inflammation. Int Immunopharmacol pii: S1567-5769(14)00033-2.
36. Montanari RM, Barbosa LC, Demuner AJ, Silva CJ, Andrade NJ, et al. (2012) Exposure to Anacardiaceae volatile oils and their constituents induces lipid peroxidation within food-borne bacteria cells. Molecules 17(8): 9728–40.
37. Xiao ZY, Zheng QY, Zhang JP, Jiang YY, Yi YH (2002) Effect of esculentoside A on autoimmunity in mice and its possible mechanisms. Acta Pharmacol Sin 23(7): 638–44.

PSMA Ligand Conjugated PCL-PEG Polymeric Micelles Targeted to Prostate Cancer Cells

Jian Jin[1], Bowen Sui[1], Jingxin Gou[2], Jingshuo Liu[1], Xing Tang[2], Hui Xu[2], Yu Zhang[2], Xiangqun Jin[1]*

[1] Department of Pharmaceutics, College of Pharmacy Sciences, Jilin University, Changchun, People's Republic of China, [2] Department of Pharmaceutics, Shenyang Pharmaceutical University, Shenyang, People's Republic of China

Abstract

In this content, a small molecular ligand of prostate specific membrane antigen (SMLP) conjugated poly (caprolactone) (PCL)-b-poly (ethylene glycol) (PEG) copolymers with different block lengths were synthesized to construct a satisfactory drug delivery system. Four different docetaxel-loaded polymeric micelles (DTX-PMs) were prepared by dialysis with particle sizes less than 60 nm as characterized by dynamic light scattering (DLS) and transmission electron microscope (TEM). Optimization of the prepared micelles was conducted based on short-term stability and drug-loading content. The results showed that optimized systems were able to remain stable over 7 days. Compared with Taxotere, DTX-PMs with the same ratio of hydrophilic/hydrophobic chain length displayed similar sustained release behaviors. The cytotoxicity of the optimized targeted DTX-PCL$_{12K}$-PEG$_{5K}$-SMLP micelles (DTX-PMs2) and non-targeted DTX-PCL$_{12K}$-mPEG$_{5K}$ micelles (DTX-PMs1) were evaluated by MTT assays using prostate specific membrane antigen (PSMA) positive prostate adenocarcinoma cells (LNCaP). The results showed that the targeted micelles had a much lower IC50 than their non-targeted counterparts (48 h: 0.87±0.27 vs 13.48±1.03 μg/ml; 72 h: 0.02±0.008 vs 1.35±0.54 μg/ml). In vitro cellular uptake of PMs2 showed 5-fold higher fluorescence intensity than that of PMs1 after 4 h incubation. According to these results, the novel nano-sized drug delivery system based on DTX-PCL-PEG-SMLP offers great promise for the treatment of prostatic cancer.

Editor: Gnanasekar Munirathinam, University of Illinois, United States of America

Funding: The authors have no funding or support to report.
Competing Interests: The authors have declared that no competing interests exist.
* Email: jinxq@jlu.edu.cn

Introduction

Polymeric micelles have received considerable attention as promising anticancer drug carriers because of their remarkable advantages, such as small size, narrow size distribution, high biocompatibility, and solubilization of hydrophobic drugs [1,2,3,4,5]. Self-assembled polymeric micelles with core/shell structures enable the system to incorporate poorly water-soluble drugs in the hydrophobic core and protect them from degradation in physiological media [6]. For example, the hydrophobic core of the micelles composed of PCL-PEG offers a reservoir for the incorporation of drugs, while the pegylated shell along with its nanoscopic size guarantees the carrier remain un-recognized by the reticuloendothelial system and undergo a long-circulation period in the blood [7,8,9].

Although polymeric micelles exhibited a number of advantages, one major challenge is their site-specific drug delivery. Ligand-modified polymeric micelle drug delivery systems are capable of site-specific drug delivery. Recently, numerous active targeting delivery systems have been designed by conjugating NPs with ligands that bind specifically to the biomarkers of extracellular domains of cancer cells. PSMA as folate hydrolase I and glutamate carboxypeptidase II, is a well-known transmembrane protein [10] over expressed on prostate cancer epithelial cells [11,12] and has been shown to have great potential for prostatic cancer (PCa) therapy. PSMA has a low expression in normal prostate epithelial cells and benign prostatic hyperplasia. It is also expressed in the neovasculature of most other solid tumors but not in the vasculature of normal tissues [13,14]. All of these characteristics make PSMA an attractive biomarker for the detection, diagnosis, and treatment of PCa [15,16]. A novel small molecular ligand ((S)-2-(3-((S)-5-amino-1-carboxypentyl) ureido) pentanedioic acid, SMLP) binding specifically to PSMA has demonstrated its potential in the treatment of cancer in recent years [17]. The urea-based PSMA inhibitor, SMLP, has a high affinity for PSMA due to strong hydrogen bonding [10]. Hrkach and Langer et al. developed ACUPA (PSMA ligand) conjugated DTX NPs composed of PEG-b-PLGA or PEG-b-PLA using a nano-emulsification method to target PSMA and evaluated the anti-tumor efficacy of the NPs in vitro and in vivo [18]. The excellent potential offered by vehicle-ligand targeting PSMA suggests the necessity in developing more diversified preparation processes and carrier-materials in this field.

In this study, a nano-sized self-assembled drug delivery system based on ligand-conjugated PEG-b-PCL micelles was found to show great promise in the field of targeted drug delivery. Copolymers of PCL and PEG are both well-known biodegradable and biocompatible materials widely used in biomedical field [19,20,21,22,23]. Due to the introduction of glycolic acid (GA) and lactic acid (LA), which disrupted the ordered structure of the molecular chains, PLGA showed low crystallinity. As a result, micelles with cores of PCL which showed higher crystallinity are more stable than those with PLGA cores. Moreover, because PLGA is a random copolymer, it is relatively difficult to control the ratio of GA to LA precisely in large-scale production. However, the ratio of the two monomers is a key factor to influence the property of PLGA [24]. So PCL was used as the core-forming block due to its better stability and ease to produce. PCL-mPEG or PCL-PEG-COOH was synthesized by ring-opening polymerization of ε-caprolactone initiated by mPEG-OH or HOOC-PEG-OH [25,26]. PCL-mPEG and PCL-PEG-SMLP micelles were prepared using DTX as a model drug to examine the cytotoxic effects on LNCaP cells. Also, a schematic illustration of preparation and endocytosis process of DTX-PCL-PEG-SMLP is shown in Figure 1.

Materials and Methods

Materials

L-glutamic acid di-tertbutyl ester hydrochloride and H-Lys(Z)-Ot-Bu hydrochloride were obtained from En lai Biological Technology Co., LTD (Chengdu, People's Republic of China). mPEG-OH (Mw: 2 kDa) and mPEG-OH (Mw: 5 kDa) (Aladdin Agent Co., Shanghai, P R China) and OH-PEG-COOH(Mw: 2 kDa),OH-PEG-COOH(Mw: 5 kDa) (Shanghai Seebio Biological Technology Co., shanghai, P R China) were dehydrated by azeotropic distillation with toluene before use. DTX (Shanghai Sanwei Pharma Ltd, Co, Shanghai, P R China) and the cellulose ester dialysis bag with a molecular cut-off of 7000 Da (Bioscience Ltd, Co, Shanghai, P R China) were used as received. ε-Caprolactone (ε-CL, Aladdin Agent Co., Shanghai, P R China) was dried over CaH_2 at room temperature for 48 h and distilled under reduced pressure. Stannous octoate was purchased from Aladdin Agent Co (Shanghai, P R China). All organic solvents used in the synthesis procedures were purchased from the National Medicine Chemical Reagent Ltd Co (Shanghai, P R China).

The prostate LNCaP and PC3 cell lines were obtained from the Type Culture Collection of the Chinese Academy of Sciences (Shanghai, China). LNCaP Cells were cultured using cell-bind culture bottles (Corning, USA).

Methods

Synthesis of PCL-mPEG (PMs1) and PCL-PEG-SMLP (PMs2) copolymers. Copolymers with a range of block lengths were prepared by ring-opening copolymerization of ε-CL initiated by hydroxyl of PEG. Briefly, a predetermined amount of ε-CL and stannous octoate were added to a reaction vessel containing mPEG-OH or OH-PEG-COOH under a dry argon atmosphere (stannous octoate/ε-CL in 1:1000 molar ratio). Then, the reaction vessel was placed in an oil bath and maintained at 120°C for 24 h. Then the crude copolymers were dissolved in DCM and precipitated in cold diethyl ether to remove the un-reacted monomer and oligomer. Then, the product was filtered and dried to obtain a white precipitate.

PCL_{12k}-PEG_{5k}-COOH (1 g, 0.059 mmol) was dissolved in 5 ml anhydrous tetrahydrofuran (THF) with 1-ethyl-3-[3-dimethylaminopropyl]-carbodiimide hydrochloride (EDC) (57.4 mg, 0.3 mmol, 5 equiv) and N-hydroxysuccinimide (NHS) (27.6 mg, 0.24 mmol, 4 equiv). Then, the solution mixture was stirred at room temperature for over 12 h under argon atmosphere. The PCL_{12k}-PEG_{5k}-NHS copolymer was precipitated in ice-cold diethyl ether to afford a white precipitate which was collected and dried to obtain the desired product as a white powder (yield, 90%). SMLP (300 mg) was dissolved in anhydrous THF (20 ml) to prepare 10 mg/ml (SMLP/THF) aqua. PCL-PEG-NHS (500 mg, 0.03 mmol) and diisopropylethylamine (0.7 ml) were added to 5 ml (SMLP/THF) aqua, and the reaction solution was stirred at room temperature for 20 h under argon. After completion of the reaction, the solution was purified by dialysis for 24 h and dried by lyophilization to obtain a white flocculent powder (yield 90%). The structure of final copolymer was characterized by ^{1}H NMR spectroscopy.

$PCL_{4.8K}$-$mPEG_{2K}$ and $PCL_{4.8k}$-PEG_{2k}-SMLP were prepared using the same method previously stated.

Polymer characterization. The ^{1}H-nuclear magnetic resonance (^{1}H NMR) spectra of all samples were recorded on a Bruker DMX 300 or 600 spectrometer (Billerica, MA). Chemical shifts (δ) were given in ppm using tetramethylsilane as the internal standard. Fourier transform infrared spectroscopy spectra were recorded on a Bruker Tensor 27 spectrometer, and samples were prepared using KBr disks (Scharlau Chemie, Barcelona, Spain).

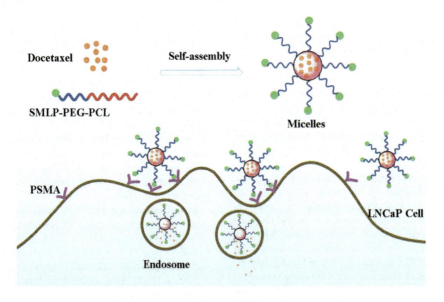

Figure 1. Schematic illustration of DTX-PCL-PEG-SMLP micelles targeted to PSMA.

Gel permeation chromatography (GPC) assay was performed on a Waters 1515 GPC instrument (Waters Corp, Milford, MA) equipped with three styragel columns (Waters Corp; 10^5, 10^4, and 103 Å) in tandem and a 2414 differential refractive index detector. DMF was selected as the eluent at a flow rate of 1.0 ml/min at 35°C. The sample concentrations were approximately 2 mg/ml. The molecular weights were calibrated using polystyrene standards.

Preparation of polymeric micelles. DTX-loaded micelles were prepared by dialysis. First, 7 mg DTX and 50 mg copolymer were completely dissolved in 2 ml THF. Then 4 ml phosphate-buffered saline (PBS; 10 mM, pH 7.4 or 10 mM, pH 5.5) was added drop-wise to the solution under continuous stirring for one hour. Then, THF was removed by dialysis against PBS (10 mM, pH 7.4 or 10 mM, pH 5.5) over 24 h using a cellulose ester dialysis bag (MWCO: 7000 Da). The outer medium was replaced three times (2, 6, and 12 hours). Finally, the mixture was passed through a 0.45 μm filter membrane to remove any precipitants.

Drug-loading content and encapsulation efficiency. To determine the drug-loading content and encapsulation efficiency, 500 μl DTX-loaded micellar solution and 5 ml THF were transferred to a 25 ml volumetric flask, sonicated at 180 W for 10 minutes in an ultrasonic bath, and then diluted with mobile phase. The concentration in the resulting solution was then determined by HPLC. Chromatographic analysis was performed using a Hitachi L-2130 pump and a Hitachi L-2400 UV-Vis detector operated at a wavelength of 230 nm, using a Unitary C18 column (5 μm, 150×4.6 mm). A mobile phase of acetonitrile and water (60/40, v/v) was selected. The flow rate was set at 1 ml/min. The peak area response versus the DTX concentration was linear over the range of 0.5–30 μg/ml ($r^2 = 0.9999$).

The drug-loading content and encapsulation efficiency were calculated from the following equations:

$$\text{Drug loading content} = \frac{\text{Weight of the drug in micelles}}{\text{Weight of the drug in micelles} + \text{Weight of the copolymers used}} \times 100\%$$

$$\text{Encapsulation efficiency} = \frac{\text{Weight of the drug in micelles}}{\text{Weight of the feeding drugs}} \times 100\%$$

Particle size measurements. The particle size and distribution of micelles were measured by DLS using NICOMP 380 Submicron Particle Sizer (Particle Sizing Systems, Santa Barbara, CA). A laser beam at a wavelength of 632.8 nm was used. The scattering angle was set at 90° when measurements were conducted.

Surface morphology. Samples for TEM observation were prepared by placing a drop of sample solution (2 mg/ml for copolymer) on to a copper grid coated with carbon. Excess solution was wiped away with filter paper. The grid was allowed to dry for a further 15 minutes. Then, the samples were examined using a Hitachi H-600 TEM operated at an accelerating voltage of 100 kV.

***In Vitro* Release.** The *in vitro* DTX release kinetics of drug-loaded micellar solutions or DTX injection (Taxotere, Sanofi-Aventis, Paris, France) containing 300 μg DTX were performed by dialysis diffusion. The drug-loaded micellar solution and free drug solution were placed in the dialysis bags (MWCO: 14000). These bags were immersed in 15 ml PBS pH 7.4 (10 mM) or pH 5.5 (10 mM) containing 0.5% w/v Tween 80. Subsequently, the bottles were placed in a shaking incubator at a shaking speed of 100 rpm under 37°C±0.5°C. All release media were replaced with fresh PBS at predetermined intervals (1 h, 2 h, 4 h, 8 h, 12 h, 24 h, 36 h, 48 h, 60 h, 72 h, 84 h and 96 h) in order to measure the drug concentration. The concentration of DTX was measured by HPLC.

Cell Culture and Cytotoxicity. The prostate LNCaP and PC3 cell lines were cultured in RPMI 1640 medium and Ham's F12K (Invitrogen, USA), supplemented with 10% fetal bovine serum (Hyclone, USA), respectively. The cultures were maintained in a 95% air humidified atmosphere containing 5% CO_2 at 37°C.

MTT assay was conducted to evaluate the cytotoxicity of DTX-PMs1 (nontargeted) and DTX-PMs2 (targeted). LNCaP cells were suspended in culture medium and seeded at 5000 cells/well in 96-well plates for 24 h. Then, dispersed DTX-PMs1, DTX-PMs2, and the DMSO solution of DTX (DSD) containing four drug concentrations (0.1, 1, 10 and 20 μg/ml) in each sample were incubated in LNCaP cells. Finally, the cell viability was determined after 48 h and 72 h using a Microplate Reader (Bio-Rad imark, USA).

The IC50 for each system was then calculated. All assays were conducted with five parallel samples.

Cellular uptake studies. In this study, coumarin 6 was used as a fluorescence probe. Androgen-dependent and androgen-independent prostate cell lines (LNCaP and PC3, respectively) were used. Cellular uptake of targeted and non-targeted PMs (200 μg/ml) carrying coumarin 6 (100 μg/ml) (PMs1 and PMs2, respectively) were conducted on LNCaP and PC3 cell lines to investigate the influence of SMLP conjugation on cellular uptake. The cells were incubated in 96-well plates with micelles for 4 h, washed with cold PBS three times, and then fixed with 70% ethanol for 2 h at −20°C. A competitive inhibition study was also conducted using free SMLP to verify whether the PMs were transported into cells in a SMLP-mediated manner. Free SMLP with three different concentrations (4 μg/ml, 20 μg/ml and 100 μg/ml) was added into the medium together with PMs2, incubated for 4 h, washed thrice with cold PBS and fixed with 70% ethanol for 2 h at −20°C. Cell nuclei were stained with Hoechst 33342.

The cells were examined using an ImageXpress Micro XL Widefield High Content Screening System (ImageXpress Micro XL, Molecular Devices, USA) with MetaXpress Software. The images of the cells were determined by the differential interference contrast channel technique and the images of coumarin 6-loaded PMs and the nuclei of the cells stained by Hoechst 33342 were recorded with the following channels: blue channel (Hoechst 33342) with excitation at 350 nm and green channel (coumarin 6) with excitation at 485 nm. Then, MetaXpress Software was used to quantify the fluorescence intensity per cell.

Statistics. All data were processed using Origin 8.5 software and presented as mean ± SD, and analyzed using Student's *t*-test. Statistical analyses were performed and $P<0.01$ was considered as the level of statistical significance.

Results and Discussion

Synthesis and characterization of PCL-mPEG and PCL-PEG-COOH copolymers

An amphiphilic block copolymer composed of a PCL block as the hydrophobic part and a PEG block as the hydrophilic part was synthesized via ring-opening polymerization using hydroxyl-terminated PEG as a macromolecular initiator.

The molecular weights of the copolymers were calculated from the ^{1}H NMR data by comparing the peak intensities of the methylene protons of PEG with the methylene protons of PCL, as shown in Figure 2E. The ratios of the hydrophobic block to the hydrophilic block were determined from the relative intensities of the PCL proton signal at 2.31 ppm and the PEG proton signal at 3.62 ppm. For GPC analysis, only one peak appeared in the GPC curve (Figure 2A), which means that the ring-opening copolymerization of ε-caprolactone with PEG-OH was complete and all the residues were removed after purification. The polydispersity of the copolymer (Mw/Mn) is outlined in Table 1.

Synthesis and characterization of PCL-PEG-SMLP

Surface functionalization of the copolymer PCL-PEG-COOH with SMLP was achieved under standard amide coupling conditions in the presence of EDC and NHS [27,28]. The coupling efficiency with amine nucleophiles can be increased by the formation of an NHS ester intermediate [29].

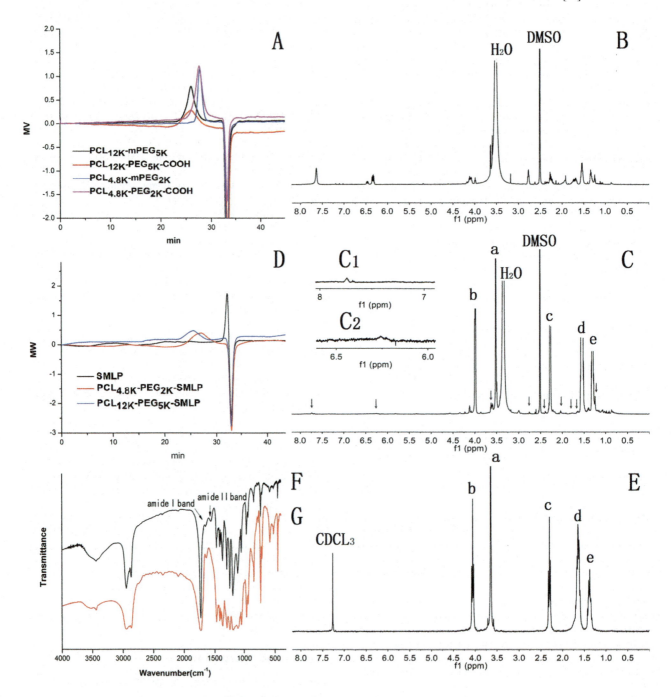

Figure 2. The gel permeation chromatography graphs of four copolymers (A) and SMLP, PCL$_{4.8K}$-PEG$_{2K}$-SMLP and PCL$_{12K}$-PEG$_{5K}$-SMLP (D), the representative ^{1}H NMR spectra of SMLP (B), copolymers PCL$_{12K}$-PEG$_{5K}$-SMLP (C) containing SMLP (black arrows) and PCL$_{12K}$-PEG$_{5K}$-COOH (E) with the peaks of PCL$_{12k}$-PEG$_{5k}$ segment (a-e) and Infrared spectra graph of PCL$_{12k}$-PEG$_{5K}$-SMLP (F) and PCL$_{12K}$-PEG$_{5K}$-COOH (G) copolymers.

Table 1. Characterization data of block copolymers and DTX-PMs.

Polymer	Feed ratio[a] (feed DP)	Final DP[b]	PDI[c]	DTX-PMs	Mean Diameter (nm)	PDI	DLC (%)	EE (%)
PCL$_{12K}$-mPEG$_{5k}$	110	104	1.08	PCL$_{12K}$-mPEG$_{5k}$	51.4±1.3	0.038±0.04	8.2±0.3	64.2±2.9
PCL$_{12K}$-PEG$_{5K}$-COOH	110	106	1.14	PCL$_{12K}$-PEG$_{5K}$-COOH	50.5±1.1	0.044±0.06	8.4±0.2	65.7±1.4
PCL$_{4.8K}$-PEG$_{2K}$	44	42	1.03	PCL$_{4.8K}$-PEG$_{2K}$	37.1±0.5	0.038±0.03	7.3±0.3	56.4±2.6
PCL$_{4.8K}$-PEG$_{2K}$-COOH	44	42	1.07	PCL$_{4.8K}$-PEG$_{2K}$-COOH	38.6±0.7	0.033±0.02	7.5±0.4	58.0±3.4

(n = 3).
Notes: [a]Calculation of feed ratio by nPCL/nPEG. [b]Degree of polymerization (DP) determined by ^{1}H NMR. [c]Molecular weight polydispersity index (PDI) determined by GPC (Mw/Mn).
Abbreviations: Drug-loading content, DLC; Encapsulation efficiency, EE.

The synthesis of polymer PCL–PEG–SMLP was accomplished by the following method. First, the carboxyl of PCL-PEG-COOH was activated with EDC and NHS to achieve the intermediate PCL-PEG-NHS. Then, the active ester (NHS) of PCL-PEG-NHS was reacted with the amine functional group of the SMLP to obtain the final polymer PCL-PEG-SMLP (Figure 3).

The polymer of PCL$_{12k}$–PEG$_{5k}$–SMLP was characterized using FT-IR, as depicted in Figure 2F. The salient peaks shown in Figure 2F at 1671 and 1557 cm^{-1} were attributed to amide band I (carbonyl group) and amide band II (amino group) respectively, while the disappearance of these peaks (Figure 2G) indicated the formation of the amide bond between SMLP and PCL$_{12k}$-PEG$_{5k}$-COOH. The structure of the conjugate was further examined by ^{1}H NMR. Figure 2C shows the ^{1}H NMR spectrum of the conjugation of the ligand and copolymer PCL$_{12k}$-PEG$_{5k}$-COOH. The characteristic signal appearing at 3.60 ppm (a) was assigned to the PEG unit. The peaks of the PCL units appear at 4.04–4.08 ppm (b), 2.28–2.33 ppm (c), 1.61–1.70 ppm (d) and 1.35–1.43 ppm (e), as shown in Figure 2C. Moreover, the signals at 2.49 ppm and 3.25–3.49 ppm were assigned to the solvent peak (DMSO) and water peak, respectively. According to Figure 2E, there are no SMLP-related signals shown in the ^{1}H NMR spectrum of unconjugated PCL$_{12k}$-PEG$_{5k}$-COOH, indicating that there is no interference with SMLP signals shown in Figure 2C. Comparing the peaks of PCL-PEG-SMLP in Figure 2C and the peaks of ligand SMLP in Figure 2B, the chemical shifts were identical. Combing the results of FT-IR and ^{1}H NMR showed that the ligand SMLP had been successfully conjugated to PCL$_{12K}$-PEG$_{5K}$-COOH. The purity of ligand conjugated polymers, which is critically related to the *in vitro* performance of the micelles, was verified by gel permeation chromatography. As shown in Figure 2D, no trace of free SMLP was observed in the chromatograms of either PCL$_{12K}$-PEG$_{5K}$-SMLP or PCL$_{4.8K}$-PEG$_{2K}$-SMLP, indicating that the excessive free ligand was completely removed.

Preparation and characterization of micelles

In this work, dialysis was employed to prepare the docetaxel-micelles, leading to the successful preparation of nontargeted [PCL$_{12K}$-mPEG$_{5k}$ (PMs1), PCL$_{4.8k}$-mPEG$_{2K}$ (PMs3)] and targeted [PCL$_{12K}$-PEG$_{5K}$-SMLP (PMs2), PCL$_{4.8K}$-PEG$_{2K}$-SMLP (PMs4)] micelles. In addition, nanoparticles with diameters larger than 100 nm are more likely to be eliminated by the reticuloendothelial system [30], while their counterparts with diameters less than 100 nm were more likely to accumulate in tumor tissues [31,32].

The average diameters of micelles (PMs1, PMs2, PMs3 and PMs4) prepared by dialysis were 51.4±1.3 nm, 50.5±1.1 nm, 37.1±0.5 nm and 38.6±0.7 nm, respectively. The polydispersity index (PDI) values of the four micelles are shown in Table 1. The DLS graphs of PMs1 and PMs2 are shown in Figure 4 (A, B). The morphology and low PDI of the micelles were further confirmed by TEM imaging. The TEM photograph (Figure 4, A$_1$ and B2) of PMs1 and PMs2 were in accordance to the results of DLS. The smaller diameters of the PMs obtained from the TEM tests compared with DLS could be ascribed to the shrinkage of the PEG shell induced by water evaporation before TEM measurement [33]. As a result, the diameter given by DLS was bigger than that of TEM due to the hydration of the PEG shell.

To evaluate the maximum drug-loading content and drug-loading efficiency of the four micelles, a simple short-term stability study of the DTX-loaded content was performed and the results are shown in Figure 5. First, excess DTX was added during the preparation of the four DTX-PMs. The over-loaded PMs were

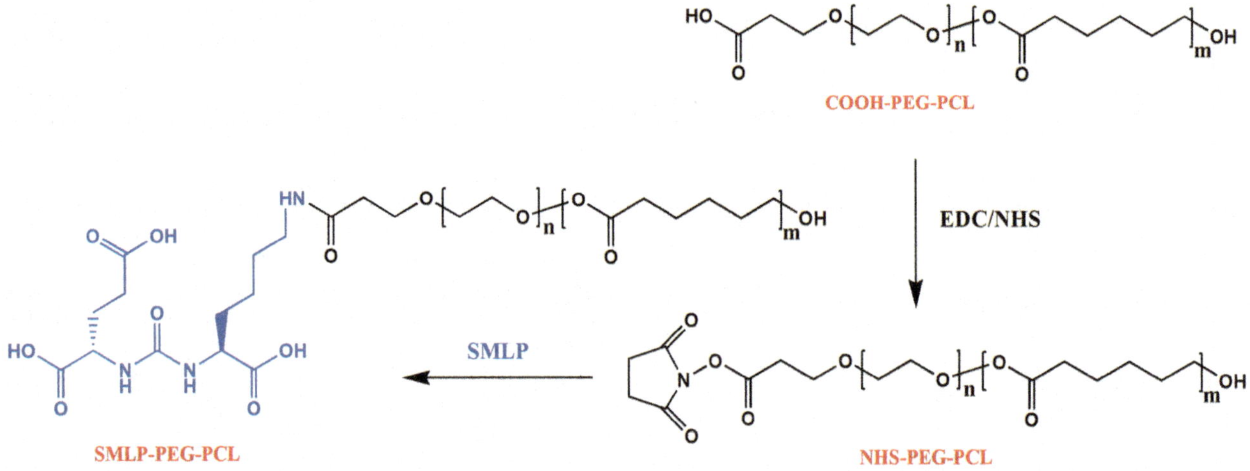

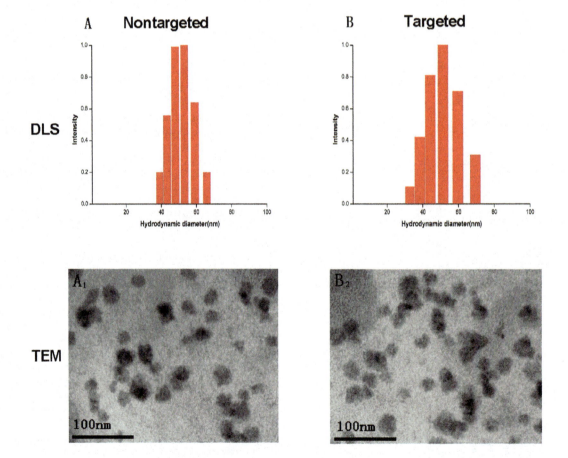

Figure 3. Synthetic representation of the chemical reaction for preparation of PCL-PEG-SMLP copolymer.

kept at room temperature and sampled at predetermined time. Then, the DTX-loading content of the samples was measured by HPLC using the method described. The profile showed that the initial DTX-loading content of the four PMs was 10.4%, 10.8%, 9.6% and 9.8%, respectively. The values of DTX-loading content fell gradually and remained constant after 12 h for PCL_{12k}-PEG_{5k} and 24 h for $PCL_{4.8k}$-PEG_{2k} (Figure 5, circled in squares). The reduction in drug-loading content may be due to the occurrence of phase separation between DTX and PCL. The drug-loading content after a 7 days test period could be deemed as the capacity of PCL for loading DTX. Also, the higher capacity of PMs1 and PMs2 compared with PMs3 and PMs4 could be ascribed to the

Figure 4. The representative DLS graphs of the DTX-PMs1 (A), and DTX-PMs2 (B), respectively. TEM graphs of DTX-PMs1 (A_1) and DTX-PMs2 (B_2).

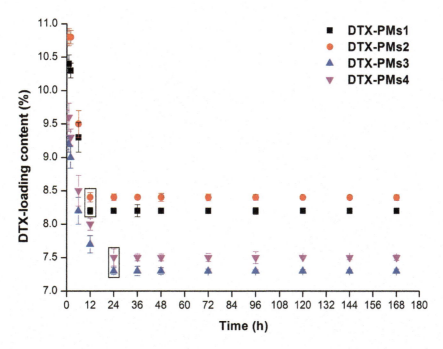

Figure 5. The short-term stability of the DLC of four DTX-PMs stored at room temperature for 7 days. (n = 3).

longer PCL chains of PMs1 and PMs2. With the same ratio of the hydrophilic block length to the hydrophobic block length, the final drug-loading content and encapsulation efficiency of the four PMs are shown in Table 1. These results showed the a good short-term stability of the DTX-loading content, the drug-loading content and efficiency, confirming that the micelles based on PCL_{12K}-PEG_{5K}-SMLP and PCL_{12K}-$mPEG_{5k}$ copolymers were optimal formulations.

In vitro release

The *in vitro* release behavior of four DTX-PMs was investigated by the dialysis diffusion method [34]. The release behavior of Taxotere was used as a control, and the DTX release profiles of the four PMs at pH 7.4 (simulated environment of normal tissues) and pH 5.5 (simulated environment of tumor tissues) are shown in Figure 6. Almost 90% of the DTX was released from Taxotere within 24 h. Unlike Taxotere, all micelles exhibited a fast release of DTX at the initial stage (first 24 h) and a sustained release over the following 72 h. Moreover, the similar release profiles of PMs1 and PMs2 indicated that ligand conjugation did not influence the release pattern.

For the four PMs, because the poly ester structure of PCL is sensitive to acid, the release of DTX from micelles was slower at pH 7.4 than that at pH 5.5. This effect promoted the release of DTX in tumor tissues and in endosomes which are more acidic than blood [35]. The amount of non-released DTX was 20–25%. This proportion of drugs existed in the micellar cores; trapped in precipitations generated by heat and tween 80 induced micellar breakdown and adsorbed on dialysis bag and glassware [36].

Cell cytotoxicity

PSMA is a validated molecular marker overexpressed by LNCaP cells [37,38]. The cytotoxicity enhancing effect of PSMA ligand (SMLP) conjugated DTX-PMs were evaluated by in vitro cytotoxicity experiments using LNCaP and PC3 cells, respectively. The biocompatibility of PCL_{12K}-$mPEG_{5K}$ and PCL_{12K}-PEG_{5K}-SMLP was confirmed by incubating drug-free micelles composed of these two polymers at various concentrations with LNCaP cells and PC3 cells, respectively. The cell viability was not affected over a 72 h incubation period which confirmed the good biocompatibility of these polymers (Figure 7). The results also demonstrated that the cells cannot be interfered in the presence of ligands.

In this study, the DMSO solution of DTX (DSD) was used instead of Taxotere as a positive control because Tween 80 in Taxotere is cytotoxic and this may influence the results [39]. According to the results of the MTT assays (Figure 8), after a 48 h incubation, the cytotoxicity of PMs1 was nearly the same as DSD. However, PMs2 showed a significantly lower LNCaP cell viability at all concentrations. In PC3 cell lines, however, no significant difference was observed in cell viability among DSD, PMs1 and PMs2 (Figure 8). This indicated that ligand conjugation is beneficial in facilitating the cellular uptake of micelles: as PMs1 and PMs2 showed similar release profiles, the decreased cell viability could be ascribed to enhanced intracellular drug accumulation via receptor-mediated endocytosis. After 72 h incubation, both PMs1 and PMs2 showed significant differences from DSD in LNCaP cell line, and PMs2 showed the greatest cytotoxicity. Moreover, significant lower cell viabilities were observed in PC3 cell lines treated with either PMs1 or PMs2 than DSD at drug concentration of 20 μg/ml, which mean that inadequate cellular uptake of micelles could be compensated by increased incubation time and drug concentration. However, there were no significant differences between PMs1 and DSD after 48h incubation for LNCaP cells. This phenomenon confirmed the sustained drug release behavior of DTX from PMs1 *in vitro*.

The cell viability of PMs2 at 20 μg/ml was almost half that of PMs1 for LNCaP cells after either 48 h or 72 h incubation. These data demonstrated that DTX-PMs2 was less effective in enhancing cytotoxicity in PC3 cells, whereas it selectively inhibits proliferation of LNCaP cells. In the other words, these results suggest the high affinity of SMLP for PSMA could enhance the cytotoxicity in LNCaP cells. After 72 h incubation on LNCaP cells with the amount of DTX given at a fixed concentration of 20 μg/ml, the

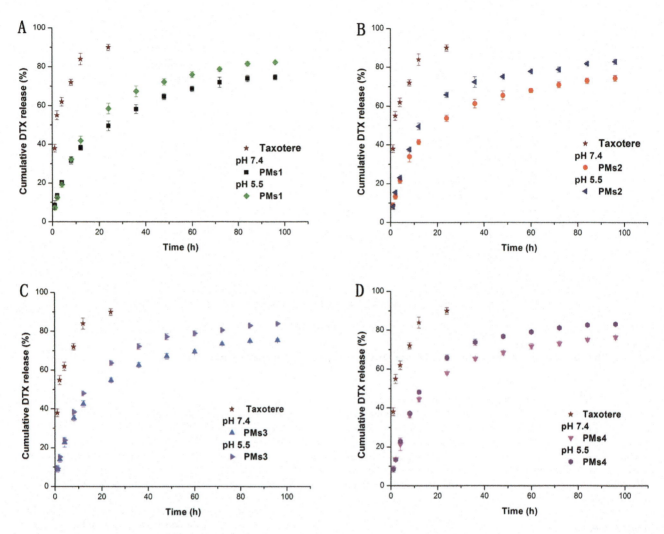

Figure 6. *In vitro* release profile of DTX from the four types of PMs solution at 37°C in PBS (10 mM, pH 7.4) or PBS(10 mM, pH 5.5), in comparison with Taxotere. (n = 3).

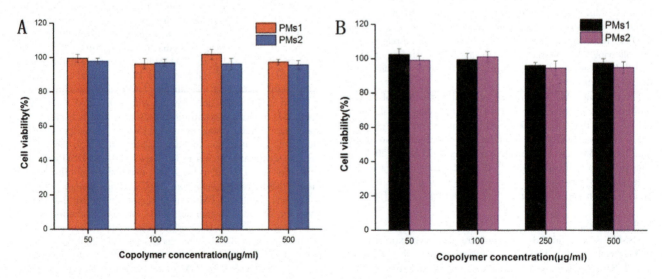

Figure 7. Different concentrations of PMs1 and PMs2 in LNCaP cells (A) and in PC3 cells (B) after incubation for 72 h. (n = 5).

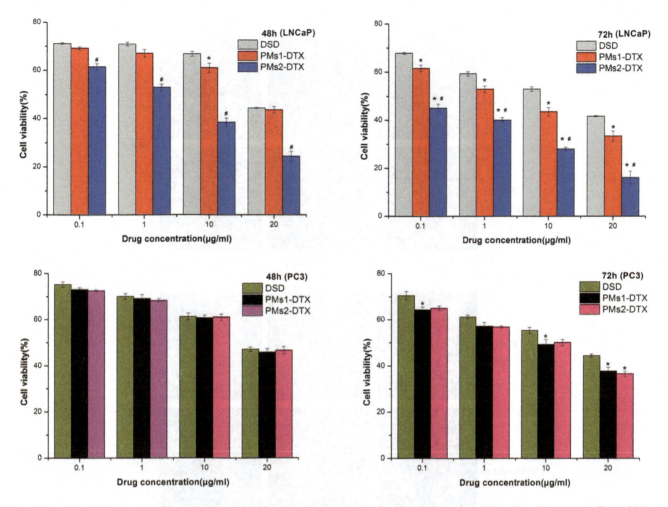

Figure 8. In vitro cytotoxicity determination of different concentrations of DSD, DTX-PMs1 and DTX-PMs2 in LNCaP cells and PC3 cells after incubation for 48 h, 72 h, respectively, using MTT assay. (*) significantly different from DSD; (#) significantly different from PMs1; (n = 5). Note: *P<0.01, #P<0.01.

cell growth inhibition rate of DSD, PMs1 and PMs2 were 58.4%, 67.7% and 83.9%, respectively.

The IC50 for each sample is shown in Table 2. For LNCaP cells, the IC50 of DTX-PMs2 was much lower than that of DTX-PMs1 and DSD after 48 h or 72 h incubation. However, the IC50 of DTX-PMs1 was almost the same as that of DSD after 48 h incubation, but was 5-fold lower after 72 h incubation with LNCaP cells, this further confirmed the compensating effect in cytotoxicity of micelles by prolonged incubation time. Although DTX-PMs2 (targeted) exhibited the highest cell-killing efficiency, the DTX-PMs1 also displayed an effect on LNCaP cells. Since the two micelles possessed similar release profiles, the differences in cytotoxicity were related to their different cell-entry ability which was reflected by the differences in affinities to PSMA.

Cellular Uptake

To study the effect of PSMA targeting ligand on the cellular uptake of the PMs, fluorescence microscopy was conducted on LNCaP cells with both targeted (PMs2) and non-targeted (PMs1) micelles labeled with coumarin-6. After 4 h incubation at 37°C, HCSS images of LNCaP cells were taken and shown in Figure 9A. The fluorescence intensity of cells incubated with targeted micelles (PMs2) was significantly higher than that of its non-targeted counterpart (PMs1), and the quantified fluorescence intensity was

Table 2. IC$_{50}$ analysis of DSD, DTX-PMs1 and DTX-PMs2 on LNCaP and PC3 cells after 48 h, 72 h incubation, respectively (n = 5).

Incubation time (h)	IC$_{50}$ values (µg/ml) of LNCaP cells			IC$_{50}$ values (µg/ml) of PC3 cells		
	DSD	DTX-PMs1	DTX-PMs2	DSD	DTX-PMs1	DTX-PMs2
48 h	14.59±2.11	13.48±1.03	0.87±0.27	19.31±3.42	18.65±3.07	19.04±2.81
72 h	7.36±1.51	1.35±0.54	0.02±0.008	11.67±1.98	3.11±0.81	3.02±0.76

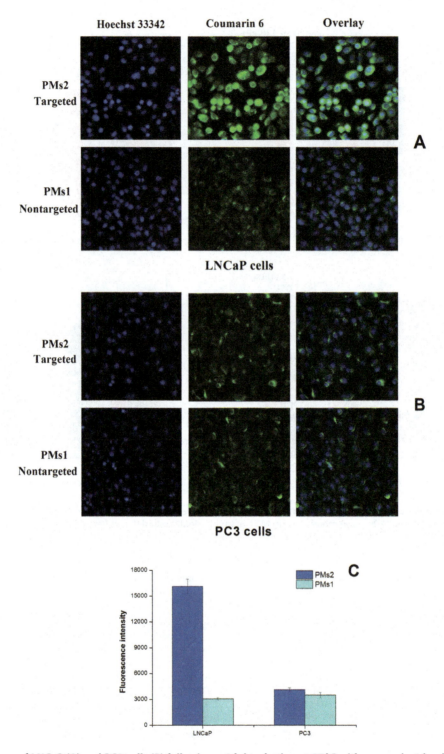

Figure 9. HCSS images of LNCaP (A) and PC3 cells (B) following a 4 h incubation at 37°C with coumarin 6-loaded PMs1 and PMs2, respectively. The cell nuclei were stained with Hoechst 33342 with the blue channel, the coumarin 6-loaded PMs are the green channel. The cellular uptake was visualized by overlaying images displayed by the nuclei channel and the PMs channel. The fluorescence intensity/cell graph of 100 µg/ml coumarin 6-loaded PMs1 and PMs2 with a concentration of 200 µg/ml after 4 h incubation with LNCaP cells and PC3 cells (C).

estimated to be 5-fold (Figure 9C). The capability of SMLP conjugation in enhancing cellular uptake could be reflected in cell viability assays. To further verify the role of SMLP in endocytosis, a ligand competing experiment was conducted. As shown in Figure 8B, addition of free ligands at various concentrations gradually decreased the uptake of PMs2, and the amount of endocytosed micelles reached a similar level to its non-targeted counterpart at high concentration of SMLP (100 µg/ml, Figure 10B), which indicated the presence of free SMLP in the medium inhibited endocytosis of PMs2 by binding to surface

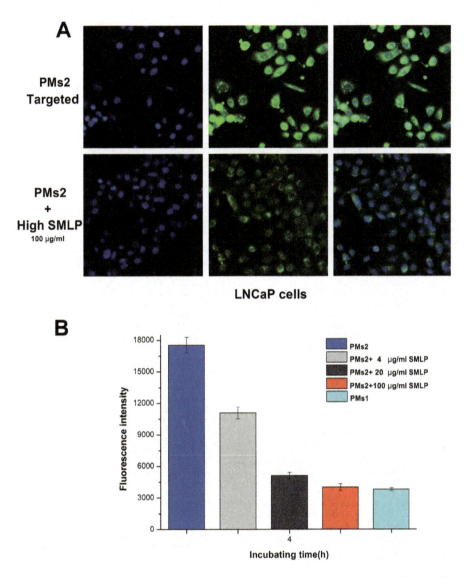

Figure 10. Competitive inhibition analysis of free SMLP (A) and fluorescence intensity/cell on LNCaP cells after 4 h incubation (B).

PSMA in a competitive manner against micelle-conjugated SMLP. To further verify the enhancement of ligand in mediating endocytosis, cellular uptake studies of both preparations with/without SMLP ligand were conducted in PC-3 cell line, which do not express the PSMA protein [40]. As shown in Figure 9 (B and C), targeted- and non-targeted micelles showed similar intracellular fluorescent intensity, which means conjugation of SMLP is a key factor in promoting cellular uptake of prepared micelles in PSMA expressing cells. Also the above results demonstrated that PMs2 was endocytosed into LNCaP cells via multiple routes: part of the micelles was taken up by LNCaP cells in a SMLP-mediated manner, while there were micelles entering cells through other pathways including caveolin-mediated endocytosis or clathrin- and caveolin-independent endocytosis [41] as the cellular uptake of micelles was not completely inhibited by SMLP addition. These results explained the higher cytotoxicity of the targeted micelles (PMs2) in MTT assays and indicated the benefit of PMs with a targeting ligand in prostate cancer therapy.

Conclusions

In this study, a novel self-assembly of DTX-PEG-PCL-SMLP micelles targeting LNCaP cells was developed. With the same hydrophilic/hydrophobic block length ratio, a series of polymeric micelles with diameters less than 60 nm were prepared by dialysis. Stable non-targeted PMs and targeted PMs with constant drug-loading content were obtained by short-term stability assays. Reliable drug loading and sustained releasing behavior were obtained due to removal of the over-loaded drugs. The cyotoxicity experiments demonstrated the advantages in LNCaP cell inhibition with a significant difference of targeted DTX-PMs > non-targeted DTX-PMs > DSD. The fluorescence intensity of coumarin 6-loaded targeted PMs were 5-fold higher than that of non-targeted PMs. Combining the cellular uptake results of both targeted- and non-targeted micelles in LNCaP and PC3 cell lines, the critical role of SMLP conjugation in facilitating micelle uptake in PSMA positive cells was demonstrated. All of these results were ascribed to the ligand targeting of PSMA that guaranteed efficient uptake of micelles composed of DTX-PCL-PEG-SMLP that exhibited highest cytotoxicity on LNCaP cells. In summary, intracellular drug delivery is crucial for the anti-tumor efficacy of poorly-permeable drugs. As shown in this study, DTX-PCL-PEG-SMLP showed remarkable cytotoxicity compared with DMSO solution of DTX. DTX-PCL-mPEG also displayed higher cyotoxicity than DMSO solution of DTX due to enhanced intracellular accumulation via endocytosis of micelles. A more positive effect could be achieved by ligand conjugation that anchored micelles to tumor cells and facilitated cellular uptake. Further investigation into other properties of this drug delivery system, such as pharmacokinetics, *in vivo* antitumor activity and tissue distribution, are still required. Moreover, PCL-PEG-SMLP as a drug carrier is expected to be used in a number of ways for PCa therapy.

Acknowledgments

Dr David B Jack is gratefully thanked for correcting the English in the manuscript.

Author Contributions

Conceived and designed the experiments: XT HX XJ. Performed the experiments: JJ BS JG. Analyzed the data: JJ YZ JL. Contributed reagents/materials/analysis tools: HX XJ. Wrote the paper: JJ XJ.

References

1. Branco MC, Schneider JP (2009) Self-assembling materials for therapeutic delivery. Acta Biomaterialia 5: 817–831.
2. Haag R (2004) Supramolecular drug-delivery systems based on polymeric core-shell architectures. Angew Chem Int Ed Engl 43: 278–282.
3. Huang W, Wang W, Wang P, Tian Q, Zhang C, et al. (2010) Glycyrrhetinic acid-modified poly(ethylene glycol)-b-poly(gamma-benzyl l-glutamate) micelles for liver targeting therapy. Acta Biomater 6: 3927–3935.
4. Saxena V, Hussain MD (2013) Polymeric Mixed Micelles for Delivery of Curcumin to Multidrug Resistant Ovarian Cancer. J Biomed Nanotechnol 9: 1146–1154.
5. Li J, He Z, Yu S, Li S, Ma Q, et al. (2012) Micelles Based on Methoxy Poly(Ethylene Glycol)/Cholesterol Conjugate for Controlled and Targeted Drug Delivery of a Poorly Water Soluble Drug. J Biomed Nanotechnol 8: 809–817.
6. Savic R, Eisenberg A, Maysinger D (2006) Block copolymer micelles as delivery vehicles of hydrophobic drugs: micelle-cell interactions. J Drug Target 14: 343–355.
7. Kazunori K, Glenn S K, Masayuki Y, Teruo O, Yasuhisa S (1993) Block copolymer micelles as vehicles for drug delivery. J Control Release 24: 119–132.
8. Gu PF, Xu H, Sui BW, Gou JX, Meng LK, et al. (2012) Polymeric micelles based on poly(ethylene glycol) block poly(racemic amino acids) hybrid polypeptides: conformation-facilitated drug-loading behavior and potential application as effective anticancer drug carriers. Int J Nanomedicine 7: 109–122.
9. Wang Y, Xu H, Liu H, Wang Y, Sun J, et al. (2012) Efficacy and Biodistribution of Tocopheryl Polyethylene Glycol Succinate Noncovalent Functionalized Single Walled Nanotubes Loading Doxorubicin in Sarcoma Bearing Mouse Model. J Biomed Nanotechnol 8: 450–457.
10. Maresca K, Hillier S, Femia F, Keith D, Barone C, et al. (2008) A series of halogenated heterodimeric inhibitors of prostate specific membrane antigen (PSMA) as radiolabeled probes for targeting prostate cancer. J Med Chem 52: 347–357.
11. Murphy GP, Elgamal AAA, Su SL, Bostwick DG, Holmes EH (1998) Current evaluation of the tissue localization and diagnostic utility of prostate specific membrane antigen. Cancer 83: 2259–2269.
12. Israeli RS, Powell CT, Corr JG, Fair WR, Heston WD (1994) Expression of the prostate-specific membrane antigen. Cancer Res 54: 1807–1811.
13. Chang SS, O'Keefe DS, Bacich DJ, Reuter VE, Heston WD, et al. (1999) Prostate-specific membrane antigen is produced in tumor-associated neovasculature. Clin Cancer Res 5: 2674–2681.
14. Ghosh A, Heston WD (2004) Tumor target prostate specific membrane antigen (PSMA) and its regulation in prostate cancer. J Cell Biochem 91: 528–539.
15. Colombatti M, Grasso S, Porzia A, Fracasso G, Scupoli MT, et al. (2009) The Prostate Specific Membrane Antigen Regulates the Expression of IL-6 and CCL5 in Prostate Tumour Cells by Activating the MAPK Pathways1. PloS one 4: e4608.
16. Wolf P, Freudenberg N, Bühler P, Alt K, Schultze-Seemann W, et al. (2010) Three conformational antibodies specific for different PSMA epitopes are promising diagnostic and therapeutic tools for prostate cancer. The Prostate 70: 562–569.
17. Sanna V, Pintus G, Bandiera P, Anedda R, Punzoni S, et al. (2011) Development of polymeric microbubbles targeted to prostate-specific membrane antigen as prototype of novel ultrasound contrast agents. Mol Pharm 8: 748–757.
18. Hrkach J, Von Hoff D, Ali MM, Andrianova E, Auer J, et al. (2012) Preclinical development and clinical translation of a PSMA-targeted docetaxel nanoparticle with a differentiated pharmacological profile. Sci Transl Med 4: 128ra139-128ra139.
19. Bae SJ, Suh JM, Sohn YS, Bae YH, Kim SW, et al. (2005) Thermogelling poly (caprolactone-b-ethylene glycol-b-caprolactone) aqueous solutions. Macromolecules 38: 5260–5265.
20. Chung Y-M, Simmons KL, Gutowska A, Jeong B (2002) Sol-gel transition temperature of PLGA-g-PEG aqueous solutions. Biomacromolecules 3: 511–516.
21. Zamani S, Khoee S (2012) Preparation of core–shell chitosan/PCL-PEG triblock copolymer nanoparticles with ABA and BAB morphologies: Effect of intraparticle interactions on physicochemical properties. Polymer 53: 5723–5736.
22. Liu C, Gong C, Pan Y, Zhang Y, Wang J, et al. (2007) Synthesis and characterization of a thermosensitive hydrogel based on biodegradable amphiphilic PCL-Pluronic (L35)-PCL block copolymers. Colloids and Surfaces A: Physicochem Eng Aspects 302: 430–438.
23. Li J, Li X, Ni X, Wang X, Li H, et al. (2006) Self-assembled supramolecular hydrogels formed by biodegradable PEO-PHB-PEO triblock copolymers and alpha-cyclodextrin for controlled drug delivery. Biomaterials 27: 4132–4140.
24. Gaucher G, Dufresne M-H, Sant VP, Kang N, Maysinger D, et al. (2005) Block copolymer micelles: preparation, characterization and application in drug delivery. J Control Release 109: 169–188.
25. Gou M, Zheng X, Men K, Zhang J, Zheng L, et al. (2009) Poly (ε-caprolactone)/poly (ethylene glycol)/poly (ε-caprolactone) nanoparticles: preparation, characterization, and application in doxorubicin delivery. J Phy Chem B 113: 12928–12933.
26. Qi R, Hu Y, Yan L, Chen X, Huang Y, et al. (2011) Synthesis of biodegradable cationic triblock copolymer mPEG-PCL-PLL for siRNA delivery. J Control Release 152: e167–e168.
27. Farokhzad OC, Cheng J, Teply BA, Sherifi I, Jon S, et al. (2006) Targeted nanoparticle-aptamer bioconjugates for cancer chemotherapy in vivo. Proc Natl Acad Sci U S A 103: 6315–6320.
28. Dhar S, Liu Z, Thomale J, Dai H, Lippard SJ (2008) Targeted single-wall carbon nanotube-mediated Pt (IV) prodrug delivery using folate as a homing device. J Am Chem Soc 130: 11467–11476.
29. Hinterwirth H, Lindner W, Lämmerhofer M (2012) Bioconjugation of trypsin onto gold nanoparticles: effect of surface chemistry on bioactivity. Anal Chim Acta 733: 90–97.
30. Torchilin V (2011) Tumor delivery of macromolecular drugs based on the EPR effect. Adv Drug Deliv Rev 63: 131–135.
31. Davis ME, Chen ZG, Shin DM (2008) Nanoparticle therapeutics: an emerging treatment modality for cancer. Nat Rev Drug Discov 7: 771–782.
32. Alexis F, Pridgen E, Molnar LK, Farokhzad OC (2008) Factors affecting the clearance and biodistribution of polymeric nanoparticles. Mol Pharm 5: 505–515.
33. Hu Y, Zhang L, Cao Y, Ge H, Jiang X, et al. (2004) Degradation Behavior of Poly(ε-caprolactone)-b-poly(ethylene glycol)-b-poly(ε-caprolactone) Micelles in Aqueous Solution. Biomacromolecules 5: 1756–1762.
34. Nie S, Hsiao WL, Pan W, Yang Z (2011) Thermoreversible Pluronic F127-based hydrogel containing liposomes for the controlled delivery of paclitaxel: in vitro drug release, cell cytotoxicity, and uptake studies. Int J Nanomedicine 6: 151–166.
35. Rofstad EK, Mathiesen B, Kindem K, Galappathi K (2006) Acidic extracellular pH promotes experimental metastasis of human melanoma cells in athymic nude mice. Cancer Res 66: 6699–6707.
36. Samarajeewa S, Shrestha R, Elsabahy M, Karwa A, Li A, et al. (2013) In vitro efficacy of paclitaxel-loaded dual-responsive shell cross-linked polymer nanoparticles having orthogonally degradable disulfide cross-linked corona and polyester core domains. Mol Pharm 10: 1092–1099.
37. Yamamichi F, Matsuoka T, Shigemura K, Kawabata M, Shirakawa T, et al. (2012) Potential establishment of lung metastatic xenograft model of androgen receptor-positive and androgen-independent prostate cancer (C4-2B). Urology 80: 951 e951–957.
38. Denmeade SR, Sokoll LJ, Dalrymple S, Rosen DM, Gady AM, et al. (2003) Dissociation between androgen responsiveness for malignant growth vs. expression of prostate specific differentiation markers PSA, hK2, and PSMA in human prostate cancer models. The Prostate 54: 249–257.
39. Esmaeili F, Dinarvand R, Ghahremani MH, Amini M, Rouhani H, et al. (2009) Docetaxel-albumin conjugates: preparation, in vitro evaluation and biodistribution studies. J Pharm Sci 98: 2718–2730.
40. Farokhzad OC, Jon S, Khademhosseini A, Tran T-NT, LaVan DA, et al. (2004) Nanoparticle-aptamer bioconjugates a new approach for targeting prostate cancer cells. Cancer Res 64: 7668–7672.
41. Conner SD, Schmid SL (2003) Regulated portals of entry into the cell. Nature 422: 37–44.

Structure-Activity Relationships of Novel Salicylaldehyde Isonicotinoyl Hydrazone (SIH) Analogs: Iron Chelation, Anti-Oxidant and Cytotoxic Properties

Eliška Potůčková[1], Kateřina Hrušková[1], Jan Bureš[1], Petra Kovaříková[1], Iva A. Špirková[1], Kateřina Pravdíková[1], Lucie Kolbabová[1], Tereza Hergeselová[1], Pavlína Hašková[1], Hana Jansová[1], Miloslav Macháček[1], Anna Jirkovská[1], Vera Richardson[2], Darius J. R. Lane[2], Danuta S. Kalinowski[2], Des R. Richardson[2], Kateřina Vávrová[1]*, Tomáš Šimůnek[1]*

1 Charles University in Prague, Faculty of Pharmacy in Hradec Králové, Hradec Králové, Czech Republic, 2 Molecular Pharmacology and Pathology Program, Bosch Institute and Department of Pathology, University of Sydney, Sydney, Australia

Abstract

Salicylaldehyde isonicotinoyl hydrazone (SIH) is a lipophilic, tridentate iron chelator with marked anti-oxidant and modest cytotoxic activity against neoplastic cells. However, it has poor stability in an aqueous environment due to the rapid hydrolysis of its hydrazone bond. In this study, we synthesized a series of new SIH analogs (based on previously described aromatic ketones with improved hydrolytic stability). Their structure-activity relationships were assessed with respect to their stability in plasma, iron chelation efficacy, redox effects and cytotoxic activity against MCF-7 breast adenocarcinoma cells. Furthermore, studies assessed the cytotoxicity of these chelators and their ability to afford protection against hydrogen peroxide-induced oxidative injury in H9c2 cardiomyoblasts. The ligands with a reduced hydrazone bond, or the presence of bulky alkyl substituents near the hydrazone bond, showed severely limited biological activity. The introduction of a bromine substituent increased ligand-induced cytotoxicity to both cancer cells and H9c2 cardiomyoblasts. A similar effect was observed when the phenolic ring was exchanged with pyridine (i.e., changing the ligating site from O, N, O to N, N, O), which led to pro-oxidative effects. In contrast, compounds with long, flexible alkyl chains adjacent to the hydrazone bond exhibited specific cytotoxic effects against MCF-7 breast adenocarcinoma cells and low toxicity against H9c2 cardiomyoblasts. Hence, this study highlights important structure-activity relationships and provides insight into the further development of aroylhydrazone iron chelators with more potent and selective anti-neoplastic effects.

Editor: Kostas Pantopoulos, Lady Davis Institute for Medical Research/McGill University, Canada

Funding: This study was supported by the Charles University in Prague (www.cuni.cz; projects GAUK 299511, SVV 260065 and 260062), the Czech Science Foundation (www.gacr.cz; grant 13-15008S), and the European Social Fund and the State Budget of the Czech Republic (www.msmt.cz; Operational Program CZ.1.07/2.3.00/30.0061). This work was also funded by a Project Grant from the National Health and Medical Research Council Australia (NHMRC; www.nhmrc.gov.au) to D.R.R. [Grant 632778]; a NHMRC Senior Principal Research Fellowship to D.R.R. [Grant 571123]; and a Cancer Institute New South Wales (cancerinstitute.org.au) Early Career Development Fellowship to D.S.K. [Grant 08/ECF/1-30]. D.J.R.L. thanks the Cancer Institute New South Wales for an Early Career Fellowship [10/ECF/2-18] and the NHMRC of Australia for an Early Career Postdoctoral Fellowship [1013810]. The funders had no role in study design, data collection and analysis, decision to publish, or preparation of the manuscript.

Competing Interests: The authors have declared that no competing interests exist.

* Email: Tomas.Simunek@faf.cuni.cz (TS); Katerina.Vavrova@faf.cuni.cz (KV)

Introduction

Iron is a crucial component of various proteins involved in oxygen transport, cellular respiration, metabolism and division [1,2,3]. The majority of cellular iron acquired by tumor cells is stored in ferritin [4,5], with smaller amounts being utilized for cellular metabolism, such as the synthesis of heme or iron-sulfur clusters [6,7]. Intracellular iron is also found within a poorly defined "labile iron pool" (LIP), in which iron may be in transit between proteins and/or low-molecular weight (M_r) ligands, or specifically transported by putative iron-chaperone proteins, such as poly(rC)-binding proteins 1–4 [8,9].

When intracellular iron is depleted, the synthesis of new iron-dependent proteins and enzymes, and the processes they regulate (e.g., cellular growth and proliferation), can be inhibited [10,11]. On the other hand, when iron is present in excess, iron-mediated oxidative stress can lead to the damage of proteins, lipids and nucleic acids and can be cytotoxic. In fact, "free" or labile redox-active iron can catalyze the Fenton and Haber-Weiss-type reactions that generate highly toxic reactive oxygen species (ROS) [2,4]. Classical iron chelators used in the clinics, such as desferrioxamine (DFO), deferiprone, and deferasirox, sequester iron and are primarily used to manage disorders with increased systemic iron levels, such as that caused by repeated blood transfusions in β-thalassemia major patients [12,13,14]. More recently, iron chelators have been also studied in pathological conditions associated with oxidative stress unrelated to iron-overload diseases [15].

Cancer cells require more iron than their neoplastic counterparts in order to support their increased rates of proliferation [1]. Indeed, iron is a key cofactor of ribonucleotide reductase, an enzyme that catalyzes the rate-limiting step in DNA synthesis [16,17]. Cancer cells up-regulate transferrin (Tf) receptor 1 (TfR1) expression on their surface to increase iron uptake from the iron transport protein, Tf [18,19]. Some cancer cells also express hepcidin, a hormone that induces the internalization of the iron-export protein, ferroportin 1, leading to reduced iron efflux from cells [19,20]. Iron chelators induce iron depletion with subsequent G_1-S cell cycle arrest and apoptosis [21] and they are increasingly studied as potential anti-neoplastic agents, with several in preclinical or clinical development [13,22,23].

N'-Salicylaldehyde isonicotinoyl hydrazone (SIH, Fig. 1) is a well-established tridentate iron chelator, which forms 2:1 complexes with both Fe^{3+} and Fe^{2+} ions [24,25]. SIH has been shown to: (*1*) protect various cell types against oxidative stress-inducing agents [15,26,27]; (*2*) prevent the cardiotoxicity of anthracycline-based antineoplastic agents both *in vitro* and *in vivo* [28]; and (*3*) act as a potential radio-protective, anti-viral and anti-cancer agent [29,30,31]. SIH has low *in vitro* and *in vivo* toxicity and good tolerability, even following prolonged administration to animals [32]. Recently, a series of new analogs of SIH were developed that have markedly enhanced hydrolytic stability compared to SIH and retain their ability to protect cells against oxidative injury [33]. In addition, these agents have increased cytotoxic activity compared to SIH [31]. The lead ligands identified in this series included (*E*)-N'-[1-(2-hydroxyphenyl)ethylidene]isonicotinoylhydrazide (HAPI; Fig. 1) and (*E*)-N'-[1-(2-hydroxyphenyl)propylidene]isonicotinoylhydrazide (HPPI; Fig. 1), which possess either a methyl or ethyl group, respectively, in proximity to the hydrazone bond [31].

To further analyze their structure-activity relationships, in the present study, we designed and synthesized derivatives of SIH, HAPI and HPPI (Fig. 1). The first modification was the reduction of the hydrazone bond leading to N'-(2-hydroxybenzyl)isonicotinoylhydrazide (redSIH; Fig. 1), N'-[1-(2-hydroxyphenyl)ethyl]isonicotinoylhydrazide (redHAPI; Fig. 1) and N'-[1-(2-hydroxyphenyl)propyl]isonicotinoylhydrazide (redHPPI; Fig. 1). These compounds were specifically synthesized to assess the importance of the hydrazone bond for the anti-oxidative and/or cytotoxic activity that has been associated with various aroylhydrazones [34,35,36].

We also studied the effects of bromination at position 5 of the phenolic ring of HAPI and HPPI, leading to (*E*)-N'-[1-(5-bromo-2-hydroxyphenyl)ethylidene]isonicotinoylhydrazide (BHAPI; Fig. 1) and (*E*)-N'-[1-(5-bromo-2-hydroxyphenyl)propylidene]isonicotinoylhydrazide (BHPPI; Fig. 1), respectively. The effect of halogenation was examined since a previous study demonstrated the high cytotoxic activity of a chloro-substituted ligand [31]. An analog, in which the phenolic ring of HAPI was exchanged for pyridine, was also prepared ((*E*)-N'-[1-(pyridin-2-yl)ethylidene]isonicotinoylhydrazide; 2API; Fig. 1) to assess the effects on its properties of changing the ligating groups from O, N, O to N, N, O. The chelation properties of 2API would be different from those of SIH because the pyridine nitrogen in 2API is a softer base relative to the hard phenolic oxygen in SIH. Considering this, 2API would be able to bind both Fe^{3+} and Fe^{2+} ions, while SIH and its analogs prefer Fe^{3+}. Thus, although 2API does not belong to the same ligand category as SIH, we aimed to explore its properties because 2API is a methyl analog of 2-pyridylcarboxaldehyde isonicotinoyl hydrazone (PCIH), which was developed for the treatment of iron overload [37,38].

An analog of HAPI with a 2C side chain as a part of an indane ring was also synthesized, leading to (*E*)-N'-(7-hydroxy-2,3-dihydro-1*H*-inden-1-ylidene)isonicotinoylhydrazide (7HII; Fig. 1). Analogs of HAPI and HPPI with varying alkyl groups adjacent to the hydrazone bond were also prepared, including derivatives containing an isopropyl substituent ((*E*)-N'-(1-(2-hydroxyphenyl)-2-methylpropylidene)isonicotinoylhydrazide; H16; Fig. 1), propyl substituent ((*E*)-N'-[1-(2-hydroxyphenyl)butylidene]isonicotinoylhydrazide; H17; Fig. 1), isobutyl substituent ((*E*)-N'-(1-(2-hydroxyphenyl)-3-methylbutylidene)isonicotinoylhydrazide; H18; Fig. 1), or cyclohexyl ring ((*E*)-N'-[cyclohexyl(2-hydroxyphenyl)methylene]isonicotinoylhydrazide; H28; Fig. 1).

To characterize these new ligands, we examined their: (*1*) stability against hydrolysis in plasma; (*2*) iron chelation and redox properties; (*3*) protective potential against oxidative injury induced by exposure of H9c2 rat embryonic cardiomyoblast cells to hydrogen peroxide (H_2O_2); (*4*) cytotoxic activity using neoplastic MCF-7 breast adenocarcinoma cells; and (*5*) selectivity by comparing their cytotoxic effects to the non-tumorigenic, cardiomyoblast cell line, H9c2. These studies are important for dissecting structure-activity relationships that are essential for the development of more effective ligands.

Materials and Methods

1 Syntheses of chelators

All chemicals were purchased from Sigma-Aldrich (St. Louis, MO, USA). Thin layer chromatography was performed on TLC sheets (silica gel 60 F254) from Merck (Darmstadt, Germany). Microwave reactions were conducted in a Milestone Micro-SYNTH Ethos 1600 URM apparatus. Melting points were measured on a Kofler apparatus and are uncorrected. All products were characterized by NMR (Varian Mercury Vx BB 300 or VNMR S500 NMR spectrometers). Chemical shifts were reported as δ values in parts per million (ppm) and were indirectly referenced to tetramethylsilane (TMS) *via* the solvent signal. All assignments were based on 1D experiments. Elemental analysis was measured on a CHNS-OCE FISONS EA 1110 apparatus.

N'-Salicylaldehyde isonicotinoyl hydrazone (SIH). SIH was synthesized as described previously [39]. Yellow crystalline solid. mp 232–234°C. ^{1}H NMR (300 MHz, DMSO-d_6): δ 12.29 (s, 1H, OH), 11.02 (s, 1H, NH), 8.80 (d, *J* = 4.4 Hz, 2H, Py), 8.68 (s, 1H, CH), 7.85 (d, *J* = 4.4 Hz, 2H, Py), 7.61 (dd, *J* = 7.7, 1.5 Hz, 1H, Ph), 7.36–7.28 (m, 1H, Ph), 6.95–6.88 (m, 2H, Ph). ^{13}C NMR (75 MHz, DMSO-d_6): δ 163.1, 157.5, 150.4, 148.9, 141.2, 131.7, 129.2, 121.5, 119.5, 116.4.

N'-(2-hydroxybenzyl)isonicotinoylhydrazide (redSIH). SIH (0.69 g, 2.8 mmol) was dissolved in 96% (v/v) ethanol (50 mL) and NaBH$_3$CN (0.36 g, 5.7 mmol) was added. The reaction mixture was adjusted to a pH of 3-5 using a 10% (v/v) solution of HCl in methanol. The reaction mixture was stirred at room temperature (RT) overnight and was then neutralized with a solution of sodium bicarbonate to pH 7. The reaction mixture was evaporated to dryness and was then partitioned against water and EtOAc. The combined organic layers were dried with anhydrous Na$_2$SO$_4$ and evaporated under reduced pressure. The product was purified with column chromatography on silica using hexane/EtOAc (1:1) as a mobile phase. The product was isolated as a white crystalline solid. Yield 0.17 g (24%). mp 143–146°C. ^{1}H NMR (300 MHz, DMSO-d_6): δ 10.43 (s, 1H, OH), 9.61 (s, 1H, NH), 8.70 (d, *J* = 5.1 Hz, 2H, Py), 7.74–7.65 (m, 2H, Py), 7.20 (dd, *J* = 7.5, 1.7 Hz, 1H, Ph), 7.12–7.02 (m, 1H, Ph), 6.84–6.67 (m, 2H, Ph), 5.65 (s, 1H, NH), 3.95 (d, *J* = 6.0 Hz, 2H, CH$_2$). ^{13}C NMR (75 MHz, DMSO-d_6): δ 163.5, 156.1, 150.4, 140.3, 130.1, 128.5, 124.1, 121.3, 118.9, 115.3, 50.7. Anal. Calcd. for C$_{13}$H$_{13}$N$_3$O$_2$: C, 64.19; H, 5.39; N, 17.27; Found: C, 64.50; H, 5.26; N, 17.56.

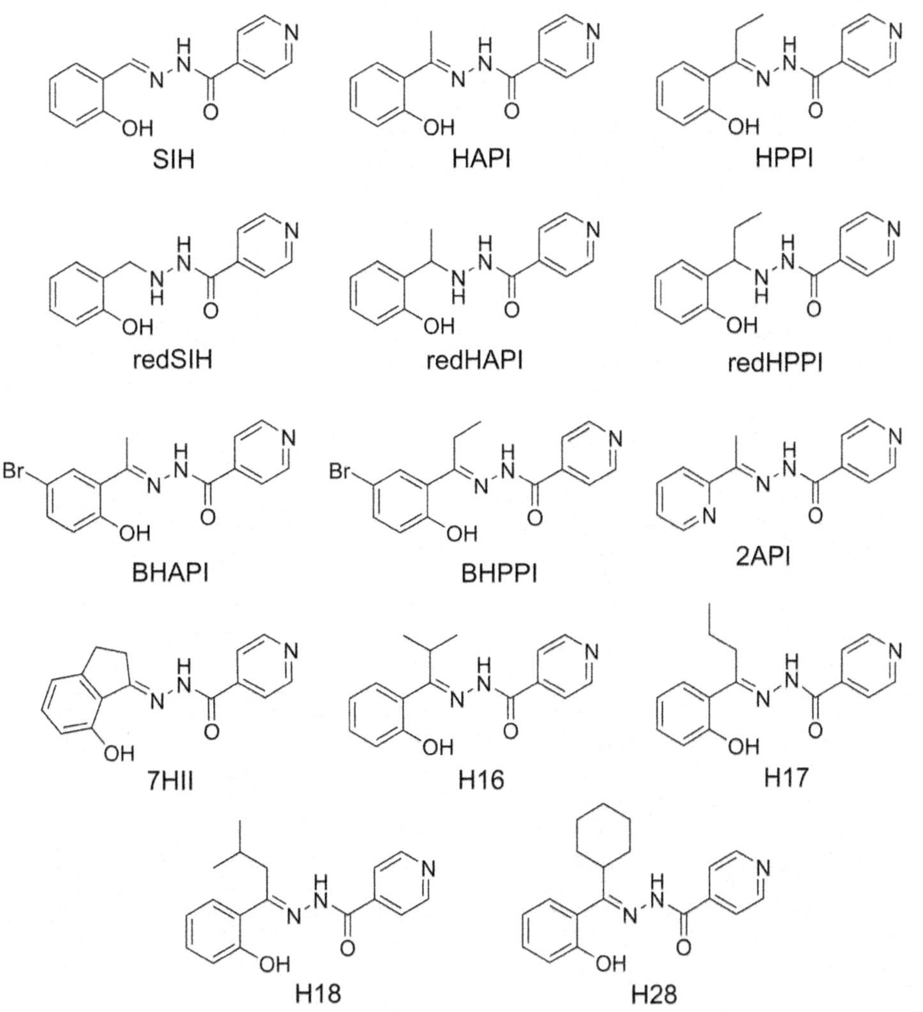

Figure 1. Line drawings of the chemical structures of the iron chelators, SIH, HAPI and HPPI, and their novel analogs.

N′-[1-(2-Hydroxyphenyl)ethyl]isonicotinoylhydrazide (redHAPI). The initial chelator, (E)-N′-[1-(2-hydroxyphenyl)ethylidene]isonicotinoylhydrazide (HAPI), was synthesized as described previously [33]. The reduced analog, redHAPI, was prepared from HAPI as described above for redSIH. The product was isolated as a yellow solid. Yield 0.18 g (26%). mp 131–134°C. ^{1}H NMR (500 MHz, DMSO-d_6): δ 10.29 (s, 1H, OH), 9.63 (s, 1H, NH), 8.70 (m, 2H, Py), 7.68 (d, J = 4.8 Hz, 2H, Py), 7.29 (dd, J = 7.8, 1.7 Hz, 1H, Ph), 7.11–7.00 (m, 1H, Ph), 6.82–6.69 (m, 2H, Ph), 5.57 (s, 1H, NH), 4.53–4.27 (m, 1H, CH), 1.28 (d, J = 6.6 Hz, 3H, CH$_3$). ^{13}C NMR (125 MHz, DMSO-d_6): δ 164.1, 155.4, 150.4, 140.3, 129.1, 127.9, 127.3, 124.9, 119.1, 115.6, 54.3, 19.7. Anal. Calcd. for C$_{14}$H$_{15}$N$_3$O$_2$: C, 65.36; H, 5.88; N, 16.33; Found: C, 64.98; H, 6.04; N, 16.53.

N′-[1-(2-Hydroxyphenyl)propyl]isonicotinoylhydrazide (redHPPI). The initial chelator, (E)-N′-[1-(2-hydroxyphenyl)propylidene]isonicotinoylhydrazide (HPPI), was synthesized as described previously [33]. The reduced analog, redHPPI was prepared from HPPI as described above for redSIH. The product was obtained as a yellow solid. Yield 0.29 g (42%). mp 115–118°C. ^{1}H NMR (500 MHz, DMSO-d_6): δ 10.21 (s, 1H, NH), 9.58 (s, 1H, NH), 8.90–8.55 (m, 2H, Py), 7.83–7.55 (m, 2H, Py), 7.27 (dd, J = 7.6, 1.7 Hz, 1H, Ph), 7.10 (m, 1H, Ph), 6.82–6.68 (m, 2H, Py), 5.62 (s, 1H, OH), 4.21 (t, J = 6.6 Hz, 1H, CH), 1.81–1.60 (m, 2H, CH$_2$), 1.14 (t, J = 7.6 Hz, 3H, CH$_3$). ^{13}C NMR (125 MHz, DMSO-d_6): δ 163.8, 155.8, 150.3, 140.3, 128.4, 127.8, 124.9, 118.9, 115.6, 60.6, 26.0, 10.7. Anal. Calcd. for C$_{15}$H$_{17}$N$_3$O$_2$: C, 66.40; H, 6.32; N, 15.49; Found: C, 66.42; H, 6.45; N, 15.55.

(E)-N′-[1-(5-Bromo-2-hydroxyphenyl)ethylidene]isonicotinoylhydrazide (BHAPI). Isoniazid (0.21 g, 1.5 mmol), 5-bromo-2-hydroxyacetophenone (0.32 g, 1.5 mmol) and acetic acid (0.25 mL) were dissolved in methanol (5 mL) and stirred for 2 h under reflux in the microwave reactor described above. The reaction mixture was then cooled to 4°C and the resulting precipitate was collected by filtration, washed with water and methanol and dried over P$_2$O$_5$ to give 0.2 g (39%) of the product as a yellow crystalline solid. mp 225–227°C. ^{1}H NMR (500 MHz, DMSO-d_6): δ 13.27 (s, 1H, OH), 11.66 (s, 1H, NH), 8.82–8.76 (m, 2H, Py), 7.86–7.79 (m, 2H, Py), 7.76 (d, J = 2.3 Hz, 1H, Ph), 7.45 (dd, J = 8.8, 2.2 Hz, 1H, Ph), 6.90 (d, J = 8.7 Hz, 1H, Ph), 2.49 (s, 3H, CH$_3$). ^{13}C NMR (125 MHz, DMSO-d_6): δ 163.3, 158.1, 158.0, 150.4, 140.1, 134.1, 131.0, 122.2, 121.5, 119.8, 109.9, 14.7. Anal. Calcd. for C$_{14}$H$_{14}$BrN$_3$O$_2$: C, 50.32; H, 3.62; N, 12.57; Found: C 50.71; H, 3.99; N, 12.88.

(E)-N′-[1-(5-Bromo-2-hydroxyphenyl)propylidene]isonicotinoylhydrazide (BHPPI). Isoniazid (0.2 g, 1.4 mmol), 5-bromo-2-hydroxypropiophenone (0.33 g, 1.4 mmol) and acetic acid (0.25 mL) were dissolved in methanol (5 mL) and stirred overnight under reflux. After cooling the reaction mixture to 4°C, the resulting precipitate was collected by filtration, washed with water and methanol and dried over P_2O_5 to give 0.32 g (64%) of the product as a yellow crystalline solid. mp 239–242°C. ^{1}H NMR (500 MHz, DMSO-d_6): δ 13.33 (s, 1H, OH), 11.69 (s, 1H, NH), 8.79 (d, J = 5.0 Hz, 2H, Py), 7.86–7.81 (m, 3H, Py, Ph), 7.45 (dd, J = 8.8, 2.4 Hz, 1H, Ph), 6.92 (d, J = 8.7 Hz, 1H, Ph), 3.01 (q, J = 7.6 Hz, 2H, CH_2), 1.09 (t, J = 7.0 Hz, 3H, CH_3). ^{13}C NMR (125 MHz, DMSO-d_6): δ 163.8, 161.2, 158.5, 150.3, 140.3, 134.0, 130.5, 122.4, 120.2, 120.1, 109.9, 19.7, 11.4. Anal. Calcd. for: $C_{15}H_{16}BrN_3O_2$: C, 51.74; H, 4.05; N, 12.07; Found: C, 51.41; H, 4.26; N, 11.74.

(*E*)-*N'*-[1-(Pyridin-2-yl)ethylidene]isonicotinoylhydrazide (**2API**). Isoniazid (0.57 g, 4.1 mmol), 2-acetylpyridine (0.5 g, 3.4 mmol) and acetic acid (0.25 mL) were dissolved in methanol (10 mL) and stirred overnight under reflux. After cooling the reaction mixture to 4°C, the resulting precipitate was collected by filtration, washed with water and methanol and dried over P_2O_5 to give 0.37 g (37%) of the product as a white crystalline solid. mp 166°C. ^{1}H NMR (500 MHz, DMSO-d_6): δ 11.10 (s, 1H, NH), 8.77 (d, J = 5.1 Hz, 2H, Py), 8.62 (d, J = 5.3 Hz, 1H, Py'), 8.12 (d, J = 8.2 Hz, 1H, Py'), 7.90–7.40 (m, 1H, Py'), 7.83–7.77 (m, 2H, Py), 7.47–7.40 (m, 1H, Py'), 2.47 (s, 3H, CH_3). ^{13}C NMR (125 MHz, DMSO-d_6): δ 163.0, 155.1, 150.3, 149.7, 141.2, 136.9, 124.7, 122.2, 121.2, 13.1. Anal. Calcd. for $C_{13}H_{12}N_4O$: C, 64.99; H, 5.03; N, 23.32; Found: C, 65.33; H, 5.31; N, 23.43.

(*E*)-*N'*-(7-Hydroxy-2,3-dihydro-1*H*-inden-1-ylidene)isonicotinoylhydrazide (**7HII**). Isoniazid (0.46 g, 3.4 mmol), 7-hydroxy-2,3-dihydro-1*H*-inden-1-one (0.5 g, 3.4 mmol) and acetic acid (0.25 mL) were dissolved in methanol (10 mL) and stirred overnight under reflux. After cooling the reaction mixture to 4°C, the resulting precipitate was collected by filtration and washed with water and methanol. The solid was suspended in toluene and was stirred for 30 min. This solution was filtered to obtain 0.37 g (66%) of the product as a yellow crystalline solid. mp 232–236°C. ^{1}H NMR (500 MHz, DMSO-d_6): δ 11.30 (s, 1H, NH), 10.15 (s, 1H, OH), 8.80–8.70 (m, 2H, Py), 7.84–7.74 (m, 2H, Py), 7.30 (dd, J = 7.8, 1.3 Hz, 1H, Ph), 6.89 (d, J = 7.4 Hz, 1H, Ph), 6.75 (d, J = 8.1 Hz, 1H, Ph), 3.13–3.00 (m, 4H, 2xCH_2). ^{13}C NMR (125 MHz, DMSO-d_6): δ 167.9, 162.5, 155.5, 150.3, 150.0, 140.8, 133.1, 122.6, 122.1, 116.6, 113.0, 28.7, 28.1. Anal. Calcd. for $C_{15}H_{13}N_3O_2$: C, 67.40; H, 4.90; N, 15.72; Found: C, 67.02; H, 5.13; N, 15.87.

(*E*)-*N'*-(1-(2-Hydroxyphenyl)-2-methylpropylidene)isonicotinoylhydrazide (**H16**). To prepare H16, 1-(2-hydroxyphenyl)-2-methylpropan-1-one was first synthesized: 2-hydroxybenzonitrile (0.36 g, 3 mmol) was dissolved in dry THF (5 mL) and a solution of isopropylmagnesium chloride in THF (2 M, 6.1 mL, 1.2 mmol) was added and the reaction mixture refluxed for 2 h. The reaction mixture was cooled in an ice bath, 10 mL of cold water was carefully added and cold concentrated H_2SO_4 added dropwise to obtain an acidic pH. The reaction mixture was then heated for 1 h at 80°C and, after cooling to RT, it was extracted twice with diethyl ether. The combined organic layer was dried with anhydrous Na_2SO_4 and evaporated under reduced pressure. The product was purified by column chromatography on silica using hexane/EtOAc (40:1) as the mobile phase. The product was obtained as a yellow oil. Yield 0.45 g (91%). ^{1}H NMR (300 MHz, CDCl$_3$): δ 12.52 (s, 1H, OH), 7.79 (dd, J = 8.1, 1.6 Hz, 1H, Ph), 7.53–7.40 (m, 1H, Ph), 7.04–6.84 (m, 2H, Ph), 3.70–3.54 (m, 1H, CH), 1.43–1.14 (m, 6H, 2xCH_3). ^{13}C NMR (75 MHz, CDCl$_3$): δ 210.9, 163.1, 136.2, 129.8, 118.8, 118.7, 118.1, 34.9, 29.7, 19.3.

1-(2-Hydroxyphenyl)-2-methylpropan-1-one (0.29 g, 1.8 mmol), isoniazid (0.24 g, 1.8 mmol) and acetic acid (0.25 mL) were dissolved in methanol (5 mL) and heated at 110°C in an autoclave for 48 h. After cooling to RT, water was added dropwise until the solution turned cloudy and the mixture was left to crystallize at 4°C for 24 h. The precipitate was collected by filtration, washed with water and methanol and dried over P_2O_5 to yield 0.07 g (14%) of H16 as a white crystalline solid. mp 228–235°C. ^{1}H NMR (300 MHz, DMSO-d_6): δ 10.08 (s, 1H, NH), 8.66 (m, 2H, Py), 7.66 (m, 2H, Py), 7.43 (d, J = 7.7 Hz, 1H, Ph), 7.35–7.22 (m, 1H, Ph), 7.13 (d, J = 7.7 Hz, 1H, Ph), 7.03–6.79 (m, 1H, Ph), 3.07–2.80 (m, 1H, CH), 1.42–0.78 (m, 6H, 2xCH_3). ^{13}C NMR (75 MHz, DMSO-d_6): δ 163.7, 163.3, 153.9, 150.4, 141.4, 130.9, 128.8, 121.2, 120.7, 119.7, 116.2, 35.9, 20.1. Anal. Calcd. for $C_{16}H_{17}N_3O_2$: C, 67.83; H, 6.05; N, 14.83; Found: C, 67.44; H, 6.37; N, 14.83.

(*E*)-*N'*-[1-(2-Hydroxyphenyl)butylidene]isonicotinoylhydrazide (**H17**). To prepare H17, 1-(2-hydroxyphenyl)butan-1-one was first synthesized: Magnesium (0.3 g, 12 mmol) was suspended in dry THF (5 mL), and propylbromide (1.5 g, 12 mmol) was added dropwise and the mixture refluxed for 2 h until the magnesium dissolved. After cooling the reaction mixture to RT, 2-hydroxybenzonitrile (0.36 g, 3 mmol) dissolved in dry THF (5 mL) was added dropwise and the reaction refluxed for 2 h. The reaction mixture was cooled in an ice bath, 10 mL of cold water was carefully added and cold concentrated H_2SO_4 added dropwise to obtain an acidic pH. The reaction mixture was then heated for 1 h at 80°C and, after cooling to RT, it was extracted twice with diethyl ether. The combined organic layer was dried with anhydrous Na_2SO_4 and evaporated under reduced pressure. The product was purified by column chromatography on silica (gradient; hexane to hexane/EtOAc 40:1). The product was obtained as a yellow oil. Yield: 0.41 g (82%). ^{1}H NMR (300 MHz, CDCl$_3$): δ 7.90–7.67 (m, 1H, Ph), 7.57–7.36 (m, 1H, Ph), 7.05–6.76 (m, 2H, Ph), 2.79 (t, J = 7.3 Hz, 2H, CH_2), 1.69–1.43 (m, 2H, CH_2), 1.03 (t, J = 7.4 Hz, 3H, CH_3). ^{13}C NMR (75 MHz, CDCl$_3$): δ 206.8, 162.5, 136.2, 130.0, 119.4, 118.8, 118.5, 40.2, 17.9, 13.8.

1-(2-Hydroxyphenyl)-butan-1-one (0.39 g, 2.4 mmol), isoniazid (0.33 g, 2.4 mmol) and acetic acid (0.25 mL) were dissolved in methanol (5 mL) and heated at 110°C in an autoclave for 72 h. After cooling to RT, water was added dropwise until the solution turned cloudy and the mixture was left to crystallize at 4°C for 24 h. The precipitate was collected by filtration, washed with water and methanol and dried over P_2O_5 to yield 0.08 g (12%) of the product as a white crystalline solid. mp 189–192°C. ^{1}H NMR (500 MHz, DMSO-d_6): δ 8.79 (d, J = 5.3, 2H, Py), 7.89–7.72 (m, 2H, Py), 7.63 (dd, J = 8.1, 1.6 Hz, 1H, Ph), 7.30 (ddd, J = 8.4, 7.1, 1.5 Hz, 1H, Ph), 7.00–6.79 (m, 2H, Ph), 3.06–2.86 (m, 2H, CH_2), 1.73–1.44 (m, 2H, CH_2), 0.99 (t, J = 7.3 Hz, 3H, CH_3). ^{13}C NMR (125 MHz, DMSO-d_6): δ 163.6, 161.7, 159.4, 150.3, 140.5, 131.6, 128.7, 122.3, 118.8, 118.3, 117.8, 27.9, 20.3, 13.9. Anal. Calcd. for $C_{16}H_{17}N_3O_2$: C, 67.83; H, 6.05; N, 14.83; Found: C, 67.42; H, 6.41; N, 14.55.

(*E*)-*N'*-(1-(2-Hydroxyphenyl)-3-methylbutylidene)isonicotinoylhydrazide (**H18**). To prepare H18, 1-(2-hydroxyphenyl)-3-methylbutan-1-one was first synthesized: Magnesium (0.41 g, 16.9 mmol) was suspended in dry THF (5 mL), and isobutylbromide (2.31 g, 16.7 mmol) was added dropwise and the mixture refluxed for 2 h until the magnesium dissolved. After cooling the reaction mixture to RT, 2-hydroxybenzonitrile (0.33 g, 2.8 mmol) dissolved in dry THF (5 mL) was added and the reaction refluxed for 2 h. The reaction mixture was cooled in an ice bath, 10 mL of cold water was carefully added and cold concentrated H_2SO_4 added dropwise to obtain an acidic pH. The reaction mixture was then heated for 1 h at 80°C and, after cooling to RT, it was extracted twice with diethyl ether. The combined organic layer was dried with anhydrous Na_2SO_4 and evaporated under reduced pressure. The product was purified by column chromatography on silica using hexane/EtOAc (40:1) as the mobile phase. The product was a yellow oil. Yield 0.45 g (91%). ^{1}H NMR (300 MHz, $CDCl_3$): δ 12.48 (s, 1H, OH), 7.89–7.63 (m, 1H, Ph), 7.59–7.40 (m, 1H, Ph), 7.08–6.83 (m, 2H, Ph), 2.92–2.74 (m, 2H, CH_2), 2.38–2.22 (m, 1H, CH), 1.13–0.94 (m, 6H, $2 \times CH_3$). ^{13}C NMR (75 MHz, $CDCl_3$): δ 206.7, 162.6, 136.2, 130.1, 119.6, 118.8, 118.5, 47.1, 25.5, 22.7.

1-(2-Hydroxyphenyl)-3-methylbutan-1-one (0.2 g, 1.1 mmol), isoniazid (0.12 g, 1.1 mmol) and acetic acid (0.25 mL) were dissolved in methanol (5 mL) and heated at 110°C in an autoclave for 72 h. After cooling to RT, water was added dropwise until the solution turned cloudy and the mixture was left to crystallize at 4°C. The precipitate was then collected by filtration, washed with water and methanol and dried over P_2O_5. The overall yield of the white crystalline product was 0.06 g (19%). mp 144–146°C. ^{1}H NMR (500 MHz, DMSO-d_6): δ 13.27 (s, 1H, OH), 11.61 (s, 1H, NH), 8.82–8.77 (m, 2H, Py), 7.81–7.73 (m, 2H, Py), 7.65 (dd, J = 8.0, 1.7 Hz, 1H, Ph), 7.42–7.19 (m, 1H, Ph), 6.97–6.86 (m, 2H, Ph), 2.99 (d, J = 7.4 Hz, 2H, CH_2), 2.02–1.93 (m, 1H, CH), 0.95 (d, J = 6.6 Hz, 6H, $2 \times CH_3$). ^{13}C NMR (125 MHz, DMSO-d_6): δ 163.3, 161.5, 159.2, 150.4, 140.4, 131.6, 129.0, 122.2, 118.7, 117.8, 34.3, 27.6, 22.2. Anal. Calcd. for $C_{17}H_{19}N_3O_2$: C, 68.67; H, 6.44; N, 14.13; Found: C, 68.28; H, 6.69; N, 13.85.

(E)-N'-[Cyclohexyl(2-hydroxyphenyl)methylene]isonicotinoylhydrazide (H28). To prepare H28, cyclohexyl(2-hydroxyphenyl)methanone was synthesized: Magnesium (0.36 g, 15 mmol) was suspended in dry THF (5 mL) and cyclohexylbromide (2.4 g, 15 mmol) was added dropwise. This reaction mixture was refluxed for 2 h until the magnesium dissolved. After cooling the reaction mixture to RT, 2-hydroxybenzonitrile (0.29 g, 2.4 mmol) dissolved in dry THF (5 mL) was added dropwise and the reaction refluxed for 3 h. The reaction mixture was cooled in an ice bath, 10 mL of cold water was added carefully and then cold concentrated H_2SO_4 was added dropwise to obtain an acidic pH. The reaction mixture was then heated overnight at 80°C and, after cooling to RT, it was extracted twice with diethyl ether. The combined organic layer was dried with anhydrous Na_2SO_4 and evaporated under reduced pressure. The product was purified by column chromatography on silica (gradient; hexane to hexane/EtOAc 40:1). The product was obtained as a yellow oil. Yield 0.49 g (97%). ^{1}H NMR (300 MHz, $CDCl_3$) δ 12.58 (s, 1H, OH), 7.88–7.69 (m, 1H, Ph), 7.55–7.32 (m, 1H, Ph), 7.07–6.95 (m, 2H, Ph), 3.43–3.12 (m, 1H, Cy), 2.03–1.06 (m, 10H, Cy). ^{13}C NMR (75 MHz, $CDCl_3$): δ 210.1, 163.1, 136.1, 129.8, 118.7, 118.7, 118.2, 45.2, 29.5, 25.8, 25.7.

Cyclohexyl(2-hydroxyphenyl)methanone (0.19 g, 0.93 mmol), isoniazid (0.13 g, 0.93 mmol) and acetic acid (0.20 mL) were dissolved in methanol (5 mL) and heated at 110°C in an autoclave for 4 days. After cooling to RT, water was added dropwise until the solution turned cloudy and the mixture was left to crystallize at 4°C for 24 h. The precipitate was collected by filtration, washed with methanol and dried over P_2O_5 to give 0.046 g (15%) of the product as a white solid. mp 251–253°C. ^{1}H NMR (300 MHz, DMSO-d_6): δ 9.27 (s, 1H, NH), 8.70–8.63 (m, 2H, Py), 7.86–7.70 (m, 2H, Py), 7.51–7.34 (m, 1H, Ph), 7.33–7.19 (m, 1H, Ph), 7.17–7.02 (m, 1H, Ph), 7.02–6.78 (m, 1H, Ph), 2.69–2.34 (m, 1H, Cy), 1.92–1.00 (m, 10H, Cy). ^{13}C NMR (75 MHz, DMSO-d_6): δ 163.0, 161.3, 150.4, 141.4, 130.8, 128.8, 121.2, 120.8, 119.7, 116.2, 30.3, 29.9, 26.0, 25.8. Anal. Calcd. for $C_{19}H_{21}N_3O_2$: C, 70.57; H, 6.55; N, 12.99; Found: C, 70.36; H, 6.91; N, 13.03.

2 Stability study

2.1 HPLC instrument and chromatographic conditions.
HPLC analyses were performed on a Prominence LC 20A chromatographic system (Shimadzu, Kyoto, Japan) consisting of a DGU-20A3 degasser, two LC-20AD pumps, SIL-20AC autosampler, a CTO-20AC column oven, SPD-20AC detector and a CBM-20AC communication module. The data were processed by LC solution software, version 1.21 SP1 (Shimadzu).

Analysis of new chelators were performed using an Ascentis C18 chromatographic column (10×3 mm, 3 μm) protected with a guard column with the same sorbent (Sigma-Aldrich). The mobile phase was composed of 1 mM EDTA in 5 mM phosphate buffer and methanol in different ratios (Table 1). The column oven was set at 25°C and the autosampler at 5°C. A flow rate of 0.3 mL/min and injection volume of 20 μL were used. Chromatographic conditions for the determination of each chelator are given in Table 1.

The linearity, precision and accuracy of the methods were examined by the analysis of plasma samples spiked with different amounts of the chelators. Selectivity was confirmed by an analysis of blank plasma samples. All evaluated parameters reached acceptable values [40]. SIH was analyzed using a previously developed and validated method [41].

2.2 Assessment of the chelator stabilities in rabbit plasma.
The drug-free plasma samples were spiked with a standard solution of each chelator (1 mg/mL in DMSO) to obtain a concentration of 100 μM. The final chelator-spiked plasma samples were maintained at 37°C and stirred at 300 rpm. Samples of the studied chelators in plasma (50 μL) were transferred into Eppendorf tubes on ice at time intervals of t = 0, 60, 120, 180, 240, 300, 360, 420, 480, 540 and 600 min from the beginning of the experiment. After this procedure, internal standards (IS) were added to the samples and then the plasma proteins were precipitated by adding methanol (200 μL). Precipitates were separated by centrifugation (10,000 rpm/10 min) and the clear supernatant was injected onto the column. In the case of redSIH, redHAPI, redHPPI and 2API, the supernatant was diluted using deionized water at a 1:1 ratio to obtain acceptable peak shapes.

3 Biological studies

3.1 Chemicals.
Constituents for various buffers as well as other chemicals (*e.g.*, various iron salts) were purchased from Sigma-Aldrich, Merck or Penta (Prague, Czech Republic) and were of the highest pharmaceutical or analytical grade available.

3.2 Cell cultures.
The MCF-7 human breast adenocarcinoma cell line was purchased from the European Collection of Cell Cultures (ECACC; Salisbury, UK), and the H9c2 cardiomyoblast cell line, derived from embryonic rat heart tissue, was obtained from the American Type Culture Collection (ATCC; Manassas, VA, USA). Cells were cultured in Dulbecco's modified Eagle's medium (DMEM; Lonza, Verviers, Belgium) with (H9c2) or without (MCF-7) phenol red and were supplemented with 10% (v/v) heat-inactivated fetal bovine serum (FBS; Lonza), 1% penicillin/streptomycin solution (Lonza) and 10 mM HEPES buffer (pH 7.0–7.6; Sigma-Aldrich). Both cell lines were cultured in 75 cm^2 tissue culture flasks (TPP, Trasadingen, Switzerland) at 37°C in a humidified atmosphere of 5% CO_2. Sub-confluent cells (70–80% confluency) were sub-cultured every 3-4 days.

3.3 Determination of iron chelating efficacy in solution.
To assess the iron chelation efficiency of the newly synthesized agents in solution, their ability to remove iron from the iron-calcein complex was examined [42]. Calcein is a fluorescent probe that readily forms iron complexes [42]. Upon formation of

Table 1. Chromatographic conditions used for the determination of the stability of the new chelators in rabbit plasma.

Chelator	Mobile phase ratio (v/v)	UV (nm)	IS
redSIH	40:60	254	redHAPI
redHAPI	40:60	254	7HII
redHPPI	40:60	254	7HII
BHAPI	30:70	254	o-108
BHPPI	30:70	254	7HII
2API	40:60	297	SIH
7HII	30:70	297	BHPPI
H16	40:60	254	o-108
H17	30:70	297	H28
H18	30:70	297	H28
H28	30:70	254	H18

the iron-calcein complex, the fluorescence of calcein is quenched. The addition of another chelating agent to the iron-calcein complex leads to the removal of iron from this complex, resulting in the formation of the new iron-chelator complex. The removal of iron from the iron-calcein complex is accompanied by an increase in fluorescence intensity (i.e., de-quenching), due to the formation of free calcein. Thus, the measurement of calcein fluorescence intensity was used to examine the iron chelation efficacy of the novel chelators [42].

A complex of calcein (free acid, 20 nM; Molecular Probes, Eugene, OR, USA) with iron derived from ferrous ammonium sulfate (200 nM) was prepared in HBS buffer (150 mM NaCl, 40 mM HEPES, pH 7.2). Calcein and ferrous ammonium sulfate were continuously stirred for 45 min in the dark, after which > 90% of the fluorescence was quenched. Then, 995 μL of the complex was pipetted into a stirred cuvette and baseline measurements were acquired. After 100 s, 5 μL of the novel chelator solution was added, yielding a final chelator concentration of 5 μM. Fluorescence intensity change was measured as a function of time at RT using a Perkin Elmer LS50B fluorimeter (Perkin Elmer, Waltham, MA, USA) at λ_{ex} = 486 nm and λ_{em} = 517 nm for 350 s. The iron chelation efficiency in solution was expressed as a percentage of the efficiency of the reference chelator, SIH (100%).

3.4 Calcein-AM assay to assess the cell membrane permeability and access to the labile iron pool. These experiments were performed according to Glickstein et al. [43] with slight modifications. MCF-7 cells were seeded in 96-well plates (10,000 cells per well). Cells were loaded with iron using the iron donor, ferric ammonium citrate (530 μg/mL), 24 h prior to the experiment, and the cells then washed. To prevent potential interference (especially with regard to various trace elements), the medium was replaced with the ADS buffer (prepared using Millipore water (18.2 MΩ/cm) supplemented with 116 mM NaCl, 5.3 mM KCl, 1 mM $CaCl_2$, 1.2 mM $MgSO_4$, 1.13 mM NaH_2PO_4, 5 mM D-glucose, and 20 mM HEPES, pH 7.4). Cells were then loaded with the membrane-permeant, calcein green acetoxymethyl ester (calcein-AM; 2 μM; Molecular Probes) for 30 min/37°C, and then washed. Cellular esterases cleave the acetoxymethyl groups to form the cell membrane-impermeant compound, calcein green, whose fluorescence is quenched upon binding iron. Intracellular fluorescence (λ_{ex} = 488 nm; λ_{em} = 530 nm) was then measured as a function of time (1 min before and 10 min after the addition of chelator) at 37°C using a Tecan Infinite 200 M plate reader (Tecan Group, Männedorf, Switzerland). The iron chelation efficiency in cells was expressed as a percentage of the efficiency of the reference chelator, SIH (100%).

3.5 Preparation of $^{59}Fe_2$-transferrin. Human Tf (Sigma-Aldrich) was labeled with Fe or ^{59}Fe (PerkinElmer) to produce Fe_2-Tf or $^{59}Fe_2$-Tf, respectively, with a final specific activity of 500 pCi/pmol Fe, as previously described [34,44]. Unbound ^{59}Fe was removed by exhaustive vacuum dialysis against an excess of 0.15 M NaCl buffered at pH 7.4 with 1.4% (w/v) $NaHCO_3$ by standard methods [34,44].

3.6 The effect of chelators on mobilizing cellular ^{59}Fe. The ability of the novel ligands to mobilize ^{59}Fe from MCF-7 cells was examined by conducting ^{59}Fe efflux experiments using established techniques [34,45]. In brief, after pre-labeling cells with $^{59}Fe_2$-Tf (0.75 μM) for 3 h/37°C, the cell cultures were washed four times with ice-cold PBS and then subsequently incubated with each chelator (25 μM) for 3 h/37°C. The overlying media containing released ^{59}Fe was then carefully separated from the cells using a Pasteur pipette. Radioactivity was measured in both the cell pellet and supernatant using a γ-scintillation counter (Wallac Wizard 3, Turku, Finland).

3.7 The effect of the chelators on the prevention of cellular ^{59}Fe uptake from $^{59}Fe2$-Tf. The ability of the chelators to prevent cellular ^{59}Fe uptake from $^{59}Fe_2$-Tf was examined using standard methods [46,47]. In brief, MCF-7 cells were incubated with $^{59}Fe_2$-Tf (0.75 μM) for 3 h/37°C in the presence of the assessed chelators (25 μM). The cells were then washed four times with ice-cold PBS and the internalized ^{59}Fe was determined via established methods by incubating the cell monolayer for 30 min/4°C with the general protease, Pronase (1 mg/mL; Sigma-Aldrich). The cells were then removed from the monolayer with a plastic spatula and centrifuged for 1 min/ 12,000×g. The supernatant represents membrane-bound, Pronase-sensitive ^{59}Fe that was released by the protease, while the Pronase-insensitive fraction represents internalized ^{59}Fe [34,46,47]. The amount of internalized ^{59}Fe was expressed as a percentage of the ^{59}Fe internalized by untreated control cells (100%).

3.8 Ascorbate oxidation assay for analysis of redox activity of iron complexes. The ability of the iron complexes of the novel ligands to mediate the oxidation of a physiological substrate, ascorbate, was examined using an established protocol [46,48]. In brief, L-ascorbic acid (100 μM) was prepared

Table 2. Molecular weights (MW) and calculated n-octanol/water coefficients (log P_{calc}) of the studied analogs.

Chelator	MW (g/mol)	log P_{calc}
SIH	241	1.5
redSIH	243	1.0
redHAPI	257	1.4
redHPPI	271	1.9
BHAPI	334	2.1
BHPPI	348	2.6
2API	240	0.7
7HII	267	1.4
H16	283	2.2
H17	283	2.2
H18	297	2.5
H28	323	3.1

The MW and log P_{calc} values were calculated using ChemBioOffice Ultra 11.0 software. The log P_{calc} is expressed as an average of the results of Crippen's and Viswanadhan's fragmentations and Broto's method.

immediately prior to the experiment and was incubated either alone or in the presence of Fe^{3+} (10 µM; as $FeCl_3$) in a 50-fold molar excess (500 µM) of citrate and chelators (1-60 µM). Chelators were assayed at iron-binding equivalents (IBE) of 0.1 (excess of iron), 1 (iron-chelator complexes with a fully saturated coordination sphere) and 3 (excess of free chelator). The iron chelators, ethylenediaminetetraacetic acid (EDTA) and DFO, were used as positive and negative controls, respectively, as their redox activity has been well characterized [49]. The decrease in absorbance at 265 nm, which is the absorption maximum of ascorbate, was measured using the plate reader described previously after 10 and 40 min of incubation at RT. The decrease in absorbance between the two time points was calculated and expressed as a percentage of the control in the absence of the chelators (100%).

3.9 Protection against oxidative injury and assessment of cytotoxicity. For these experiments, cells were seeded in 96-well plates (TPP) at a density of 10,000 cells/well (H9c2 rat cardiomyoblast) or 5,000 cells/well (MCF-7). H9c2 cells were seeded in the plates 48 h prior to addition of the studied ligands and 24 h prior to the experiments, the medium was changed to serum- and pyruvate-free DMEM (Sigma-Aldrich). The ability of the ligands to protect against oxidative injury was assessed by a simultaneous 24 h incubation with H_2O_2 (200 µM) in the presence and absence of varying concentrations of the chelators. The inherent cytotoxicity of the ligands was studied using the H9c2 cell line after a 72 h incubation. For proliferation studies, MCF-7 cells were seeded 24 h prior to addition of the chelators. The cytotoxic effects of the various iron chelators were then studied at different concentrations after a 72 h incubation. To dissolve the lipophilic agents, dimethyl sulfoxide (DMSO; Sigma-Aldrich) was utilized leading to a final DMSO concentration of 0.1% (v/v) in the culture medium of all groups. At this concentration, DMSO had no effect on cytotoxicity (data not shown). The viability of the H9c2 and MCF-7 cells was determined using the neutral red (NR; Sigma) uptake assay, which is based on the ability of viable cells to incorporate NR into lysosomes [33,50]. The optical density of soluble NR was measured at $\lambda = 540$ nm using the Tecan Infinite 200 M plate reader. The viability or proliferation of the experimental groups was expressed as a percentage of the untreated controls (100%). Control experiments using viable cell counts demonstrated a direct correlation to NR uptake.

3.10 Data analysis and statistics. The values of the molecular weights (MW) and n-octanol/water coefficients (log P_{calc}; Table 2) were calculated using ChemBioOffice Ultra 11.0 software (CambridgeSoft, Cambridge, MA, USA). The log P_{calc} is expressed as an average of the results of Crippen's [51], Viswanadhan's [52], and Broto's [53] method. SigmaStat for Windows 3.5 (Systat Software, San Jose, CA, USA) statistical software was used for data analyses. The data are expressed as the mean ±S.D. of at least 3 experiments. Statistical significance was determined using a one-way ANOVA with a Bonferroni *post-hoc* test (comparisons of multiple groups against the relevant control). The results were considered to be statistically significant when $p < 0.05$. The EC_{50} (half-maximal effective concentration) and IC_{50} (half-maximal inhibitory concentration) values were calculated using CalcuSyn 2.0 software (Biosoft, Cambridge, UK). Raw data underlying the findings in this study are in Data S1.

Results

1 Stability of the chelators in plasma

The stabilities of the newly prepared chelators in rabbit plasma were studied using HPLC analysis following a 600 min (10 h) incubation *in vitro*. The results were expressed as a percentage of the initial concentration of chelators at time $t = 0$ min. In our previous studies, SIH showed low stability, with less than 10% of SIH remaining intact after 180 min [33] and this was confirmed in our present investigation (Fig. 2A). The methylated and ethylated analogs of SIH, namely HAPI and HPPI, were markedly more resistant than SIH to hydrolysis in plasma. In fact, HAPI and HPPI were present at 26% and 41% of their original concentration at $t = 600$ min [33].

The reduction of the hydrazone bond of SIH caused a marked increase in the stability of redSIH, with 30% of the intact ligand remaining at $t = 600$ min (Fig. 2B). On the other hand, the reduction of the hydrazone bond of HAPI and HPPI, led to comparable or slightly decreased stability relative to SIH, with 23% of redHAPI and 25% of redHPPI remaining intact in plasma at $t = 600$ min (Fig. 2C, D). The bromination of HAPI increased the stability of BHAPI relative to SIH, with 45% of the ligand

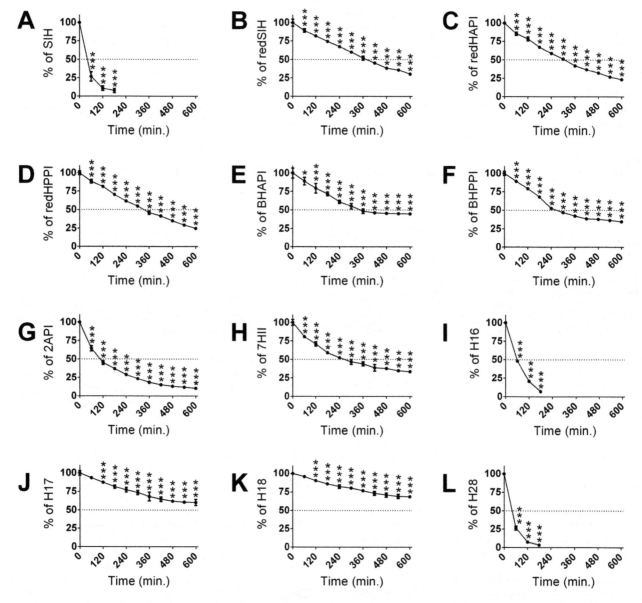

Figure 2. Stabilities of SIH and its novel analogs in rabbit plasma. SIH (**A**), redSIH (**B**), redHAPI (**C**), redHPPI (**D**), BHAPI (**E**), BHPPI (**F**), 2API (**G**), 7HII (**H**), H16 (**I**), H17 (**J**), H18 (**K**) and H28 (**L**) were incubated at 37°C in rabbit plasma and their concentrations were analyzed using HPLC every 60 min until $t = 600$ min. Results are expressed as a percentage of the concentration at $t = 0$ min (100 μM). Results are Mean ±SD ($n = 3$ experiments). Statistical significance (ANOVA): * $p<0.05$, ** $p<0.01$, *** $p<0.001$ compared to the concentration at $t = 0$ min (100%).

remaining intact, while the bromination of HPPI had no significant effect relative to SIH (i.e., 35% of BHPPI remained intact at the end of the 600 min incubation period; Fig. 2E, F).

The 2-acetylpyridine derivative, 2API, showed better stability than the parent chelator, SIH, but was less stable than HAPI, with 10% of 2API remaining intact after the 600 min incubation (Fig. 2G). The cyclic ligand, 7HII, possessed comparable stability to HPPI, with 34% of 7HII remaining at the end of incubation (Fig. 2H). The introduction of a bulky isopropyl or cyclohexyl group to analogs H16 and H28, respectively, resulted in a surprisingly short half-life in plasma, with almost complete decomposition of these ligands at $t = 180$ min (Fig. 2I, L). Pilot experiments showed that the rapid decomposition of H16 was only partially due to hydrolysis of the hydrazone bond (only 10% of the expected ketone was found in plasma), with the instability probably also involving the hydrazine bond. Nevertheless, this remains to be carefully elucidated by using additional advanced analytical methods. In contrast, the introduction of an unbranched propyl or terminally-branched isobutyl moiety (ligands H17 and H18, respectively) led to a pronounced increase of their stability in plasma relative to SIH (Fig. 2J, K), with 60% of H17 and 69% of H18 remaining intact in plasma after a 10 h incubation.

2. Determination of the iron chelating efficacy in solution and in MCF-7 cells

To assess the iron chelation efficacy of the ligands in solution, the iron complexes of the weak iron chelator, calcein, were used. In this assay, the examined chelators compete with calcein for iron and the fluorescence of the free, dequenched calcein is proportional to their chelation efficacy in comparison to calcein. The iron chelation efficacy of the novel ligands was expressed as a percentage of the level of calcein de-quenching caused by the parent chelator, SIH (100%).

The reduction of the hydrazone bond in redSIH, redHAPI and redHPPI resulted in significantly ($p<0.001$) reduced iron chelating efficacies in solution (Fig. 3A). The brominated ligands, BHAPI and BHPPI, and the alkylated analogs, 7HII, H17 and H18 exhibited iron chelating activity similar to the reference agent, SIH (Fig. 3A). The 2-acetylpyridine derivative, 2API, was observed to have poor iron chelating efficacy in this assay relative to SIH. However, this may be due to the ability of the iron complex of 2API to oxidize calcein [54], as the iron complex of 2API was identified to act as a pro-oxidant (see below), and thus, resulted in decreased calcein fluorescence. Additionally, low chelation efficacy was also observed for the ligands, H16 and H28 (Fig. 3A), that possess an isopropyl or cyclohexyl group, respectively, adjacent to the hydrazone bond.

The efficacy of the ligands to permeate the cell membrane to gain access to the LIP was examined using the calcein-AM assay in iron-loaded MCF-7 cells (Fig. 3B). In these studies, the iron chelation efficacy of the synthesized ligands was expressed as a percentage of the efficiency of the parent chelator, SIH (100%). The ability of the chelators, BHPPI, 7HII and H17 to permeate the cell membrane and to bind iron from the calcein-AM detectable LIP did not significantly ($p>0.05$) differ from that of SIH (Fig. 3B). This was well correlated with their high chelation efficacy in solution (Fig. 3A). The ligands, redSIH, BHAPI, 2API, H18 and H28, exhibited moderate (50–80% relative to SIH), but significantly ($p<0.05-0.001$) decreased iron chelation efficacy in MCF-7 cells relative to SIH (Fig. 3B). In contrast, redHAPI, redHPPI and H16 displayed the poorest ability (<50% relative to SIH) to access and bind iron from the LIP (Fig. 3B) and this was in good correlation to their chelation activity in solution (Fig. 3A).

3. The effect of the chelators on the mobilization of cellular 59Fe and prevention of cellular 59Fe uptake from 59Fe2-Tf

To examine the ability of the novel ligands to mobilize intracellular ^{59}Fe from MCF-7 cells, ^{59}Fe efflux experiments were performed using established techniques [34,45]. The novel ligands were compared to control medium containing no added chelator and also to the parent analog, SIH (Fig. 4A). The control medium showed limited ability to mobilize cellular ^{59}Fe, resulting in the release of 8% of cellular ^{59}Fe (Fig. 4A). In contrast, SIH displayed high ^{59}Fe mobilization efficacy, mediating the release of 55% of cellular ^{59}Fe (Fig. 4A). The ligands, BHAPI, BHPPI, 2API, 7HII, H17 and H18 were highly effective in mediating ^{59}Fe mobilization and resulted in the release of 43–58% of cellular ^{59}Fe (Fig. 4A). The agents, redSIH and H28 demonstrated significantly ($p<0.001$) increased ^{59}Fe mobilization compared to the control. However, their ^{59}Fe mobilization efficacy was approximately half that of SIH (Fig. 4A). The ^{59}Fe mobilization efficacy of redHAPI, redHPPI and H16 were poor and comparable to the untreated control (Fig. 4A). In general, the results of this assay correlated well with the observed iron-chelation efficacies of these analogs in solution (Fig. 3A) and in the cell-based calcein-AM assay (Fig. 3B). The only notable exception was 2API, which demonstrated high activity at mobilizing cellular ^{59}Fe (Fig. 4A), which was in contrast to the iron chelation assay in solution (Fig. 3A). As noted previously, this could be due to its pro-oxidative effects on calcein [54].

As the iron chelation efficacy and cytotoxic activity of a ligand are due to both its ability to mobilize cellular Fe, but also, inhibit Fe uptake from Tf [34], the ability of the chelators to prevent the

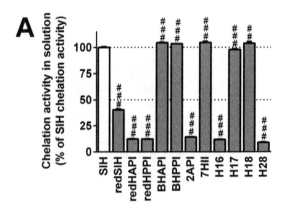
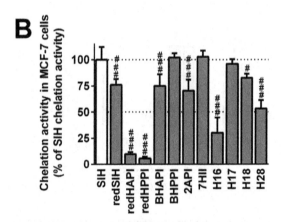

Figure 3. Iron chelation properties of the novel analogs in solution (A) and in MCF-7 cells (B). (A) The chelation dynamics of the new agents in solution were observed for 360 s using the calcein assay, and the agent was applied at $t=100$ s. The fluorescence intensity of free calcein at $t=360$ s was expressed as a percentage of that observed using the reference iron chelator, SIH. (B) The ability of the analogs to chelate "free" iron from the LIP in MCF-7 cells was measured using the calcein-AM assay. The fluorescence intensity of free calcein at $t=600$ s was expressed as a percentage of that observed in the presence of SIH. Results are Mean ±SD ($n\geq3$ experiments). Statistical significance (ANOVA): # $p<0.05$, ## $p<0.01$, ### $p<0.001$ compared to the reference chelator, SIH.

cellular uptake of ^{59}Fe from ^{59}Fe$_2$-Tf was determined and expressed as a percentage of the untreated control (Fig. 4B). As observed in the ^{59}Fe mobilization experiments, the parent chelator, SIH, demonstrated high ^{59}Fe chelation efficacy and inhibited ^{59}Fe uptake to 15% of the control (Fig. 4B).

Importantly, those ligands that showed high ^{59}Fe mobilization efficacy (Fig. 4A) were also highly effective at inhibiting the uptake of ^{59}Fe from ^{59}Fe$_2$-Tf (Fig. 4B). For example, the ligands, BHAPI, BHPPI, 2API, 7HII, H17 and H18, that demonstrated high ^{59}Fe mobilization activity, were able to limit ^{59}Fe uptake to 10–26% of the control (Fig. 4B). In contrast, the compounds, redSIH, redHAPI, redHPPI, H16, and H28, showed limited ability to prevent ^{59}Fe uptake, inhibiting it to >70% of the control (Fig. 4B).

4. Examination of the ability of the iron-chelator complexes to catalyze the oxidation of ascorbate

It has been previously observed that the cytotoxic effects of some iron chelators is due not only to their ability to bind cellular iron, but also to form redox-active iron complexes [12,46,55]. Thus, we examined whether the iron complexes of our novel

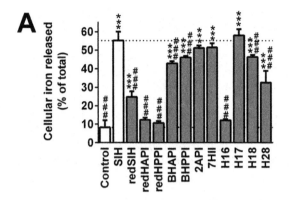

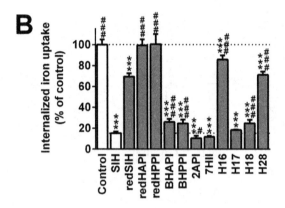

Figure 4. The effect of SIH and its analogs on ^{59}Fe mobilization from pre-labeled MCF-7 cells (A) and on internalized ^{59}Fe uptake from ^{59}Fe$_2$-transferrin (Tf) by MCF-7 cells (B). (A) The ability of the ligands to promote ^{59}Fe mobilization from MCF-7 cells was performed by first prelabeling the cells with ^{59}Fe$_2$-Tf (0.75 μM) for 3 h/37°C, followed by washing and then reincubation for 3 h/37°C with either control medium alone, or control medium containing the chelator (25 μM). (B) Inhibition of ^{59}Fe uptake from ^{59}Fe$_2$-Tf by MCF-7 cells by chelators was performed by incubating cells for 3 h/37°C with ^{59}Fe$_2$-Tf (0.75 μM) in the presence or absence of the chelator (25 μM). Results are Mean ±SD (n≥3 experiments). Statistical significance (ANOVA): * $p<0.05$, ** $p<0.01$, *** $p<0.001$ compared to the control (untreated) group, and # $p<0.05$, ## $p<0.01$, ### $p<0.001$ compared to the reference chelator, SIH.

ligands were able to redox cycle by assessing their ability to mediate the oxidation of ascorbate by standard methods [46,48]. The ability of the iron complexes to catalyze the oxidation of ascorbate was expressed as a percentage of the control (ascorbate with "free" Fe^{3+}).

The chelators, DFO and EDTA, were used as negative (anti-oxidative) and positive (pro-oxidative) controls, respectively [46,49]. As previously observed, the Fe complex of DFO demonstrated a typical anti-oxidative profile [56], resulting in decreased levels of ascorbate oxidation at an IBE of 3 (excess DFO) than at an IBE of 0.1 (excess iron; Fig. 5). In contrast, the iron complex of EDTA exhibited a pro-oxidative effect and mediated higher levels of ascorbate oxidation at an IBE of 3 relative to that at 0.1 (Fig. 5). In fact, at an IBE of 3, the iron complex of EDTA increased the oxidation of ascorbate to 924% of the control.

The iron complex of the parent chelator, SIH, exhibited anti-oxidant activity similar to that of the iron complex of DFO (Fig. 5). All of the iron complexes of the novel ligands, with the exception of 2API, demonstrated neither anti-oxidant nor pro-oxidative effects and were comparable to the control. The iron complex of the pyridine derivative, 2API, was the only Fe complex that showed pro-oxidative effects and significantly ($p<0.001$) increased ascorbate oxidation to 256% relative to the control at an IBE of 3 (Fig. 5).

5. Prevention of oxidative injury induced by hydrogen peroxide

The ability of the ligands to act as protective agents in a model of oxidative stress was then examined by assessing the cellular viability of H9c2 cardiomyoblast cells upon a 24 h co-incubation of the chelators with H_2O_2 (200 μM). These results are shown in Fig. 6 and summarized in Table 3. In these experiments, the EC_{50} value is calculated which represents the concentration that reduced the cytotoxicity induced by hydrogen peroxide (200 μM) to 50% of the untreated control after a 24 h/37°C incubation with H9c2 cells. SIH was used as a positive control and resulted in an EC_{50} value of 7.63±1.38 μM (Table 3).

Of all the novel ligands synthesized, the analog that displayed the highest level of cytoprotective activity was 7HII, with an EC_{50} value of 2.68±1.30 μM (Table 3). In fact, 7HII demonstrated significantly ($p<0.001$) greater protection against hydrogen peroxide-induced cytotoxicity than the parent chelator, SIH. Although the iron chelators, BHAPI, BHPPI, 2API, H17 and H18 also prevented peroxide-induced cytotoxicity (EC_{50}: 8.48–42.57 μM), their EC_{50} values were higher than that of SIH. The ligands, redSIH, redHAPI, redHPPI, H16 and H28 did not display protective activity against peroxide-induced cytotoxicity in the concentration range examined.

6. Cytotoxicity studies in H9c2 cardiomyoblast cells

The selectivity of the novel ligands was then examined after a 72 h incubation with the non-tumorigenic H9c2 cardiomyoblast cell line (Fig. 7; Table 3). The parent chelator, SIH, was examined as a control and demonstrated an IC_{50} value of 49.47±1.77 μM (Table 3).

Of the synthesized analogs, redHAPI, redHPPI, H16 and H28 were the least toxic agents, with IC_{50} values>80 μM. The ligands, redSIH and H17, showed comparable cytotoxicity to H9c2 cardiomyoblasts as the parent chelator, SIH. The other studied ligands, BHAPI, BHPPI, 2API, 7HII, H18, were more toxic than the chelator, SIH, with IC_{50} values ranging from 0.62 μM to 7.40 μM. The most cytotoxic agent was 7HII with an IC_{50} value of 0.62±0.17 μM (Table 3; Fig. 7).

7. Cytotoxic effects of SIH derivatives on MCF-7 cells

The cytotoxic effects of the SIH derivatives were studied in MCF-7 breast adenocarcinoma cells following a 72 h incubation. The parent chelator, SIH, was used as a control and demonstrated moderate cytotoxic activity (IC_{50}: 4.21±1.05 μM; Table 3; Fig. 8), similar to that previously observed [31].

The analogs containing a reduced hydrazone bond (redSIH, redHAPI and redHPPI) or an isopropyl group adjacent to this bond (H16) exhibited poor cytotoxic activity (IC_{50}>100 μM). The chelator, H28, with a bulky cyclohexyl group in close proximity to the hydrazone bond demonstrated intermediate cytotoxic effects, with an IC_{50} of 42.41±3.15 μM. The remaining agents, BHAPI, BHPPI, 2API, 7HII, H17 and H18, showed increased cytotoxic activity (IC_{50}: 0.38–2.92 μM; Table 3) relative to SIH (Table 3). The greatest level of cytotoxic activity was observed with the indanone derivative, 7HII (IC_{50} = 0.38±0.11 μM).

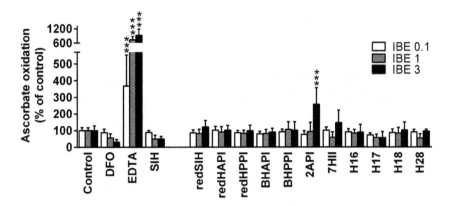

Figure 5. Effects of SIH and its analogs on iron-induced oxidation of ascorbic acid in a buffered solution (pH 7.4). Chelators were assayed at iron binding equivalents (IBE) of 0.1 (excess of Fe), 1 (iron-chelator complexes with a fully filled coordination sphere) and 3 (excess of free chelator). DFO and EDTA were used as negative and positive control chelators, respectively. The results are expressed as a percentage of the control group in the absence of chelator (100%). Results are Mean ±SD ($n \geq 3$ experiments). Statistical significance (ANOVA): * $p<0.05$, ** $p<0.01$, *** $p<0.001$ as compared to the control group (iron with ascorbate).

To provide insight into the selectivity of the cytotoxic effects of the novel ligands, which is crucial for potential anti-cancer agents, their IC_{50} values in H9c2 cells and their IC_{50} values in MCF-7 cells were compared by calculating a "selectivity ratio", namely IC_{50} H9c2/IC_{50} MCF-7 cells (Table 3). SIH had a selectivity ratio of 11.75. The analogs, redSIH and redHAPI, with reduced hydrazone bonds had lower IC_{50} values in H9c2 cardiomyoblasts than in MCF-7 cancer cells, indicating greater cytotoxic activity in the former. Relative to SIH, this resulted in a marked decrease in the selectivity ratio to 0.14 and 0.63, respectively (Table 3). The ligands, redHPPI, 2API, 7HII and H28, showed somewhat similar cytotoxic activity in both the MCF-7 and H9c2 cell-types leading to selectivity ratios that were far less than SIH, and which ranged between 1.05 and 2.01. On the other hand, the bromine-substituted chelators (BHAPI and BHPPI) demonstrated selective activity against MCF-7 breast cancer cells relative to the H9c2 cell-type, although their selectivity ratios were approximately half that observed for SIH, viz., 6.59 and 7.60, respectively (Table 3). The analogs that demonstrated the greatest selectivity profile against MCF-7 cells relative to H9c2 cells were the propyl (H17) and isobutyl (H18) derivatives of SIH, which were more active than SIH itself, demonstrating selectivity ratios of 14.36 and 15.10, respectively (Table 3).

Discussion

Aroylhydrazones represent an intriguing group of chelators that exhibit a variety of biological effects associated with their ability to influence cellular iron levels [27,33,57]. The aim of the present study was to synthesize and evaluate the biological activity of a series of new analogs of the well-established iron-binding ligand, SIH, with respect to their: (*1*) stability in plasma, (*2*) cytotoxic effects; (*3*) ability to protect cells against oxidative injury; and (*4*) cytotoxicity to H9c2 non-tumorigenic cardiomyoblast cells. The iron chelation activity, ability to mobilize cellular ^{59}Fe, efficacy to inhibit ^{59}Fe uptake from ^{59}Fe$_2$-Tf, and the redox activity of the iron complexes of the novel analogs were also determined, as these properties are crucial factors involved in their biological activity [34,35]. The primary goal was to further characterize the structure-activity relationships of SIH-related aroylhydrazones for the future rational design of compounds with therapeutic potential.

1. Reduction of the hydrazone bond

First, we probed the role of the hydrazone bond itself, as it is prone to hydrolysis and is a site of instability in this class of compounds [58]. Previous studies suggested that structurally-related compounds with a reduced $C=N$ bond retained their chelation properties [59]. In fact, these reduced compounds inhibited the iron-induced generation of hydroxyl radicals and protected murine dermal fibroblasts against UV-induced lipid peroxidation and UV-induced cytotoxicity [59]. Thus, we examined the effect of the reduction of the hydrazone bond of the chelators, SIH, HAPI and HPPI, as these ligands previously exhibited cardioprotective [33] and cytotoxic [31] activity.

The results of the present study revealed that the reduced analogs were relatively non-toxic against both tumorigenic MCF-7 cells and non-tumorigenic H9c2 cardiomyoblasts (Table 3). The cytotoxicity of redHAPI and redHPPI were approximately one order of magnitude lower than those of the parent chelators (HAPI and HPPI, respectively) [31,33], while the cytotoxic activity of redSIH towards H9c2 cells was similar to that of SIH (Table 3). This effect could be caused by the increased stability of redSIH (Fig. 2B) compared to SIH (Fig 2A), and therefore, the prolonged exposure of cells to intact redSIH compensated for the reduced (yet significant) iron chelation activity. Reduction of the hydrogen bond in redSIH, redHAPI and redHPPI led to a marked decrease in their selectivity ratios (0.14–1.14) relative to SIH (11.75; Table 3). In fact, these agents containing a reduced hydrazone bond had the lowest selectivity ratios of all analogues examined in this investigation. Furthermore, these latter compounds lost the ability to protect H9c2 cells against oxidative stress relative to SIH (Table 3) [33]. This lack of protection against oxidative stress is likely due to their limited iron chelation (Fig. 3) and ^{59}Fe mobilization efficacy (Fig. 4A). Of the reduced analogs, only redSIH retained limited chelation activity (Figs. 3 and 4). Therefore, the presence of the hydrazone bond is an important criterion for the cardioprotective and cytotoxic effects of these aroylhydrazones. The loss of iron chelation efficacy of the reduced analogs may be a result of the altered molecular spatial arrangement of the ligating groups due to the free rotation of the single C-N bond, or the decreased electron density on the chelating nitrogen due to its transition from sp^2 to sp^3 orbital hybridization.

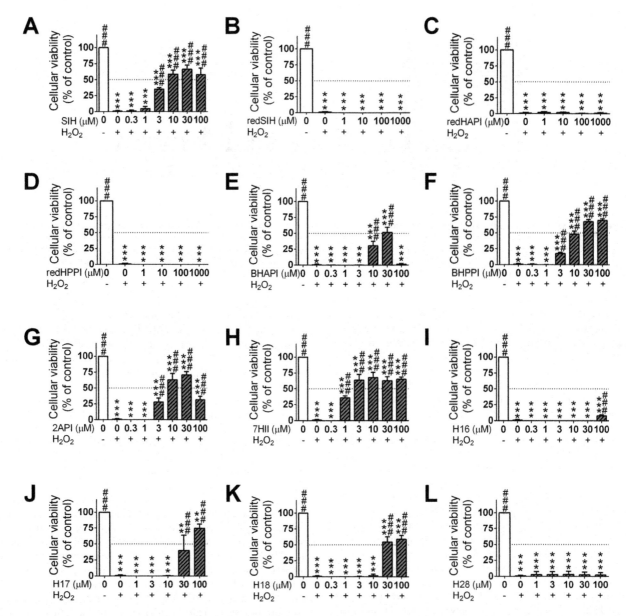

Figure 6. Protective effects of the chelator, SIH (A), and the new analogues (B–L). The ability of the SIH derivatives to protect H9c2 cardiomyoblast cells against oxidative injury were evaluated using a 24 h/37°C incubation of the cells with H_2O_2 (200 μM) and the novel analogs (0.3–1000 μM). Results are Mean ±SD ($n \geq 4$ experiments). Statistical significance (ANOVA): * $p<0.05$, ** $p<0.01$, *** $p<0.001$ compared to the control (untreated) group, and # $p<0.05$, ## $p<0.01$, ### $p<0.001$ compared to the H_2O_2 group.

2. Bromination of the phenyl ring

The introduction of a halogen into the structure of a molecule enhances its lipophilicity (Table 2), which can potentially facilitate its permeation into cells. The halogen substitution, due to its inductive electron-withdrawing effects, may also influence the stability of the hydrazone bond and the ability of the compound to chelate metal ions. Indeed, a previously synthesized chlorinated HAPI derivative (i.e., (E)-N′-[1-(5-chloro-2-hydroxyphenyl)ethylidene]isonicotinoylhydrazide; CHAPI), showed greater hydrolytic stability than HAPI and moderate cytotoxic activity ($IC_{50} = 0.65 \pm 0.07$ μM against MCF-7 cells) [31]. Therefore, the brominated analog, BHAPI, bearing a bromine instead of chlorine, and its homolog, BHPPI (Fig. 1), was prepared to evaluate the influence of halogenation on the cardioprotective and cytotoxic activity of these chelators. The stability of BHAPI and BHPPI was similar to the chloro derivative, CHAPI. However, the presence of bromine instead of the chlorine substituent increased the chelating efficiency of these compounds in cells from approximately 50% for CHAPI, to 75% and 100% for BHAPI and BHPPI, respectively. Both BHAPI and BHPPI showed comparable iron chelation efficacy to SIH in solution, as well as in cells (Fig. 3). The cytotoxic activity of these brominated analogs against MCF-7 cells was greater than that found for SIH (Table 3). Further, both BHAPI and BHPPI showed greater cytotoxic activity against MCF-7 breast cancer cells relative to non-tumorigenic, H9c2 cardiomyoblasts, although their selectivity ratios were approximately half that observed for SIH (Table 3). In addition, BHAPI and BHPPI were less effective than SIH when assessing the ability of these agents to prevent the cytotoxicity

Table 3. Protective and cytotoxic effects of the synthesized SIH derivatives and their calculated "selectivity ratios".

Chelator	EC$_{50}$ H9c2 (µM)	IC$_{50}$ H9c2 (µM)	IC$_{50}$ MCF-7 (µM)	Selectivity Ratio
SIH	7.63±1.38	49.47±1.77	4.21±1.05	11.75
redSIH	N/A	39.59±5.11	279.97±53.17	0.14
redHAPI	N/A	83.96±2.76	133.47±28.76	0.63
redHPPI	N/A	226.12±6.31	197.86±13.09	1.14
BHAPI	30.34±7.23	6.99±0.82	1.06±0.46	6.59
BHPPI	17.18±4.39	6.31±0.59	0.83±0.50	7.60
2API	8.48±3.11	3.07±0.55	2.92±0.67	1.05
7HII	2.68±1.30	0.62±0.17	0.38±0.11	1.63
H16	N/A	>100	153.67±24.20	-
H17	42.57±7.94	32.60±1.09	2.27±0.14	14.36
H18	27.76±3.90	7.40±2.13	0.49±0.18	15.10
H28	N/A	85.37±12.90	42.41±3.15	2.01

The EC$_{50}$ values (concentration that reduced the cytotoxicity induced by H$_2$O$_2$ (200 µM) to 50% of the untreated control) were calculated after a 24 h incubation with non-tumorigenic H9c2 cardiomyoblasts. The IC$_{50}$ values (concentration that reduced the cellular viability or proliferation to 50% of the untreated control) were calculated after a 72 h incubation with H9c2 cardiomyoblasts or MCF-7 breast cancer cells. Selectivity ratios were calculated via IC$_{50}$ H9c2 cells/IC$_{50}$ MCF-7 cells. Mean ± SD; n≥4 experiments. N/A - the EC$_{50}$ value was not achieved within the studied concentration range (no protection).

induced by H$_2$O$_2$ in H9c2 cardiomyoblasts (Table 3). Similar results were previously observed for the chlorine derivative, CHAPI [33].

3. Exchange of phenol for pyridine

The ligand, 2API, which contains a pyridine nitrogen as a donor atom instead of the phenolic oxygen, was prepared to examine the effect of alterations of the donor atom set from O, N, O to N, N, O on their biological activity. The main reason for this structural modification was that exchanging a hard base ligand (phenolic oxygen) for a softer base (nitrogen) could markedly alter the ability of such a compound to bind Fe^{3+}/Fe^{2+}. In addition, structurally similar hydrazones derived from pyridine-2-carbaldehyde gained attention in the treatment of iron overload diseases [37,38]. The cytotoxic activity of 2API was similar in MCF-7 breast cancer cells and non-tumorigenic H9c2 cells, with the selectivity ratio decreasing markedly (to 1.05) relative to that observed with SIH (11.75; Table 3). This observation may be explained by the redox activity of 2API, as it was the only analog that exhibited significant pro-oxidative activity in the ascorbate oxidation assay (Fig. 5). In fact, previous studies reported the reversible Fe$^{2+/3+}$ redox couple of the iron complex of 2API [60] and the current investigation demonstrates its ability to oxidize ascorbate.

The iron chelation efficacy and ^{59}Fe mobilization activity of 2API in cells was marked, with the ligand being generally comparable to SIH (Figs. 3B, 4A, 4B). In contrast, the iron chelation activity of 2API in solution did not correlate with the results of cellular experiments (Fig. 3A), which may be explained by the pro-oxidative effects of 2API. It is possible the ability of the 2API iron complex to redox cycle may have interfered in the solution-based calcein assay, as it is known that the fluorescence of free calcein decreases in an oxidative environment [54]. Whereas the unaltered sensitivity of the calcein-AM assay in cells (Fig. 3B) with regards to 2API, may be due to the redox buffering capacity provided by glutathione and other intracellular anti-oxidative systems [61] that maintain calcein sensitivity. In summary, the alteration of the donor atom set from O, N, O to N, N, O in 2API resulted in the formation of a redox active iron complex with decreased selectivity against MCF-7 breast cancer cells. However, the exact mechanism of action of this compound remains to be elucidated.

4. Branching, prolongation or cyclization of the alkyl chain adjacent to the hydrazone bond

In a previous investigation, we found that the presence of an alkyl chain adjacent to the hydrazone bond did not significantly increase the cytotoxic activity of the ketone-derived hydrazones, HAPI and HPPI, compared to SIH [31]. In the current study, we synthesized the analogs, 7HII, H16, H17, H18 and H28, to evaluate the influence of alkyl chain length and branching on biological activity.

The 7-hydroxyindanone derivative, 7HII, contains an extra five-membered ring relative to SIH and showed comparable iron chelating and ^{59}Fe mobilization efficacy (Figs. 3, 4). The cyclization of the alkyl chain, and hence, its increased rigidity, improved its hydrolytic stability (Fig 2H) and also its ability to protect cells against oxidative stress compared to SIH, with 7HII being the most effective ligand screened in this regard (Table 3). However, this structural change in 7HII resulted in significantly higher cytotoxicity towards H9c2 cells and a marked drop in the selectivity ratio relative to SIH (Table 3). Therefore, this structural modification resulted in unfavorable biological activity.

The ligand, H16, bears an additional isopropyl chain at the α-position from the hydrazone bond relative to SIH (Fig. 1). This modification was intended to: (**1**) protect the hydrazone bond against hydrolysis [62]; and (**2**) increase lipophilicity, which is known to enhance cellular permeability of aroylhydrazone ligands [34]. However, this structural modification in H16 resulted in similar stability in plasma as SIH and a marked loss of its iron chelation activity relative to SIH. This effect may be due to steric hindrance around the hydrazone bond mediated by the bulky branched isopropyl group that potentially reduces binding to iron. Notably, consistent with the loss of iron-binding, the cytotoxic activity of H16 was very low in H9c2 and MCF-7 cells and did not show any protective effects against H$_2$O$_2$ (Table 3).

To examine whether the effect of the isopropyl chain of H16 was caused by steric hindrance close to the hydrazone bond,

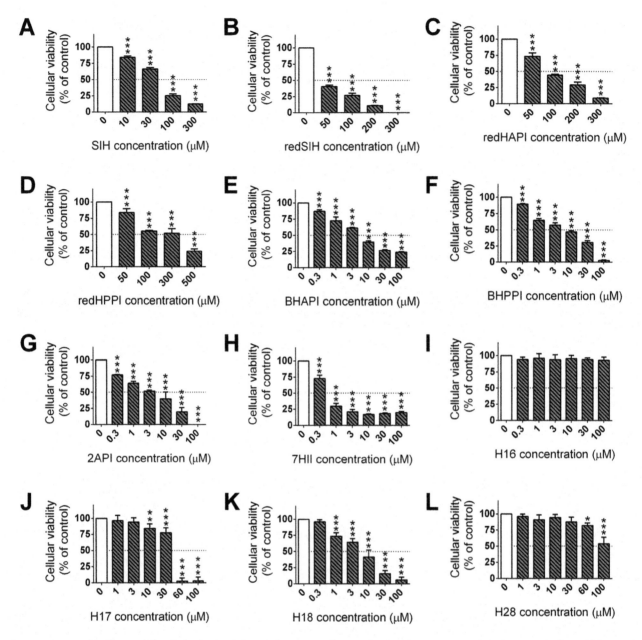

Figure 7. Cytotoxic effects of the chelator, SIH (A), and the new analogues (B–L), using non-tumorigenic H9c2 cardiomyoblasts. The effect of the analogs (0.3–300 μM) on the cellular viability of H9c2 cardiomyoblasts were performed using a 72 h/37°C incubation. Results are Mean ±SD ($n \geq 4$ experiments). Statistical significance (ANOVA): * $p<0.05$, ** $p<0.01$, *** $p<0.001$ as compared to the control (untreated) group.

compound H17, with an unbranched propyl chain, was prepared. Interestingly, this ligand was even more stable in plasma (Fig. 2J) than its homolog HPPI [33]. Furthermore, the iron chelation and ^{59}Fe mobilization efficacy of H17 was similar to SIH, with the compound showing selective cytotoxic activity against MCF-7 cancer cells relative to non-tumorigenic H9c2 cardiomyoblasts [31,33]. In fact, the selectivity ratio of H17 (14.36) was greater than that found for SIH (11.75), demonstrating its potential. We were also interested to examine whether H18, with an isobutyl substituent adjacent to the hydrazone bond (Fig. 1), would retain the favorable activity of H17. In contrast to H16, H18 is branched at the β-position in relation to the imine carbon and led to the ligand maintaining hydrolytic stability, iron chelation efficacy in solution and also in cells relative to SIH (Figs. 2J, 3, 4). This structural change increased the cytotoxic activity of H18 against both MCF-7 tumor cells and H9c2 cardiomyoblasts relative to SIH and H17 (Table 3). However, notably, H18 had the best selectivity ratio of all the studied compounds (i.e., 15.10).

To further examine the structure-activity relationships of bulky substituents close to the hydrazone bond, compound H28, with a cyclohexyl group, was prepared. As in the case of H16, this modification did not improve the low hydrolytic stability observed with SIH (Fig. 2L). Also, the iron chelation efficacy of H28 was markedly decreased (Figs. 3, 4). Furthermore, in comparison with H16, the cytotoxic activity of H28 was greater in both MCF-7 and H9c2 cells, leading to an unfavorable selectivity ratio of 2.01 which was much less than SIH. In addition, the cardioprotective activity

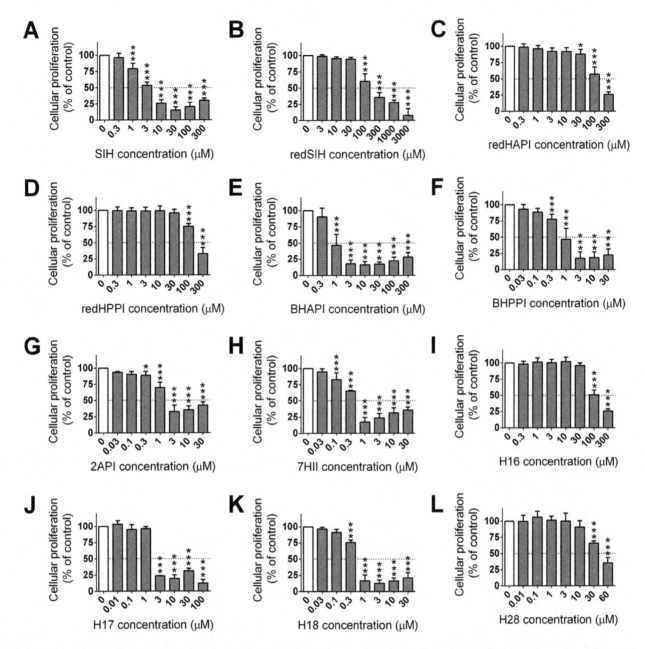

Figure 8. Cytotoxic effects of the chelator, SIH (A), and the new analogues (B–L) against MCF-7 breast cancer cells. For the determination of their cytotoxic activity, MCF-7 breast adenocarcinoma cells were incubated with the analogs (0.01–3000 µM) for 72 h/37°C. Results are Mean ±SD ($n \geq 4$ experiments). Statistical significance (ANOVA): * $p<0.05$, ** $p<0.01$, *** $p<0.001$ as compared to the control (untreated) group.

of H28 against H_2O_2 was completely abolished, which is consistent with the low iron chelation efficacy of H28.

Thus, the alkyl chain on the imine carbon markedly influenced the activity of such hydrazones. Prolonged linear or iso-branched alkyl groups increased their anti-cancer potential, while branching or cyclization in close proximity to the hydrazone bond dramatically decreased their chelation ability and, consequently, decreased their cytotoxic activity against MCF-7 cells and their ability to protect H9c2 cells against oxidative injury.

5. Conclusions

In this study, we identified several structural parameters important for the design of aroylhydrazone iron chelators. First, the hydrazone bond is essential for chelation activity. Second, bromination of the phenyl ring does not have any beneficial effect due to increased non-selective cytotoxic activity against non-tumorigenic H9c2 cardiomyoblasts. Third, exchange of the chelating phenolic hydroxyl (a hard base) for a pyridine nitrogen (softer base) resulted in increased non-selective cytotoxic activity, the mechanism of which is not exactly known. Finally, and most significantly, the exchange of the aldimine hydrogen in SIH for a longer unbranched or iso-branched alkyl group is a favorable modification to increase the stability and anti-cancer potential of such hydrazones. The most promising compounds identified in this study are the propyl-containing analog, H17, and isobutyl-containing derivative, H18, which possessed the highest selectivity ratios. These compounds warrant further investigation.

Author Contributions

Conceived and designed the experiments: EP KH JB PK PH DJRL DSK DRR KV TŠ. Performed the experiments: EP KH JB PK IAŠ KP LK TH PH HJ MM AJ VR DJRL. Analyzed the data: EP KH JB PK KV TŠ. Wrote the paper: EP KH JB PK PH DJRL DSK DRR KV TŠ.

References

1. Wang J, Pantopoulos K (2011) Regulation of cellular iron metabolism. Biochem J 434: 365–381.
2. Lawen A, Lane DJ (2013) Mammalian iron homeostasis in health and disease: uptake, storage, transport, and molecular mechanisms of action. Antioxid Redox Signal 18: 2473–2507.
3. Dunn LL, Suryo Rahmanto Y, Richardson DR (2007) Iron uptake and metabolism in the new millennium. Trends Cell Biol 17: 93–100.
4. Hentze MW, Muckenthaler MU, Andrews NC (2004) Balancing acts: molecular control of mammalian iron metabolism. Cell 117: 285–297.
5. Richardson DR, Baker E (1991) The release of iron and transferrin from the human melanoma cell. Biochim Biophys Acta 1091: 294–302.
6. Napier I, Ponka P, Richardson DR (2005) Iron trafficking in the mitochondrion: novel pathways revealed by disease. Blood 105: 1867–1874.
7. Richardson DR, Lane DJ, Becker EM, Huang ML, Whitnall M, et al. (2010) Mitochondrial iron trafficking and the integration of iron metabolism between the mitochondrion and cytosol. Proc Natl Acad Sci U S A 107: 10775–10782.
8. Arredondo M, Nunez MT (2005) Iron and copper metabolism. Mol Aspects Med 26: 313–327.
9. Leidgens S, Bullough KZ, Shi H, Li F, Shakoury-Elizeh M, et al. (2013) Each member of the poly-r(C)-binding protein 1 (PCBP) family exhibits iron chaperone activity toward ferritin. J Biol Chem 288: 17791–17802.
10. Cooper CE, Lynagh GR, Hoyes KP, Hider RC, Cammack R, et al. (1996) The relationship of intracellular iron chelation to the inhibition and regeneration of human ribonucleotide reductase. J Biol Chem 271: 20291–20299.
11. Lane DJ, Mills TM, Shafie NH, Merlot AM, Saleh Moussa R, et al. (2014) Expanding horizons in iron chelation and the treatment of cancer: Role of iron in the regulation of ER stress and the epithelial-mesenchymal transition. Biochim Biophys Acta 1845: 166–181.
12. Kalinowski DS, Richardson DR (2005) The evolution of iron chelators for the treatment of iron overload disease and cancer. Pharmacol Rev 57: 547–583.
13. Merlot AM, Kalinowski DS, Richardson DR (2013) Novel chelators for cancer treatment: where are we now? Antioxid Redox Signal 18: 973–1006.
14. Richardson DR, Kalinowski DS, Lau S, Jansson PJ, Lovejoy DB (2009) Cancer cell iron metabolism and the development of potent iron chelators as anti-tumour agents. Biochim Biophys Acta 1790: 702–717.
15. Bendova P, Mackova E, Haskova P, Vavrova A, Jirkovsky E, et al. (2010) Comparison of clinically used and experimental iron chelators for protection against oxidative stress-induced cellular injury. Chem Res Toxicol 23: 1105–1114.
16. Torti SV, Torti FM (2013) Iron and cancer: more ore to be mined. Nat Rev Cancer 13: 342–355.
17. Kolberg M, Strand KR, Graff P, Andersson KK (2004) Structure, function, and mechanism of ribonucleotide reductases. Biochim Biophys Acta 1699: 1–34.
18. Walker RA, Day SJ (1986) Transferrin receptor expression in non-malignant and malignant human breast tissue. J Pathol 148: 217–224.
19. Jiang XP, Elliott RL, Head JF (2010) Manipulation of iron transporter genes results in the suppression of human and mouse mammary adenocarcinomas. Anticancer Res 30: 759–765.
20. Pinnix ZK, Miller LD, Wang W, D'Agostino R, Jr., Kute T, et al. (2010) Ferroportin and iron regulation in breast cancer progression and prognosis. Sci Transl Med 2: 43ra56.
21. Le NT, Richardson DR (2002) The role of iron in cell cycle progression and the proliferation of neoplastic cells. Biochim Biophys Acta 1603: 31–46.
22. Whitnall M, Howard J, Ponka P, Richardson DR (2006) A class of iron chelators with a wide spectrum of potent antitumor activity that overcomes resistance to chemotherapeutics. Proc Natl Acad Sci U S A 103: 14901–14906.
23. Lovejoy DB, Sharp DM, Seebacher N, Obeidy P, Prichard T, et al. (2012) Novel second-generation di-2-pyridylketone thiosemicarbazones show synergism with standard chemotherapeutics and demonstrate potent activity against lung cancer xenografts after oral and intravenous administration in vivo. J Med Chem 55: 7230–7244.
24. Vitolo LMW, Hefter GT, Clare BW, Webb J (1990) Iron Chelators of the Pyridoxal Isonicotinoyl Hydrazone Class.2. Formation-Constants with Iron(Iii) and Iron(Ii). Inorganica Chimica Acta 170: 171–176.
25. Dubois JE, Fakhrayan H, Doucet JP, Chahine JME (1992) Kinetic and Thermodynamic Study of Complex-Formation between Iron(Ii) and Pyridoxal Isonicotinoylhydrazone and Other Synthetic Chelating-Agents. Inorganic Chemistry 31: 853–859.
26. Horackova M, Ponka P, Byczko Z (2000) The antioxidant effects of a novel iron chelator salicylaldehyde isonicotinoyl hydrazone in the prevention of H(2)O(2) injury in adult cardiomyocytes. Cardiovasc Res 47: 529–536.
27. Simunek T, Boer C, Bouwman RA, Vlasblom R, Versteilen AM, et al. (2005) SIH–a novel lipophilic iron chelator–protects H9c2 cardiomyoblasts from oxidative stress-induced mitochondrial injury and cell death. J Mol Cell Cardiol 39: 345–354.
28. Simunek T, Sterba M, Popelova O, Kaiserova H, Adamcova M, et al. (2008) Anthracycline toxicity to cardiomyocytes or cancer cells is differently affected by iron chelation with salicylaldehyde isonicotinoyl hydrazone. Br J Pharmacol 155: 138–148.
29. Berndt C, Kurz T, Selenius M, Fernandes AP, Edgren MR, et al. (2010) Chelation of lysosomal iron protects against ionizing radiation. Biochem J 432: 295–301.
30. Fillebeen C, Pantopoulos K (2010) Iron inhibits replication of infectious hepatitis C virus in permissive Huh7.5.1 cells. J Hepatol 53: 995–999.
31. Mackova E, Hruskova K, Bendova P, Vavrova A, Jansova H, et al. (2012) Methyl and ethyl ketone analogs of salicylaldehyde isonicotinoyl hydrazone: novel iron chelators with selective antiproliferative action. Chem Biol Interact 197: 69–79.
32. Klimtova I, Simunek T, Mazurova Y, Kaplanova J, Sterba M, et al. (2003) A study of potential toxic effects after repeated 10-week administration of a new iron chelator—salicylaldehyde isonicotinoyl hydrazone (SIH) to rabbits. Acta Medica (Hradec Kralove) 46: 163–170.
33. Hruskova K, Kovarikova P, Bendova P, Haskova P, Mackova E, et al. (2011) Synthesis and initial in vitro evaluations of novel antioxidant aroylhydrazone iron chelators with increased stability against plasma hydrolysis. Chem Res Toxicol 24: 290–302.
34. Richardson DR, Tran EH, Ponka P (1995) The potential of iron chelators of the pyridoxal isonicotinoyl hydrazone class as effective antiproliferative agents. Blood 86: 4295–4306.
35. Chaston TB, Lovejoy DB, Watts RN, Richardson DR (2003) Examination of the antiproliferative activity of iron chelators: multiple cellular targets and the different mechanism of action of triapine compared with desferrioxamine and the potent pyridoxal isonicotinoyl hydrazone analogue 311. Clin Cancer Res 9: 402–414.
36. Chaston TB, Richardson DR (2003) Redox chemistry and DNA interactions of the 2-pyridyl-carboxaldehyde isonicotinoyl hydrazone class of iron chelators: Implications for toxicity in the treatment of iron overload disease. J Biol Inorg Chem 8: 427–438.
37. Becker EM, Lovejoy DB, Greer JM, Watts R, Richardson DR (2003) Identification of the di-pyridyl ketone isonicotinoyl hydrazone (PKIH) analogues as potent iron chelators and anti-tumour agents. Br J Pharmacol 138: 819–830.
38. Richardson DR, Ponka P (1994) The iron metabolism of the human neuroblastoma cell: lack of relationship between the efficacy of iron chelation and the inhibition of DNA synthesis. J Lab Clin Med 124: 660–671.
39. Edward JT, Gauthier M, Chubb FL, Ponka P (1988) Synthesis of New Acylhydrazones as Iron-Chelating Compounds. Journal of Chemical and Engineering Data 33: 538–540.
40. Administration FaD (2001) Available: http://www.fda.gov/downloads/Drugs/GuidanceComplianceRegulatoryInformation/Guidances/UCM070107.pdf. Accessed 2014 September 15.
41. Kovarikova P, Mrkvickova Z, Klimes J (2008) Investigation of the stability of aromatic hydrazones in plasma and related biological material. J Pharm Biomed Anal 47: 360–370.
42. Esposito BP, Epsztejn S, Breuer W, Cabantchik ZI (2002) A review of fluorescence methods for assessing labile iron in cells and biological fluids. Anal Biochem 304: 1–18.
43. Glickstein H, El RB, Link G, Breuer W, Konijn AM, et al. (2006) Action of chelators in iron-loaded cardiac cells: Accessibility to intracellular labile iron and functional consequences. Blood 108: 3195–3203.
44. Richardson DR, Milnes K (1997) The potential of iron chelators of the pyridoxal isonicotinoyl hydrazone class as effective antiproliferative agents II: the mechanism of action of ligands derived from salicylaldehyde benzoyl hydrazone and 2-hydroxy-1-naphthylaldehyde benzoyl hydrazone. Blood 89: 3025–3038.
45. Baker E, Richardson D, Gross S, Ponka P (1992) Evaluation of the iron chelation potential of hydrazones of pyridoxal, salicylaldehyde and 2-hydroxy-1-naphthylaldehyde using the hepatocyte in culture. Hepatology 15: 492–501.
46. Richardson DR, Sharpe PC, Lovejoy DB, Senaratne D, Kalinowski DS, et al. (2006) Dipyridyl thiosemicarbazone chelators with potent and selective antitumor activity form iron complexes with redox activity. J Med Chem 49: 6510–6521.
47. Becker E, Richardson DR (1999) Development of novel aroylhydrazone ligands for iron chelation therapy: 2-pyridylcarboxaldehyde isonicotinoyl hydrazone analogs. J Lab Clin Med 134: 510–521.

48. Mladenka P, Kalinowski DS, Haskova P, Bobrovova Z, Hrdina R, et al. (2009) The novel iron chelator, 2-pyridylcarboxaldehyde 2-thiophenecarboxyl hydrazone, reduces catecholamine-mediated myocardial toxicity. Chem Res Toxicol 22: 208–217.
49. Chaston TB, Watts RN, Yuan J, Richardson DR (2004) Potent antitumor activity of novel iron chelators derived from di-2-pyridylketone isonicotinoyl hydrazone involves fenton-derived free radical generation. Clin Cancer Res 10: 7365–7374.
50. Repetto G, del Peso A, Zurita JL (2008) Neutral red uptake assay for the estimation of cell viability/cytotoxicity. Nat Protoc 3: 1125–1131.
51. Ghose AK, Crippen GM (1987) Atomic physicochemical parameters for three-dimensional-structure-directed quantitative structure-activity relationships. 2. Modeling dispersive and hydrophobic interactions. J Chem Inf Comput Sci 27: 21–35.
52. Viswanadhan VN, Ghose AK, Revankar GR, Robins RK (1989) Atomic physicochemical parameters for three dimensional structure directed quantitative structure-activity relationships. 4. Additional parameters for hydrophobic and dispersive interactions and their application for an automated superposition of certain naturally occurring nucleoside antibiotics. J Chem Inf Comput Sci 29: 163–172.
53. Broto P, Moreau G, Vandycke C (1984) Molecular Structures: Perception, Autocorrelation Descriptor and SAR Studies. System of Atomic Contributions for the Calculation of the n-Octanol/Water Partition Coefficients. Eur J Med Chem Chim Theor 19: 71–78.
54. Zhang XZ, Li M, Cui Y, Zhao J, Cui ZG, et al. (2012) Electrochemical Behavior of Calcein and the Interaction Between Calcein and DNA. Electroanalysis 24: 1878–1886.
55. Yuan J, Lovejoy DB, Richardson DR (2004) Novel di-2-pyridyl-derived iron chelators with marked and selective antitumor activity: in vitro and in vivo assessment. Blood 104: 1450–1458.
56. Gutteridge JM, Richmond R, Halliwell B (1979) Inhibition of the iron-catalysed formation of hydroxyl radicals from superoxide and of lipid peroxidation by desferrioxamine. Biochem J 184: 469–472.
57. Ponka P, Borova J, Neuwirt J, Fuchs O (1979) Mobilization of iron from reticulocytes. Identification of pyridoxal isonicotinoyl hydrazone as a new iron chelating agent. FEBS Lett 97: 317–321.
58. Kalia J, Raines RT (2008) Hydrolytic stability of hydrazones and oximes. Angew Chem Int Ed Engl 47: 7523–7526.
59. Kitazawa M, Iwasaki K (1999) Reduction of ultraviolet light-induced oxidative stress by amino acid-based iron chelators. Biochim Biophys Acta 1473: 400–408.
60. Bernhardt PV, Wilson GJ, Sharpe PC, Kalinowski DS, Richardson DR (2008) Tuning the antiproliferative activity of biologically active iron chelators: characterization of the coordination chemistry and biological efficacy of 2-acetylpyridine and 2-benzoylpyridine hydrazone ligands. J Biol Inorg Chem 13: 107–119.
61. Sies H (1993) Strategies of antioxidant defense. Eur J Biochem 215: 213–219.
62. Richardson D, Vitolo LW, Baker E, Webb J (1989) Pyridoxal isonicotinoyl hydrazone and analogues. Study of their stability in acidic, neutral and basic aqueous solutions by ultraviolet-visible spectrophotometry. Biol Met 2: 69–76.

Celastrol Stimulates Hypoxia-Inducible Factor-1 Activity in Tumor Cells by Initiating the ROS/Akt/p70S6K Signaling Pathway and Enhancing Hypoxia-Inducible Factor-1α Protein Synthesis

Xiaoxi Han[1,9], Shengkun Sun[2,9], Ming Zhao[3], Xiang Cheng[3], Guozhu Chen[3], Song Lin[3], Yifu Guan[1]*, Xiaodan Yu[3]*

1 Department of Biochemistry and Molecular Biology, China Medical University, Shenyang, China, 2 Department of Urology, The General Hospital of PLA, Beijing, China, 3 Department of Cognitive Science, Institute of Basic Medical Sciences, Cognitive and Mental Health Research Center, Beijing, China

Abstract

Celastrol, a tripterine derived from the traditional Chinese medicine plant *Tripterygium wilfordii* Hook F. ("Thunder of God Vine"), has been reported to have multiple effects, such as anti-inflammation, suppression of tumor angiogenesis, inhibition of tumor growth, induction of apoptosis and protection of cells against human neurodegenerative diseases. However, the mechanisms that underlie these functions are not well defined. In this study, we reported for the first time that Celastrol could induce HIF-1α protein accumulation in multiple cancer cell lines in an oxygen-independent manner and that the enhanced HIF-1α protein entered the nucleus and promoted the transcription of the HIF-1 target genes VEGF and Glut-1. Celastrol did not influence HIF-1α transcription. Instead, Celastrol induced the accumulation of the HIF-1α protein by inducing ROS and activating Akt/p70S6K signaling to promote HIF-1α translation. In addition, we found that the activation of Akt by Celastrol was transient. With increased exposure time, inhibition of Hsp90 chaperone function by Celastrol led to the subsequent depletion of the Akt protein and thus to the suppression of Akt activity. Moreover, in HepG2 cells, the accumulation of HIF-1α increased the expression of BNIP3, which induced autophagy. However, HIF-1α and BNIP3 did not influence the cytotoxicity of Celastrol because the main mechanism by which Celastrol kills cancer cells is through stimulating ROS-mediated JNK activation and inducing apoptosis. Furthermore, our data showed that the dose required for Celastrol to induce HIF-1α protein accumulation and enhance HIF-1α transcriptional activation was below its cytotoxic threshold. A cytotoxic dose of Celastrol for cancer cells did not display cytotoxicity in LO2 normal human liver cells, which indicated that the novel functions of Celastrol in regulating HIF-1 signaling and inducing autophagy might be used in new applications, such as in anti-inflammation and protection of cells against human neurodegenerative diseases. Future studies regarding these applications are required.

Editor: Kasper Rouschop, Maastricht University, Netherlands

Funding: This work was supported in part by Grant 2012CB518200 from the "973" Program of the Ministry of Science and Technology of China (to X. Yu) and by Grants 31371434 (to X. Yu) from the National Natural Science Foundation of China. The funders had no role in study design, data collection and analysis, decision to publish, or preparation of the manuscript.

Competing Interests: The authors have declared that no competing interests exist.

* Email: yfguan@mail.cmu.edu.cn (YG); yuxd@bmi.ac.cn (XY)

[9] These authors contributed equally to this work.

Introduction

Hypoxia-inducible factor 1 (HIF-1) is the key regulator of the hypoxia response. HIF-1 is a heterodimer composed of HIF-1α and HIF-1β [1]. Unlike the constitutively expressed HIF-1β, HIF-1α is induced by hypoxia, and this oxygen-sensitive induction occurs by decreasing protein degradation instead of enhancing mRNA expression. In normoxia, the HIF-1α protein is barely detectable because the Von Hippel Lindau gene (VHL) mediates its ubiquitination and rapid degradation through the proline hydroxylases (PHDs) and the proteasome pathway. The activities of PHDs are dependent on oxygen, and the binding of pVHL to HIF-1α requires the PHD-mediated modification of the oxygen-dependent degradation domain (ODD) of the protein. Therefore, HIF-1α cannot be hydroxylated and degraded during hypoxia [2]. In hypoxic circumstances, HIF-1α accumulates, translocates to the nucleus and binds to HIF-1β to form the active transcription factor HIF-1. The HIF-1 complex then binds to hypoxia response element (HRE) sequences in the promoters of HIF-1 target genes to initiate gene expression [1]. Many genes regulated by HIF-1α are involved in glycolysis, glucose metabolism, mitochondrial function, angiogenesis, cell survival, apoptosis and resistance to oxidative stress. In this regard, HIF-1 activation may play different roles in triggering cellular protection and metabolic alterations because of the consequences of oxygen deprivation or apoptosis in the presence of different environmental factors.

Celastrol, a triterpenoid from the Celastracae family that is extracted from the plant *Tripterygium Wilfordii* [3], has been reported to have multiple biological functions. In addition to treating autoimmune and neurodegenerative diseases by its anti-oxidative and anti-inflammatory effects [4,5], Celastrol is frequently investigated for its potential anti-cancer activities *in vitro* and *in vivo*, including inhibiting tumor cell proliferation, inducing apoptosis in different types of cancer cells [6–9] and synergistically enhancing the cytotoxicity of radiotherapy and some chemotherapeutic agents [10–13]. Although previous studies have reported that Celastrol has the potential to inhibit HIF-1α mRNA transcription and suppress hypoxia-induced angiogenesis and tumor metastasis [14,15], in this study, we found that a short amount of time exposure of Celastrol did not affect the HIF-1α mRNA levels. Instead, we found that Celastrol could induce HIF-1α protein accumulation in multiple cancer cell lines in an oxygen-independent manner and that the enhanced HIF-1α protein entered the nucleus and promoted the transcription of the HIF-1 target genes VEGF and Glut-1. Celastrol induced the accumulation of the HIF-1α protein by inducing ROS, which initiates the activation of Akt/p70S6K signaling to promote HIF-1α translation. These new data indicate that the full effect and function of Celastrol in regulating HIF-1 signaling may require further evaluation.

Materials and Methods

Cell culture

The human hepatocarcinoma cell line HepG2, the cervical carcinoma cell line HeLa, the breast cancer cell line MCF-7, the prostate cancer cell line PC-3 and the non-small cell lung cancer cell line H1299 were obtained from the American Tissue Culture Collection (Manassas, VA, USA). The normal liver LO2 cell line was kindly offered by Dr. Yan Wang (Beijing Institute of Basic Medical Sciences). The cells were cultured with Dulbecco's modified Eagle medium (Gibco, Grand Island, NY, USA) containing 10% fetal bovine serum (FBS, HyClone, Logan, UT, USA). For the hypoxia experiments, the cells were cultured in a hypoxia chamber with 3% O_2 and 5% CO_2 (with the balance being N_2). Alternatively, to mimic hypoxia, 100 μM Cobalt chloride ($CoCl_2$) was added to the culture medium [16], and the cells were cultured for the indicated hours.

Reagents and antibodies

Celastrol was purchased from Calbiochem (San Diego, CA, USA) and dissolved in DMSO. Cobalt chloride, N-acetylcysteine (NAC) and cycloheximide (CHX) were purchased from Sigma (St Louis, MO, USA). LY294002 was purchased from Alexis (San Diego, CA, USA). The antibodies used were as follows: anti-HIF-1α and anti-HIF-1β (BD Transduction Laboratories, San Jose, CA, USA); anti-Raf, anti-Akt, anti-p-Akt (S473), anti-p-p70S6K (T389) and anti-PARP (Cell Signaling, Beverly, MA, USA); anti-BNIP3, anti-p53 and anti-p21 (Santa Cruz, Dallas, TX, USA); and anti-Bcl2, anti Bcl-xL and anti-β-actin (Calbiochem, San Diego, CA, USA). The dual-Luciferase reporter assay system was purchased from Promega (Madison, WI, USA).

Cell viability assay

Cell viability was analyzed using the MTT assay. The cells were seeded in a 96-well plate at a density of 1×10^4 and were treated with the indicated concentrations of Celastrol for 6 or 24 h. After each time point, 20 μl MTT (0.5 mg/ml) was added to each well, and the cells were cultured for another 4 h. Then, the medium was removed and 100 μl DMSO was added. The absorbance was read using a microplate reader (Tecan Infinite F50).

Cell cycle assay

HepG2 cells were collected after treatment with Celastrol for 24 h and then washed with PBS twice. The cells were fixed with 70% ethanol/PBS at −20°C overnight. After washing with PBS, the cells were treated with RNase for 30 min at 37°C, and the cell cycle distribution was analyzed by fluorescence-activated cell sorting (FACS) of propidium iodide-stained cells.

Isolation of nuclei

Nuclei were isolated using a Nuclei Isolation Kit (Applygen Technologies Beijing, China) according to the manufacturer's suggestions. Briefly, cells were collected by trypsinization and resuspended with the cytosol extraction reagent provided in the kit. The cells were homogenized using a grinder until less than 5% of the cells were intact, and the homogenate was centrifuged at $1000 \times g$ for 10 min at 4°C. The supernatant and pellet were retained as the cytosolic fraction and nuclear fraction, respectively. The nuclei were washed twice with the nuclear extraction reagent provided in the kit, centrifuged at $4,000 \times g$ for 5 min and then lysed with Laemmli buffer.

Western blotting

For western blotting, the cells were washed with PBS and suspended in Laemmli Buffer (Bio-Rad Laboratories, Hercules, CA, USA). The protein concentration was quantified using a BCA Protein Assay Kit (Pierce, Rockford, IL, USA), and the proteins were separated by SDS-polyacrylamide gel electrophoresis (SDS-PAGE), with 50–100 μg of protein loaded into each lane, and then transferred to a polyvinylidene difluoride membrane (Bio-Rad). The membrane was blocked in 5% skim milk, blotted with primary antibodies for 12–15 h at 4°C and then incubated with a horseradish peroxidase-conjugated secondary antibody for 1 h at room temperature. The proteins were detected using a Super Enhanced Chemiluminescence Detection Kit (Applygen Technologies, Beijing, China).

Transfection and luciferase assays

HepG2 cells were co-transfected with pGL3-HRE-Luc and pRL-CMV plasmids using Mega Tran 1.0 (OriGene, MD, USA) according to the suggested protocol. Twenty-four hours after transfection, the cells were treated with Celastrol for 6 h, and the luciferase activity was then measured using the Dual-Luciferase Reporter Assay System according to the manufacturer's instructions.

Real-time PCR

Total RNA was isolated from HepG2 cells using TRIzol Reagent (Invitrogen, Carlsbad, CA, USA) following a standard protocol. RNA was reverse transcribed into cDNA using the RevertAid First Strand cDNA Synthesis Kit (Fermentas, Glen Burnie, MD, USA) according to the manufacturer's instructions, and the resulting cDNA was used for qRT-PCR reactions with SYBR Green PCR Master Mix (Fermentas) and the Stratagene Mx3000P QPCR System. The primers used for amplification were as follows:

VEGF sense primer, 5′-ATGAACTTTCTGCTGTCTTG-3′; VEGF antisense primer 5′- TGAACTTCACCACTTCGT −3′; Glut-1 sense primer, 5′- GCTGTCTGGCATCAACGCTGTCTT −3′; Glut-1 antisense primer, 5′-GCCTGCTCGCTCCACCACAA −3′;

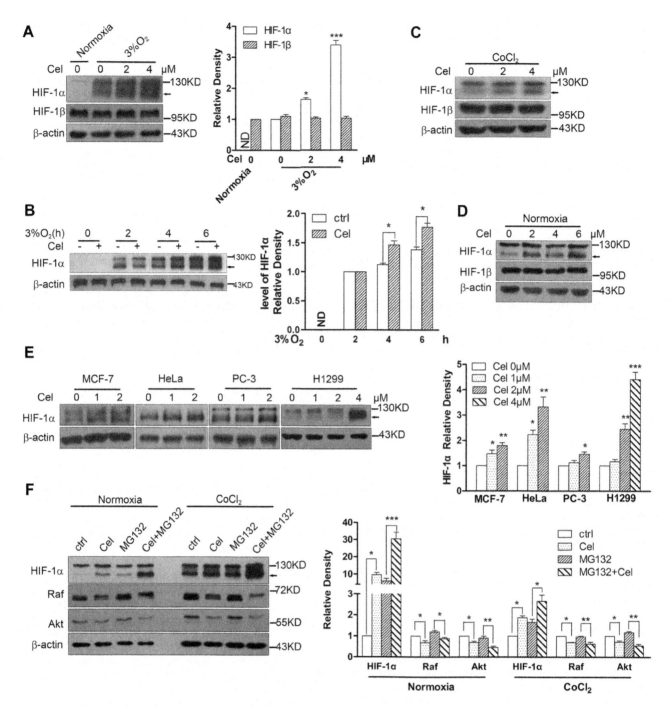

Figure 1. Celastrol increases the protein level of HIF-1α. 1a. Celastrol dose-dependently enhanced HIF-1α expression under hypoxia. HepG2 cells were cultured in either normoxia or 3% hypoxia and treated with the indicated doses of Celastrol for 6 h. Western blotting was used to detect the expression of HIF-1α and HIF-1β, and β-actin was used as a loading control; an arrow shows the position of HIF-1α. The histogram results are representative of the mean ± SD of three independent experiments. 1b. Celastrol time-dependently enhanced HIF-1α expression under hypoxia. HepG2 cells were cultured with 4 μM Celastrol for the indicated time in hypoxia. 1c. Celastrol enhanced HIF-1α expression in HepG2 cells under mimetic hypoxia induced by 100 μM $CoCl_2$ and treated for 6 h. 1d. Celastrol dose-dependently enhanced HIF-1α expression under normoxia. HepG2 cells were treated with the indicated doses of Celastrol under normoxia for 6 h, and 100 μg of total protein was used for western blotting to detect HIF-1 proteins with a long exposure. 1e. Celastrol enhanced HIF-1α expression in multiple cell lines. MCF-7, HeLa, PC-3 and H1299 cells were treated with the indicated doses of Celastrol for 12 h under 3% hypoxia, and western blotting was used to detect the HIF-1 proteins. 1f. Celastrol decreased the levels of other Hsp90 client proteins but increased that of HIF-1α. HepG2 cells were treated with normal medium, 4 μM Celastrol for 6 h, 5 μM MG132 for 6 h or pretreated with MG132 for 1 h then treated with Celastrol for 6 h. Protein expression was determined by western blotting with the corresponding antibodies.

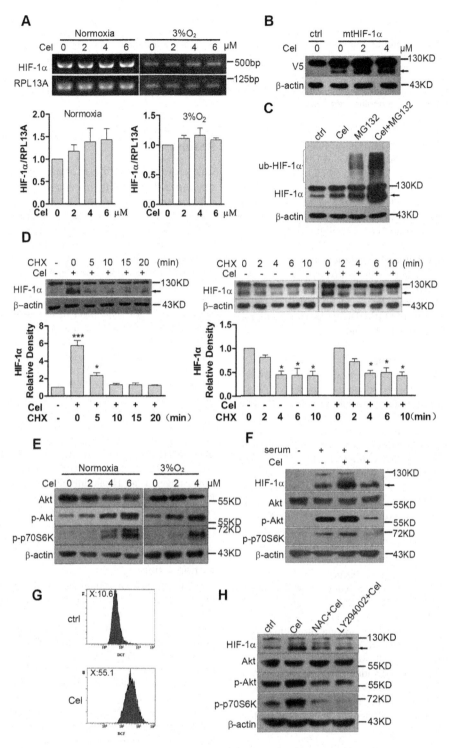

Figure 2. Celastrol increases the HIF-1α protein level by enhancing its translation. 2a. Celastrol did not affect HIF-1α transcription. After treatment with different concentrations of Celastrol for 6 h, total RNA was extracted, and the mRNA levels of HIF-1α and RPL13A were determined by RT-PCR. The relative expression of HIF-1α was normalized to that of RPL13A. The values are presented as the means ± SD of three independent experiments. 2b. Celastrol enhanced the expression of the HIF-1α P402A/P564A mutant. HeLa cells were seeded in 6-well plates and transiently transfected with either pcDNA-V5 empty vector (ctrl) or pcDNA3-P402A/P564A-HIF-1α-V5 (mtHIF-1). Twenty-four hours later, the cells were treated with 1–2 μM Celastrol for 6 h under normoxia. Mutant HIF-1α expression was analyzed by western blotting with the anti-V5 antibody. 2c. Celastrol did not affect HIF-1α ubiquitination. HepG2 cells were treated separately with 4 μM Celastrol, 10 μM MG132 or Celastrol plus MG132 for 4 h under normoxia, and the ub-HIF-1α protein level was determined by western blotting using the anti-HIF-1α antibody. 2d. The effect of the protein synthesis inhibitor CHX on Celastrol-induced HIF-1α accumulation. HepG2 cells were treated with or without 4 μM Celastrol for 6 h. Then, 10 μM CHX was added to the culture medium, and the cells were collected at the indicated times (left). HepG2 cells were cultured in medium containing 100 μM $CoCl_2$ with or without 4 μM Celastrol for 4 h, then 10 μM CHX was added, and the cells were collected at the indicated times (right). The HIF-1α protein level was analyzed by western blot analysis. 2e. Celastrol induced AKT/p70S6K activation under normoxia and hypoxia. HepG2 cells were

challenged with the indicated doses of Celastrol for 6 h under normoxia or hypoxia. The protein levels were analyzed by western blotting with the corresponding antibodies. 2f. Celastrol induced AKT/p70S6K activation under serum starvation. HepG2 cells were cultured in serum-free medium for 24 h. Then, 10% FBS, 4 μM Celastrol or both were added, and the cells were cultured for another 6 h. The protein expression was analyzed by western blotting with the corresponding antibodies. 2 g. Celastrol induced the accumulation of ROS. HepG2 cells were treated with 4 μM Celastrol for 12 h under normoxia. The levels of ROS were measured by DCFH-DA staining and subsequently assayed by flow cytometry. 2 h. The effect of Celastrol-induced HIF-1α accumulation depends on ROS-mediated AKT activation. HepG2 cells were pretreated with 5 mM NAC or 10 μM LY294002 for 1 h. Then, 4 μM Celastrol was added to the culture medium, and the cells were cultured for another 6 h. The protein expression was determined by western blotting with the corresponding antibodies.

RPL13A sense primer 5′- CGCTCTGGACCGTCTCAA −3′; RPL13A antisense primer 5′- AGATAGGCAAACTTTCTTG-TAGGC −3′.

Standard curve reactions and melt curves were routinely run to validate the primer pairs and PCR reactions. The expression of the genes of interest was normalized and analyzed using RPL13A as an internal reference according to the Pfaffl method [17].

Measurement of intracellular ROS generation

Intracellular ROS generation was measured by flow cytometry with a 2′,7′-dichlorodihydrofluorescein diacetate (DCFH-DA) probe (Applygen Technologies, Beijing, China). Untreated or treated cells were stained with 20 μM DCFH-DA for 30 min in the dark and subsequently assayed by flow cytometry.

Immunofluorescence microscopy

Cells cultured on glass coverslips were treated with Celastrol for the indicated time, fixed with 4% paraformaldehyde in PBS for 10 min at room temperature and permeabilized with PBS plus 0.5% Triton X-100 for 10 min. The cells were incubated with PBS containing 1% bovine serum albumin for 30 min at room temperature and then washed three times with PBS. The cells were labeled with different primary antibodies for 1 h at room temperature or overnight at 4°C, followed by a 1-h incubation with FITC-conjugated secondary antibodies. DNA was counterstained with DAPI or Hoechst 33258, and the coverslips were examined by fluorescence microscopy at 1000×magnification under an immersion oil lens with a Zeiss 510 META microscope.

Small interfering RNA

The siRNAs for HIF1α (target sequence of 5′-AGTTAT-GATTGTGAAGTTA-3′) and BNIP3 (target sequence of 5′-TTCATGACGCTCGTGTTCCT-3′) and a control siRNA (target sequence of 5′-UUCUCCGAACGUGUCACGU-3′) were synthesized by Shanghai GeneChem (Shanghai, China), and siRNA knockdown was performed according to the manufacturer's protocol. Aliquots of 2×10^5 cells were plated in 6-well plates, incubated for 24 h and transfected with 100 nM target siRNA or control siRNA using Entranster-R (Engreen Biosystem, Beijing, China). After 24 h, the cells were treated with Celastrol for another 24 h, and the cells were collected and analyzed by western blotting.

Statistical analysis

The results are presented as the means ± SD of at least three separate experiments. The differences between groups were evaluated by Student's t-test or one-way analysis of variance (ANOVA) followed by Dunnett's test for multiple comparisons. Analyses were done with GraphPad Prism software (Graphpad; La Jolla, CA, USA). The significance level was defined as * $P<0.05$, ** $P<0.01$, and *** $P<0.001$.

Results

Celastrol increases the protein level of HIF-1α in an oxygen-independent manner

Unexpectedly, when we used Celastrol to treat HepG2 cells under 3% hypoxia for 6 h, we noticed that the protein level of HIF-1α increased in a time- and dose-dependent manner, but Celastrol did not affect the protein level of HIF-1β (Figs. 1a, 1b). Additionally, when using cobalt chloride ($CoCl_2$) to mimic hypoxia, Celastrol also enhanced HIF-1α accumulation (Fig. 1c). More importantly, when the cells were treated with 2–6 μM Celastrol under normoxia, enhanced HIF-1α expression still occurred (Fig. 1d). The effect of Celastrol in enhancing HIF-1α expression was not cell-type specific because we also detected the same changes in human mammary carcinoma MCF-7 cells, cervical cancer HeLa cells, prostate cancer PC-3 cells and non-small cell lung cancer H1299 cells (Fig. 1e). These results supported the finding that Celastrol increased HIF-1α expression in an oxygen-independent manner. In addition, although the activation of the p53 gene has been reported to promote proteasomal degradation of the HIF-1α protein [18], the influence of p53 on this process was excluded because Celastrol could increase HIF-1α protein in MCF-7 cells, which have wild type p53, and in PC-3 and H1299 cells, which are p53 null. Interestingly, as an Hsp90 inhibitor, Celastrol could decrease the levels of Hsp90 client proteins, such as Raf and Akt from HepG2 cells; however, it increased the level of HIF-1α protein, though HIF-1α is also an Hsp90 client protein (Fig. 1f).

Celastrol increases the HIF-1α protein level by enhancing its translation

Because it is known that the enhanced expression of HIF-1α under hypoxia is regulated at the protein level rather than at the mRNA level, we also excluded the possibility that Celastrol increased HIF-1α protein levels by promoting HIF-1α transcription, as Celastrol did not affect the mRNA expression of HIF-1α in HepG2 cells under normoxia or hypoxia (Fig. 2a). The most common mechanism for hypoxia-induced HIF-1α protein accumulation is mediated by prolyl hydroxylases (PHDs) that control HIF-1α by maintaining it at low levels under normal conditions; under hypoxia, PHDs activity drops and HIF-1α accumulates [2]. To investigate whether Celastrol increased the HIF-1α protein level by affecting PHDs activity, we transiently transfected the pcDNA3-V5 and pcDNA-P402/564A-HIF-1α-V5 vectors into HeLa cells separately. Because PHDs recognize the P402/564 sites of the HIF-1α protein, those sites were mutated to make the mutant HIF-1α protein resistant to PHD-VHL mediated degradation; therefore, the HIF-1α protein could be easily detected under normoxia. We then treated the cells with Celastrol, and the result showed that Celastrol still induced the accumulation of the mutated HIF-1α protein (Fig. 2b), which excluded the possibility that Celastrol enhanced HIF-1α expression by inhibiting PHDs. Previously, Celastrol has been identified as a proteasome inhibitor [19,20]; therefore, we wondered whether Celastrol increased HIF-

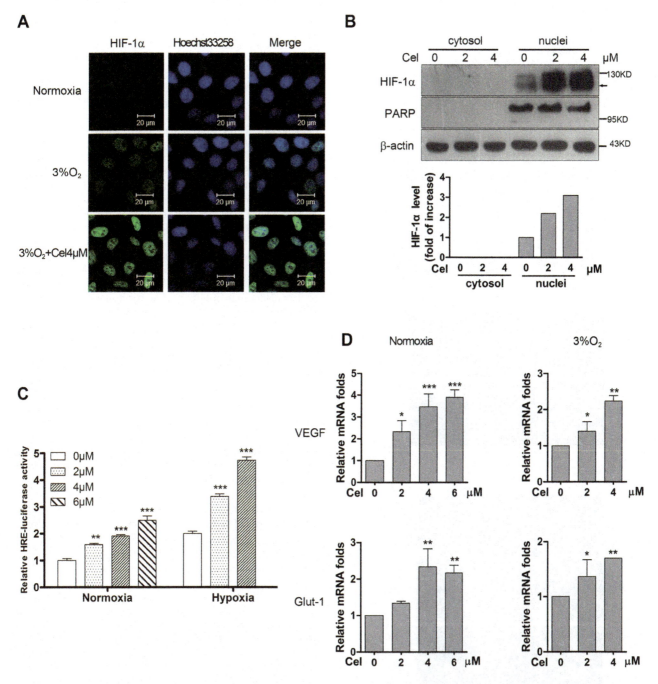

Figure 3. Celastrol promotes the hypoxia-induced accumulation of the HIF-1α protein in the nucleus, which increases the transcriptional activity of HIF-1α target genes. 3a. Celastrol enhances HIF-1α protein expression, which was localized in the nucleus. HepG2 cells were cultured in medium with or without 4 μM Celastrol for 6 h under normoxia or hypoxia. The subcellular localization of HIF-1α was determined by immunofluorescent staining using the anti-HIF-1α antibody, and the nucleus was immunolabeled with Hoechst 33258. 3b. HepG2 cells were treated with the indicated dose of Celastrol for 6 h, protein was extracted from the nucleus and cytosol, and the protein expression levels were revealed by western blot analysis. PARP served as the nuclear protein loading control. 3c. Celastrol promotes HIF-1α transcriptional activation activity. After transient transfection with the HRE-luciferase reporter plasmids for 24 h, HepG2 cells were challenged with the indicated doses of Celastrol in normoxia or hypoxia for another 6 h. Then, the HIF-1α transcriptional activation activity was analyzed by luciferase assay. The values are presented as the means ± SD of three independent experiments. 3d. Celastrol promotes the transcription of the HIF-1α target genes VEGF and Glut-1. The VEGF and Glut-1 mRNA levels were evaluated by real-time PCR. The values are presented as the means±SD of three independent experiments.

1α protein levels by enhancing its ubiquitination and blocking its degradation. We thus treated HepG2 cells separately with Celastrol, the proteasome inhibitor MG132 or Celastrol plus MG132 and detected the ubiquitination of HIF-1α by western blotting. The result showed that, unlike MG132, Celastrol alone did not increase the ubiquitination of HIF-1α, but Celastrol showed a remarkable, synergistic effect in enhancing MG132-induced ubiquitination of HIF-1α (Fig. 2c). These results excluded

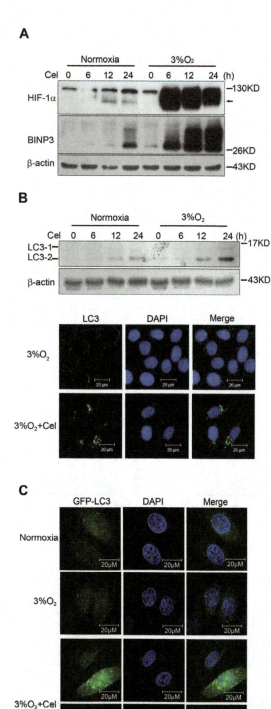

Figure 4. Celastrol-mediated HIF-1α accumulation stimulates BNIP3 expression and induces mitochondrial autophagy. 4a. Celastrol time-dependently enhanced the expression of HIF-1α and BNIP3. HepG2 cells were treated with 4 μM Celastrol in normoxia or hypoxia for the indicated times. The protein levels were determined by western blot analysis. 4b. Celastrol enhances LC3-II expression and the formation of LC-3 aggregates. HepG2 cells were treated with 4 μM Celastrol under normoxia or hypoxia for the indicated times. The LC3I/II protein levels were determined by western blot analysis (upper), and the LC3 aggregates were stained by indirect immunofluorescence and observed by confocal microscopy. 4c. Celastrol induced autophagy. HepG2 cells were transiently transfected with GFP-LC3, and 24 h later, the cells were treated with 4 μM Celastrol for another 24 h. GFP fluorescence was then observed by confocal microscopy.

the possibility that Celastrol induced HIF-1α accumulation by promoting HIF-1α mRNA transcription or by inhibiting HIF-1α protein degradation. In addition, HIF-1α can be regulated at the translational level. Previous studies have reported that some types of stimulation, such as cytokines or serum, could upregulate the HIF-1α protein level via the activation of Akt/mTOR and inhibition of GSK3, which led to increased HIF-1α translation [21,22]. To evaluate whether Celastrol enhanced HIF-1α protein levels via this mechanism, we first treated cells with or without Celastrol under normoxia and then added the protein synthesis inhibitor cycloheximide (CHX). The results showed that Celastrol-induced HIF-1α accumulation indeed required new protein synthesis because CHX could completely block this effect (Fig. 2d). Then, HepG2 cells were treated with 100 μM $CoCl_2$ with or without 4 μM Celastrol for 4 h, and CHX was added to observe the degradation rate of HIF-1α. The result showed that Celastrol did not affect the degradation rate of the HIF-1α protein (Fig. 2d). Then, we treated HepG2 cells with Celastrol and confirmed that Celastrol dose-dependently induced the activation of Akt/p70S6K under normoxic and hypoxic conditions (Fig. 2e). In addition, we observed that Celastrol could induce the activation of Akt/p70S6K under serum starvation, which was also coincident with HIF-1α accumulation (Fig. 2f). Moreover, Celastrol induced ROS production (Fig. 2 g), which was coincident with the Celastrol-induced activation of Akt/p70S6K, and HIF-1α accumulation could be blocked by the PI3K inhibitor LY294002 and ROS scavenger NAC (Fig. 2 h). These results indicate that Celastrol may indirectly activate Akt by inducing ROS, and the activation of Akt further promotes HIF-1α translation.

Celastrol promotes the hypoxia-induced, nuclear accumulation of the HIF-1α protein and increases the transcriptional activity of HIF-1α-target genes

The effect of Celastrol in enhancing HIF-1α expression led us to further determine whether the enhanced expression of HIF-1α represented HIF-1 signal activation. First, we detected the cellular localization of the HIF-1α protein using immunofluorescent staining. As in Fig. 3a, immunofluorescent staining illustrated that the exposure of HepG2 cells to 3% hypoxia induced the HIF-1α protein to accumulate in the nucleus, and Celastrol-treated cells showed an obvious increase in HIF-1α protein levels in the nucleus. This result was further confirmed by detecting HIF-1α by western blotting in the cytosolic and nuclear fractions. As Fig. 3b shows, Celastrol-induced the nuclear localization of nearly all of the HIF-1α present in the cell, indicating that Celastrol did induce the activation of HIF-1α. This conclusion was reconfirmed using an HRE-luciferase assay to detect the transcriptional activation activity of HIF-1α and using real-time PCR to evaluate the transcriptional activity of its target genes, such as VEGF and Glut-1. The results showed that Celastrol oxygen-independently but dose-dependently enhanced the transcriptional activation activity of HIF-1α (Fig. 3c) and promoted the transcription of its target genes (Fig. 3d).

Celastrol-mediated HIF-1α accumulation stimulates BNIP3 expression and induces autophagy

Previously, many studies have reported that HIF-1α induces the expression of Bcl2/adenovirus E1B 19 kD-interacting protein 3

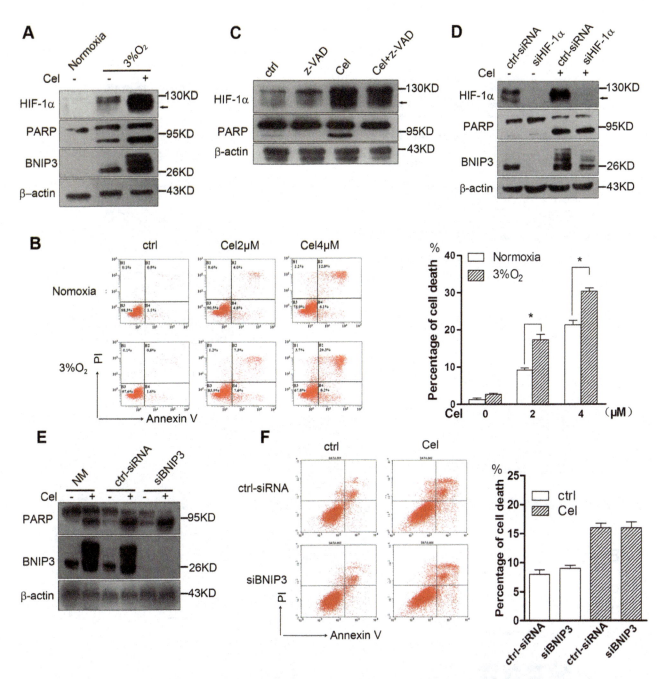

Figure 5. Knockdown of HIF-1α or BNIP3 did not influence Celastrol-induced cell apoptosis under hypoxia. 5a. Celastrol enhanced the HIF-1α and BNIP3 expression that was accompanied by increased PARP cleavage under hypoxia. HepG2 cells were cultured under normoxia or hypoxia with or without 4 μM Celastrol for 24 h. Western blotting was used to detect protein expression. 5b. The cytotoxicity of Celastrol was enhanced under hypoxia. HepG2 cells were cultured under normoxia or hypoxia with or without 2–4 μM Celastrol for 24 h. The cells were then stained with Annexin-V/PI and analyzed by flow cytometry. The data are presented as the mean values obtained from three independent experiments. 5c. Z-VAD blocked Celastrol-induced PARP cleavage but did not affect HIF-1α accumulation. HepG2 cells were pre-treated with 10 μM zVAD for 1 h then exposed to 4 μM Celastrol for another 6 h. The proteins were detected by western blot analysis. 5d. Knockdown of HIF-1α did not affect Celastrol-induced PARP cleavage. HepG2 cells were transfected with a non-silencing siRNA or HIF-1α siRNA for 24 h, and the cells were then treated with 4 μM Celastrol for 24 h. The proteins were detected by western blot analysis. 5e, 5f. Knockdown of BNIP3 did not affect Celastrol-induced cell death. HepG2 cells were transfected with non-silencing siRNA or BNIP3 siRNA for 24 h, and the cells were then treated with 4 μM Celastrol for 24 h. Cell death was measured by Annexin-V/PI staining and flow cytometry, and the proteins were detected by western blotting.

(BNIP3), which triggers selective mitochondrial autophagy [23,24]. Therefore, we analyzed the influence of Celastrol-induced HIF-1α accumulation on BNIP3 expression. Western blotting demonstrated that Celastrol time-dependently enhanced the protein level of BNIP3, which was coincident with enhanced HIF-1α (Fig. 4a). The microtubule-associated protein 1 light chain 3 (LC3) has been used as a marker for autophagy because, upon induction of autophagy, some LC3-I is converted into LC3-II. We

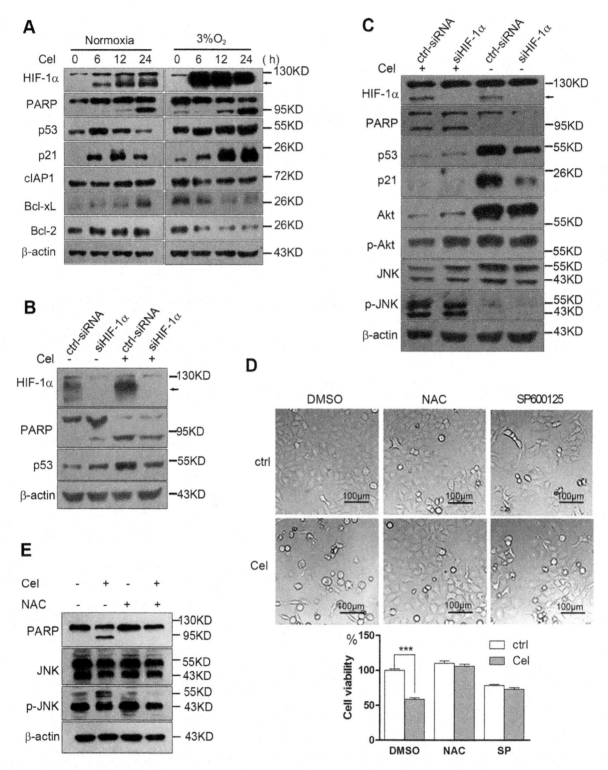

Figure 6. Celastrol kills HepG2 cells via ROS-mediated JNK activation. 6a. Celastrol transiently activates p53 under normoxia but persistently activates p53 under hypoxia. HepG2 cells were cultured in normoxia or hypoxia with or without 4 μM Celastrol for the indicated times. The proteins were detected by western blotting. 6b. The effect of HIF1α knockdown on p53 expression under hypoxia. HepG2 cells were transfected with control or HIF1α siRNA for 24 h and then treated with or without 4 μM Celastrol under hypoxia for 24 h. The proteins were detected by western blotting. 6c. The effect of HIF1α knockdown on Celastrol-induced p53 expression and Akt and JNK activation under normoxia. HepG2 cells were transfected with control or HIF1α siRNA for 24 h and then treated with or without 4 μM Celastrol under normoxia for 24 h. The proteins were detected by western blotting. 6d, 6e. Suppression of ROS-induced JNK activity could prevent Celastrol-mediated cell death. HepG2 cells were pretreated with either the ROS scavenger 5 mM NAC or the JNK kinase inhibitor 40 μM SP600125 for 1 h and then treated with or without 4 μM Celastrol under normoxia for 24 h. Cell death was examined by microscopy (200×), as based on morphological changes, and quantified using the MTT assay. The proteins were detected by western blotting.

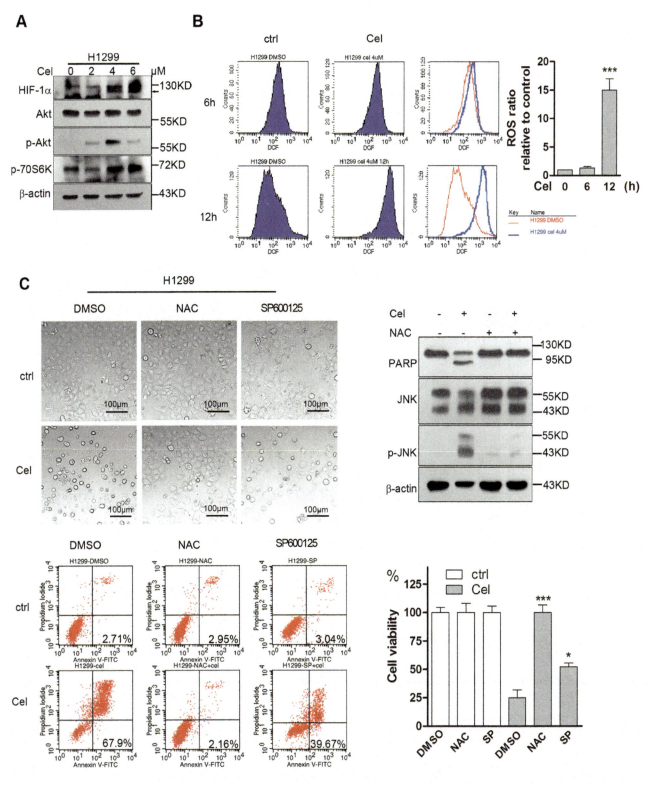

Figure 7. Celastrol kills p53-null H1299 cells via ROS-mediated JNK activation. 7a. Celastrol enhances HIF-1α expression and induces Akt activation in H1299 cells. H1299 cells were treated with the indicated doses of Celastrol for 6 h, and the proteins were detected by western blotting. 7b. Celastrol time-dependently induces ROS accumulation in H1299 cells. H1299 cells were treated with 4 μM Celastrol for the indicated times. The levels of ROS were measured by DCFH-DA staining and subsequently assayed by flow cytometry. 7c. Suppression of ROS-induced JNK activity could prevent Celastrol-mediated H1299 cell death. H1299 cells were pretreated with either the ROS scavenger 5 mM NAC or the JNK kinase inhibitor 40 μM SP600125 for 1 h and then treated with or without 4 μM Celastrol under normoxia for 24 h. Cell death was examined by microscopy (200×) and measured by Annexin-V/PI staining and flow cytometry. The proteins were detected by western blotting.

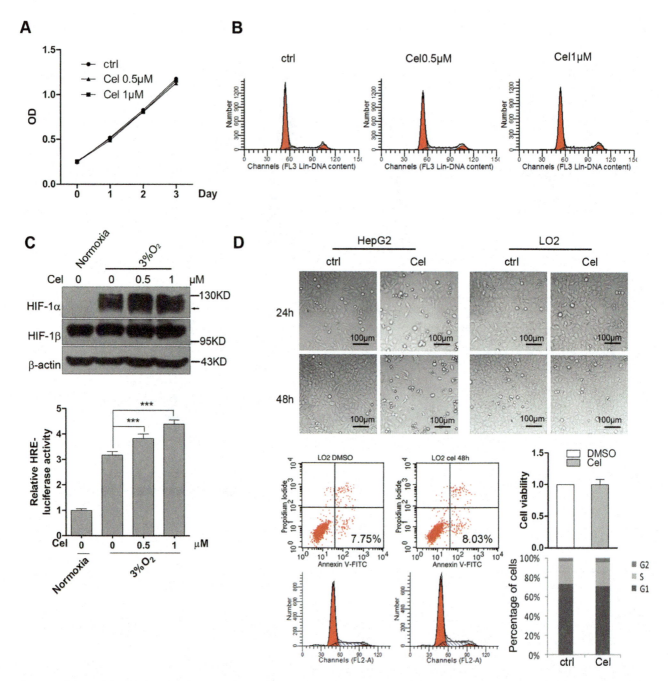

Figure 8. Celastrol could stimulate HIF-1α accumulation with a dose below its cytotoxic threshold. 8a. Low dose of Celastrol stimulated HIF-1α accumulation. HepG2 cells were treated with 0.5–1 μM Celastrol for 24 h in normoxia and hypoxia, and the viability of the cells was then detected by the MTT assay. 8b. 0.5–1 μM Celastrol did not arrest the cell cycle. HepG2 cells were treated with 0.5–1 μM Celastrol for 12 h in normoxia, and cell cycle analysis was performed using PI staining and flow cytometry. 8c. The effects of a low dose of Celastrol on HIF-1α protein expression and its transcriptional activation activity. HepG2 cells were treated with 0.5–1 μM Celastrol for 12 h in normoxia, and protein expression was determined using western blotting (upper). The transcriptional activation activity of HIF-1 was determined by transient transfection of HepG2 cells with HRE-luciferase reporter plasmids for 24 h followed by Celastrol exposure under normoxia for another 12 h. Then, HRE activity was analyzed using the luciferase assay (lower). The values are presented as the means ± SD of three independent experiments. 8d. The effect of Celastrol on LO2 normal liver cells. LO2 cells and HepG2 cells were treated with 4 μM Celastrol for 24–48 h, and the cytotoxicity of Celastrol was observed by microscopy (200×). Cell death and the cell cycle progression of the LO2 cells were measured by flow cytometry.

detected the expression of LC3 by indirect immunofluorescence staining and western blotting, and the results showed that Celastrol time-dependently increased LC3-II expression, and followed Celastrol exposure, the formation of LC3 aggregates became significant (Fig. 4b). To further confirm this change, HepG2 cells were transfected with the GFP-LC3 plasmid, and the cells were treated with or without Celastrol for 24 h and then observed using a confocal microscope. As Fig. 4c shows, in control cells, GFP-LC3 was evenly distributed throughout the entire cytoplasm; however, following Celastrol treatment, the formation of GFP-

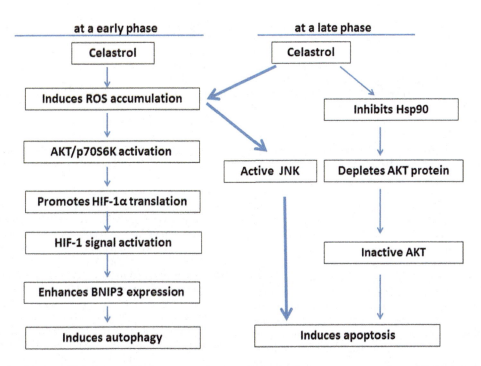

Figure 9. The mechanism by which Celastrol induces autophagy and apoptosis. In our system, we showed that Celastrol could induce ROS-mediated autophagy and apoptosis. Celastrol-induced autophagy occurred at an early phase and was initiated by ROS to stimulate AKT/p70S6K signal activation, which promotes HIF-1α translation and BNIP3 expression, leading to autophagy. Apoptosis occurred at a late phase, and the main mechanism by which Celastrol killed HepG2 and H1299 cells was through the ROS-mediated activation of JNK and inhibition of Hsp90 chaperone function, which led to Akt protein depletion and a decrease in Akt activity, finally resulting in the induction of apoptosis.

LC3 aggregates also became significant, indicating the formation of LC3-II, and more vacuole-like structures appeared, indicating that Celastrol induced autophagy.

Knockdown of HIF-1α or BNIP3 did not influence Celastrol-induced cell apoptosis under hypoxia

Previous studies have reported that hypoxia-mediated expression of BNIP3 has the potential to protect cells [25] [26]; however, we observed that, under hypoxia, although Celastrol significantly increased the expression of HIF-1α and BNIP3, it still enhanced the expression of the cleaved-PARP protein (Fig. 5a). Annexin V/PI staining and flow cytometry analysis also showed that the cytotoxicity of Celastrol was enhanced under hypoxia (Fig. 5b). Using the caspase inhibitor Z-VAD to pretreat HepG2 cells completely blocked Celastrol-induced PARP cleavage, but it did not affect HIF-1α accumulation (Fig. 5c). To confirm whether the Celastrol-induced accumulation of HIF-1α or BNIP3 could affect cell death, we evaluated the effect of knockdown of HIF-1α or BNIP3 on Celastrol-induced cell death using siRNAs. The result showed that knocking down HIF-1α expression completely inhibited BNIP3 expression, but it did not affect PARP cleavage induced by 4 µM Celastrol (Fig. 5d). Similarly, knockdown of BNIP3 did not affect Celastrol-induced PARP cleavage or cell death (Figs. 5e, 5f). These data indicated that the accumulation of HIF-1α and HIF-1α-mediated BNIP3 protein did not involve Celastrol-induced cell death.

Celastrol kills cancer cells via ROS-mediated JNK activation

To further investigate the possible mechanism by which Celastrol kills cancer cells, we detected the expression of several proteins in HepG2 cells after 4 µM Celastrol exposure for the indicated times. We found that Celastrol induced the activation of p53, but the dynamic changes in p53 expression were different under normoxia and hypoxia. Under normoxia, Celastrol transiently enhanced the expression of the p53 protein at 6 h, but the p53 protein level declined at 24 h (Fig. 6a). In contrast, under hypoxia, Celastrol persistently enhanced the expression of p53 and its target protein p21 (Fig. 6a). As a key mediator of cellular stress responses, HIF1α has been reported to either stimulate or suppress p53 depending on the oxygen conditions [27]. Our results showed that siRNA knockdown of HIF1α under hypoxia could enhance p53 expression; however, Celastrol-induced p53 activation was weakened, indicating that Celastrol-induced p53 activation is at least partially dependent on HIF-1 (Fig. 6b). In contrast, under normoxia, HIF1α knockdown decreased the intrinsic expression of p53 and p21 (Fig. 6c), and similar to the results shown in Fig. 6a, treating HepG2 cells with Celastrol under normoxia for 24 h obviously suppressed p53 activation, reduced p21 expression and, at the same time, induced PARP cleavage (Fig. 6c). These data do not support that the transient or lasting activation of p53 that is induced by Celastrol in normoxia or hypoxia involves cell killing. In addition to p53, we observed that Celastrol induced remarkable JNK activation, which was not affected by HIF-1α knockdown (Fig. 6c). More importantly, unlike Celastrol-induced Akt activation at 6 h (Fig. 2e, 2f, 2 h), treating cells with Celastrol for 24 h induced a remarkable depletion of the total Akt protein and reduced phosphor-Akt (Fig. 6c). HIF-1α knockdown lessened the inhibition of Akt activation, but it did not save the cells from Celastrol-induced apoptosis, as the cells showed the same amount of PARP cleavage as the control (Fig. 6c). Next, we used the ROS scavenger NAC or the JNK kinase inhibitor SP600125 to treat HepG2 cells incubated with or without 4 µM Celastrol for 24 h and observed their effects on Celastrol-induced cell death. The results showed that NAC could completely block the cytotoxicity of Celastrol, whereas SP600125 inhibited cell proliferation and rescued the cells from cell death (Fig. 6d). Western blotting also showed that NAC could completely inhibit Celastrol-induced JNK activation and block PARP cleavage (Fig. 6e), indicating that Celastrol-induced ROS accumulation and JNK activation were the important mechanisms for cell killing. To further support this conclusion, we repeated these experiments in H1299 cells, which are p53-null cells. Like HepG2 cells, H1299 cells treated with 2–6 μM Celastrol for 6 h could activate Akt and induce HIF-1α protein accumulation (Fig. 7a). Celastrol also time-dependently induced ROS production (Fig. 7b), and NAC blocked Celastrol-induced JNK activation and rescued cell death (Fig. 7c).

Celastrol could stimulate HIF-1α accumulation with a dose below its cytotoxic threshold

To investigate whether HIF-1α signal activation by Celastrol is correlated with cytotoxicity, we treated HepG2 cells with 0.5–1 μM Celastrol for 0–72 h and detected the cell-growth rate using the MTT assay. The result showed that Celastrol did not inhibit cell proliferation with a dose of less than 1 μM (Fig. 8a), and this conclusion was further confirmed by flow cytometric analysis of the cell cycle (Fig. 8b). Subsequently, we treated the cells with the indicated low dose of Celastrol and detected the accumulation of the HIF-1α protein and its transcription activity under hypoxia using the methods described above. The results showed that Celastrol could still enhance HIF-1α expression and active HIF-1 signaling at this dose without causing cytotoxicity (Fig. 8c). In addition, we observed the cytotoxicity of Celastrol in a normal liver cell line, LO2. It is interesting to note that, unlike in cancer cells, treating the cells with 4 μM Celastrol for as long as 48 h did not arrest the cell cycle or induce cell death (Fig. 8d).

Discussion

In this study, we found, for the first time, that Celastrol could induce accumulation of the HIF-1α protein in an oxygen-independent manner, and the accumulation of HIF-1α increased the expression of BNIP3, which induced autophagy. A previous study showed that treating HepG2 cells with Celastrol for 16 h decreased the HIF-1α mRNA level under normoxia and hypoxia and inhibited hypoxia-induced accumulation of the HIF-1α protein in the nuclei of HepG2 cells [15]; however, in our study, exposure of HepG2 cells for a shorter amount of time yielded the opposite result. In our system, treating cells with Celastrol for 6 h did not influence HIF-1α transcription, as its mRNA level did not change after Celastrol treatment under normoxia or hypoxia. Furthermore, Celastrol induced HIF-1α protein accumulation, which then entered the nucleus and promoted HIF-1 target-gene transcription. The difference in exposure time could explain these discrepant results. The effect of Celastrol in enhancing HIF-1α expression was not specific to HepG2 cells because this effect could be observed in other cell lines, including MCF-7, HeLa, PC-3 and H1299 cells. Secondly, we demonstrated that the mechanism by which Celastrol induces the accumulation of the HIF-1α protein is inducing ROS and activating Akt/p70S6K signaling to promote HIF-1α translation.

Although the protein level of HIF-1α is normally regulated by oxygen-dependent, pVHL-mediated ubiquitination and degradation [28], other molecules, such as p53 and Hsp90, have also been identified to regulate the stability of HIF-1α [18,29]. Celastrol has been reported to be a potent proteasome [19] and Hsp90 inhibitor [30,31]; however, these two functions should theoretically have opposing effects on the stability of HIF-1α. Therefore, the mechanism by which Celastrol affects HIF-1 signaling is unclear. In this study, we found that Celastrol did not enhance HIF-1α ubiquitination, as did the proteasome inhibitor MG132. Furthermore, as an Hsp90 inhibitor, Celastrol depleted other Hsp90 client proteins, such as Raf-1 and Akt, but it enhanced HIF-1α expression, though HIF-1α is also a client of Hsp90 [32]. Moreover, the enhancement of HIF-1α protein levels caused by Celastrol was independent of p53 and pVHL-mediated hydroxylation, but it required new protein synthesis, which indicated that the regulation of HIF-1α by Celastrol did not involve inhibition of HIF-1α degradation.

In addition to oxygen-dependent regulation, it is known that HIF-1 is activated or influenced through oxygen-independent mechanisms via the PI3K/AKT/mTOR pathways [22,33–35]. The activation of Akt was reported to augment HIF-1α expression by increasing its translation under normoxic and hypoxic conditions [36], and the Akt/mTOR-dependent translation of HIF-1α was reported to play a critical role in the post-irradiation up-regulation of intratumoral HIF-1 activity [22]. Although a previous study showed that mitochondrial ROS produced under hypoxia played an important role in stabilization of the HIF-1α protein by inhibiting prolyl hydroxylase enzymes [37], further studies revealed that mitochondrial ROS-upregulated HIF-1α expression is dependent upon PI3K/AKT activity [38–40]. Previously, we reported that Celastrol targets mitochondrial respiratory chain complex I to induce ROS-dependent cytotoxicity in tumor cells [41]. In this study, we showed that the enhancement of HIF-1α expression by Celastrol was ROS- and PI3K/AKT-dependent. This finding supported the hypothesis that the promotion of HIF-1α expression by Celastrol is correlated with ROS-initiated AKT activation, which enhances HIF-1α translation. As an important transcriptional factor, the accumulation of HIF-1α may affect multiple signaling pathways and regulate various biological functions, such as inducing autophagy [42,43], promoting tumor cell invasion and metastasis [44–46] and protecting cells of the brain, liver, kidney and heart from cellular oxidative stress and ischemia/reperfusion-induced injury [47–49]. Although Celastrol induced the transient accumulation of HIF-1α and VEGF, whether it can promote tumor angiogenesis and metastasis is a remaining question. Previous studies have shown that Celastrol could suppress tumor invasion and metastasis [14,50–52]; however, when considering that radiation-induced HIF-1α activation plays a crucial role in triggering tumor radioresistance [53,54], the effects of Celastrol on tumor angiogenesis and vasculogenesis may warrant further investigation.

BNIP3 is an atypical BH3-only family member that has been implicated in the pathogenesis of cancer and heart disease. Previous studies have reported that mitochondrial autophagy induced by hypoxia requires the HIF-1-dependent expression of BNIP3, which plays a protective role by disrupting the Bcl-2-Beclin1 complex without inducing cell death in tumor cells [42,43]. Similarly, in heart muscle, the expression of BNIP3 that is regulated by hypoxia is associated with decreased myocardial function via the induction of autophagy [26,55]. Previous studies have found that Celastrol induces autophagy, but the mechanism is unclear [56,57]. Our data showed that the activation of HIF-1/BNIP3 signaling is an important mechanism for Celastrol to induce autophagy. Because the dose required for Celastrol to induce accumulation of the HIF-1α protein and enhance HIF-1α transcriptional activation is below its cytotoxic threshold and because normal cells are very resistant to Celastrol, using a low dose of Celastrol to activate the HIF-1-mediated autophagic pathway could be a good strategy for utilizing the neuroprotective effects of Celastrol while avoiding its cytotoxicity. A recent study has demonstrated that Celastrol protects human neuroblastoma SH-SY5Y cells from rotenone-induced injuries only through the induction of autophagy [56].

Previous studies have demonstrated that Celastrol exerts its anticancer effects by suppressing Akt activation in tumor cells [14,58]. In this study, we observed that Celastrol induced Akt activation and enhanced HIF-1α expression, which seems contradictory to the previous conclusion. However, it is worth noting that the effect of Celastrol on Akt activation was transient and occurred early (exposure for 2–6 h) and that Celastrol continually inhibited Hsp90 chaperone function; therefore, the Akt protein was remarkably depleted, and the activity of Akt was finally inhibited (Fig. 6c), which is consistent with previous studies. Because knockdown of HIF-1α partially relieved Celastrol-induced Akt suppression but failed to reduce cell death, we believe that suppression of Akt activation only partially contributed to Celastrol-induced HepG2 cell death. ROS-mediated JNK activation has been reported to lead to cancer cell apoptosis [58]. In our experiments in both HepG2 and H1299 cells, Celastrol induced remarkable ROS accumulation, and ROS scavenging suppressed ROS-induced JNK activation and prevented cell death, which supported that mitochondrial targeting and ROS induction are the important mechanisms by which Celastrol kills cancer cells, as previously reported [41]. Based on these discoveries, we have summarized the main mechanism for the induction of autophagy or apoptosis by Celastrol in a schematic diagram (Fig. 9).

Acknowledgments

We thank Dr. Thilo Hagen (Department of Biochemistry, Yong Loo Lin School of Medicine, National University of Singapore) for kindly providing the pcDNA3-V5 and pcDNA3-P402A/P564A HIF-1α-V5 plasmids. We are also grateful to Dr. Voest EE (University Medical Center Utrecht, the Netherlands) for providing the pGL3-HRE-Luc reporter plasmid.

Author Contributions

Conceived and designed the experiments: XY YG XH. Performed the experiments: XH SS MZ GC XC SL. Analyzed the data: XH MZ XC. Contributed to the writing of the manuscript: XY XH MZ.

References

1. O'Rourke JF, Dachs GU, Gleadle JM, Maxwell PH, Pugh CW, et al. (1997) Hypoxia response elements. Oncol Res 9: 327–332.
2. D'Angelo G, Duplan E, Boyer N, Vigne P, Frelin C (2003) Hypoxia up-regulates prolyl hydroxylase activity: a feedback mechanism that limits HIF-1 responses during reoxygenation. J Biol Chem 278: 38183–38187.
3. Calixto JB, Campos MM, Otuki MF, Santos ARS (2004) Anti-inflammatory compounds of plant origin. Part II. Modulation of pro-inflammatory cytokines, chemokines and adhesion molecules. Planta Med 70: 93–103.
4. Venkatesha SH, Yu H, Rajaiah R, Tong L, Moudgil KD (2011) Celastrus-derived celastrol suppresses autoimmune arthritis by modulating antigen-induced cellular and humoral effector responses. J Biol Chem 286: 15138–15146.
5. Faust K, Gehrke S, Yang Y, Yang L, Beal MF, et al. (2009) Neuroprotective effects of compounds with antioxidant and anti-inflammatory properties in a Drosophila model of Parkinson's disease. BMC Neurosci 10: 109.
6. Ge P, Ji X, Ding Y, Wang X, Fu S, et al. (2010) Celastrol causes apoptosis and cell cycle arrest in rat glioma cells. Neurol Res 32: 94–100.
7. Dai Y, Desano J, Tang W, Meng X, Meng Y, et al. (2010) Natural proteasome inhibitor celastrol suppresses androgen-independent prostate cancer progression by modulating apoptotic proteins and NF-kappaB. PLoS One 5: e14153.
8. Mou H, Zheng Y, Zhao P, Bao H, Fang W, et al. (2011) Celastrol induces apoptosis in non-small-cell lung cancer A549 cells through activation of mitochondria- and Fas/FasL-mediated pathways. Toxicol In Vitro 25: 1027–1032.
9. Sha M, Ye J, Zhang LX, Luan ZY, Chen YB (2013) Celastrol induces apoptosis of gastric cancer cells by miR-146a inhibition of NF-kappaB activity. Cancer Cell Int 13: 50.
10. Sethi G, Ahn KS, Pandey MK, Aggarwal BB (2007) Celastrol, a novel triterpene, potentiates TNF-induced apoptosis and suppresses invasion of tumor cells by inhibiting NF-kappaB-regulated gene products and TAK1-mediated NF-kappaB activation. Blood 109: 2727–2735.
11. Dai Y, DeSano JT, Meng Y, Ji Q, Ljungman M, et al. (2009) Celastrol potentiates radiotherapy by impairment of DNA damage processing in human prostate cancer. Int J Radiat Oncol Biol Phys 74: 1217–1225.
12. Jo H, Loison F, Hattori H, Silberstein LE, Yu H, et al. (2010) Natural product Celastrol destabilizes tubulin heterodimer and facilitates mitotic cell death triggered by microtubule-targeting anti-cancer drugs. PLoS One 5: e10318.
13. Zhu H, Ding WJ, Wu R, Weng QJ, Lou JS, et al. (2010) Synergistic anti-cancer activity by the combination of TRAIL/APO-2L and celastrol. Cancer Invest 28: 23–32.
14. Pang X, Yi Z, Zhang J, Lu B, Sung B, et al. (2010) Celastrol suppresses angiogenesis-mediated tumor growth through inhibition of AKT/mammalian target of rapamycin pathway. Cancer Res 70: 1951–1959.
15. Huang L, Zhang Z, Zhang S, Ren J, Zhang R, et al. (2011) Inhibitory action of Celastrol on hypoxia-mediated angiogenesis and metastasis via the HIF-1alpha pathway. Int J Mol Med 27: 407–415.
16. Liu XH, Kirschenbaum A, Yao S, Stearns ME, Holland JF, et al. (1999) Upregulation of vascular endothelial growth factor by cobalt chloride-simulated hypoxia is mediated by persistent induction of cyclooxygenase-2 in a metastatic human prostate cancer cell line. Clin Exp Metastasis 17: 687–694.
17. Pfaffl MW (2001) A new mathematical model for relative quantification in real-time RT-PCR. Nucleic Acids Res 29: e45.
18. Kaluzova M, Kaluz S, Lerman MI, Stanbridge EJ (2004) DNA damage is a prerequisite for p53-mediated proteasomal degradation of HIF-1alpha in hypoxic cells and downregulation of the hypoxia marker carbonic anhydrase IX. Mol Cell Biol 24: 5757–5766.
19. Yang H, Chen D, Cui QC, Yuan X, Dou QP (2006) Celastrol, a triterpene extracted from the Chinese "Thunder of God Vine," is a potent proteasome inhibitor and suppresses human prostate cancer growth in nude mice. Cancer Res 66: 4758–4765.
20. Walcott SE, Heikkila JJ (2010) Celastrol can inhibit proteasome activity and upregulate the expression of heat shock protein genes, hsp30 and hsp70, in Xenopus laevis A6 cells. Comp Biochem Physiol A Mol Integr Physiol 156: 285–293.
21. Schnitzer SE, Schmid T, Zhou J, Eisenbrand G, Brune B (2005) Inhibition of GSK3beta by indirubins restores HIF-1alpha accumulation under prolonged periods of hypoxia/anoxia. FEBS Lett 579: 529–533.
22. Harada H, Itasaka S, Kizaka-Kondoh S, Shibuya K, Morinibu A, et al. (2009) The Akt/mTOR Pathway Assures the Synthesis of HIF-1 alpha Protein in a Glucose- and Reoxygenation-dependent Manner in Irradiated Tumors. Journal of Biological Chemistry 284: 5332–5342.
23. Zhang H, Bosch-Marce M, Shimoda LA, Tan YS, Baek JH, et al. (2008) Mitochondrial autophagy is an HIF-1-dependent adaptive metabolic response to hypoxia. J Biol Chem 283: 10892–10903.
24. Band M, Joel A, Hernandez A, Avivi A (2009) Hypoxia-induced BNIP3 expression and mitophagy: in vivo comparison of the rat and the hypoxia-tolerant mole rat, Spalax ehrenbergi. FASEB J 23: 2327–2335.
25. Tracy K, Macleod KF (2007) Regulation of mitochondrial integrity, autophagy and cell survival by BNIP3. Autophagy 3: 616–619.
26. Hamacher-Brady A, Brady NR, Gottlieb RA, Gustafsson AB (2006) Autophagy as a protective response to Bnip3-mediated apoptotic signaling in the heart. Autophagy 2: 307–309.
27. Obacz J, Pastorekova S, Vojtesek B, Hrstka R (2013) Cross-talk between HIF and p53 as mediators of molecular responses to physiological and genotoxic stresses. Mol Cancer 12: 93.
28. Wei W, Yu XD (2007) Hypoxia-inducible factors: crosstalk between their protein stability and protein degradation. Cancer Lett 257: 145–156.
29. Minet E, Mottet D, Michel G, Roland I, Raes M, et al. (1999) Hypoxia-induced activation of HIF-1, role of HIF-1 alpha-Hsp90 interaction. Febs Letters 460: 251–256.
30. Zhang T, Li Y, Yu Y, Zou P, Jiang Y, et al. (2009) Characterization of celastrol to inhibit hsp90 and cdc37 interaction. J Biol Chem 284: 35381–35389.
31. Chadli A, Felts SJ, Wang Q, Sullivan WP, Botuyan MV, et al. (2010) Celastrol inhibits Hsp90 chaperoning of steroid receptors by inducing fibrillization of the Co-chaperone p23. J Biol Chem 285: 4224–4231.
32. Liu YV, Baek JH, Zhang H, Diez R, Cole RN, et al. (2007) RACK1 competes with HSP90 for binding to HIF-1 alpha and is required for O-2-independent and HSP90 inhibitor-induced degradation of HIF-1 alpha. Molecular Cell 25: 207–217.
33. Xie SR, Wang Y, Liu CW, Luo K, Cai YQ (2012) Liquiritigenin Inhibits Serum-induced HIF-1a and VEGF Expression via the AKT/mTOR-p70S6K Signalling Pathway in HeLa Cells. Phytotherapy Research 26: 1133–1141.
34. Majumder PK, Febbo PG, Bikoff R, Berger R, Xue Q, et al. (2004) mTOR inhibition reverses Akt-dependent prostate intraepithelial neoplasia through regulation of apoptotic and HIF-1-dependent pathways. Nature Medicine 10: 594–601.

35. Agani F, Jiang BH (2013) Oxygen-independent Regulation of HIF-1: Novel Involvement of PI3K/AKT/mTOR Pathway in Cancer. Curr Cancer Drug Targets 13: 245–251.
36. Pore N, Jiang ZB, Shu HK, Bernhard E, Kao GD, et al. (2006) Akt1 activation can augment hypoxia-inducible factor-1 alpha expression by increasing protein translation through a mammalian target of rapamycin-independent pathway. Molecular Cancer Research 4: 471–479.
37. Chandel NS, McClintock DS, Feliciano CE, Wood TM, Melendez JA, et al. (2000) Reactive oxygen species generated at mitochondrial complex III stabilize hypoxia-inducible factor-1 alpha during hypoxia - A mechanism of O-2 sensing. Journal of Biological Chemistry 275: 25130–25138.
38. Gao N, Ding M, Zheng JZ, Zhang Z, Leonard SS, et al. (2002) Vanadate-induced expression of hypoxia-inducible factor 1 alpha and vascular endothelial growth factor through phosphatidylinositol 3-kinase/Akt pathway and reactive oxygen species. Journal of Biological Chemistry 277: 31963–31971.
39. Koshikawa N, Hayashi JI, Nakagawara A, Takenaga K (2009) Reactive Oxygen Species-generating Mitochondrial DNA Mutation Up-regulates Hypoxia-inducible Factor-1 alpha Gene Transcription via Phosphatidylinositol 3-Kinase-Akt/Protein Kinase C/Histone Deacetylase Pathway. Journal of Biological Chemistry 284: 33185–33194.
40. Guo LL, Li L, Wang WQ, Pan ZH, Zhou QH, et al. (2012) Mitochondrial reactive oxygen species mediates nicotine-induced hypoxia-inducible factor-1 alpha expression in human non-small cell lung cancer cells. Biochimica Et Biophysica Acta-Molecular Basis of Disease 1822: 852–861.
41. Chen G, Zhang X, Zhao M, Wang Y, Cheng X, et al. (2011) Celastrol targets mitochondrial respiratory chain complex I to induce reactive oxygen species-dependent cytotoxicity in tumor cells. BMC Cancer 11: 170.
42. Mazure NM, Pouyssegur J (2009) Atypical BH3-domains of BNIP3 and BNIP3L lead to autophagy in hypoxia. Autophagy 5: 868–869.
43. Bellot G, Garcia-Medina R, Gounon P, Chiche J, Roux D, et al. (2009) Hypoxia-induced autophagy is mediated through hypoxia-inducible factor induction of BNIP3 and BNIP3L via their BH3 domains. Mol Cell Biol 29: 2570–2581.
44. Lin MT, Kuo IH, Chang CC, Chu CY, Chen HY, et al. (2008) Involvement of hypoxia-inducing factor-1alpha-dependent plasminogen activator inhibitor-1 up-regulation in Cyr61/CCN1-induced gastric cancer cell invasion. J Biol Chem 283: 15807–15815.
45. Kurokawa T, Miyamoto M, Kato K, Cho Y, Kawarada Y, et al. (2003) Overexpression of hypoxia-inducible-factor 1 alpha(HIF-1 alpha) in oesophageal squamous cell carcinoma correlates with lymph node metastasis and pathologic stage. British Journal of Cancer 89: 1042–1047.
46. Whitney LK, Williams KJ, Stratford IJ, Lunt SJ, Brown L (2004) The role of hypoxia and the transcription factor HIF-1 in the development of metastasis. British Journal of Cancer 91: S50–S50.
47. Bernhardt WM, Campean V, Kany S, Jurgensen JS, Weidemann A, et al. (2006) Preconditional activation of hypoxia-inducible factors ameliorates ischemic acute renal failure. Journal of the American Society of Nephrology 17: 1970–1978.
48. Philipp S, Jurgensen JS, Fielitz J, Bernhardt WM, Weidemann A, et al. (2006) Stabilization of hypoxia inducible factor rather than modulation of collagen metabolism improves cardiac function after acute myocardial infarction in rats. European Journal of Heart Failure 8: 347–354.
49. Sen Banerjee S, Thirunavukkarasu M, Rishi MT, Sanchez JA, Maulik N, et al. (2012) HIF-prolyl hydroxylases and cardiovascular diseases. Toxicol Mech Methods 22: 347–358.
50. Zhou YX, Huang YL (2009) Antiangiogenic effect of celastrol on the growth of human glioma: an in vitro and in vivo study. Chin Med J (Engl) 122: 1666–1673.
51. Zhu H, Liu XW, Cai TY, Cao J, Tu CX, et al. (2010) Celastrol acts as a potent antimetastatic agent targeting beta1 integrin and inhibiting cell-extracellular matrix adhesion, in part via the p38 mitogen-activated protein kinase pathway. J Pharmacol Exp Ther 334: 489–499.
52. Kim Y, Kang H, Jang SW, Ko J (2011) Celastrol inhibits breast cancer cell invasion via suppression of NF-kB-mediated matrix metalloproteinase-9 expression. Cell Physiol Biochem 28: 175–184.
53. Lerman OZ, Greives MR, Singh SP, Thanik VD, Chang CC, et al. (2010) Low-dose radiation augments vasculogenesis signaling through HIF-1-dependent and -independent SDF-1 induction. Blood 116: 3669–3676.
54. Harada H, Kizaka-Kondoh S, Li G, Itasaka S, Shibuya K, et al. (2007) Significance of HIF-1-active cells in angiogenesis and radioresistance. Oncogene 26: 7508–7516.
55. Hamacher-Brady A, Brady NR, Logue SE, Sayen MR, Jinno M, et al. (2007) Response to myocardial ischemia/reperfusion injury involves Bnip3 and autophagy. Cell Death Differ 14: 146–157.
56. Deng YN, Shi J, Liu J, Qu QM (2013) Celastrol protects human neuroblastoma SH-SY5Y cells from rotenone-induced injury through induction of autophagy. Neurochem Int 63: 1–9.
57. Lee HW, Jang KS, Chun KH (2014) Celastrol inhibits gastric cancer growth by induction of apoptosis and autophagy. BMB Rep.
58. Kannaiyan R, Manu KA, Chen L, Li F, Rajendran P, et al. (2011) Celastrol inhibits tumor cell proliferation and promotes apoptosis through the activation of c-Jun N-terminal kinase and suppression of PI3 K/Akt signaling pathways. Apoptosis 16: 1028–1041.

Mechanisms by Which Low Glucose Enhances the Cytotoxicity of Metformin to Cancer Cells Both *In Vitro* and *In Vivo*

Yongxian Zhuang[1]*[☯], Daniel K. Chan[2][☯], Allison B. Haugrud[1], W. Keith Miskimins[1]

1 Cancer Biology Research Center, Sanford Research/USD, Sioux Falls, South Dakota, United States of America, **2** Sanford School of Medicine, The University of South Dakota, Vermillion, South Dakota, United States of America

Abstract

Different cancer cells exhibit altered sensitivity to metformin treatment. Recent studies suggest these findings may be due in part to the common cell culture practice of utilizing high glucose, and when glucose is lowered, metformin becomes increasingly cytotoxic to cancer cells. In low glucose conditions ranging from 0 to 5 mM, metformin was cytotoxic to breast cancer cell lines MCF7, MDAMB231 and SKBR3, and ovarian cancer cell lines OVCAR3, and PA-1. MDAMB231 and SKBR3 were previously shown to be resistant to metformin in normal high glucose medium. When glucose was increased to 10 mM or above, all of these cell lines become less responsive to metformin treatment. Metformin treatment significantly reduced ATP levels in cells incubated in media with low glucose (2.5 mM), high fructose (25 mM) or galactose (25 mM). Reductions in ATP levels were not observed with high glucose (25 mM). This was compensated by enhanced glycolysis through activation of AMPK when oxidative phosphorylation was inhibited by metformin. However, enhanced glycolysis was either diminished or abolished by replacing 25 mM glucose with 2.5 mM glucose, 25 mM fructose or 25 mM galactose. These findings suggest that lowering glucose potentiates metformin induced cell death by reducing metformin stimulated glycolysis. Additionally, under low glucose conditions metformin significantly decreased phosphorylation of AKT and various targets of mTOR, while phospho-AMPK was not significantly altered. Thus inhibition of mTOR signaling appears to be independent of AMPK activation. Further in vivo studies using the 4T1 breast cancer mouse model confirmed that metformin inhibition of tumor growth was enhanced when serum glucose levels were reduced via low carbohydrate ketogenic diets. The data support a model in which metformin treatment of cancer cells in low glucose medium leads to cell death by decreasing ATP production and inhibition of survival signaling pathways. The enhanced cytotoxicity of metformin against cancer cells was observed both in vitro and in vivo.

Editor: Viji Shridhar, Mayo Clinic College of Medicine, United States of America

Funding: This work was supported through grant KG100497 (W.K. Miskimins) from Susan G. Komen for the Cure. Seahorse XF24 experiments were supported by COBRE award 5P20GM10358 (W.K Miskimins) from the National Institute of General Medical Sciences at the National Institutes of Health. The project was also supported in part by a COBRE pilot award (Y. Zhuang) and PHS grant 1R01CA180033-01 (W.K. Miskimins) from the National Cancer Institute. The funders had no role in study design, data collection and analysis, decision to publish, or preparation of the manuscript.

Competing Interests: The authors have declared that no competing interests exist.

* Email: Yongxian.Zhuang@sanfordhealth.org

☯ These authors contributed equally to this work.

Introduction

In the transformation to cancer, cells undergo reprogramming of their ordinary metabolic functions to facilitate rapid growth potential. Otto Warburg reported high rates of glycolysis in cancer cells even in aerobic conditions. This paradoxical change is one mechanism by which cancer cells have adapted for rapid proliferation. As a result of this altered metabolism, cancer cells use large amounts of glucose and generate high amounts of lactate. Glucose metabolism through glycolysis contributes to ATP synthesis and provides intermediates for other biosynthetic processes. Thus, cancer cells are dependent on the high rates of glucose uptake and metabolism for survival [1,2].

Current methods of *in vitro* cancer cell culture commonly use high glucose, 25 mM (450 mg/dL), in the growth medium. While high glucose medium creates an optimal environment for cancer cell proliferation, these glucose levels may complicate the interpretation of drug efficacy studies. High glucose alone has the ability to activate proliferation pathways in a cancer cell [2], and the constant availability of glucose places little of the normal stress cancer cells experience *in vivo*. In pancreatic cancer cells, Sinnett-Smith *et al.* [3] found that metformin's actions on AMPK activation were enhanced through use of 5 mM glucose media in cultured cells.

Normal serum glucose is usually maintained between 4 and 6 mM (approximately 72–108 mg/dL). In cases of low nutrient availability, serum glucose levels may drop to 2.5 mM (45 mg/dL), with tissue levels of glucose commonly lower. Reducing glucose availability has also been attempted as a cancer treatment by a variety of methods. Modifying diet by direct caloric restriction or fasting has been investigated as a method of reducing cancer growth with some promising results [4–6]. Generally, fasting appears to be more effective than constant caloric restriction at reducing cancer growth [5]. Besides diet modification, anti-diabetic drugs are another means of lowering plasma glucose. In a clinical trial comparing metformin's efficacy to existing type II diabetes medications, metformin was found to lower plasma glucose concentrations by approximately 3 mM (55 mg/dL) from pretreatment levels [7]. However, it is worth noting that metformin did not have significant effects on reduction of plasma glucose in non-diabetics [8].

Recently metformin has gained renewed interest as a potential cancer therapeutic and chemotherapy adjuvant. Metformin's potential anti-cancer activity was implicated by the lower incidence of cancer in type II diabetics versus other glucose controlling drugs [9]. This effect was initially attributed to metformin's systemic glucose and insulin regulating properties. Later metformin was also found to inhibit cancer growth at the cellular level. The anti-oncogenic action for metformin is likely a combination of systemic insulin control effects and direct cellular effects. Many groups have demonstrated metformin's action *in vitro* in a variety of cancer types [10–14]. However, to mimic the effects of metformin *in vitro* that are observed *in vivo*, high concentrations, commonly 5–20 mM, of metformin are necessary. Recent studies suggest these findings may be due in part to the common cell culture practice of utilizing high glucose, and when glucose is lowered, metformin becomes increasingly cytotoxic to cancer cells [15,16]. Additionally, the carbon source for cancer cells was found to significantly alter anti-cancer effects of metformin when comparing glucose to glutamine [17]. In this study cancer cells exposed to high glutamine in the absence of glucose were much more sensitive to inhibition by metformin.

While the precise mechanism for metformin's cancer cytotoxicity remains unidentified, metformin's systemic actions likely combine with the direct cellular action to enhance its effect on cancer cell growth inhibition and cancer cell death. Here we show that low to normal glucose levels, as opposed to high glucose conditions, potentiate the effect of metformin in breast and ovarian cancer cell lines. The possible mechanisms for this activity are explored. These observations may reveal both more relevant cell culture techniques for studying metformin in cancer as well as provide insight into clinical use of metformin as an adjuvant cancer therapy.

Methods

Chemicals and reagents

The following chemicals were used in this study: metformin (1, 1-dimethylbiguanide,), D-(−)-fructose, D-(+)-galactose, 2-deoxy-D-glucose, oligomycin (Sigma Chemical Co). Dulbecco's modified Eagle's Medium (DMEM) with high glucose (Hyclone), Gibco DMEM without glucose (Life Technology), SYTOX Green Nucleic Acid Stain (Invitrogen), and ATP Assay kit (Invitrogen).

Cell culture

Human cancer cell lines MCF7, MDAMB231, OVCAR3, PA-1, SKRB3, and human mammary epithelial MCF10A cells were all purchased from ATCC and maintained in DMEM containing 10% fetal bovine serum with varying glucose levels and 1% penicillin-streptomycin at 37°C under a humidified atmosphere containing 5% CO_2. All the cell lines were used within passage ten after receiving from ATCC to ensure cell line authentication.

Cell death assay using Sytox Green Nucleic Acid Stain

Cells were plated into 96 well plates and treated with the indicated treatment for one or two days. Sytox Green nucleic acid stain (10 μM) was added directly to cells in 96 well plates and incubated for 10 minutes. The plate was read at excitation/emission of 485 nm and 530 nm, respectively, with a 515 nm cutoff using a fluorescence plate reader (SpectraMax M5 Multi-Mode Microplate Reader, Molecular Devices, LLC). Fluorescence was measured to obtain number of dead cells. Subsequently, to determine total cell number, 0.4% Triton-X100 was added to each sample and it was incubated for 30 minutes at room temperature to permeabilize all the cells, and fluorescence at 485/530 nm was measured again to obtain the total cell number.

ATP assay

Cells were seeded into 6 well plates followed by incubation for 24 hours. Treatment was given with fresh medium for 24 hours. Equal numbers of cells were lysed in each treatment group and 10 μl was used from each sample following the manufacturer's protocol for ATP assays (Invitrogen, ATP Determination Kit, A22066). Briefly, 100 μl of the standard reaction solution was measured in a luminometer for background luminescence. Then 10 μl of the lysate supernatant was added to the reaction solution and the luminescence was again measured. Background luminescence was subtracted from sample luminescence and results were plotted as fold change from control samples.

Western blotting

Cells in 35 mm dishes were rinsed once with PBS and lysed by addition of sodium dodecylsulfate (SDS) sample buffer [2.5 mM Tris-HCl (pH 6.8), 2.5% SDS, 100 mM dithiothreitol, 10% glycerol, 0.025% pyronine Y]. Equal amounts of protein from each treatment group were separated on 10% or 15% SDS-polyacrylamide gels. Proteins were transferred to Immobilon P membranes (Millipore) using a semi-dry Bio-Rad Trans-blot apparatus with a transfer buffer of 48 mM Tris-HCl and 39 mM glycine. The membranes were blocked with 5% non-fat dry milk or 5% BSA in Tris-buffered saline [10 mM Tris-HCl (pH 7.5), 150 mM NaCl] containing 0.1% Tween-20 (TBS-T) for one hour at room temperature. The membrane was then incubated with the appropriate antibody in TBS-T containing 5% non-fat dry milk or 5% BSA for 1 hour at room temperature or overnight at 4°C. After washing in TBS-T the membrane was incubated with the appropriate horseradish peroxidase (HRP)-conjugated secondary antibody. Proteins were detected using the Super Signal West Pico chemiluminescent substrate (Pierce Biochemical). Anti-β-actin monoclonal antibody (A5441, used at 1:10,000) was purchased from Sigma. Antibodies against phosphorylated AKT at threonine 473 (#05-669 used at 1:1000) was purchased from Upstate Biotechnologies. Antibodies against AKT phosphorylated at threonine 308 (#4056, used at 1:1000), ATK (#4691, used at 1:1000), phosphorylated S6K (#9206, used at 1:2000), S6K (#9202, used at 1:2000), PARP (#9542, used at 1:2000), cleaved PARP (#9541, used at 1:2000), AMPK phosphorylated at threonine 172 (#2535, used at 1:1000), and AMPK (#2532, used at 1:1000), Cleaved Caspase 7 (#9491, used at 1:1000) were purchased from Cell Signalling Technology. Secondary horseradish peroxidase-linked anti-mouse (#31430, used at 1:5000) and anti-rabbit (#31460, used at 1:5000) IgG antibodies were purchased from Pierce Biochemical.

Lactate assay

MCF7 were plated in 96 well plates and treated as indicated for 15 hours. Medium from each treatment was collected and tested for lactate concentration using an L-Lactate Assay Kit (Eton Biosciences Inc.). Cells were counted using Sytox Green staining method as described previously. Relative lactate levels were obtained after normalizing by total cell number.

Measurement of Extra Cellular Acidification Rate (ECAR) and Oxygen Consumption Rate (OCR)

ECAR and OCR were measured using a Seahorse XF24 analyzer according to manufacturer's instructions (Seahorse Bioscience). Briefly, MCF7 cells were plated at 40,000 cells/well in XF24-well plates. Cells were treated as indicated the next day. Before being processed with the Seahorse XF24 analyzer, cells were washed and equilibrated with buffer free medium (D5030, Sigma) at 37°C in a CO_2-free incubator for one hour. Initial measurements of ECAR and OCR were obtained followed by addition of different concentrations of glucose (2.5 mM or 25 mM), fructose (25 mM) or galactose (25 mM). ECAR and OCR were further measured following injection of oligomycin and 2-deoxyglucose. Cell number was obtained by trypsinizing cells and counting using a hemocytometer. ECAR and OCR were plotted after normalizing by total cell number.

In vivo mouse studies

All experiments were performed in accord with institutional and national guidelines and regulations; the protocol was approved by the institutional animal care and use committee at Sanford Research. Briefly, using a 25-gauge needle, Balb/C mice were subcutaneously injected with 1×10^5 cells in the flank (10 mice per treatment condition). Four days after tumor cell injection, the mice were switched to a calorie restricted low carbohydrate ketogenic diet (BioServ P3666) for the KD group (see below for details of diets). The control groups remained on normal mouse chow (Teklad Global 18% Protein Rodent Diet) and were fed as libitum. Metformin (2 mg/mouse) was administered intraperitoneally daily starting 7 days after tumor injection. Tumor volume was estimated using $A^2 \times B$ where A is the larger diameter and B is the smaller diameter. Animals were euthanized when the tumor size was greater than 15 mm in its greatest dimension, or tumor volumes reach 3000 mm³, or when the animal was substantially emaciated.

Serum glucose measurement

Serum glucose levels were measured using tail vein blood after puncturing the tail with a 25 gauge needle to produce one drop of blood for each test. Glucose was measured using a Bayer Contour Glucometer and glucose test strips.

Diet information

The low carbohydrate ketogenic diet was purchased from BioServ (#F3666). This diet provides calories from protein, fat and carbohydrates at approximately 4.6%, 93.4%, and 2%, respectively. All mice being fed this diet were subjected to 30% calorie restriction (7 kCal/day/mouse) starting the 4th day after tumor cell injection. Calorie restriction was determined by measuring the weight of food consumed each day. The appropriate amount of the ketogenic diet was provided every day on a petri dish within the cage. Calories were increased to 7.5 kCal/day/mouse (25% restriction) at day 7 after initiation of the ketogenic diet to prevent weight loss. Calories were further increased to 8 kCal/day/mouse at day 11 after the initiation of ketogenic diet and maintained at this level until the end of the experiment. The control diet groups were fed ad libitum on standard mouse chow (Teklad Global 18% protein rodent diet) which provides calories from protein, fat and carbohydrates at approximately 24%, 18%, and 58%, respectively.

Statistical analysis

Error bars shown are standard deviations from the mean of at least three replicates. Two-tailed pairwise Student's t tests were used to compare two groups. P values less than or equal to 0.05 were considered to have significance.

Results

Our previous research has demonstrated that metformin is cytotoxic to many breast and ovarian cancer cell lines. However, some cell lines such as the breast cell lines MDAMB231 and SKBR3 exhibited resistance to metformin cytotoxicity [14,18,19]. Previous experiments were carried out in DMEM containing 25 mM glucose, which is significantly higher than normal physiological conditions of 4–8 mM. To determine the influence glucose concentration has on the cytotoxicity of metformin, we tested the effects of different concentrations of glucose in the culture medium of cancer cells exposed to metformin treatment. All cell cultures were initially maintained in high glucose medium (25 mM glucose) and plated into 96 well plates for one day, the next day cells were treated with metformin (0 mM, 2 mM, 4 mM, 8 mM and 16 mM) in medium containing different concentrations of glucose (0 mM, 2.5 mM, 5 mM, 10 mM, 15 mM and 25 mM) for one day. As glucose levels in the medium decrease, metformin treatment significantly increased the percentage of dead cells in MDAMB231, MCF7, and SKBR3 cells (Figure 1A, 1B, 1C). Previous data show that, in high glucose medium, both MDAMB231 and SKBR3 cells are resistant to metformin treatment (8 mM) for up to three days [14,18,19]. In high glucose conditions these cell lines, MDAMB231 and SKBR3, continued to be resistant to metformin treatments up to 16 mM concentrations of the drug. However, when the glucose levels were reduced to 2.5 mM or less both MDAMB231 and SKBR3 show a cytotoxic response to metformin treatment from 4 mM to 16 mM.

Concurrently, the effects of metformin at different concentrations of glucose were examined in the non-cancer human mammary epithelial cell line MCF10A (Figure 1D). In contrast to the cancer cell cultures, reduction of glucose concentration did not significantly sensitize MCF10A to metformin treatment over this time period. This difference may be a result of underlying differences in glucose metabolism between normal mammary epithelial cells and cancer cells.

In order to test whether these effects on metformin cytotoxicity applied to other cancer cell types, we also examined ovarian cancer cells. In a similar fashion, lowering the glucose was found to increase the cytotoxicity of metformin in the ovarian cancer cell lines OVCAR3 and PA-1 (Figure 2). This suggests that lowering the glucose flux in cancer cells could significantly enhance the cytotoxicity of metformin, and that this effect may be broadly relevant to various cancer cell types.

Other known cellular actions of metformin include inhibition of complex I of the electron transport chain and oxidative phosphorylation [20]. This action can result in deceased production of ATP and other cellular intermediates. The cellular ATP levels of MCF7, MDAMB231, and PA-1 were examined after metformin treatment (24 hours) in either high glucose (25 mM) or low glucose (2.5 mM) tissue culture medium (Figure 3). The results show that metformin strongly decreases ATP levels only in low glucose medium. In high glucose

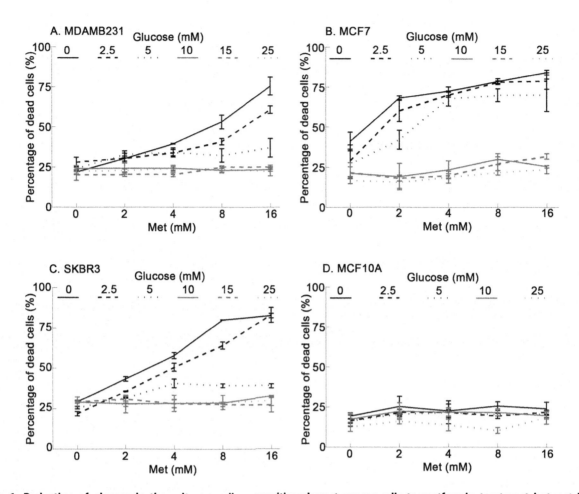

Figure 1. Reduction of glucose in the culture medium sensitizes breast cancer cells to metformin treatment but not human mammary epithelial MCF10A cells. All cells were treated with different concentrations of metformin (0, 2, 4, 8, 16 mM) in medium containing different levels of glucose (0, 2.5, 5, 10, 15, 25 mM) for one day. Percentage of dead cells was determined using Sytox Green staining. Metformin significantly increased percentage of dead cells with decreasing glucose concentration in (**A**) MDAMB231 cells, (**B**) MCF7 cells, and (**C**) SKBR3 cells but not in (**D**) MCF10A cells. Data were presented as mean ± standard deviation.

conditions, at this time point, metformin tended to increase ATP but not to a level of significance.

In high glucose conditions, metformin treated cells potentially maintain ATP levels by activation of AMPK and enhancing glycolysis [21,22]. To test this, MCF7 cells were treated with metformin (8 mM) for 15 hours, cellular oxygen consumption (OCR) and extracellular acidification rate (ECAR) were measured using the XF24 seahorse analyzer. As expected, metformin significantly inhibited oxygen consumption of MCF7 cells in medium containing either 25 mM or 2.5 mM glucose (Figure 4A). Enhanced glycolysis in metformin treated cells in 25 mM glucose containing medium was confirmed by increased acidification of the extracellular medium (Figure 4B) and lactate secretion (Figure 4C). However, in low glucose treated cancer cells showed diminished augmentation of ECAR and lactate production by metformin, indicating a reduced ability to promote an increase in glycolysis (Figure 4B, 4C). Thus, failure to sufficiently promote glycolysis correlates with an inability to maintain intracellular ATP under these conditions.

AMPK is known to regulate glycolysis by enhancing glucose uptake and regulation of several key enzymes in the pathway [21–25]. Our previous data showed that metformin could activate AMPK by enhancing the phosphorylation of AMPK at Threonine 172 in medium containing 25 mM glucose [14]. Therefore, the levels of AMPK activation with metformin treatment in both high glucose and low glucose were examined. MCF7 and MDAMB231 cells were treated with metformin (8 mM) for one day in either 25 mM or 2.5 mM glucose containing medium. Western blotting was performed to detect phosphorylated AMPK and total AMPK. In both cell lines metformin enhanced the levels of phosphorylated of AMPK, the active form of the enzyme, in medium containing 25 mM glucose, but not in medium containing 2.5 mM glucose after one day treatment (Figure 4D). In contrast, while low glucose, itself, increased phosphorylation of AMPK, the addition of metformin in these conditions appeared to decrease both phospho-AMPK and total levels of the enzyme. This is further demonstrated by densitometry of western blots of MCF7 cells to quantify the ratio of phosphorylated AMPK to total AMPK and the ratio of phosphorylated AMPK to actin (Figure 4D). In medium containing 2.5 mM glucose, metformin still enhanced the activation of AMPK compared to control, demonstrated by the increased ratio of phosphorylated AMPK to total AMPK. However, because of the strong reduction of total AMPK, total phosphorylated AMPK was decreased with metformin treatment compared to control. The reduction of AMPK levels with metformin treatment in medium containing 2.5 mM glucose was associated with significant apoptotic cell death as demonstrated by increased cleaved caspase 7 (Figure 4D lower panel). The variance

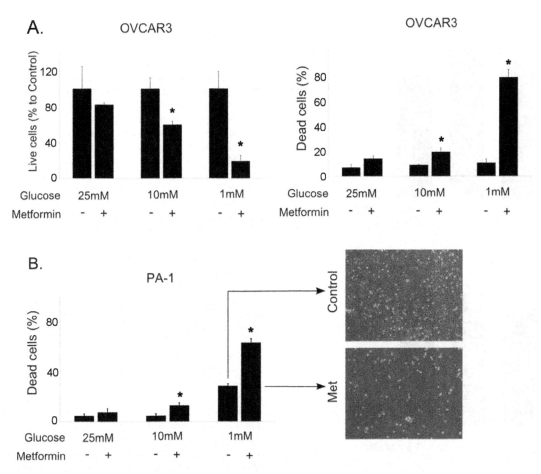

Figure 2. Metformin treatment of ovarian cancer cells is enhanced by low glucose conditions. A. After 48 hour treatments with metformin (5 mM, +) or control vehicle (H$_2$O, −), live OVCAR3 cell number was determined by counting trypan blue negative cells and dead cell number was determined by counting trypan blue positive cells. **B.** PA-1 cell death was determined as described in A. Phase contrast images (40x) of the cells cultured with (lower image) or without (upper image) metformin treatment. Bar graphs represented mean ± standard deviation. All metformin treated groups in medium containing low glucose (1 mM) were significantly different from their control groups. *Indicates significant difference between groups.

in levels of active AMPK between high and low glucose containing medium could be the underlying cause of the difference in glycolytic metabolism stimulation by metformin treatment. To further confirm the role of AMPK in promoting glycolysis, MCF7 cells were treated with or without compound C (10 μM), a specific inhibitor of AMPK. After 15 hours in medium containing 25 mM glucose with or without metformin, ECAR as well as lactate measurements were obtained. The extent of ECAR augmentation and accumulation of lactate with metformin treatment was partially blocked by cotreatment with compound C (Figure 4E, 4F). This supports a role for metformin-induced AMPK activation in stimulating glycolysis in high glucose containing medium. In addition, these findings support the conclusion that failure to activate or maintain AMPK activation by metformin in low glucose containing medium leads to depletion of ATP.

To better understand the intracellular changes that occur with metformin treatment in high and low glucose media, protein levels of several kinases were examined. Both MCF7 and MDAMB231 cells were treated with metformin (8 mM) for one day in medium containing either 25 mM or 2.5 mM glucose. Western blotting was performed to test phosphorylation of AKT and targets of mTOR signaling. The response to metformin was greatly considerably altered in low glucose conditions. In low glucose conditions metformin was found to substantially reduce the phosphorylation of AKT and decrease the phosphorylation levels of targets of mTOR (S6K and 4EBP1), compared to high glucose conditions (Figure 5A, 5B). Since these pathways are known to promote cell survival as well as glycolytic metabolism, their inhibition by metformin may contribute to reduced glycolysis, subsequent depletion of ATP, and ultimately cell death.

In order to further investigate the role of glucose in protecting cells from metformin-induced death, the effects of glucose were compared to those of related sugars, including the hexoses fructose and galactose. It has previously been reported that fructose and galactose do not contribute significantly to glycolytic metabolism in cancer cells [26,27]. Furthermore, processing of galactose through glycolysis results in no net ATP synthesis. Based on these finding we predicted that fructose and galactose would be unable to support ATP synthesis in the presence of metformin. To test this, glucose-free cell culture medium was supplemented with glucose, fructose, or galactose and cultures were again analyzed for cell death (Figure 6A, 6B). Breast cancer cell lines MCF7 and MDAMB231 were treated with or without metformin for 1.5 days in DMEM containing glucose (0 or 25 mM), fructose (25 mM), galactose (25 mM), or fructose plus galactose (12.5 mM each). Similar to previous results, increasing the glucose concentration

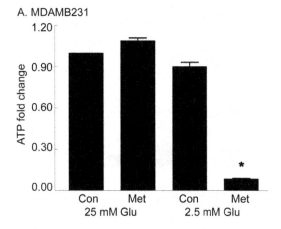
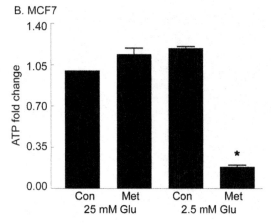
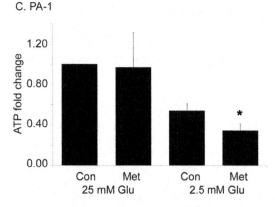

Figure 3. Metformin decreases ATP levels in medium containing low glucose (2.5 mM). MDAMB231 (**A**) and (**B**) MCF7 cells were treated with metformin (8 mM) in either 25 mM glucose or 2.5 mM glucose for one day and ATP levels were measured and fold change of ATP compared with control was plotted. **C.** ATP measurements in PA-1 cells after 12 hours with or without metformin. This time point was chosen because of the rapid rate of PA-1 growth under control culture conditions. Data were presented as mean ± standard deviation. All metformin treated groups in medium containing low glucose (2.5 mM) were significantly different from their control groups. *Indicates significant difference between groups.

substantially reduced the cytotoxicity of metformin in both MCF7 and MDAMB231 cells. However, fructose and galactose were not effective in preventing the cytotoxicity of metformin. ATP levels were also examined in cells treated with metformin in medium containing the various hexoses. Metformin treatment led to significantly decreased ATP levels in low glucose, high fructose, or high galactose conditions, but not in high glucose (25 mM) conditions. The reduction in ATP despite high fructose or galactose may explain why these sugars are unable to rescue the cells from metformin induced cytotoxicity.

To further examine glucose as a specific carbon source for maintaining glycolysis and the production of ATP in the presence of metformin, we next tested the effects of the drug on oxidative phosphorylation and glycolysis by measuring OCR and ECAR in 25 mM glucose, 25 mM fructose, or 25 mM galactose media. Metformin inhibited OCR in all three conditions (Figure 7A, 7C), consistent with its effects on electron transport. However, metformin stimulated glycolysis, as measured by ECAR, only in high glucose. Glycolytic metabolism was reduced with either fructose or galactose alone and was not enhanced by metformin treatment (Figure 7B, 7D). This further confirms the role of enhanced glycolysis in maintaining ATP levels and cell survival after oxidative phosphorylation was inhibited by metformin in high glucose containing medium. Failure to maintain highly activated glycolysis in medium containing low glucose, high fructose or high galactose contributes to the depletion of ATP and eventually to cell death caused by metformin.

The cell culture experiments described above suggest that limiting the availability of glucose to tumors would enhance the anti-cancer effects of metformin in vivo. To test this a calorie restricted low carbohydrate ketogenic diet was used to lower serum glucose in Balb/c mice. Tumors were established from mouse mammary cancer 4T1 cells and tumor growth was monitored. The low carbohydrate ketogenic diet (KD) significantly reduced serum glucose levels (Figure 8A) from ~6 mM to below 3 mM. Metformin appeared to induce a slight reduction in serum glucose levels in both diets. Metformin had no effect on tumor growth in mice being fed the control diet (CD). The ketogenic diet alone slowed tumor growth and the slowest tumor growth was observed in mice on the ketogenic diet that were treated with metformin (Figure 8B, 8C). This suggests that lowering glucose in vivo enhances metformin cytotoxicity to cancer cells.

Discussion

A common criticism of current metformin research is that in vitro concentrations are unattainable *in vivo*. While previous groups have shown that metformin is concentrated within cells, especially the mitochondria [28,29], the current work also suggests that the use of high glucose media masks some of the effects of metformin, requiring higher doses to mimic the effects observed *in vivo*. While commonly used glucose concentration is 25 mM in cell culture growth media, plasma levels of glucose are usually maintained in a range of 5–7 mM. Using low concentrations of glucose in vitro may also be more relevant to metformin's mechanism *in vivo*. Using low glucose concentrations can mimic the systemic glucose modulation effects of metformin and potentially provide a more accurate view of the pathways activated within cancer cells.

Our results support and extend previous observations of enhanced effects of glucose deprivation on metformin activity against tumor cells. Several groups have found synergism between metformin or other biguanides and 2-deoxyglucose, a compound that blocks glycolysis and has similar effects as glucose deprivation [16,30–32]. Menendez et al. [15] reported increased cell death of breast cancer cells when treated with metformin in the absence of glucose. Our data suggest that similar increases in cell death are observed when glucose is reduced to physiologic levels of

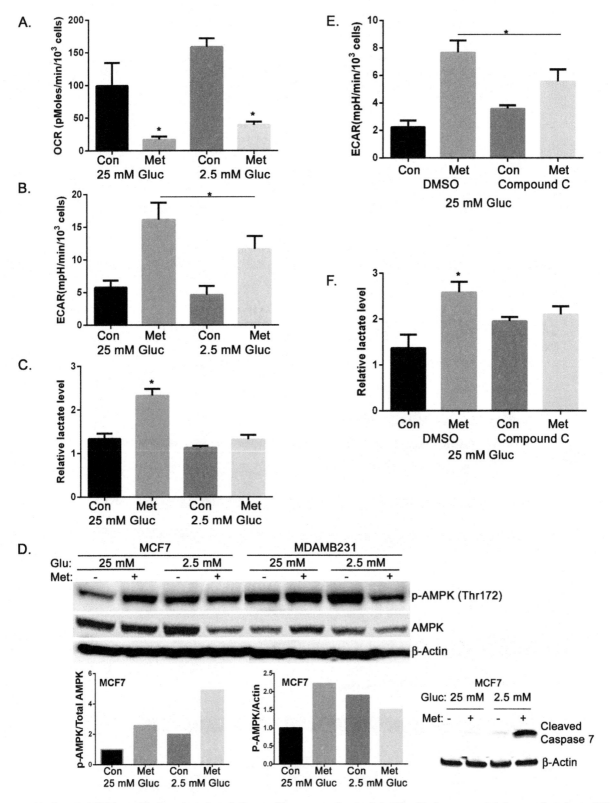

Figure 4. Metformin inhibits oxidative phosphorylation and increases glycolysis in 25 mM glucose containing medium in an AMPK-dependent manner. A. MCF7 cells were treated with metformin (8 mM) for 15 hours in either 25 mM or 2.5 mM glucose containing media. Oxygen consumption rate (OCR) was determined using the FX24 instrument for metabolic flux analysis. Metformin treated groups were significantly different from their control groups. **B.** MCF7 cells were treated with metformin (8 mM) for 15 hours. Extracellular acidification rate (ECAR) was determined using the FX24 instrument for metabolic flux analysis. Metformin treated groups were significantly different from each other and their control groups. **C.** MCF7 cells were treated with metformin (8 mM) for 15 hours, and medium lactate levels were measured as an indicator of glycolytic flux. Metformin treated groups were significantly different from each other. **D.** Extracts of MCF7 and MDAMB231 cells harvested one day treatment with metformin in either 25 or 2.5 mM glucose were used for Western blotting detection of phosphorylated AMPK and total AMPK. β-Actin was detected

as a loading control. Densitometry of p-AMPK/AMPK or p-AMPK/Actin for MCF7 cells is presented as a bar graph. Cleaved capsase 7 in MCF7 cells was detected with western blotting. β-Actin was detected as a loading control. **E.** MCF7 cells in high glucose were treated with metformin (8 mM) and compound C (10 μM) as indicated for 15 hours. DMSO is the vehicle control for compound C. ECAR was determined as described in B. Metformin treated groups were significantly different from each other. **F.** MCF7 cells in high glucose were treated with metformin (8 mM) and compound C (10 μM) as indicated for 15 hours. Medium lactate levels were determined as in C. Metformin treated groups were significantly different from each other. All bar graphs represent mean ± standard deviation. *Indicates significant difference between groups.

metformin and does not require complete elimination of the sugar. Saito et al. [33] also demonstrated that the cytotoxic effects of metformin and other biguanides to cancer cells are dramatically enhanced in glucose-free conditions. This same group went on to show that biguanides inhibit the unfolded protein response (UPR) that is induced by glucose deprivation. They found that this effect was mediated by hyperactivation of 4EBP1 through mTOR inhibition and that this was likely to be independent of AMPK [16]. Our data also show that metformin, in low glucose conditions, causes a dramatic decrease in phosphorylation of 4EBP1 and other mTOR targets, while at the same time failing to increase phosphorylated (active) AMPK. Javeshghani et al. [17] observed that the sensitivity of colon cancer cells to metformin was dependent on the fuel source. They found that the effects of metformin were enhanced by a lack of glucose but not by a lack of glutamine, which requires mitochondrial metabolism for production of ATP. As in our studies, they observed a drop in ATP levels when cells were treated with metformin under glucose deprivation. They also found that metformin could enhance lactate production only in cells cultured in high glucose conditions. Our results confirm these finding and also show that enhanced lactate production in metformin treated cells under high glucose

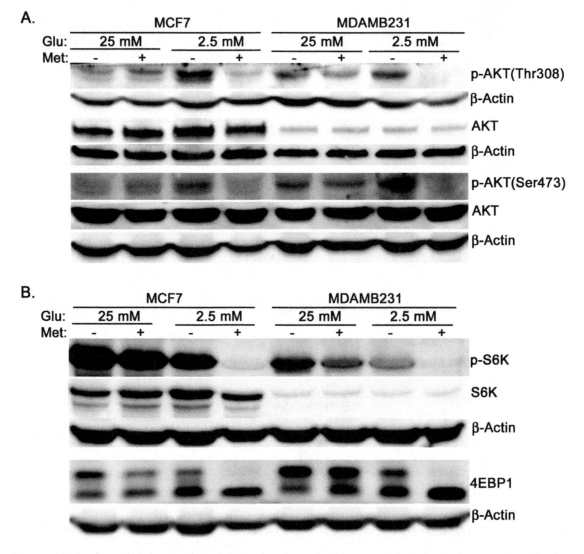

Figure 5. In low glucose medium metformin inhibits AKT phosphorylation and mTOR activation. MCF7 and MDAMB231 cells were treated with metformin in DMEM containing either 25 mM glucose or 2.5 mM glucose for one day. Western blotting was used to estimate the levels of p-AKT (Thr308), p-AKT (Thr473), total AKT, p-S6K, total S6K, 4EBP1 (lower bands represent hypophosphorylated and higher bands represent hyperphosphorylated), and β-actin as loading control.

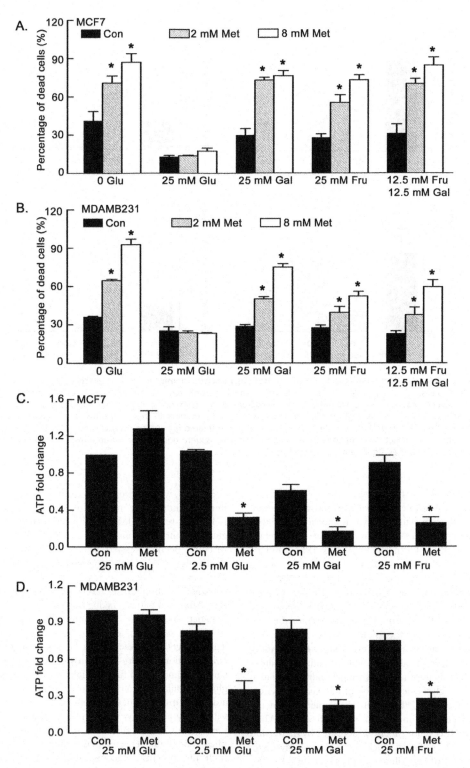

Figure 6. **Replacement of glucose with fructose or galactose does not prevent metformin induced cell death or metformin induced ATP reduction.** MCF7 (**A**) and MDAMB231 (**B**) cells were treated with metformin in DMEM without glucose, with 25 mM glucose, with 25 mM galactose, 25 mM fructose, or 12.5 mM fructose plus 12.5 mM galactose for 1.5 days. Percentage of dead cells was determined by Sytox Green staining. Metformin treated groups in 25 mM galactose, 25 mM fructose and 12.5 mM fructose plus 12.5 mM galactose were significantly different from metformin treated groups in 25 mM glucose. MCF7 (**C**) and MDAMB231 (**D**) cells were treated in the indicated medium with or without metformin (8 mM) for one day and ATP levels were measured. Metformin treated groups in 2.5 mM glucose, 25 mM galactose and 25 mM fructose were significantly different from their control groups. Results were displayed as fold change compared with control. Data are presented as mean ± standard deviation. *Indicates significant difference between groups.

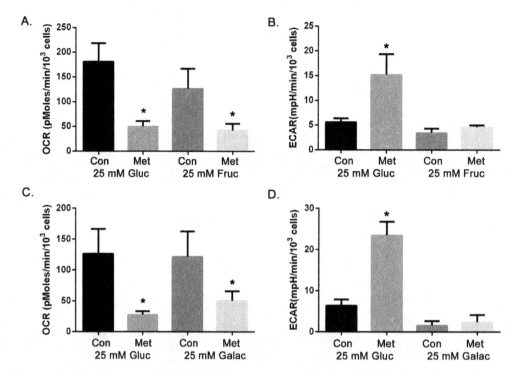

Figure 7. High fructose (25 mM) and galactose (25 mM) do not support metformin enhanced glycolysis as observed in high glucose medium (25 mM). MCF7 cells were treated with metformin (8 mM) in medium containing 25 mM glucose, 25 mM fructose or 25 mM galactose for 15 hours. OCR and ECAR were measured. **A.** OCR in either high glucose or fructose conditions, metformin treated groups were significantly different from their control groups, **B.** ECAR in either high glucose or fructose conditions, metformin treated groups were significantly different from each other, **C.** OCR in either high glucose or galactose containing media, metformin treated groups were significantly different from their control groups, **D.** ECAR in either high glucose or galactose conditions, metformin treated groups were significantly different from each other. Data are presented as mean ± standard deviation. *Indicates significant difference between groups.

conditions is associated with activation of AMPK. We have also found that the alternative hexose fuels fructose and galactose are unable to prevent metformin cytotoxicity. It is known that neither fructose or galactose contributes significantly to glycolytic metabolism in cancer cells [27]. Furthermore, the AMPK inhibitor compound C reduces the ability of metformin to promote glycolysis. This last observation is consistent with the findings of Shackelford et al. [34] who showed that loss of LKB1, a tumor suppressor that phosphorylates and activates AMPK, selectively enhances the anticancer effects of the biguanide phenformin.

Based on our results and the discussion above we propose that high glucose protects against metformin cytotoxicity by providing a fuel source for glycolytic metabolism, which maintains cellular ATP levels even when metformin blocks mitochondrial oxidative metabolism. Enhanced glycolytic metabolism induced by metformin requires activation of AMPK and the availability of glucose allows glycolytic metabolism to run at high efficiency. When glucose is limiting, AMPK is not effectively activated by metformin and cancer cells lack sufficient fuel to maintain glycolytic metabolism. Also, mTOR signalling is blocked in an AMPK-independent manner, further enhancing the metabolic deficiency. Cellular ATP becomes depleted, leading to energy collapse and cell death. This is consistent with previous reports of the ability of AMPK signalling to maintain ATP levels in response to hypoxia, fuel deprivation, and other stressors [35]. Interestingly, non-cancer cells do not appear to be sensitized to the cytotoxic effects of metformin by glucose deprivation (see Fig. 1D). It is likely that normal cells are less dependent on glucose as a fuel source and are able to maintain ATP levels by utilizing other glycolytic substrates.

Notably, when glucose concentration is lowered, the pH change in media induced by metformin treatment no longer occurs. This is likely a result of less lactate production when normal to low glucose concentrations are used. High lactate production has recently been proposed as a protective factor to glucose deprivation [36]. High glucose concentrations with metformin treatment may have increased lactate production and lactic acidosis in cell culture to levels that do not occur in patients. In type 2 diabetes patients taking metformin, the risk of lactic acidosis in patients with normal renal function is minimal and was found to be no greater than any other anti-hyperglycemic agent [37]. Taken together, these results suggest modifications in glucose concentration *in vitro* may provide a more accurate model of studying cancer, and further highlight the importance of reducing glucose availability to cancer cells. Despite a long history of use as a diabetes medication, the precise cellular actions of metformin are still largely a mystery. Furthermore, the mechanism of action for metformin's cancer inhibition and killing effects remains unidentified. The results reported in this study contribute to evidence that both the systemic glucose lowering effects and direct cancer cellular effects contribute to metformin's mechanism of action. The increased cancer cytotoxicity when glucose concentrations were lowered may also be evidence that the multiple pathways affected by metformin enhance one another to promote cancer cell death. As discussed above, alternative carbon energy sources such as fructose and galactose did not alter metformin's cancer inhibitory and cell death effects in the same manner as increasing glucose concentrations. This suggests that the altered cancer cell metabolism has sacrificed flexibility in carbon source in order to maintain rapid proliferation [26,27]. Thus, attempting to lower

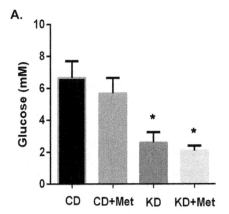

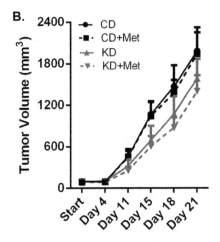

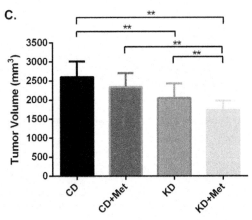

Figure 8. Ketogenic diets reduced serum glucose concentration and enhanced metformin effects on reducing 4T1 breast tumor growth in Balb/c mice. A. Serum glucose was measured and demonstrated as bar graph. Data are presented as mean ± standard deviation. Groups on Ketogenic diets are significant different from groups on control diets. **B.** Tumor growth was measured at indicated time for CD (control diet), CD+Met (control diet plus metformin), KD (ketogenic diet) and KD+Met (ketogenic diet plus metformin). CD+Met treatment group was significantly different from KD+Met treatment group after day 11. **C.** Tumor volume at day 23. Data are presented as mean ± standard deviation (**indicates significant difference between groups).

available glucose through methods such as diet may simultaneously enhance metformin treatment and inhibit cancer growth.

Zhou et al. showed that calorically restricted ketogenic diet could significantly lower plasma glucose level and was an effective therapeutic alternative for malignant brain tumor [38]. We used a similar commercially available ketogenic diet with calories restriction and successfully obtained serum glucose reduction from ~6 mM to below 3 mM in Balb/c mice. Mice on a ketogenic diet and metformin treatment showed the slowest tumor growth. This further emphasizes the importance of glucose deprivation in determining metformin cytotoxicity.

Oleksyszyn proposed using a ketogenic diet with metformin as anti-cancer therapy to control glucose levels [39]. This is based on the theory that systemically lowering serum glucose is associated with decreased tumor growth. In that proposal, the focus is the effects of metformin on controlling glucose levels by inhibiting gluconeogenesis rather than direct cytotoxicity to cancer cells. In the mouse model that we have used, metformin only slightly decreases glucose levels in mice on either the control or ketogenic diet. Therefore, the observed tumor growth inhibition with metformin treatment was most likely not due to its effects on glucose regulation but direct cytotoxicity on cancer cells. 4T1 tumor cells are known for their aggressive growth and metastasis in vivo [40]. This limits metformin treatment time before mice have to be euthanized due to emaciation or large tumor burden. This also explains why metformin has not shown effects on slowing tumor growth in mice on control diet with normal serum glucose and limited treatment time. Future studies might be done to evaluate the effects of a ketogenic diet without calorie restriction but with metformin treatment on tumor growth.

These results may also impact clinical use of metformin in cancer patients, as ketogenic diets may be utilized to promote low glucose states while still providing necessary energy for many normal cell types. Ketotic states are common in diets focused on carbohydrate reduction, and fasting states do not appear to be harmful to normal cells. Moreover, metformin and caloric restriction have both been shown to increase lifespan in mice [41] and caloric restriction trials for improved longevity in humans are gaining increased interest. In related studies, Zhu et al. [18] found that metformin combined with dietary energy restriction protected against new tumor occurrence in a rat mammary cancer model.

With metformin's extensive safety data from decades of use as a diabetic medication, another role for the drug may be as an adjuvant between other courses of therapy such as surgery, radiation, or traditional chemotherapy. In cancers that are difficult to screen and follow such as ovarian cancer, metformin could potentially have use as a relatively low side effect adjuvant therapy following surgical debulking. Because of metformin's low side effect profile, therapy could potentially be initiated much sooner following surgery and would generally not interfere with the standard chemotherapy schedule. In patients with lower risk stratification, where chemotherapy is generally not indicated, adjuvant therapies such as metformin may be a useful addition to routine surveillance. Metformin could potentially play a similar role in cancers as tamoxifen maintenance therapy in estrogen receptor positive breast cancers. While metformin's effect may not be as strong as tamoxifen's, metformin is also not limited by estrogen receptor status. Past metformin research has shown many benefits: from promising epidemiological data for cancer reduction [42] to direct cancer stem cell killing [11]. This research provides additional evidence that metformin has direct cancer cytotoxic effects, and that these effects are enhanced with lower glucose concentrations. Future research will help to better define metformin's role as a potential cancer therapy.

Acknowledgments

We thank Joseph D. Coppock for insight on experimental design and assistance with mouse study.

Author Contributions

Conceived and designed the experiments: YZ DKC ABH WKM. Performed the experiments: YZ DKC ABH. Analyzed the data: YZ DKC. Contributed reagents/materials/analysis tools: YZ DKC ABH WKM. Contributed to the writing of the manuscript: YZ DKC ABH WKM.

References

1. Sandulache VC, Ow TJ, Pickering CR, Frederick MJ, Zhou G, et al. (2011) Glucose, not glutamine, is the dominant energy source required for proliferation and survival of head and neck squamous carcinoma cells. Cancer.
2. Han L, Ma Q, Li J, Liu H, Li W, et al. (2011) High glucose promotes pancreatic cancer cell proliferation via the induction of EGF expression and transactivation of EGFR. PLoS One 6: e27074.
3. Sinnett-Smith J, Kisfalvi K, Kui R, Rozengurt E (2013) Metformin inhibition of mTORC1 activation, DNA synthesis and proliferation in pancreatic cancer cells: dependence on glucose concentration and role of AMPK. Biochem Biophys Res Commun 430: 352–357.
4. De Lorenzo MS, Baljinnyam E, Vatner DE, Abarzua P, Vatner SF, et al. (2011) Caloric restriction reduces growth of mammary tumors and metastases. Carcinogenesis 32: 1381–1387.
5. Lee C, Longo VD (2011) Fasting vs dietary restriction in cellular protection and cancer treatment: from model organisms to patients. Oncogene 30: 3305–3316.
6. Seyfried TN, Kiebish MA, Marsh J, Shelton LM, Huysentruyt LC, et al. (2011) Metabolic management of brain cancer. Biochim Biophys Acta 1807: 577–594.
7. DeFronzo RA, Goodman AM (1995) Efficacy of metformin in patients with non-insulin-dependent diabetes mellitus. The Multicenter Metformin Study Group. N Engl J Med 333: 541–549.
8. Rizkalla SW, Elgrably F, Tchobroutsky G, Slama G (1986) Effects of metformin treatment on erythrocyte insulin binding in normal weight subjects, in obese non diabetic subjects, in type 1 and type 2 diabetic patients. Diabete Metab 12: 219–224.
9. Knowler WC, Barrett-Connor E, Fowler SE, Hamman RF, Lachin JM, et al. (2002) Reduction in the incidence of type 2 diabetes with lifestyle intervention or metformin. N Engl J Med 346: 393–403.
10. Gotlieb WH, Saumet J, Beauchamp MC, Gu J, Lau S, et al. (2008) In vitro metformin anti-neoplastic activity in epithelial ovarian cancer. Gynecol Oncol 110: 246–250.
11. Hirsch HA, Iliopoulos D, Tsichlis PN, Struhl K (2009) Metformin selectively targets cancer stem cells, and acts together with chemotherapy to block tumor growth and prolong remission. Cancer Res 69: 7507–7511.
12. Buzzai M, Jones RG, Amaravadi RK, Lum JJ, DeBerardinis RJ, et al. (2007) Systemic treatment with the antidiabetic drug metformin selectively impairs p53-deficient tumor cell growth. Cancer Res 67: 6745–6752.
13. Vazquez-Martin A, Oliveras-Ferraros C, Menendez JA (2009) The antidiabetic drug metformin suppresses HER2 (erbB-2) oncoprotein overexpression via inhibition of the mTOR effector p70S6K1 in human breast carcinoma cells. Cell Cycle 8: 88–96.
14. Zhuang Y, Miskimins WK (2008) Cell cycle arrest in Metformin treated breast cancer cells involves activation of AMPK, downregulation of cyclin D1, and requires p27Kip1 or p21Cip1. J Mol Signal 3: 18.
15. Menendez JA, Oliveras-Ferraros C, Cufi S, Corominas-Faja B, Joven J, et al. (2012) Metformin is synthetically lethal with glucose withdrawal in cancer cells. Cell Cycle 11: 2782–2792.
16. Matsuo J, Tsukumo Y, Saito S, Tsukahara S, Sakurai J, et al. (2012) Hyperactivation of 4E-binding protein 1 as a mediator of biguanide-induced cytotoxicity during glucose deprivation. Mol Cancer Ther 11: 1082–1091.
17. Javeshghani S, Zakikhani M, Austin S, Bazile M, Blouin MJ, et al. (2012) Carbon source and myc expression influence the antiproliferative actions of metformin. Cancer Res 72: 6257–6267.
18. Zhu Z, Jiang W, Thompson MD, McGinley JN, Thompson HJ (2011) Metformin as an energy restriction mimetic agent for breast cancer prevention. J Carcinog 10: 17.
19. Zhuang Y, Miskimins WK (2011) Metformin induces both caspase-dependent and poly(ADP-ribose) polymerase-dependent cell death in breast cancer cells. Mol Cancer Res 9: 603–615.
20. Batandier C, Guigas B, Detaille D, El-Mir MY, Fontaine E, et al. (2006) The ROS production induced by a reverse-electron flux at respiratory-chain complex 1 is hampered by metformin. J Bioenerg Biomembr 38: 33–42.
21. Marsin AS, Bertrand L, Rider MH, Deprez J, Beauloye C, et al. (2000) Phosphorylation and activation of heart PFK-2 by AMPK has a role in the stimulation of glycolysis during ischaemia. Curr Biol 10: 1247–1255.
22. Wu SB, Wei YH (2012) AMPK-mediated increase of glycolysis as an adaptive response to oxidative stress in human cells: implication of the cell survival in mitochondrial diseases. Biochim Biophys Acta 1822: 233–247.
23. Andrade BM, Cazarin J, Zancan P, Carvalho DP (2012) AMP-activated protein kinase upregulates glucose uptake in thyroid PCCL3 cells independent of thyrotropin. Thyroid 22: 1063–1068.
24. Habibollahi P, van den Berg NS, Kuruppu D, Loda M, Mahmood U (2013) Metformin-an adjunct antineoplastic therapy-divergently modulates tumor metabolism and proliferation, interfering with early response prediction by 18F-FDG PET imaging. J Nucl Med 54: 252–258.
25. Smith TA, Zanda M, Fleming IN (2013) Hypoxia stimulates 18F-fluorodeoxyglucose uptake in breast cancer cells via hypoxia inducible factor-1 and AMP-activated protein kinase. Nucl Med Biol 40: 858–864.
26. Marroquin LD, Hynes J, Dykens JA, Jamieson JD, Will Y (2007) Circumventing the Crabtree effect: replacing media glucose with galactose increases susceptibility of HepG2 cells to mitochondrial toxicants. Toxicol Sci 97: 539–547.
27. Reitzer LJ, Wice BM, Kennell D (1979) Evidence that glutamine, not sugar, is the major energy source for cultured HeLa cells. J Biol Chem 254: 2669–2676.
28. El-Mir MY, Nogueira V, Fontaine E, Averet N, Rigoulet M, et al. (2000) Dimethylbiguanide inhibits cell respiration via an indirect effect targeted on the respiratory chain complex I. J Biol Chem 275: 223–228.
29. Owen MR, Doran E, Halestrap AP (2000) Evidence that metformin exerts its anti-diabetic effects through inhibition of complex 1 of the mitochondrial respiratory chain. Biochem J 348 Pt 3: 607–614.
30. Ben Sahra I, Laurent K, Giuliano S, Larbret F, Ponzio G, et al. (2010) Targeting cancer cell metabolism: the combination of metformin and 2-deoxyglucose induces p53-dependent apoptosis in prostate cancer cells. Cancer Res 70: 2465–2475.
31. Sandulache VC, Ow TJ, Pickering CR, Frederick MJ, Zhou G, et al. (2011) Glucose, not glutamine, is the dominant energy source required for proliferation and survival of head and neck squamous carcinoma cells. Cancer 117: 2926–2938.
32. Lea MA, Chacko J, Bolikal S, Hong JY, Chung R, et al. (2011) Addition of 2-deoxyglucose enhances growth inhibition but reverses acidification in colon cancer cells treated with phenformin. Anticancer Res 31: 421–426.
33. Saito S, Furuno A, Sakurai J, Sakamoto A, Park HR, et al. (2009) Chemical genomics identifies the unfolded protein response as a target for selective cancer cell killing during glucose deprivation. Cancer Res 69: 4225–4234.
34. Shackelford DB, Abt E, Gerken L, Vasquez DS, Seki A, et al. (2013) LKB1 inactivation dictates therapeutic response of non-small cell lung cancer to the metabolism drug phenformin. Cancer Cell 23: 143–158.
35. Bonini MG, Gantner BN (2013) The multifaceted activities of AMPK in tumor progression-why the "one size fits all" definition does not fit at all? IUBMB Life 65: 889–896.
36. Wu H, Ding Z, Hu D, Sun F, Dai C, et al. (2011) Central role of lactic acidosis in cancer cell resistance to glucose deprivation-induced cell death. J Pathol.
37. Salpeter SR, Greyber E, Pasternak GA, Salpeter EE (2010) Risk of fatal and nonfatal lactic acidosis with metformin use in type 2 diabetes mellitus. Cochrane Database Syst Rev: CD002967.
38. Zhou W, Mukherjee P, Kiebish MA, Markis WT, Mantis JG, et al. (2007) The calorically restricted ketogenic diet, an effective alternative therapy for malignant brain cancer. Nutr Metab (Lond) 4: 5.
39. Oleksyszyn J (2011) The complete control of glucose level utilizing the composition of ketogenic diet with the gluconeogenesis inhibitor, the anti-diabetic drug metformin, as a potential anti-cancer therapy. Med Hypotheses 77: 171–173.
40. Aslakson CJ, Miller FR (1992) Selective events in the metastatic process defined by analysis of the sequential dissemination of subpopulations of a mouse mammary tumor. Cancer Res 52: 1399–1405.
41. Martin-Montalvo A, Mercken EM, Mitchell SJ, Palacios HH, Mote PL, et al. (2013) Metformin improves healthspan and lifespan in mice. Nat Commun 4: 2192.
42. Evans JM, Donnelly LA, Emslie-Smith AM, Alessi DR, Morris AD (2005) Metformin and reduced risk of cancer in diabetic patients. BMJ 330: 1304–1305.

Putrescine-Dependent Re-Localization of TvCP39, a Cysteine Proteinase Involved in *Trichomonas vaginalis* Cytotoxicity

Bertha Isabel Carvajal-Gamez[1], Laura Itzel Quintas-Granados[1], Rossana Arroyo[2], Laura Isabel Vázquez-Carrillo[1], Lucero De los Angeles Ramón-Luing[2], Eduardo Carrillo-Tapia[1], María Elizbeth Alvarez-Sánchez[1]*

[1] Genomic Sciences Postgraduate, Autonomous University of Mexico City (UACM), Mexico City, Mexico, [2] Department of Infectomics and Molecular Pathogenesis, Center for Research and Advanced Studies, IPN, Mexico City, Mexico

Abstract

Polyamines are involved in the regulation of some *Trichomonas vaginalis* virulence factors such as the transcript, proteolytic activity, and cytotoxicity of TvCP65, a cysteine proteinase (CP) involved in the trichomonal cytotoxicity. In this work, we reported the putrescine effect on TvCP39, other CP that also participate in the trichomonal cytotoxicity. Parasites treated with 1,4-diamino-2-butanone (DAB) (an inhibitor of putrescine biosynthesis), diminished the amount and proteolytic activity of TvCP39 as compared with untreated parasites. Inhibition of putrescine biosynthesis also reduced ~80% the *tvcp39* mRNA levels according to RT-PCR and qRT-PCR assays. Additionally, actinomycin D-treatment showed that the *tvcp39* mRNA half-life decreased in the absence of putrescine. However, this reduction was restored by exogenous putrescine addition, suggesting that putrescine is necessary for *tvcp39* mRNA stability. TvCP39 was localized in the cytoplasm but, in DAB treated parasites transferred into exogenous putrescine culture media, TvCP39 was re-localized to the nucleus and nuclear periphery of trichomonads. Interestingly, the amount and proteolytic activity of TvCP39 was recovered as well as the *tvcp39* mRNA levels were restored when putrescine exogenous was added to the DAB-treated parasites. In conclusion, our data show that putrescine regulate the TvCP39 expression, protein amount, proteolytic activity, and cellular localization.

Editor: Heidar-Ali Tajmir-Riahi, University of Quebect at Trois-Rivieres, Canada

Funding: The work was supported by grants from Universidad Autónoma de la Ciudad de México (UACM) and by grants from Consejo Nacional de Ciencia y Tecnología (CONACyT) (83808) and Instituto de Ciencia y Tecnología del Distrito Federal (ICyT-DF) (PIFUTP08-150) to MEAS. BICG was supported by a scholarship from ICyT-DF Mexico. The funders had no role in study design, data collection and analysis, decision to publish, or preparation of the manuscript.

Competing Interests: The authors have declared that no competing interests exist.

* Email: elizbethalvarezsanchez@yahoo.com.mx

Introduction

Trichomonosis is the most common non-viral sexually transmitted infection (STI) caused by *Trichomonas vaginalis*. This infection mainly affects women, causing vaginitis, cervictis, urethritis, and infertility [1,2]. It also causes low birth weight infants, preterm delivery [3], and a predisposition to cervical neoplasia [4]. It is also considered as a cofactor in the transmission of the human immunodeficiency virus [5]. According to the genome sequence this parasite contains an expanded degradome of more than 400 peptidases such as metallo, cysteine, serine, threonine, and aspartic peptidases [6]. The *T. vaginalis* cysteine proteinases (CPs) play important roles in trichomonad pathogenesis such as cytoadherence, immune evasion, haemolysis, and cytotoxicity [7–12]. The synthesis and proteolytic activity of certain CPs are regulated by environmental factors such as iron, pH, oxidation-reduction capacity, temperature, and polyamines [9,11,13–15]. The 39 kDa CP (TvCP39), which was found in vaginal washes from patients with trichomonosis and it is localized in the parasite surface, is involved in cytotoxicity to HeLa, DU145 and vaginal epithelial cells (VECs). Interestingly, this CP is *in vivo* and *in vitro* secreted by *T. vaginalis*, and is active in the pH range found in human vagina and prostate [11].

Recently, it has been shown that polyamines are essential nutrient for pathogens that can regulate a variety of trichomonal properties such as cytoadherence and cytotoxicity [14,16]. A link between trichomonosis infection and polyamines has been suggested by the presence of putrescine in the vaginal fluid of trichomonosis patients [17–19]. Quantitative analyses of polyamines in vaginal washes from patients with trichomonosis showed that putrescine and cadaverine are present at high concentrations (0.27 and 0.96 mM, respectively). However, other polyamines as spermine, and spermidine were undetectable [20]. Interestingly, spermine and spermidine are present in the semen at high concentration levels (2.29 and 251 µM, respectively), suggesting that the main contribution of these polyamines is through this fluid [21]. However, the amount of putrescine and other diamines in vaginal secretions were undetectable in patients after get cured [20], suggesting that parasite metabolism is the primary source of putrescine during women infection. Putrescine is synthesized by the ornithine decarboxylase enzyme (ODC), which can be inhibited by polyamine analogues such as 1,4-diamino-2-butanone

(DAB) or by 2-difluoromethyl ornithine (DFMO) [19]. Previous studies showed that *T. vaginalis* treated with 20 mM DAB resulted in growth arrest. Additionally, the amount of adhesins involved in trichomonal adherence did not change in DAB-treated parasites; however, an increase in *T. vaginalis* adherence was observed [16]. Interestingly, the addition of 40 mM putrescine to DAB-treated trichomonads was used to rescue growth arrest, and reduced the elevated levels of adherence [16].

Since in TvCP65 is involved in trichomonal cytotoxicity and the expression, protein amount, and proteolytic activity of this CP were reduced in DAB-treated parasites, we suggested that probably exist a relationship between the parasite virulence and polyamines concentration in *T. vaginalis* [14]. However, the polyamines effect on TvCP39 another cysteine protease involved in trichomonal cytotoxicity is still unknown. In this study, we focused on determinate the effect of putrescine on TvCP39 and we found that these cations regulate the *tvcp39* expression, mRNA stability and proteolytic activity, but also the TvCP39 cellular localization.

Materials and Methods

1. *T. vaginalis* culture and inhibition/restoration of putrescine metabolism

Late-logarithmic-phase trophozoites of *T. vaginalis* isolate CNCD147 grown for 24 h in Diamond's trypticase-yeast extract-maltose (TYM) medium pH 6.2 with 10% heat-inactivated horse serum (Gibco) (normal media) at 37°C were used for all assays. The putrescine metabolism inhibition was performed as previously reported [14,22]. Parasite viability after these treatments was checked by the trypan blue (Sigma) exclusion method [23].

2. RNA extraction and cDNA synthesis

Total RNA from 2×10^7 parasites grown in the absence or presence of 20 mM DAB in TYM medium for 24 h, and DAB-treated parasites transferred into 40 mM exogenous putrescine medium for 30 min at 37°C and into TYM medium (as a control). The RNA was extracted using TRizol reagent (Invitrogen), according to the manufacturer's protocol. Purified RNA was digested with DNase I (Invitrogen) to discard the DNA contaminant, according to the manufacturer's protocol. RNA concentration and purity were determined by measuring absorbance using NanoDrop 2000 (Thermo Scientific); all 260/280 ratios were between 1.8 and 2.1. Then, 1 μg of total RNA was reverse-transcribed using the Superscript II Reverse Transcriptase Kit (Invitrogen), according to the manufacturer's protocol using the oligo-dT (dT_{18}) (10 pmol/μl) primer.

3. Analysis of *tvcp39* expression by semi-quantitative and quantitative RT-PCR

To validate the expression of *tvcp39* in different putrescine conditions, RT-PCR analysis were performed using 50 ng cDNA from parasites grown in the absence or presence of 20 mM DAB, or DAB-treated parasites transferred into 40 mM exogenous putrescine medium, 10 pmol of each primer pair and 0.25 U of Taq DNA polymerase (Invitrogen). PCR was carried out in a GeneAmp PCR System 9700 thermal cycler (Applied Biosystems Inc., Foster City, CA, USA). Specific primer pairs were designed using Primer3 software version 3.0 (www.primer3.sourceforge.net). We used the following primer pairs to amplify: 110 bp of the *tvcp39* gene (accession number XM_001316379), sense (CP39-FRT) 5' CAGTATGCTATCACAACAGG 3' and antisense (CP39-RRT) 5' CGCCCTGGTGCTTGACAACAT 3'; and 112 bp of the *β-tubulin* gene as reported [24]. The amplified products were analyzed on 2% agarose gels and visualized by ethidium bromide staining. Gene expression densitometry analyses were performed using the Quantity One Software (BioRad). Data from densitometry quantification of the housekeeping gene (*β-tubulin*) were used to normalize the results.

To further support the semi-quantitative data, qRT-PCR was performed using the SYBR Green (QIAGEN) stain, according to the manufacturer's instructions. Specific primers pairs were used: sense CP39-FRT and antisense CP39-RRT. The reaction was carried out in optical 96-well standard plates (Applied Biosystems). PCR was performed with an initial incubation at 94°C for 3 min, followed by 40 cycles at 94°C for 30 s, 60°C for 30 s, and 72°C for 30 s. The reaction was terminated by a final incubation at the dissociation temperatures. The relative quantification of *tvcp39* expression was calculated after the threshold cycle (Ct) and was normalized with the Ct of *β-tubulin* (*β-tub*) gene. Furthermore, the expression of *tvcp39* in different putrescine conditions was expressed as normalized Ct values. All reactions including no-template and RT minus controls for each mRNA were run in triplicate. All experimental data were expressed as means ± standard deviation (SD) from three separate biological experiments. The significance of the difference between means was determined by ANOVA with Prisma Firewall 1.53 software. The level of significance was also determined by the Bonferroni multiple comparisons test.

4. Actinomycin D Half-Life Experiments

tvcp39 mRNA stability was monitored in DAB-treated, DAB-putrescine-treated, and untreated parasites using the transcriptional inhibitor actinomycin D (Sigma). Trichomonads were incubated in TYM medium with 50 μg/ml actinomycin D in dimethyl sulfoxide [25] at 37°C. Parasites (2.0×10^7) were taken at different time-points (0, 1, 3, 6, 8, 12, and 24 h) after transcriptional blockage. Total RNA from trichomonads was extracted by TRIzol, followed by semi-quantitative RT-PCR analysis to detect the presence and stability of *tvcp39* mRNA. The *tvcp39* and *β-tub* mRNA levels were analyzed on ethidium bromide–stained agarose gels and quantified by densitometric analysis with the Quantity One software (BioRad). The *tvcp39* mRNA levels were normalized with the *β-tub* mRNA. The experiment was performed by triplicate and the data were used to calculate the half life. The pixels produced by the *tvcp39* transcript in trichomonads cultured without treatment (t_0) were defined as 100% for each condition to determine the stability time of *tvcp39* transcript. The experimental *tvcp39* mRNA half-life (the time at which 50% of mRNA molecules remained intact) was determined by the quantity of *tvcp39* mRNA at different times. The theoretical half-life of *tvcp39* mRNA was obtained from the logarithmically transformed best-fit line by linear regression analysis using the decay equation $t½ = \ln 2/K$, where K corresponds to the decay constant, using the Sigmaplot program.

5. Western Blot assays

Cytoplasmic, nuclear and total protein extract obtained from (2×10^7) DAB-putrescine-treated and untreated parasites were loaded on a 12% polyacrylamide gel with an equivalent of 4×10^5 parasites/lane. Proteins were transferred to nitrocellulose membranes (BioRad) for 20 min at 20 V using a semi-dry transfer electroblotting system (Trans-blot SD Semi-Dry Transfer Cell, BioRad). The membranes were blocked with 5% skim milk in PBS pH 7.0 –0.05%Tween solution at 4°C for 18 h and subsequently incubated at 4°C overnight with distinct antibodies anti-CP39 (1:1000 dilution), anti-PCNA (1:3000) [26], anti-nucleoporin antibody (1:1000), anti-TveIF-5A antibody (1:100) [22] or anti-α tubulin (1:3000)(Zymed Laboratories, South San Francisco, CA) used as a control. After 3 washes with PBS, the peroxidase conjugated secondary antibody (1:3000) was added to the membrane and incubated at room temperature for 1 h, washed with PBS, developed by the enhanced chemiluminescence ECL Plus Western Blotting Detection System (GE Healthcare), using a Kodak AR film (Kodak, Rochester, NY) exposed for 5 min.

6. Indirect immunofluorescence assays

Parasites grown in the presence or absence of 20 mM DAB were fixed using 4% paraformaldehyde for 1 h at 37°C and washed with PBS pH 7.0. Half of the fixed parasites were permeabilized using 1 M HCl for 2 h at room temperature, blocked with 0.2 M glycine for 1 h at 37°C followed by 0.2% fetal bovine serum for 15 min. Then trichomonads were incubated with polyclonal mouse anti-TvCP39 antibody (1:100 dilution) or preimmune sera (PI) for 18 h at 4°C, washed with PBS, incubated with fluorescein isothiocyanate-conjugated anti-mouse immunoglobulins (1:90 dilution, Jackson ImmunoResearch) for 40 min at room temperature, washed and mounted with Vectashield-DAPI mounting solution (Vector Lab).

For re-localization assays, parasites grown in the presence of DAB and transferred into 40 mM exogenous putrescine were fixed, permeabilized, and blocked as previously described. Trichomonads were then incubated with polyclonal rabbit anti-TvCP39 antibody (1:100 dilution) and polyclonal mouse HSP70 antibody (1:150) for 18 h at 4°C. Parasites were incubated with fluorescein isothiocyanate-conjugated anti-rabbit and tetra-methylrhodamine isothiocyanate (TRITC) anti-mouse immunoglobulins (both 1:90 dilution, Jackson ImmunoResearch) for 1 h at room temperature, and Vectashield-DAPI mounting solution was added. All samples were observed and analyzed using a Leica, DMLS laser-scanning confocal microscopy, and all photographs were taken at the same exposure time.

7. Translational blockage by cycloheximide treatment

Translational inhibition in trichomonads cultured in normal and DAB-treated conditions was obtained by adding 10 μg/ml of cycloheximide (Sigma) into the culture medium at time 0 of growth at 37°C [25] and monitored at different time-points (0, 4, 8, 12, and 24). Normal and DAB-treated parasites were transferred into 40 mM putrescine containing medium and incubated at 37°C for extra time (15, 30, and 60 min). After that, total protein extract was obtained from 2×10^7 parasites by 10% TCA-precipitation as previously described [9]. Solubilized proteins were boiled in sample buffer [27], separated by SDS-PAGE in a 12% polyacrylamide gel, transferred onto nitrocellulose membranes, and western blot assays were performed to detect TvCP39 using the anti-TvCP39 antibody [28]. The anti-tubulin antibody was used as a loading control. Three independent experiments were performed for each time interval, and each measurement was in duplicate.

8. Proteinase activity and cell-binding assay

The cell-binding assay to detect proteinases with affinity to the host cell surface was performed as previously described [29]. Parasites (2×10^7) grown in the absence or presence of DAB, and DAB-treated parasites recovered by exogenous putrescine addition were incubated for 18 h at 4°C with 1×10^6 fixed HeLa cells. Then trichomonad proteinases bound to the surface of fixed cells were eluted in Laemmli buffer [27] for 20 min at 37°C. Released proteinases were separated on 10% SDS-PAGE gel copolymerized with 2% gelatin. Gels were washed with 10% Triton X-100 for 10 min with gentle agitation and proteinase activation was performed in 100 mM sodium acetate buffer pH 4.5 with 0.1% β-mercaptoethanol for 18 h at 4°C. The gels were further stained with Coomassie Brilliant Blue for a visualization in which clear bands against a dark background indicate proteolytic activity. In addition, we analyzed the proteinase activity of total protein extracts from all conditions as controls. Densitometry analyses of activity bands were performed in triplicate using the software Quantity One version 4.6.3 (BioRad).

Furthermore, the proteolytic activity of the cytoplasmic and nuclear extract was determinate as described above.

Results

The putrescine effect on the TvCP39 proteolytic activity

The TvCP39 proteolytic activity was analyzed by zymograms. Fig. 1A shows the proteolytic activity of total protein extract from trichomonads grown in normal media (N) (Fig. 1A, lane 1), 20 mM DAB-treated trichomonads (D) (Fig. 1A, lane 2) and DAB-treated parasites and transferred into exogenous putrescine medium (DP) (Fig. 1A, lane 3). In addition the proteinase activity pattern from DAB-treated trichomonad transferred into normal medium (DN) (Fig. 1A, lane 4) and trichomonads grown in normal media and transferred into exogenous putrescine media (NP) (Fig. 1A, lane 5) were used as controls. The zymograms showed that no major changes were observed on total lysates from the DAB-treated parasites (Fig. 1A, lane 2), as compared with untreated control parasites (Fig. 1A, lane 1). These results are consistent with the previously reported [14]. These extracts were also used for cell-binding assays using fixed HeLa cells followed by substrate gel electrophoresis to analyze the proteolytic activity of the TvCP39 bound to HeLa cells (Fig. 1B). The proteolytic activity from TvCP39 bound to the surface of HeLa cells (N) (Fig. 1B, lane 1) was taken as 100% for comparison. Figure 1C showed the densitometric analyses of the TvCP39 proteolytic activity. Interestingly, the proteolytic activity of TvCP39 decreased ~80% in DAB-treated parasites (D) (Fig. 1B, lane 2 and Fig. 1C). In DAB-treated parasites transferred to exogenous putrescine (DP) (Fig. 1B, lane 3), the TvCP39 activity was ~90% restored (Fig. 1C) but not in those parasites transferred into a normal media (DN) (20%) (Fig. 1B, lane 4 and Fig. 1C), suggesting that the activity restoration was due to the exogenous putrescine addition. In the control trichomonads grown in normal media transferred into an exogenous putrescine media (NP)(Fig. 1B, lane 5), the TvCP39 activity was similar to that observed in normal-grown parasites (100%)(Fig. 1C).

TvCP39 transcript levels, protein amount and localization depend on putrescine

Moreover, to determine whether the *tvcp39* mRNA levels and protein amount correlate with the TvCP39 proteolytic activity, we performed RT-PCR, qRT-PCR and Western blot assays. Consistently, the *tvcp39* mRNA levels decreased in DAB-treated parasites (D)(Fig. 2A, lane 2), and this effect was reverted by the addition of exogenous putrescine (DP)(Fig. 2A, lane 3). In DAB-treated parasites transferred into normal medium a partial recovery of the *tvcp39* mRNA levels was observed (DN)(Fig. 2A, lane 4) and in parasites grown in normal culture medium and transferred into a exogenous putrescine medium, the *tvcp39* mRNA levels (NP)(Fig. 2A, lane 5) were similar to levels observed in parasites grown in normal culture medium (N)(Fig. 2A, lane 1). As a loading control, the 112-bp product from *β-tubulin* was amplified and no changes were observed (Fig. 2A, lanes 1 to 5). Furthermore, qRT-PCR assay showed that the *tvcp39* mRNA

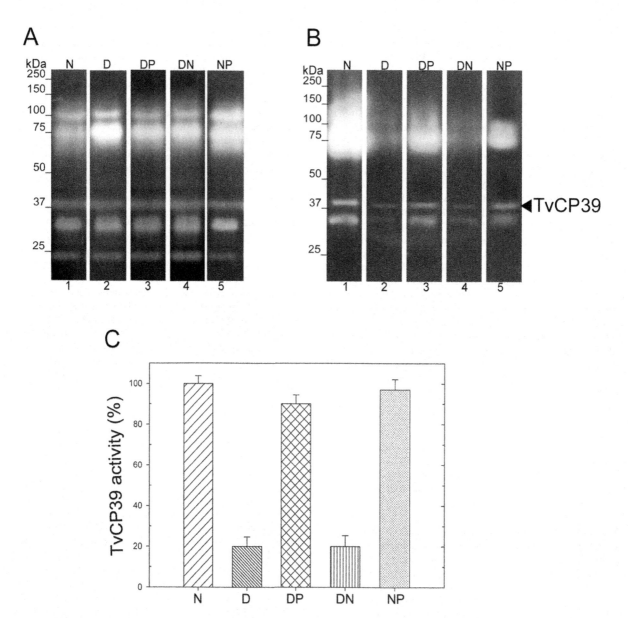

Figure 1. Putrescine effect on the TvCP39 activity from *T. vaginalis*. A) Putrescine effect on the proteolytic activity of *T. vaginalis*. Zimograms using total proteinases from parasites grown in normal media (N)(lane 1), DAB-treated parasites (D)(lane 2), DAB-treated parasites transferred into exogenous putrescine (DP)(lane 3), DAB-treated trichomonads transferred into a normal medium (DN)(lane 4) and parasites grown in normal medium transferred into an exogenous putrescine media (NP)(lane 5). B) Polyamine effect on the proteinases activity bound to HeLa cells. Ligand-proteinases assays using untreated parasites grown in normal medium (N)(lane 1); DAB-treated parasites (D)(lane 2); DAB-treated parasites transferred into exogenous putrescine media (DP)(lane 3), DAB-treated parasites transferred into normal media (DN)(lane 4) and parasites grown in normal media and transferred into an exogenous putrescine media (NP)(lane 5). Arrowhead shows the TvCP30 proteolytic activity. C) Densitometry analyses of TvCP39 proteolytic activity bands from panel B. Bars indicate the average of the intensity of TvCP39 activity bands from three independent ligand-proteinases assays and error bars represent the standard deviations.

expression decreased about 80% ($p<0.05$) in DAB-treated parasites (Fig 2B, bar D), and addition of exogenous putrescine restored the expression of *tvcp39* mRNA in about 70% ($p<0.05$)(Fig. 2B, bar DP), compared with trichomonad grown in normal culture medium (Fig. 2B, bar N).

We also analyzed whether the reduction in TvCP39 proteolytic activity correlated with the protein amount by western blot assay using the anti-TvCP39 antibody (1: 6000) [28]. The amount of TvCP39 decreased in DAB-treated parasites (D)(Fig. 2C, lane 2) compared with the amount observed in parasites grown in normal culture media (N)(Fig. 2C, lane 1). However, it was recovered in ~90 in DAB-treated parasites transferred into exogenous putrescine media (DP)(Fig. 2C, lane 3). In contrast, in DAB-treated parasites transferred into a normal media (DN)(Fig. 2C, lane 4) a partial recovery of TvCP39 amount was observed. In parasites grown in normal culture medium and transferred into a exogenous putrescine medium (NP)(Fig. 2C, lane 5), the TvCP39 amount was similar to the amount observed in parasites grown in normal culture medium (N)(Fig. 2C, lane 1). All this data suggested that the restoration TvCP39 amount and transcript levels were due to the exogenous putrescine addition.

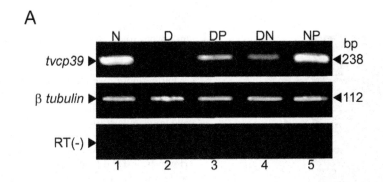

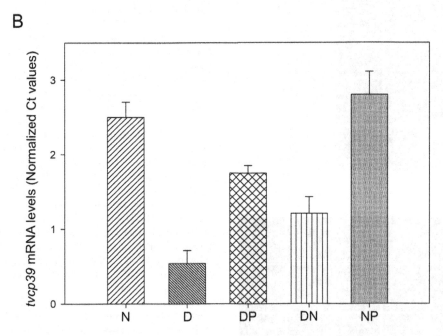

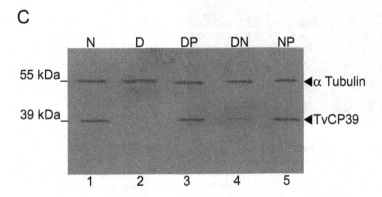

Figure 2. Putrescine effect on TvCP39 transcript and protein. A) Semi-quantitative RT-PCR analysis performed with total RNA from untreated parasites grown in normal medium (N)(lane 1); DAB-treated parasites (D)(lane 2,); DAB-treated trichomonads transferred into 40 mM exogenous putrescine medium (DP)(lane 3); DAB-treated trichomonads transferred to normal medium (DN)(lane 4), and trichomonads grown in normal medium and transferred into 40 mM exogenous putrescine medium (NP)(lane 5) to amplify 238 bp from the *tvcp39*. A 112 pb amplicon from *β-tubulin* was amplify as a loading control. B) qRT-PCR of samples described in A. The Ct levels of *tvcp39* mRNA in trichomonads after DAB treatment (bar D) decreased at 20% but the *tvcp39* mRNA were restored (70%) by adding 40 mM exogenous putrescine to DAB-treated parasites (bar DP). C) Total protein extract from *T. vaginalis* grown in normal media (N)(lane 1); DAB-treated parasites (D)(lane 2); DAB-treated trichomonads transferred into exogenous putrescine media (DP)(lane 3); DAB-treated parasites transferred into normal medium (DN)(lane 4) and trichomonads grown in normal medium transferred to medium with 40 mM exogenous putrescine (NP)(lane 5) were blotted onto nitrocellulose membranes and incubated with anti-TvCP39 and anti-α-tubulin (loading control) antibodies. Arrowheads indicate the immunodetected protein for each antibody employed.

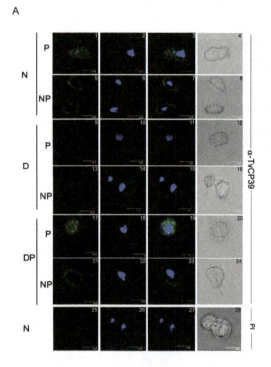

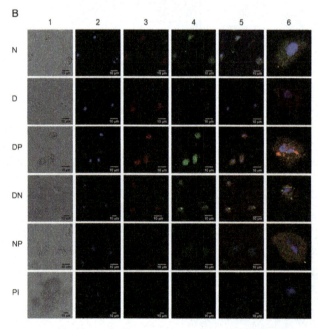

Figure 3. Putrescine effect on TvCP39 localization. A) TvCP39 localization in the polyamine presence. Immunofluorescence analysis of fixed, permeabilized (P; 1-4, 9-12, and 17-20) and Non permeabilized (NP; 5-8, 13-16, and 21,24) parasites untreated (N) (1-8), DAB-treated (D) (9-16), or DAB-treated transferred into exogenous putrescine media (DP) (17-24) incubated with the anti-TvCP39 antibody (1-24) or preimmune sera (PI; 25-28) followed by secondary anti-mouse conjugated to a fluorescein isothiocyanate (Jackson) antibody (1:90 dilution) and mounted with Vectashield-DAPI. Photographs were taken under laser confocal microscopy (Leica, DMLS). B) Re-localization of TvCP39. Immunofluorescence analyses of fixed and permeabilized parasites that were untreated (Panel N1 to N6) or DAB-treated (Panel D1 to D6), or DAB-treated transferred into exogenous putrescine media (Panel DP1 to DP6), or normal culture parasites that were transferred into exogenous putrescine media (Panel NP1 to NP6). The parasites were incubated with the antibody raised against TvCP39 (green) and anti-HSP70 (red) or with preimmune sera (Panel PI). Nuclei are labeled with DAPI (blue). Photographs were taken under laser confocal microscopy (Leica, DMLS). Scale bar = 10 µm.

Furthermore, we analyzed the putrescine effect over the TvCP39 location by indirect immunofluorescence assays using fixed and permeabilized and non-permeabilized in DAB-treated and untreated parasites. TvCP39 was located in the cytoplasm and at the surface of permeabilized and non-permeabilized parasites, respectively (Fig. 3A, panels 1-8) in normal-grown parasites (N). However, in DAB-treated parasites (D), the TvCP39 fluorescence signal was very low in both types of parasites (Fig. 3A, panels 9–16). Interestingly, the addition of exogenous putrescine (DP) restored the TvCP39 fluorescence signal in the cytoplasm and at the surface of parasites in vesicular forms (Fig. 3A, panels 17–24). Interestingly and unexpectedly, TvCP39 was also observed in the parasite nucleus (Fig. 3A, panels 17–20), suggesting an uncharacterized TvCP39 nuclear function.

In order to confirm the TvCP39 nuclear localization, as a control, we localize HSP70 in the same parasites (Fig. 3B). The TvCP39 was located in the nucleus and nuclear periphery only in DAB-treated parasites transferred into exogenous putrescine media (DP) (Fig. 3B, panels DP1 to DP6) as compared with normal-grown trichomonad (Fig. 3B, panels N1 to N6) and DAB-treated parasites (Fig. 3B, panel D1 to D6), used as controls. HSP70 (red chanel) was localized dispersed in the cytoplasm, nuclear periphery and nucleus in the all conditions (Fig. 3B, panels N3, D3, DP3, DN3, and NP3). Interestingly, in DAB-treated trichomonads that were transferred into exogenous putrescine media, TvCP39 co-localized with HSP70 (Fig. 3B, panel DP6), showed a portion of the protein in the nucleus. These results suggest that TvCP39 is re-localized by the addition of putrescine after DAB treatment.

Furthermore, cytoplasmic (Cyt) and nuclear (Nuc) protein fractions obtained from parasites grown in the putrescine depleted conditions were analyzed by Western blot assays using the anti-TvCP39 antibody (Fig. 4A).

TvCP39 was localized in the cytoplasmic fraction in normal culture trichomonads (N)(Fig. 4A, panel TvCP39 lane 3) but not in the nuclear fraction (Fig. 4A, panel TvCP39 lane 4). Interestingly, TvCP39 was localized in the nuclear fraction in DAB-treated parasites transferred into exogenous putrescine media (DP)(Fig. 4A, panel TvCP39, lane 2) and in the cytoplasmic fraction (Fig. 4A, panel TvCP39 lane 1). Antibodies anti-TveIF-5A (cytoplasmic protein, 20 kDa), anti-nucleoporin (nuclear pore protein, 53 kDa), and anti-PCNA (proliferating cellular nuclear antigen, 28 kDa) were used as fractionation controls [22,26]. TveIF-5A was observed in the cytoplasm (Fig. 4A, panel TveIF-5A lanes 1 and 3), consistent with previous report [30]. The nucleoporin protein was immunodetected in the nuclear fraction (Fig. 4A, panel nucleoporin lanes 2 and 4) as previously reported [31]. On the other hand, PCNA has a nuclear localization (Fig. 4A, panel PCNA lanes 2 and 4), this result is in agreement to *Entamoeba histolytica* PCNA protein localization [26]. According to these results, the fractionation was reliable, suggesting that TvCP39 is located in the nucleus only after DAB treatment and restoration with exogenous putrescine addition.

In order to determinate if TvCP39 was an active proteinase when it is localized in the nucleus, we performed zymograms using the cytoplasmic and nuclear fractions described above (Fig. 4B). In normal culture trichomonads (N), we observed the TvCP39 proteolytic activity band in the cytoplasmic (Fig. 4B, lane 3) but not in the nuclear fraction (Fig. 4B, lane 4). Interestingly, in DAB-treated parasites transferred into exogenous putrescine media (DP), we observed a proteolytic activity band corresponding to TvCP39 activity in the nuclear (Fig. 4B, lane 2) and cytoplasmic fractions (Fig. 4B, lane 1).

The *tvcp39* mRNA stability depends on putrescine

Furthermore, we evaluate the putrescine effect over the mRNA stability. In untreated parasites, the *tvcp39* mRNA stability was 12 h after the transcription blockage (Fig. 5A, panel N tvcp39, lanes 1 to 6). In contrast, in DAB-treated parasites, the mRNA stability diminished up to 3 h after transcriptional blockage (Fig. 5, panel D tvcp39, lanes 1 to 3). Interestingly, the *tvcp39* RNAm stability is restored in DAB-treated parasites transferred into putrescine medium (Fig. 5A, panel DP tvcp39, lanes 1 to 4). In DAB-treated parasites transferred into normal medium, no *tvcp39* mRNA stability recovery was observed (Fig. 5A, panel DN tvcp39, lanes 1 to 3). Besides, in parasites grown in normal medium and transferred into exogenous putrescine (Fig. 5A, panel NP tvcp39, lanes 1 to 6), the *tvcp39* stability observed was similar from parasites grown in normal culture media. The *β-tubulin* transcript was used as a loading control (Fig. 5A, panels N βtub, D βtub, DP βtub, DN βtub, and NP βtub) and its stability (>24 h) did not change in all tested conditions.

The *tvcp39* mRNA half-life was estimated to be ~2.5±0.5 h in parasites grown in normal culture medium (Fig. 5B, N). In DAB-treated parasites, the transcript half-life was 45±10 min (Fig. 5B, D). Interestingly, the *tvcp39* mRNA half-life in DAB-treated parasites transferred into exogenous putrescine media was ~2.3±0.5 h (Fig. 5B, DP). The DAB-treated parasites transferred into normal medium, and parasites grown in normal medium and transferred into exogenous putrescine medium were used as controls (Fig. 5B, DN and NP).

Putrescine is necessary for TvCP39 stability

Finally, we compared the effects of actinomycin D and cycloheximide on TvCP39 protein stability in parasites grown in the presence or absence of putrescine using western blot assay (Fig. 5C). In normal culture conditions (N), TvCP39 protein was present up to 12 h (Fig. 5C, lanes 1 to 4); however, at 24 h its amount decreased considerably (Fig. 5C, lane 5). In contrast, in DAB-treated parasites (D) the TvCP39 protein amount started to decrease at 4 h (Fig. 5C, lane 7) and it was continued decreasing until 24 h (Fig. 5C, lanes 8 to 10).

Interestingly, in DAB-treated parasites transferred into exogenous putrescine medium (DP), a TvCP39 amount restoration was observed (Fig. 5C, lanes 11 to 14). These results suggest that putrescine is necessary for TvCP39 protein stability after DAB treatment. No changes were observed in the immunodetection of αtubulin protein (loading control) in all tested conditions (Fig. 5C, lanes 1 to 14). The densitometric analysis (Fig. 5D) performed using biological triplicates are in agreement with the results described above.

Discussion

T. vaginalis contains multiple cysteine proteinases [6], and TvCP65 is well described as a virulence factor of this parasite [9,14,32]. Moreover, another CP with a molecular mass of 39 kDa (TvCP39) participates in the cellular damage caused by *T. vaginalis* [28]. TvCP39 specifically binds to host cell surfaces and is immunogenic in patient with trichomonosis [12,28,33]. In this work, we show that TvCP39 proteolytic activity was up regulated by exogenous putrescine addition after DAB treatment. Our finding suggest that TvCP39 proteolytic activity might vary

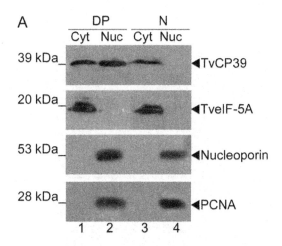

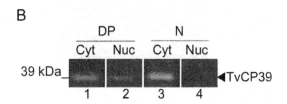

Figure 4. TvCP39 re-localization after DAB treatment and putrescine restoration. A) Cytoplasmic (Cyt) and nuclear (Nuc) protein extract from DAB-treated parasites transferred into exogenous putrescine media (DP) (lanes 1 and 2) and from untreated parasites grown in normal media (N)(lanes 3 and 4) were blotted into a nitrocellulose membrane and incubated with anti-TvCP39, anti-TvelF-5A (control of cytoplasmic protein), anti-nucleoporin (control of nuclear protein) and anti-PCNA (control of nuclear protein) antibodies. Arrowheads show TvCP39 (39 kDa), the TvelF-5A (20 kDa), the nucleoporin (53 kDa), and the PCNA (28 kDa) protein bands. B) Zymograms from Cytoplasmic (Cyt) and nuclear (Nuc) protein extract from DAB-treated parasites transferred into exogenous putrescine media (DP) (lanes 1 and 2) and from untreated parasites grown in normal media (N)(lanes 3 and 4). Arrowhead indicates the TvCP39 proteolytic activity.

during infection, probably by the fluctuations in putrescine concentrations in the vaginal environment [34]. Interestingly, TvCP39 is down regulated by iron [11]; therefore, we suggest that *T. vaginalis* virulence factors, such as TvCP39, are regulated by several environmental host factors.

Our data show that the decreasing in the TvCP39 proteolytic activity correlated with its amount. These results are similar to those reported for TvCP65 [14]. According to our results, putrescine in *T. vaginalis* play important role in the regulation of TvCP39. In other organisms these polycations also regulate basic functions such as replication, transcription, translation, post-translation modifications. In *Plasmodium falciparum* the polyamines depletion arrested the invasion in the early trophozoite stage [35]. In *Leishmania donovani* the ODC activity is necessary for human infections and survival in the host [36]. These data show the important role of the polyamines metabolism in protozoan. DAB acts as an antiparasitic in others protozoan inhibiting the virulence properties [37,38], but the mechanism is still unknown. The 39 kDa CP is just one of several CP involved in the cellular damage caused by *T. vaginalis*. Others include the TvCP65 that also requires polyamines for expression [14].

TvCP39 is localized in the cytoplasm and parasite membrane [12,28]. Interestingly, in DAB-treated parasites and after exoge-

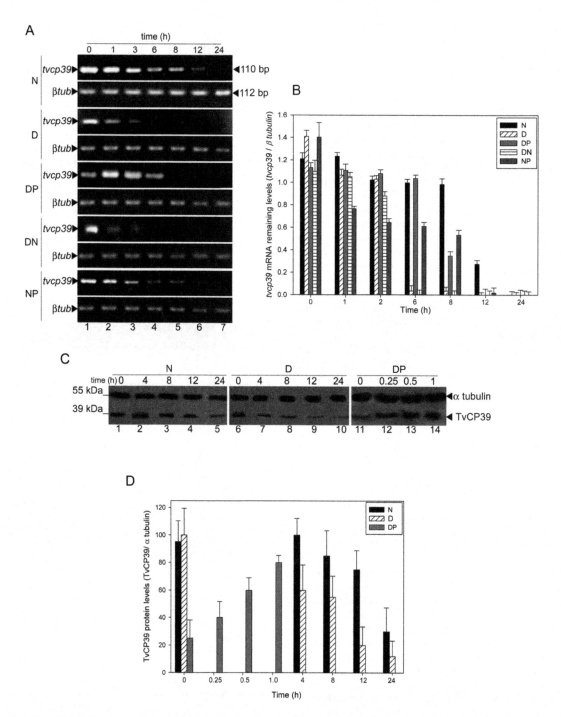

Figure 5. The *tvcp39* mRNA and protein stabilities are regulated by putrescine. A) RNAm levels of *tvcp39* by semi-quantitative RT-PCR analysis using total RNA from parasites treated with actinomycin D and grown in normal culture media (N); or DAB-treated parasites (D); or DAB-treated trichomonads transferred into 40 mM exogenous putrescine medium (DP); or DAB-treated trichomonads transferred to normal medium (DN); or trichomonads grown in normal medium and transferred into 40 mM exogenous putrescine medium (NP). Samples were taken at 0, 1, 3, 6, 8, 12 and 24 h for amplification of 110 pb of *tvcp39* mRNA and 112 bp of β-tubulin mRNA (β-tub)(loading control). Arrowheads indicate the amplification products obtained. B) Transcriptional blockade using actinomycin D. Trichomonads grown in normal medium (N), DAB-treated trichomonads (D), DAB-treated trichomonads transferred into 40 mM exogenous putrescine medium (DP), DAB-treated trichomonads transferred into normal medium (DN), and trichomonads grown in normal medium and transferred into an exogenous putrescine medium (NP) were treated with actinomycin D. Samples taken at several times (0, 1, 2, 6, 8, 12, and 24 h) were use to amplified the *tvcp39* mRNA which was quantified by densitometric analysis and normalized. Bars represent the mean of each sample and the standard errors were included. C) Blockage of protein synthesis by cycloheximide. Trichomonads were treated with 10 μg of cycloheximide and grown in normal culture media (N); or DAB-treated parasites (D); or DAB-treated trichomonads transferred into 40 mM exogenous putrescine medium (DP). Samples were taken at several times for Western blot analysis using anti-TvCP39 (dilution 1: 1000) and α-tubulin (dilution 1:100) antibodies. Arrowheads indicate the TvCP39 and α-tubulin proteins. D) Densitometric analysis of the samples described in C. The bands corresponded to TvCP39 were quantified and normalized to α tubulin. Bars represent the mean of three biological triplicates.

nous putrescine addition, TvCP39 was also detected in the nucleus. This re-localization might be related to a novel TvCP39 function, further studies are necessary to elucidate it.

However, nuclear localization of a CP is not unusual for example; EhCP4 of *Entamoeba histolytica* was localized into cytoplasmic vesicles, the nuclear region and perinuclear endoplasmic reticulum [39]. Interestingly, EhCP4 plays a key role in disrupting the colonic epithelial barrier and the innate host immune response during invasion.

Moreover, the mammalian cathepsin L isoform responsible for proteolytic processing of the N-terminal histone 3 (H3) tail, also has a nuclear localization and this proteinase is an active enzyme in the nucleus [40,41]. This cathepsin L was originally described as a lysosomal protease; however, in the nucleus plays an important role as a chromosomal regulator in the proteolytic processing of the transcriptional factor CDP/Cux and histone H3 [40,41]. In addition, serpin A3G (SpiA3G), a proteinase that under a proinflammatory stimulus macrophages it was relocalized into the nucleolus that co-localizes with cathepsin L, and only the stimulus induce increased nucleolar localization of SpiA3G. Interestingly, the SpiA3g translocation into the nucleolus might be important in host defense against pathogens [42]. The nuclear localization of all these CPs is usually associated with cell cycle or differentiation. The nuclear localization of TvCP39 might be related to an environmental stress caused by putrescine depletion. Although, the nuclear TvCP39 is an active enzyme, the specific role of this proteinase in the nucleus and its transport mechanism remain unknown. Work is in progress to elucidate them.

On the other hand, the TvCP39 protein and *tvcp39* mRNA stability also were affected by putrescine depletion. Moreover, polyamines depletion decreased the mRNA levels, stability and protein amount of TveIF-5A, a polyamine-dependent protein due polyamines are required for the unique posttranslational modification called hypusination [22], suggesting an autoregulatory mechanism in which TveIF-5A modulates the stability of its own transcript [22].

In conclusion, putrescine affects virulence factors of *T. vaginalis*, such as TvCP39. In putrescine absence, the protein and mRNA stability and also the protein amount decreased. However, the putrescine-depletion effect was reverted by the putrescine exogenous addition.

Acknowledgments

We want to thank Dr. Luis Brieba for donating the *Entamoeba histolytica*. anti-PCNA antibody. We appreciate the excellent technical support of Alfredo Padilla.

Author Contributions

Conceived and designed the experiments: MEAS. Performed the experiments: BICG LIQG. Analyzed the data: BICG LIQG ECT. Contributed reagents/materials/analysis tools: RA. Wrote the paper: BICG LIQG. LIVC LARL.

References

1. Schwebke JR, Burgess D (2004) Trichomoniasis. Clin Microbiol Rev 17: 794–803.
2. El-Shazly AM, El-Naggar HM, Soliman M, El-Negeri M, El-Nemr HE, et al. (2001) A study on *Trichomoniasis vaginalis* and female infertility. J Egypt Soc Parasitol 31: 545–553.
3. Cotch MF, Pastorek II JG, Nugent RP, Hillier SL (1997) *Trichomonas vaginalis* associated with low birth weight and preterm delivery. Sexually Trans Dis 24: 353–360.
4. Viikki M, Pukkala E, Nieminen P, Hakama M (2000) Gynaecological infections as risk determinants of subsequent cervical neoplasia. Acta Oncol 9: 71–75.
5. Guenthner PC, Secor WE, Dezzutti CS (2005) *Trichomonas vaginalis*-Induced Epithelial Monolayer Disruption and Human Immunodeficiency Virus Type 1 (HIV-1) Replication: Implications for the Sexual Transmission of HIV-1. Infect Immun 73: 4155–4160.
6. Carlton JM, Hirt RP, Silva JC, Delcher AL, Schatz M, et al. (2007) Draft Genome Sequence of the Sexually Transmitted Pathogen *Trichomonas vaginalis*. Science 315: 207–212.
7. Neale KA, Alderete JF (1990) Analysis of the proteinases of representative Trichomonas vaginalis isolates. Infect Immun 58: 157–162.
8. Provenzano D, Alderete JF (1995) Analysis of human immunoglobulin-degrading cysteine proteinase of *Trichomonas vaginalis*. Infect Immun 63: 3388–3395.
9. Alvarez-Sanchez ME, Avila-Gonzalez L, Becerril-Garcia C, Fattel-Facenda LV, Ortega-Lopez J, et al. (2000) A novel cysteine proteinase (CP65) of *Trichomonas vaginalis* involved in cytotoxicity. Microbial Pathogenesis 28: 193–202.
10. Mendoza-Lopez MR, Becerril-Garcia C, Fattel-Facenda LV, Avila-Gonzalez L, Ruiz-Tachiquin ME, et al. (2000) CP30, a Cysteine Proteinase Involved in *Trichomonas vaginalis* Cytoadherence. Infect Immun 68: 4907–4912.
11. Hernandez-Gutierrez R, Ortega-López J, Arroyo R (2003) A 39-kDa Cysteine Proteinase CP39 from *Trichomonas vaginalis*, Which Is Negatively Affected by Iron May Be Involved in Trichomonal Cytotoxicity. J Euk Microbiol 50: 696–698.
12. Hernández-Gutiérrez R, Avila-González L, Ortega-López J, Cruz-Talonia F, Gómez-Gutierrez G, et al. (2004) *Trichomonas vaginalis*: characterization of a 39-kDa cysteine proteinase found in patient vaginal secretions. Exp Parasitol 107: 125–135.
13. Bozner P, Demes P (1990) Proteinases in *Trichomonas vaginalis* and *Tritrichomonas mobilensis* are not exclusively of cysteine type. Parasitology 102.
14. Alvarez-Sanchez ME, Carvajal-Gamez BI, Solano-Gonzalez E, Martinez-Benitez M, Garcia AF, et al. (2008) Polyamine depletion down-regulates expression of the *Trichomonas vaginalis* cytotoxic CP65, a 65-kDa cysteine proteinase involved in cellular damage. International J of Biochem and Cell Biol 40: 2442–2451.
15. Coombs GH, North MJ (1983) An analysis of the proteinases of *Trichomonas vaginalis* by polyacrylamide gel electrophoresis. Parasitology 86: 1–6.
16. Garcia AF, Benchimol M, Alderete JF (2005) *Trichomonas vaginalis* Polyamine Metabolism Is Linked to Host Cell Adherence and Cytotoxicity. Infection and Immunity 73: 2602–2610.
17. Reis IA, Martinez MP, Yarlett N, Johnson PJ, Silva-Filho FC, et al. (1999) Inhibition of Polyamine Synthesis Arrests Trichomonad Growth and Induces Destruction of Hydrogenosomes. Antimicrob Agents Chemother 43: 1919–1923.
18. Yarlett N, Bacchi CJ (1988) Effect of dl-[alpha]-difluoromethylornithine on polyamine synthesis and interconversion in *Trichomonas vaginalis* grown in a semi-defined medium. Mol Biochem Parasitol 31: 1–9.
19. Yarlett N, Bacchi CJ (1994) Parasite polyamine metabolism: targets for chemotherapy. Biochem Soc Trans 4: 875–879.
20. Chen KC, Forsyth PS, Buchanan TM, Holmes KK (1979) Amine content of vaginal fluid from untreated and treated patients with nonspecific vaginitis. The Journal of Clinical Investigation 63: 828–835.
21. Rui H, Gerhardt P, Mevåg B, Thomassen Y, Purvis K (1984) Seminal plasma characteristics during frequent ejaculation. Int J Androl 7: 119–128.
22. Carvajal-Gamez BI, Arroyo R, Camacho-Nuez M, Lira R, Martínez-Benitez M, et al. (2011) Putrescine is required for the expression of eif-5a in *Trichomonas vaginalis*. Mol Biochem Parasitol 180: 8–16.
23. Alvarez-Sánchez ME, Solano-González E, Yañez-Gómez C, Arroyo R (2007) Negative iron regulation of the CP65 cysteine proteinase cytotoxicity in *Trichomonas vaginalis*. Microbes Infect 9: 1597–1605.
24. Leon-Sicairos CR, Leon-Felix J, Arroyo R (2004) tvcp12: a novel *Trichomonas vaginalis* cathepsin L-like cysteine proteinase-encoding gene. Microbiol 150: 1131–1138.
25. Lehker MW, Arroyo R, Alderete JF (1991) The regulation by iron of the synthesis of adhesins and cytoadherence levels in the protozoan *Trichomonas vaginalis*. J Exp Med 174: 311–318.
26. Cardona-Felix CS, Lara-Gonzalez S, Brieba LG (2011) Structure and biochemical characterization of proliferating cellular nuclear antigen from a parasitic protozoon. Acta Crystallographica Section D 67: 497–505.
27. Laemmli UK (1970) Cleavage of structural proteins during the assembly of the head of bacteriophage T4. Nature 227: 680–685.
28. Ramón-Luing LdlÁ, Rendón-Gandarilla FJ, Puente-Rivera J, Ávila-González L, Arroyo R (2011) Identification and characterization of the immunogenic cytotoxic TvCP39 proteinase gene of Trichomonas vaginalis. The International Journal of Biochemistry & Cell Biology 43: 1500–1511.
29. Arroyo R, Alderete JF (1995) Two *Trichomonas vaginalis* surface proteinases bind to host epithelial cells and are related to levels of cytoadherence and cytotoxicity. Arch Med Res 26: 279–285.
30. Carvajal-Gamez B, Arroyo R, Lira R, López-Camarillo C, Alvarez-Sánchez ME (2010) Identification of two novel *Trichomonas vaginalis* eif-5a genes. Infection, Genetics and Evolution 10: 284–291.
31. Grünwald D, Singer RH, Rout M (2011) Nuclear export dynamics of RNA-protein complexes. Nature 475: 333–341.

32. Solano-González E, Alvarez-Sánchez ME, Avila-González L, Rodríguez-Vargas VH, Arroyo R, et al. (2006) Location of the cell-binding domain of CP65, a 65 kDa cysteine proteinase involved in *Trichomonas vaginalis* cytotoxicity. International J of Biochem and Cell Biol 38: 2114–2127.
33. Ramon-Luing LA, Rendon-Gandarilla FJ, Cardenas-Guerra RE, Rodrıguez-Cabrera NA, Ortega-Lopez J, et al. (2010) Immunoproteomics of the active degradome to identify biomarkers for *Trichomonas vaginalis*. Proteomics 10: 435–444.
34. Sanderson BE, White E, Baldson MJ (1983) Amine content of vaginal fluid from patients with trichomoniasis and gardnerella associated non-specific vaginitis. Br J Vener Dis 59: 302–305.
35. Becker J, Mtwisha L, Crampton B, Stoychev S, van Brummelen A, et al. (2010) *Plasmodium falciparum* spermidine synthase inhibition results in unique perturbation-specific effects observed on transcript, protein and metabolite levels. BMC Genomics 11: 235.
36. Boitz JM, Yates PA, Kline C, Gaur U, Wilson ME, et al. (2009) *Leishmania donovani* Ornithine Decarboxylase Is Indispensable for Parasite Survival in the Mammalian Host. Infection and Immunity 77: 756–763.
37. Calvo-Méndez C, Villagómez-Castro JC, López-Romero E (1993) Ornithine decarboxylase activity in *Entamoeba invadens*. International Journal for Parasitology 23: 847–852.
38. Arteaga-Nieto P, Villagómez-Castro JC, Calvo-Méndez C, López-Romero E (1996) Partial purification and characterization of ornithine decarboxylase from *Entamoeba histolytica*. International Journal for Parasitology 26: 253–260.
39. He C, Nora GP, Schneider EL, Kerr ID, Hansell E, et al. (2010) A Novel *Entamoeba histolytica* Cysteine Proteinase, EhCP4, Is Key for Invasive Amebiasis and a Therapeutic Target. Journal of Biological Chemistry 285: 18516–18527.
40. Goulet B, Baruch A, Moon N-S, Poirier M, Sansregret LL, et al. (2004) A Cathepsin L Isoform that Is Devoid of a Signal Peptide Localizes to the Nucleus in S Phase and Processes the CDP/Cux Transcription Factor. Molecular cell 14: 207–219.
41. Duncan EM, Muratore-Schroeder TL, Cook RG, Garcia BA, Shabanowitz J, et al. (2008) Cathepsin L Proteolytically Processes Histone H3 During Mouse Embryonic Stem Cell Differentiation. Cell 135: 284–294.
42. Konjar Š, Yin F, Bogyo M, Turk B, Kopitar-Jerala N (2010) Increased nucleolar localization of SpiA3G in classically but not alternatively activated macrophages. FEBS Letters 584: 2201–2206.

Methyllycaconitine Alleviates Amyloid-β Peptides-Induced Cytotoxicity in SH-SY5Y Cells

XiaoLei Zheng[1], ZhaoHong Xie[1], ZhengYu Zhu[1], Zhen Liu[1], Yun Wang[1], LiFei Wei[1], Hui Yang[1], HongNa Yang[1], YiQing Liu[1], JianZhong Bi[1,2,3]*

[1] Department of Neural Medicine, Second Hospital of Shandong University, Jinan, China, [2] Institute of Neurology, Shandong University, Jinan, China, [3] Key Laboratory of Translational Medicine on Neurological Degenerative Disease in Universities of Shandong (Shandong University), Jinan, China

Abstract

Alzheimer's disease (AD) is a chronic progressive neurodegenerative disorder. As the most common form of dementia, it affects more than 35 million people worldwide and is increasing. Excessive extracellular deposition of amyloid-β peptide (Aβ) is a pathologic feature of AD. Accumulating evidence indicates that macroautophagy is involved in the pathogenesis of AD, but its exact role is still unclear. Although major findings on the molecular mechanisms have been reported, there are still no effective treatments to prevent, halt, or reverse Alzheimer's disease. In this study, we investigated whether $A\beta_{25-35}$ could trigger an autophagy process and inhibit the growth of SH-SY5Y cells. Furthermore, we examined the effect of methyllycaconitine (MLA) on the cytotoxicity of $A\beta_{25-35}$. MLA had a protective effect against cytotoxicity of Aβ, which may be related to its inhibition of Aβ-induced autophagy and the involvement of the mammalian target of rapamycin pathway. Moreover, MLA had a good safety profile. MLA treatment may be a promising therapeutic tool for AD.

Editor: James A. Duce, The University of Melbourne, Australia

Funding: This research was supported by the National Natural Science Foundation of China (No. 81171214, 81371420), Shandong Province Natural Science Foundation (ZR2011HM064) and Jinan Science and Technology Development Foundation (201202048). The funders had no role in study design, data collection and analysis, decision to publish, or preparation of the manuscript.

Competing Interests: The authors have declared that no competing interests exist.

* Email: bjz@sdu.edu.cn.

Introduction

Alzheimer's disease (AD), the most prevalent form of dementia in older adults, is a chronic progressive neurodegenerative disorder [1]. AD patients have severe progressive cognitive dysfunction, memory impairment, behavioral symptoms and loss of independence [2]. According to Alzheimer's Disease International (ADI), at least 35.6 million people had dementia in 2010, with the numbers nearly doubling every 20 years [3]. Many factors contribute to the etiology of AD, elevated amyloid-β peptide (Aβ) and loss of nicotinic acetylcholine receptors (nAChRs) being prominent [4]. Extracellular amyloid plaques, predominantly consisting of Aβ, and intracellular neurofibrillar tangles, formed by hyperphosphorylated tau, are the major pathological hallmarks in the brain of AD patients [5]. Abnormal Aβ protein accumulation represents a key feature and is the triggering mechanism of subsequent cerebral degradation in AD [6].

Aβ is generated predominantly as a 40- or 42-amino acid peptide from amyloid precursor protein (APP) on sequential cleavage by β-secretase and the γ-secretase complex [7]. $A\beta_{1-42}$ has a strong ability to oligomerize to form diffusible dimers and trimers as well as larger oligomers, which induces early synaptotoxic effects and progressive dendritic-spine loss in AD [8]. $A\beta_{25-35}$ is neurotoxic when forming oligomers, which is similar to $A\beta_{1-42}$ [9]. Aβ plays a critical role in the pathogenesis of AD and is associated with energy failure, neuronal apoptosis and neuron loss in the AD brain [10]. The mechanism of Aβ in AD pathogenesis is still unclear. However, suppressing Aβ-induced cytotoxicity has become the focus of much AD research.

Macroautophagy (hereafter referred to as autophagy) is an evolutionarily conserved lysosomal-dependent pathway degrading long-lived or misfolded proteins and damaged organelles. It is an intracellular self-defense process by providing an adaptive strategy for cell survival in eukaryotes [11]. Specific membrane segments elongate, encapsulate part of the cytoplasm, and form double-membrane structures to generate an autophagosome. Autophagosomes become autolysosomes by fusion with endosome or lysosome containing proteases (autophagic maturation), and their inner-membrane and contents undergo clearance [12]. In autophagy studies, LC3 is proposed to act during elongation and expansion of the phagophore membrane. LC3 is cleaved to generate the cytosolic LC3-I with a C-terminal glycine residue, which is conjugated to phosphatidylethanolamine. The lipidated form of LC3 (LC3-II) is attached to both faces of the phagophore membrane but is ultimately removed from the autophagosome outer membrane, which is followed by fusion of the autophagosome with a late endosome/lysosome [13]. Mammalian target of rapamycin (mTOR) is a master controller of autophagy. Activated mTORC1 enhances protein translation by directly phosphorylating 4E-binding protein 1 and p70S6K to negatively regulate autophagy, which is involved in normal physiological processes, including aging, and the pathogenesis of diverse diseases, such as certain types of neuronal degeneration and cancer [14]. Autophagy pathology has been observed in AD. A massive accumulation of autophagic vacuoles was observed in dystrophic neurites in an animal model of AD and in postmortem brains from AD patients, which colocalized intimately with β-secretase complexes, APP, and γ-secretase-derived C-terminal fragment (γ-CTF). Here, autophagy seems to be abnormal because of alteration in the endolysosomal pathway, which impairs fusion of autophagosomes with lysosomes [15]. It is indicated that abnormal Aβ-related autophagic vacuoles accumulation may closely cause neuron dysfunction and neuron loss, thereby leading to Alzheimer's neurodegeneration [16,17].

Neuronal nicotinic acetylcholine receptors (nAChRs) are a family of ligand gated ion channels widely distributed in the human brain. Multiple subtypes of these receptors are involved in a wide range of physiological and behavioral processes, including cognitive enhancement, increased arousal and decreased anxiety and neuroprotection [18]. AD is characterized by a loss of neurons, particularly those expressing nAChRs. The loss of nAChRs has been detected in several regions of the brains of patients with AD, which is thought to underlie memory impairment and cognitive deficits in AD [19]. In our previous study, we found that granulocyte colony-stimulating factor could improve the learning and memory deficits of APP transgenic mice by up-regulating α7nAChR in the brain [20]. $Aβ_{1-42}$ co-immunoprecipitated with α7nAChR in postmortem samples of hippocampal tissue from patients with AD [21]. This suggests that Aβ and α7nAChR may have a high affinity and binding interaction. All the evidences have revealed that α7nAChR may play an important role in the Aβ-induced pathogenic process of AD.

Methyllycaconitine (MLA), a norditerpenoid alkaloid isolated from the seeds of Delphinium brownii, is one of the most potent and specific α7nAChR ligands that bind to neuronal α-bungarotoxin sites. Because of its specific, concentration-dependent, reversible, and voltage-independent antagonism, it could inhibit acetylcholine- and anatoxin-induced whole-cell currents in cultured fetal rat hippocampal neurons [22]. One recent report showed that MLA and the weak (<10%) agonist NS6740 reduced lipopolysaccharide-induced tumor necrosis factor α release, so α7nAChR antagonism may confer anti-inflammatory properties on microglia. As well, antagonism of α7nAChRs may reduce neuroinflammation, which is beneficial to AD [23]. Observations of the crystal structure of a complex between MLA and an AChBP isolated from the salt-water snail, Aplysia californica, revealed that MLA interacted with AChBP at the molecular level [24]. Thus, MLA might affect the pathogenic process of AD caused by Aβ.

In this study, we treated the human neuroblastoma cell line SH-SY5Y cell line with $Aβ_{25-35}$ to observe the neurotoxicity of $Aβ_{25-35}$ and analyzed the role of autophagy in Aβ-induced cytotoxicity. Furthermore, we evaluated the effect of MLA on Aβ-induced cytotoxicity and its underlying mechanisms.

Materials and Methods

Reagents, chemicals and the preparation of drugs

Fetal bovine serum (FBS; SH300088.03) and RPMI-1640 (SH30809.01B) were obtained from Hyclone. Amyloid β-protein fragment 25–35 ($Aβ_{25-35}$; A4559), methyllycaconitine (MLA; M168), rapamycin (R0395), dansylcadaverine (MDC; 30432), Hoechst 33258 (B2883), dimethyl sulfoxide (DMSO; D5879) and protease inhibitor cocktail (P8340) were from Sigma-Aldrich. Thiazolyl blue tetrazolium bromide (MTT; 0793) was from Amresco. $Aβ_{25-35}$ was prepared as described [25]. Briefly, $Aβ_{25-35}$ was initially dissolved in double-distilled water to 1 mM. The peptide solution was divided into aliquots and stored at −20°C. Before use, the $Aβ_{25-35}$ solution was incubated at 37°C for 7–10 days to form aggregated diffusible oligomers, then diluted in medium to the indicated concentration. MLA was dissolved in double-distilled water as a stock solution at 1 mM. Then the stock solution was divided into aliquots and stored at −20°C.

Antibodies

LC3B (2775), p70S6K (9202), p-p70S6K (9206) and Beclin1 (3495P) antibodies were purchased from Cell Signaling Technology. β-actin (sc-47778) antibody was from Santa Cruz Biotechnology. P62 (610833) was from Biosciences.

Cell culture and drug treatment

The human neuroblastoma cell line SH-SY5Y was purchased from the Cell Resource Center, IBMS, CAMS/PUMC. Cells were cultured in RPMI-1640 supplemented with 10% FBS at 37°C. Cells at 60–70% confluence were treated with concentrations of $Aβ_{25-35}$, MLA, rapamycin or $Aβ_{25-35}$ with or without MLA. Control cells were cultured under normal conditions.

Cell viability assay

Cells were plated in 96-well plates containing complete medium and cultured for 24 h. Then cells were treated with compounds at the indicated concentrations for specified times. After drug treatment, cell viability was measured by MTT assay [26]. Briefly, 10 μl of the MTT solution (5 mg/mL) was added to each well and incubated for 4 h at 37°C. After removing the supernatant, 100 μL DMSO was added into each well. The absorbance was measured at 570 nm with a microplate reader (Thermo, MULTISKAN MK3, USA). All experiments were repeated 3 times.

Monodansylcadaverine staining (MDC)

To detect autophagy in SH-SY5Y cells, cells were plated on coverslips in 6-well plates. After 24 h, cells were treated with compounds at the indicated concentrations, fixed with 4% paraformaldehyde for 15 min at room temperature, then stained with MDC (1 μg/mL in phosphate buffered saline [PBS]) at 37°C in the dark, and observed immediately with fluorescence microscopy. To quantify the number of cells with acidic vesicles, cells were seeded into 6-well plates and cultured overnight, then stained with 1 μg/mL MDC at 37°C for 15 min. After incubation, cells were washed with PBS and removed with trypsin-EDTA, resuspended, and analyzed by flow cytometry.

Apoptosis detection by Hoechst 33258 staining

Hoechst 33258 staining was used to detect apoptotic nuclei. Cells were plated in 24-well plates. After drug treatment, cells were stained with 10 μg/mL Hoechst 33258 for 15 min. After being gently washed with PBS once, cells were observed and photographed under a fluorescence microscopy (NIKON ECLIPSE 90i, LH-M100CB-1, Japan).

Apoptosis detection by flow cytometry

Cells were plated in six-well plates and incubated for 24 h, exposed to desired concentrations of $Aβ_{25-35}$ for 24 h, then harvested by trypsinization, and washed twice in PBS. After staining with a combination of AnnexinV/fluorescein isothiocyanate (FITC) and propidium iodide (PI) (Annexin V: FITC Apoptosis Detection Kit, BD Pharmingen), cells were immediately analyzed by flow cytometry (FACS Calibur, Becton Dickinson).

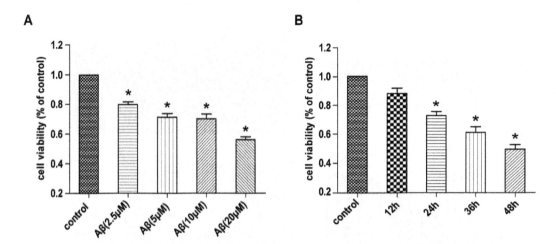

Figure 1. Amyloid-β peptide 25–35 (Aβ$_{25-35}$) inhibits the growth of SH-SY5Y cells. Cell viability was examined by MTT assay in SH-SY5Y cells. Cells were treated with various doses of Aβ$_{25-35}$ for 24 h (A) and 10 μM Aβ$_{25-35}$ for various times (B).

Immunocytochemistry

Immunocytochemical staining was performed as described [27]. Briefly, cells were seeded on cover slips over night. After drug treatment, cells were fixed for 30 min in 4% paraformaldehyde. After blocking, cells were incubated with primary antibody (anti-LC3) overnight at 4°C. After being washed with PBS, cells were incubated with PE-labeled secondary antibodies (1:500; Invitrogen) at room temperature for 1 h, then counterstained with 4-6-diamidino-2-phenylindole (DAPI) for 10 minutes. Images were obtained by laser scanning microscopy (NIKON ECLIPSE 90i, LH-M100CB-1, Japan).

Western blot analysis

After treatment, cells were collected and washed gently with PBS twice, then lysed with protein lysis buffer (1% SDS in 25 mM Tris-HCl, pH 7.5, 4 mM EDTA, 100 mM NaCl, 1 mM PMSF, 1% cocktail protease inhibitor). Samples were centrifuged at 12,000 g for 15 min at 4°C, and supernatants were collected. The concentration of the protein was determined by Coomassie brilliant blue protein assay. Equal amounts of protein (50 μg) were resolved by SDS-PAGE and transferred onto nitrocellulose membrane, which was blocked with 5% non-fat dry milk in TBS for 1 h at room temperature, and then incubated with primary antibodies (1:1000) overnight at 4°C. Membranes were washed and treated with appropriate secondary antibodies for 1 h at room temperature. The immunocomplexes were detected with an enhanced chemiluminescence plus kit.

Electron microscopy (EM)

Cells were postfixed with 2% osmium tetroxide, followed by an increasing gradient dehydration step with ethanol and propylene oxide. Cells were then embedded in LX-112 medium (Ladd), and sections were cut ultrathin (90 nm), placed on uncoated copper grids, and stained with 0.2% lead citrate and 1% uranyl acetate. Images were examined under a JEOL-1010 electron microscope (JEOL) at 80 kV.

RNA interference of beclin 1 expression

Cells were seeded in 6-well plates and incubated overnight. Control scramble small interfering RNA (siRNA) or beclin 1-targeted siRNA was transfected by use of Lipofectamine 2000 (Invitrogen) according to the manufacturer's protocol. After 48 h transfection, cells were treated with Aβ$_{25-35}$, then collected and cell lysates underwent immunoblotting for Beclin 1 and LC3 protein level. Cells were also processed for cell viability analysis.

Data analysis

Data were analyzed by use of SPSS 15.0 (SPSS Inc.). Data were expressed as mean ± SE. Differences between groups were analyzed by t test. P<0.05 was considered statistically significant.

Results

Aβ25–35 inhibits the growth of SH-SY5Y cells

Growing evidence suggests that Aβ has neurotoxic effects both in vitro [28] and in vivo [29,30], which contributes to cognitive deficits in the pathogenesis of AD. To determine the cytotoxicity of Aβ in SH-SY5Y cells, we pretreated Aβ$_{25-35}$ so that it formed oligomers and then examined the effect of Aβ$_{25-35}$ on the viability of SH-SY5Y cells by MTT assay. Consistent with previous observations [26], we observed the cytotoxic effect of Aβ in SH-SY5Y cells. Cell viability was significantly decreased after exposure to 5, 10 and 20 μM Aβ$_{25-35}$ for 24 h, and cell growth was inhibited by 10 μM Aβ$_{25-35}$ after treatment for 24, 36 and 48 h (Fig. 1A and 1B). Thus, Aβ$_{25-35}$ could inhibit cell growth dose- and time-dependently.

Aβ25–35 induces autophagy in SH-SY5Y cells

Autophagosomes developed in the brains of the AD model mice [31], so we tested whether Aβ$_{25-35}$ could induce autophagy in SH-SY5Y cells. After exposure to exogenous Aβ$_{25-35}$ (5, 10, 20 uM), the level of LC3-II increased in SH-SY5Y cells, and the LC3-II/LC3-I ratio increased (Fig. 2A). To visualize autophagosome formation, the distribution of LC3 was measured by immunocytochemistry with an LC3-specific antibody after administration of Aβ$_{25-35}$ (10 μM). Control SH-SY5Y cells showed a diffuse and weak LC3-associated red fluorescence. The SH-SY5Y cells treated with Aβ$_{25-35}$ exhibited characteristic punctate pattern of LC3, which suggests that Aβ$_{25-35}$ can induce autophagosome accumulation in SH-SY5Y cells (Fig. 2B). Electron micrographs of Aβ$_{25-35}$-treated SH-SY5Y cells also showed abnormal accumulation of large double-membrane vesicles (Fig. 2C), which indicates that Aβ$_{25-35}$ could induce autophagy.

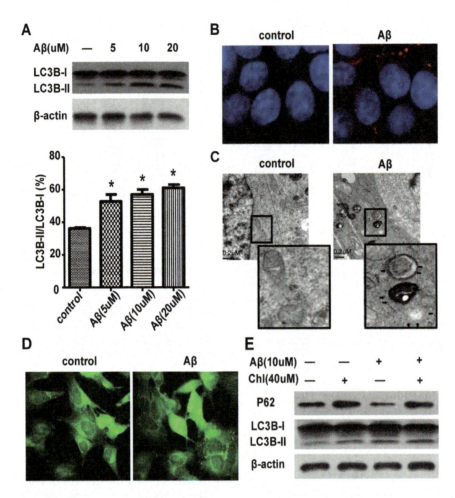

Figure 2. Aβ25–35 induces autophagy in SH-SY5Y cells. (A) Western blot analysis of LC3 protein expression in SH-SY5Y cells treated with different doses of Aβ$_{25-35}$ and quantification, β-actin was a loading control. (B) Immunofluorescence microscopy of punctate pattern of LC3 localization in SH-SY5Y cells treated with Aβ$_{25-35}$. (C) Electron micrographs of SH-SY5Y cells treated with Aβ$_{25-35}$ for 24 h. (D) Fluorescence microscopy of the formation of acidic vesicles after MDC staining in SH-SY5Y cells treated with Aβ$_{25-35}$ for 4 h. (E)Western blot analyses of the protein expression of LC3 and p62 in cells treated with Aβ$_{25-35}$ with and without chloroquine.

To confirm the cause of Aβ-induced autophagosome accumulation, we analyzed autolysosomal maturation in SH-SY5Y cells with MDC staining. MDC is a lysosomotropic compound used for identifying of acidic vesicles [32]. Thus, MDC staining was used to detect autolysosomes by fluorescence microscopy or flow cytometry. The accumulation of MDC-labeled vacuoles increased with Aβ$_{25-35}$ treatment (Fig. 2D), which suggests that Aβ does not impair autolysosomal maturation. To examine autophagosomal formation in greater detail, we measured the degradation of p62, an autophagy-specific substrate. The degradation of p62 increased in Aβ$_{25-35}$-treated SH-SY5Y cells (Fig. 2E), which suggests that there was no defective clearance of autophagosomes. Thus, Aβ$_{25-35}$ induced autophagy in SH-SY5Y cells, particularly autophagosome formation.

Aβ25–35-induced growth inhibition of SH-SY5Y cells is mediated by autophagy

To identify the causes of Aβ-induced growth inhibition of SH-SY5Y cells, we tested the effect of Aβ$_{25-35}$ on apoptosis of SH-SY5Y cells by flow cytometry and Hoechst 33258 staining. The SH-SY5Y cells administrated with Aβ$_{25-35}$ for 24 h didn't induce obvious apoptosis (Fig. 3A and 3B). Therefore, cytotoxicity induced by Aβ could not be attributed to apoptosis.

The role of autophagy in Aβ-mediated growth inhibition was further studied by siRNA knockdown of the expression of beclin 1, a component of the class III phosphatidy-linositol 3-kinase complex essential for autophagosome formation. The expression of beclin 1 was markedly suppressed in SH-SY5Y cells transfected with beclin 1 siRNA but not scramble siRNA (Fig. 3C). Accordingly, siRNA knockdown of beclin 1 expression reduced LC3-II accumulation after Aβ treatment as compared with the siRNA control (Fig. 3C). Although the result did not reach statistical significance, it showed that the growth inhibition effect of Aβ could be decreased by siRNA knockdown of beclin 1 expression as compared with the siRNA control (Fig. 3D, $P = 0.0522$). These data suggest that autophagy is required for Aβ-induced growth inhibition.

MLA alleviates the toxic effect of Aβ25–35 in SH-SY5Y cells

Many studies have shown that α7nAChR could be an important therapeutic target for treatment of AD, because α7nAChR is involved in Aβ-induced neurotoxic effects both in vitro and in vivo [18,19]. Here, we studied the effect of MLA, a selective α7nAChR antagonist, on Aβ-induced neurotoxicity in SH-SY5Y cells. Pretreatment with 5 and 10 μM MLA inhibited the decreased

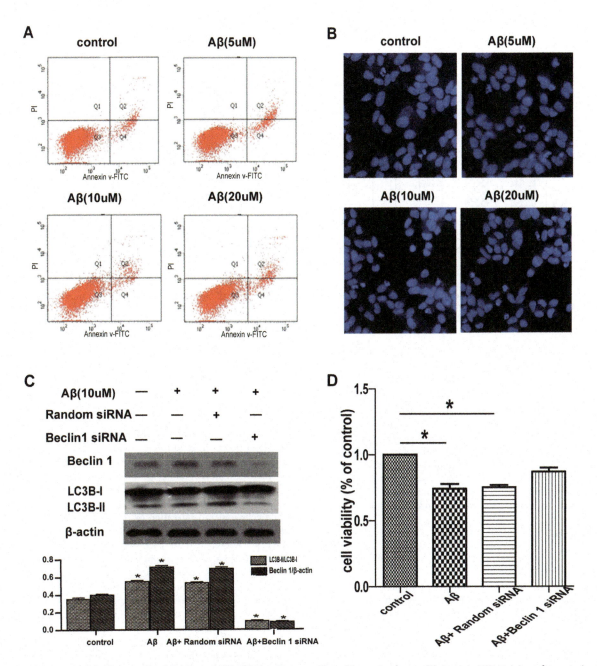

Figure 3. Aβ25–35-induced growth inhibition of SH-SY5Y cells is mediated by autophagy. (A) Annexin V/PI staining of apoptosis of SH-SY5Y cells treated with different doses of $Aβ_{25-35}$ for 24 h. (B) Hoechst staining of apoptosis of SH-SY5Y cells treated with different doses of $Aβ_{25-35}$ for 24 h. (C) Immunoblotting of Beclin 1 and LC3 expression with SH-SY5Y cell lysates. Cells were treated with 10 μM $Aβ_{25-35}$ for additional 24 h after transfection with random siRNA or beclin 1 siRNA for 48 h. (D) MTT assay of cell viability of SH-SY5Y cells treated with 10 μM $Aβ_{25-35}$ for 24 h after transfection with random siRNA or beclin 1 siRNA for 48 h.

cell viability induced by $Aβ_{25-35}$ (Fig. 4B), which suggested that MLA had a protective effect against Aβ-induced cytotoxicity. Furthermore, cell viability did not decrease after exposure to MLA (2.5, 5, 10, 20 uM), which suggests a good safety profile (Fig. 4A).

MLA inhibits Aβ-induced autophagy in SH-SY5Y cells

To determine the mechanism by which MLA treatment improves the viability of SH-SY5Y cells exposed to $Aβ_{25-35}$, we examined the effect of MLA on Aβ-induced autophagy. $Aβ_{25-35}$ treatment increased LC3-II levels, which was inhibited by administration of MLA (Fig. 5A). To visualize autophagosome formation, LC3 protein was measured by immunocytochemistry with an LC3-specific antibody (Fig. 5B). MLA also inhibited Aβ-induced autophagosome accumulation in SH-SY5Y cells. Furthermore, MDC staining was used to evaluate the effect of MLA on the accumulation of acidic vacuoles induced by $Aβ_{25-35}$. The result showed that $Aβ_{25-35}$ treatment increased MDC-labeled vacuoles, which was inhibited by administration of MLA (Fig. 5C). Flow cytometry also demonstrated decreased MDC-labeled vacuoles with MLA treatment (Fig. 5D). Therefore, MLA could inhibit Aβ-induced autophagy in SH-SY5Y cells, which may contribute to alleviating the cytotoxic effect of $Aβ_{25-35}$.

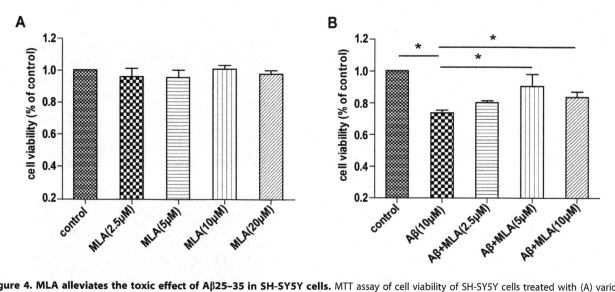

Figure 4. MLA alleviates the toxic effect of Aβ25–35 in SH-SY5Y cells. MTT assay of cell viability of SH-SY5Y cells treated with (A) various doses of MLA for 24 h or (B) 10 μM Aβ$_{25-35}$ with various doses of MLA.

MLA inhibition of Aβ-induced autophagy is mediated by mTOR signaling in SH-SY5Y cells

In recent years, several signaling pathways were found to regulate autophagy, with the mTOR pathway playing a key role [11]. We measured the phosphorylation of P70S6K, an mTORC1 downstream substrate, to identify the signaling pathways mediating Aβ-induced autophagy. Aβ$_{25-35}$ treatment dose-dependently decreased the phosphorylation of p70S6K (Fig. 6A). However, Aβ-decreased p70S6K phosphorylation was attenuated by administration of MLA (Fig. 6B), which may contribute to suppress Aβ-activated autophagy. Therefore, MLA may inhibit Aβ-induced autophagy via an mTOR signaling pathway in SH-SY5Y cells.

Discussion

One of the main histopathological features of AD is the presence of extracellular proteinaceous deposits in the brain, identified as senile plaques, which are enriched in Aβ. It is widely accepted that AD onset can be initially triggered by interaction of Aβ oligomers with the brain parenchyma [33]. In agreement with this, the levels of soluble Aβ oligomers appear to correlate well with the severity of AD dysfunction [34,35]. In vitro [28] and in vivo [29,30] studies have shown that these soluble oligomers produced toxicity leading to neuron dysfunction or loss. Consistent with previous studies, we also observed the neurotoxicity of Aβ oligomers on the SH-SY5Y cells. Cell growth was remarkably inhibited by Aβ oligomers treatment. MLA, a norditerpenoid alkaloid isolated from the seeds of Delphinium brownii, had a protective effect against the cytotoxicity of Aβ, which may be related to its inhibition of Aβ-induced autophagy and the involvement of the mTOR pathway. Moreover, it had a good safety profile. MLA treatment may be a promising therapeutic tool for AD.

Although AD has been discovered for 100 years, the disease continues to affect millions of patients. Although multiple drugs have now been approved, their expected benefits are modest. Therefore, numerous efforts have been made to develop more potent AD drugs. To date, emphasis has been on strategies to reduce the pathogenicity of amyloid-β (Aβ) peptides [36], widely believed to play a key role in AD. As an antagonist selective for α-bungarotoxin-sensitive α7nAChR, MLA alleviated Aβ-induced cytotoxicity in our SH-SY5Y cells. Pretreatment with MLA could significantly inhibit the decreased cell viability induced by Aβ$_{25-35}$, which indicates a protective effect of MLA against Aβ-induced cytotoxicity. Of note, MLA from 5 to 20 μM alone did not have any significant anti-proliferative effect on SH-SY5Y cells. MLA is a relatively small reversible-binding compound that can easily across the blood-brain barrier in vivo [37,38]. Considering the low cytotoxicity and the ability to pass the blood-brain barrier, MLA may be a potent drug in the treatment of AD.

Autophagy is a lysosome degradation process that turns over cytoplasmic materials and helps the cell maintain homeostasis. It is usually maintained at low levels under normal conditions for cell survival but can be augmented rapidly as a cytoprotective response when cells undergo starvation or damaging components, such as oxidative stress, infection, or protein aggregate accumulation [11,12]. Dysregulated or excessive autophagy can lead to cell death. Autophagosomes accumulate abnormally in the brain in several neurodegenerative disorders including AD [39]. Here, we found that Aβ could induce autophagy in SH-SY5Y cells. Aβ treatment could increase LC3II expression, punctate fluorescent signals in SH-SY5Y cells, the formation of acidic vesicular organelles and the accumulation of autophagosomes. These results are consistent with our previous study of PC12 cells in vitro [40].

To investigate the possible mechanism by which MLA pretreatment alleviated the cytotoxicity of Aβ in SH-SY5Y cells, we examined the effect of MLA on Aβ-induced autophagy. Aβ-induced upregulation of LC3BII levels and accumulation of autophagosomes or autolysosomes was inhibited by administration of MLA, which suggests that MLA could inhibit Aβ-induced autophagy in SH-SY5Y cells. Autophagy can be a pro-survival response or contribute to cell death; whether it is detrimental or protective remains unclear in AD [41]. It was reported that beclin-1, a protein with a key role in autophagy, was decreased in level in patients with AD and in APP transgenic mice early in the disease process, beclin 1 deficiency disrupted neuronal autophagy and promoted neurodegeneration in mice [42]. Another report showed that rapamycin administration could reduce Aβ levels in neurons and improve cognitive deficits by enhancing autophagy [43]. This evidence indicates that increasing autophagy may be helpful to AD. However, excessive Aβ can activate autophagy, thus resulting in cell dysfunction or death in vitro [44] and in vivo [45,46], and suppression of autophagy may alleviate Aβ-induced cell death or

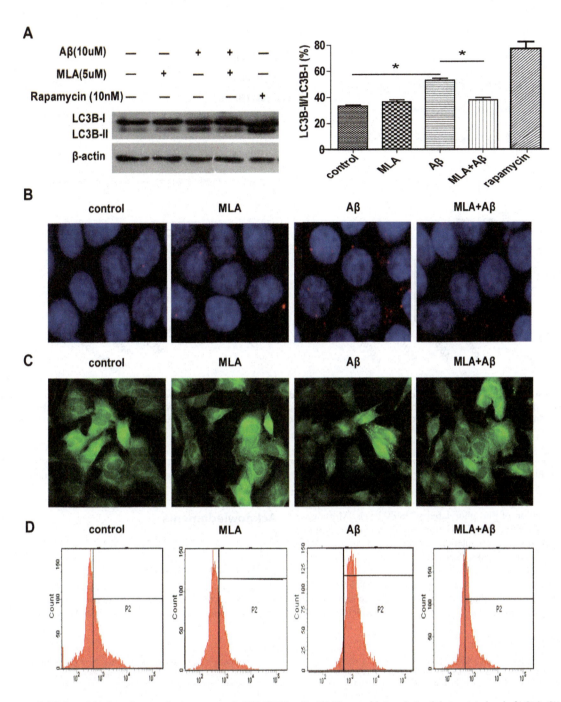

Figure 5. MLA inhibits Aβ-induced autophagy process in SH-SY5Y cells. (A) Western blot analysis of the protein level of LC3 in SH-SY5Y cells treated with 10 μM Aβ$_{25-35}$ with or without MLA. (B) Immunofluorescence microscopy of punctate pattern of LC3 localization in SH-SY5Y cells treated with 10 μM Aβ$_{25-35}$ with or without MLA. (C) Fluorescence microscopy of the formation of acidic vesicles with MDC staining in SH-SY5Y cells treated with 10 μM Aβ$_{25-35}$ with or without MLA. (D) Flow cytometry of the formation of acidic vesicles after MDC staining in SH-SY5Y cells treated with 10 μM Aβ$_{25-35}$ with or without MLA.

cognitive deficits. Aβ generation was found linked to autophagy, which is activated and abnormal in AD, and suppressing autophagy by 3-MA could decrease Aβ$_{1-40}$ secretion [47]. Furthermore, an AD drug, galanthamine hydrochloride, and an AD drug candidate, Ghrelin, could inhibit autophagy, which suggests that decreasing input into the lysosomal system may help reduce cellular stress in AD [48]. This evidence suggests that augmented autophagy in AD may be harmful; suppressing augmented autophagy could be an effective therapy for AD. Here, we found that MLA could inhibit Aβ-induced autophagy in SH-SY5Y cells. The suppression of autophagy by MLA may contribute to its protective effect against the cytotoxity of Aβ.

Several signaling pathways regulate the autophagy process with the mTOR pathway playing a key role. We paid attention to the downstream targets. 4E-binding protein 1 and p70S6K are directly phosphorylated by activated mTORC1 to negatively

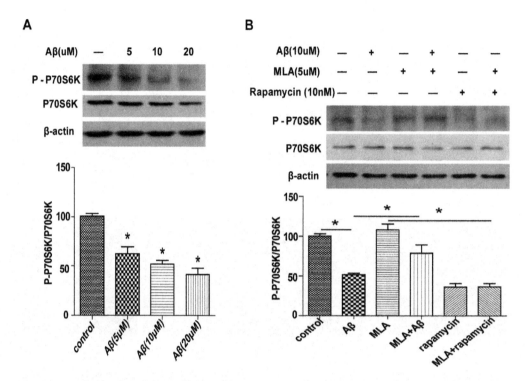

Figure 6. MLA inhibition of Aβ-induced autophagy is mediated by mTOR signal pathway in SH-SY5Y cells. (A) After exposure to different doses of Aβ$_{25-35}$, the level of phosphorylated p70S6K, a mTOR complex 1 substrate, was evaluated by western blot analysis. Signals were quantified by densitometry. (B) Western blot analysis of level of phosphorylated p70S6K after exposure to 10 μM Aβ$_{25-35}$ with or without MLA.

regulate autophagy [14]. In our previous study, we showed that Aβ could induce autophagy in PC12 cells through an mTOR-dependent pathway [40]. Here, we also found that Aβ induced autophagy in SH-SY5Y cells via mTOR signaling as evidenced by the downregulation of phosphorylated p70S6K levels. Moreover, Aβ-decreased p70S6K phosphorylation was attenuated by administration of MLA. The upregulation of mTOR signaling by MLA may inhibit Aβ-induced autophagy and contribute to its protective effect against Aβ-related cytotoxicity.

In conclusion, we showed that Aβ$_{25-35}$ inhibited SH-SY5Y cell growth and induced autophagy. Furthermore, MLA could provide neuroprotection against the cytotoxicity of Aβ, which may be related to its inhibition of Aβ-induced autophagy via an mTOR pathway. MLA may be a safe and promising drug candidate for treatment of AD.

Acknowledgments

We thank Dr. TongGang Qi for his assistance with western blot analysis.

Author Contributions

Conceived and designed the experiments: JB. Performed the experiments: XZ Hui Yang ZZ. Analyzed the data: LW HongNa Yang YL. Contributed reagents/materials/analysis tools: ZX ZL YW. Wrote the paper: XZ.

References

1. Mancuso M, Orsucci D, LoGerfo A, Calsolaro V, Siciliano G (2010) Clinical features and pathogenesis of Alzheimer's disease: Involvement of mitochondria and mitochondrial DNA. Adv Exp Med Biol 685: 34–44. PubMed: 20687493.
2. Förstl H, Kurz A (1999) Clinical features of Alzheimer's disease. Eur Arch Psychiatry Clin Neurosci 249: 288–290. PubMed: 10653284.
3. Cumming T, Brodtmann A (2010) Dementia and stroke: The present and future epidemic. Int J Stroke 5: 453–454. doi: 10.1111/j.1747-4949.2010.00527.x. PubMed: 21050400.
4. Buckingham SD, Jones AK, Brown LA, Sattelle DB (2009) Nicotinic acetylcholine receptor signalling: roles in Alzheimer's disease and amyloid neuroprotection. Pharmacol Rev 61: 39–61. doi: 10.1124/pr.108.000562. PubMed: 19293145.
5. Perl DE (2010) Neuropathology of Alzheimer's disease. Mt Sinai J Med 77: 32–42. doi: 10.1002/msj.20157. PubMed: 20101720.
6. Huang Y, Mucke L (2012) Alzheimer mechanisms and therapeutic strategies. Cell 148: 1204–1222. doi: 10.1016/j.cell.2012.02.040. PubMed: 22424230.
7. Sinha S, Lieberburg I (1999) Cellular mechanisms of beta-amyloid production and secretion. Proc Natl Acad Sci USA 96: 11049–11053. PubMed: 10500121.
8. Murphy MP, LeVine H 3rd (2010) Alzheimer's disease and the amyloid-beta peptide. J Alzheimers Dis 19: 311–23. doi: 10.3233/JAD-2010-1221. PubMed: 20061647.
9. Frozza RL, Horn AP, Hoppe JB, Simão F, Gerhardt D et al. (2009) A comparative study of beta-amyloid peptides Abeta1-42 and Abeta25-35 toxicity in organotypic hippocampal slice cultures. Neurochem Res 34: 295–303. doi: 10.1007/s11064-008-9776-8. PubMed: 18686032.
10. Selkoe DJ (1994) Alzheimer's disease: a central role for amyloid. J Neuropathol Exp Neurol 53: 438–447. PubMed: 8083687.
11. Glick D, Barth S, Macleod KF (2010) Autophagy: cellular and molecular mechanisms. J Pathol 221: 3–12. doi: 10.1002/path.2697. PubMed: 20225336.
12. Klionsky DJ (2007) Autophagy: from phenomenology to molecular understanding in less than a decade. Nat. Rev. Mol. Cell Biol 8: 931–937. PubMed: 17712358.
13. Yang Z, Klionsky DJ (2009) An overview of the molecular mechanism of autophagy. Curr Top Microbiol Immunol 335:1–32. doi: 10.1007/978-3-642-00302-8_1. PubMed: 19802558.
14. Kim J, Kundu M, Viollet B, Guan KL (2011) AMPK and mTOR regulate autophagy through direct phosphorylation of Ulk1. Nature cell biology 13 (2):132–41. doi: 10.1038/ncb2152. PubMed: 21258367.
15. Nixon RA, Wegiel J, Kumar A, Yu WH, Peterhoff C et al. (2005) Extensive involvement of autophagy in Alzheimer disease: an immuno-electron microscopy study. J Neuropathol Exp Neurol 64: 113–122. PubMed: 15751225.
16. Shacka JJ, Roth KA, Zhang J (2008) The autophagy-lysosomal degradation pathway: role in neurodegenerative disease and therapy. Front Biosci 13: 718–736. PubMed: 17981582.
17. Ling D, Salvaterra PM (2011) Brain aging and Aβ1–42 neurotoxicity converge via deterioration in autophagy-lysosomal system: a conditional Drosophila

17. model linking Alzheimer's neurodegeneration with aging. Acta Neuropathol 121: 183–191. doi: 10.1007/s00401-010-0772-0. PubMed: 21076961.
18. Paterson D, Nordberg A (2000) Neuronal nicotinic receptors in the human brain. Prog Neurobiol 61: 75–111. PubMed: 10759066.
19. Nordberg A (2001) Nicotinic receptor abnormalities of Alzheimer's disease: therapeutic implications. Biol Psychiatry 49: 200–210. PubMed: 11230871.
20. Jiang H, Liu CX, Feng JB, Wang P, Zhao CP et al. (2010) Granulocyte colony-stimulating factor attenuates chronic neuroinflammation in the brain of amyloid precursor protein transgenic mice: an Alzheimer's disease mouse model. J Int Med Res 38: 1305–1312. PubMed: 20926003.
21. Wang HY, Lee DH, D'Andrea MR, Peterson PA, Shank RP et al. (2000) beta-Amyloid(1–42) binds to alpha7 nicotinic acetylcholine receptor with high affinity. Implications for Alzheimer's disease pathology. J Biol Chem 275: 5626–5632. PubMed: 10681545.
22. Alkondon M, Pereira EF, Wonnacott S, Albuquerque EX (1992) Blockade of nicotinic currents in hippocampal neurons defines methyllycaconitine as a potent and specific receptor antagonist. Mol Pharmacol 41: 802–808. PubMed: 1569927.
23. Thomsen MS, Mikkelsen JD (2012) The $\alpha 7$ nicotinic acetylcholine receptor ligands methyllycaconitine, NS6740 and GTS-21 reduce lipopolysaccharide-induced TNF-α release from microglia. J Neuroimmunol 251: 65–72. doi: 10.1016/j.jneuroim.2012.07.006. PubMed: 22884467.
24. Hansen SB, Sulzenbacher G, Huxford T, Marchot P, Taylor P et al. (2005) Structures of Aplysia AChBP complexes with nicotinic agonists and antagonists reveal distinctive binding interfaces and conformations. EMBO J 24: 3635–3646. PubMed: 16193063.
25. Liu RT1, Zou LB, Lü QJ (2009) Liquiritigenin inhibits Abeta(25–35)-induced neurotoxicity and secretion of Abeta(1–40) in rat hippocampal neurons. Acta Pharmacol Sin 30(7):899–906. doi: 10.1038/aps.2009.74.
26. Luo S, Lan T, Liao W, Zhao M, Yang H (2012) Genistein inhibits Aβ25-35-induced neurotoxicity in PC12 cells via PKC signaling pathway. Neurochem Res 37: 2787–2794. doi: 10.1007/s11064-012-0872-4. PubMed: 22949092.
27. Cho HJ, Son SM, Jin SM, Hong HS, Shin DH et al. (2009) RAGE regulates BACE1 and Abeta generation via NFAT1 activation in Alzheimer's disease animal model. FASEB J 23: 2639–2649. doi: 10.1096/fj.08-126383. PubMed: 19332646.
28. Puttfarcken PS, Manelli AM, Neilly J, Frail DE (1996) Inhibition of age-induced beta-amyloid neurotoxicity in rat hippocampal cells. Exp Neurol 138: 73–81. PubMed: 8593898.
29. Walsh DM, Klyubin I, Fadeeva JV, Cullen WK, Anwyl R et al. (2002) Naturally secreted oligomers of amyloid beta protein potently inhibit hippocampal long-termpotentiation in vivo. Nature 416: 535–539. PubMed: 11932745.
30. Shankar GM, Li S, Mehta TH, Garcia-Munoz A, Shepardson NE et al. (2008) Amyloid-beta protein dimers isolated directly from Alzheimer's brains impair synaptic plasticity and memory. Nat Med 14: 837–842. doi: 10.1038/nm1782. PubMed: 18568035.
31. Son SM, Jung ES, Shin HJ, Byun J, Mook-Jung I (2012) Aβ-induced formation of autophagosomes is mediated by RAGE-CaMKKβ-AMPK signaling. Neurobiology of Aging 33: 1006.e11–e23. doi: 10.1016/j.neurobiolaging.2011.09.039. PubMed: 22048125.
32. Mizushima N (2004) Methods for monitoring autophagy. Int J Biochem Cell Biol 36: 2491–502. PubMed: 15325587.
33. Masters CL, Simms G, Weinman NA, Multhaup G, McDonald BL et al. (1985) Amyloid plaque core protein in Alzheimer disease and Down syndrome. Proc Natl Acad Sci USA 82: 4245–4249. PubMed: 3159021.
34. McLean CA, Cherny RA, Fraser FW, Fuller SJ, Smith MJ et al. (1999) Soluble pool of Ab amyloid as a determinant of severity of neurodegeneration in Alzheimer's disease. Ann Neurol 46: 860–866. PubMed: 10589538.
35. McLean CA, Cherny RA, Fraser FW, Fuller SJ, Smith MJ et al. (1999) Soluble pool of Abeta amyloid as a determinant of severity of neurodegeneration in Alzheimer's disease. Ann Neurol 46: 860–866. PubMed: 10589538.
36. Citron M (2004) Strategies for disease modification in Alzheimer's disease. Nat Rev Neurosci 5: 677–85. PubMed: 15322526.
37. Navarro HA, Zhong D, Abraham P, Xu H, Carroll FI (2000) Synthesis and pharmacological characterization of [125I] iodomethyllycaconitine ([125I] Iodo-MLA). A new ligand for the $\alpha 7$ nicotinic acetylcholine receptor. Journal of medicinal chemistry 43, 142–145. PubMed: 10649969.
38. Lockman PR, Van der Schyf CJ, Abbruscato TJ, Allen DD (2005) Chronic nicotine exposure alters blood-brain barrier permeability and diminishes brain uptake of methyllycaconitine. J Neurochem 2005 Jul;94(1):37–44. DOI: 10.1111/j.1471-4159.2005.03162.x. PubMed: 15953347.
39. Funderburk SF, Marcellino BK, Yue Z (2010) Cell "self-eating" (autophagy) mechanism in Alzheimer's disease. MtSinai J Med 77: 59–68. doi: 10.1002/msj.20161. PubMed: 20101724.
40. Yang S, Wang S, Peng N, Xie Z, Wang P et al. (2012) Butyrolactone derivative 3-benzyl-5-((2-nitrophenoxy) methyl)-dihydrofuran-2(3H)-one protects against amyloid-β peptides-induced cytotoxicity in PC12 cells. J Alzheimers Dis 28: 345–356. doi: 10.3233/JAD-2011-110863. PubMed: 21988929.
41. Barnett A, Brewer GJ (2011) Autophagy in aging and Alzheimer's disease: pathologic or protective? J Alzheimers Dis 25: 85–94. doi: 10.3233/JAD-2011-101989. PubMed: 21422527.
42. Pickford F, Masliah E, Britschgi M, Lucin K, Narasimhan R et al. (2008) The autophagy-related protein beclin1 shows reduced expression in early Alzheimer disease and regulates amyloid beta accumulation in mice. J Clin Invest 118: 2190–2199. doi: 10.1172/JCI33585. PubMed: 18497889.
43. Spilman P, Podlutskaya N, Hart MJ, Debnath J, Gorostiza O et al. (2010) Inhibition of mTOR by rapamycin abolishes cognitive deficits and reduces amyloid-beta levels in a mouse model of Alzheimer's disease. PLoS One 5: e9979. doi: 10.1371/journal.pone.0009979. PubMed: 20376313.
44. Wang H, Ma J, Tan Y, Wang Z, Sheng C et al. (2010) Amyloid-beta1–42 induces reactive oxygen species-mediated autophagic cell death in U87 and SH-SY5Y cells. J Alzheimers Dis 21: 597–610. doi: 10.3233/JAD-2010-091207. PubMed: 20571221.
45. Maycotte P, Guemez-Gamboa A, Moran J (2010) Apoptosis and autophagy in rat cerebellar granule neuron death: Role of reactive oxygen species. J Neurosci Res 88: 73–85. doi: 10.1002/jnr.22168. PubMed: 19598251.
46. Ling D, Song HJ, Garza D, Neufeld TP, Salvaterra PM (2009) Abeta42-induced neurodegeneration via an age-dependent autophagic-lysosomal injury in Drosophila. PLoS One 4: e4201. doi: 10.1371/journal.pone.0004201. PubMed: 19145255.
47. Yu WH, Cuervo AM, Kumar A, Peterhoff CM, Schmidt SD et al. (2005) Macroautophagy – a novel Beta-amyloid peptide-generating pathway activated in Alzheimer's disease. J Cell Biol 171: 87–98. PubMed: 16203860.
48. Lipinski MM, Zheng B, Lu T, Yan Z, Py BF et al. (2010) Genome-wide analysis reveals mechanisms modulating autophagy in normal brain aging and in Alzheimer's disease. Proc Natl Acad Sci USA 107: 14164–14169. doi: 10.1073/pnas.1009485107. PubMed: 20660724.

Permissions

All chapters in this book were first published in PLOS ONE, by The Public Library of Science; hereby published with permission under the Creative Commons Attribution License or equivalent. Every chapter published in this book has been scrutinized by our experts. Their significance has been extensively debated. The topics covered herein carry significant findings which will fuel the growth of the discipline. They may even be implemented as practical applications or may be referred to as a beginning point for another development.

The contributors of this book come from diverse backgrounds, making this book a truly international effort. This book will bring forth new frontiers with its revolutionizing research information and detailed analysis of the nascent developments around the world.

We would like to thank all the contributing authors for lending their expertise to make the book truly unique. They have played a crucial role in the development of this book. Without their invaluable contributions this book wouldn't have been possible. They have made vital efforts to compile up to date information on the varied aspects of this subject to make this book a valuable addition to the collection of many professionals and students.

This book was conceptualized with the vision of imparting up-to-date information and advanced data in this field. To ensure the same, a matchless editorial board was set up. Every individual on the board went through rigorous rounds of assessment to prove their worth. After which they invested a large part of their time researching and compiling the most relevant data for our readers.

The editorial board has been involved in producing this book since its inception. They have spent rigorous hours researching and exploring the diverse topics which have resulted in the successful publishing of this book. They have passed on their knowledge of decades through this book. To expedite this challenging task, the publisher supported the team at every step. A small team of assistant editors was also appointed to further simplify the editing procedure and attain best results for the readers.

Apart from the editorial board, the designing team has also invested a significant amount of their time in understanding the subject and creating the most relevant covers. They scrutinized every image to scout for the most suitable representation of the subject and create an appropriate cover for the book.

The publishing team has been an ardent support to the editorial, designing and production team. Their endless efforts to recruit the best for this project, has resulted in the accomplishment of this book. They are a veteran in the field of academics and their pool of knowledge is as vast as their experience in printing. Their expertise and guidance has proved useful at every step. Their uncompromising quality standards have made this book an exceptional effort. Their encouragement from time to time has been an inspiration for everyone.

The publisher and the editorial board hope that this book will prove to be a valuable piece of knowledge for researchers, students, practitioners and scholars across the globe.

List of Contributors

Sang Y. Lee, Becky Slagle-Webb, Elias Rizk, Akshal Patel and James R. Connor
Department of Neurosurgery, Pennsylvania State University College of Medicine, Penn State M.S. Hershey Medical Center, Hershey, Pennsylvania, United States of America

Patti A. Miller
Department of Radiology, Pennsylvania State University College of Medicine, Penn State M.S. Hershey Medical Center, Hershey, Pennsylvania, United States of America

Shen-Shu Sung
Department of Pharmacology, Pennsylvania State University College of Medicine, Penn State M.S. Hershey Medical Center, Hershey, Pennsylvania, United States of America

Meiyan Jiang, Qi Wang, Takatoshi Karasawa, Hongzhe Li and Peter S. Steyger
Oregon Hearing Research Center, Oregon Health & Science University, Portland, Oregon, United States of America

Ja-Won Koo
Oregon Hearing Research Center, Oregon Health & Science University, Portland, Oregon, United States of America
Department of Otorhinolaryngology, Seoul National University College of Medicine, Bundang Hospital, Seongnam, Gyeonggi, Republic of Korea

Ján Vančo, Jana Gáliková, Jan Hošek and Zdeněk Trávníček
Regional Centre of Advanced Technologies and Materials & Department of Inorganic Chemistry, Faculty of Science, Palacky´ University, Olomouc, Czech Republic

Zdeněk Dvořák
Regional Centre of Advanced Technologies and Materials & Department of Cell Biology and Genetics, Faculty of Science, Palacký University, Olomouc, Czech Republic

Lenka Paráková
Department of Human Pharmacology and Toxicology, Faculty of Pharmacy, University of Veterinary and Pharmaceutical Sciences Brno, Brno, Czech Republic

Sohyun Yun, Hae Young Song, Young Kyeung Kim, Haiyoung Jung, Young-Jun Park and Suk Ran Yoon
Immunotherapy Research Center, Korea Research Institute of Bioscience and Biotechnology, Daejeon, Republic of Korea

Sei-Ryang Oh, Su Ui Lee and Hyun-Jun Lee
Natural Medicine Research Center, Korea Research Institute of Bioscience and Biotechnology, Ochang-eup, Republic of Korea

Jung Min Kim
NAR Center, Inc., Daejeon Oriental Hospital of Daejeon University, Daejeon, Republic of Korea

Tae-Don Kim and Inpyo Choi
Immunotherapy Research Center, Korea Research Institute of Bioscience and Biotechnology, Daejeon, Republic of Korea
Department of Functional Genomics, Korea University of Science and Technology, Daejeon, Republic of Korea

Xiao-hua Shi, Shao-liang Wang, Yi-ming Zhang, Xin Zhou, Zeyuan Lei and Dong-li Fan
Department of Plastic and Cosmetic Surgery, Xinqiao Hospital, the Third Military Medical University, Chongqing, 400037, People's Republic of China

Yi-cheng Wang
Department of Plastic and Cosmetic Surgery, Chongqing Armed Police Corps Hospital, Chongqing, 400061, People's Republic of China

Zhi Yang
Department of War Trauma care, Hainan branch of PLA General Hospital, Sanya, Hainan, 572013, People's Republic of China

Huize Chen and Rong Han
Higher Education Key Laboratory of Plant Molecular and Environmental Stress Response (Shanxi Normal University) in Shanxi Province, Linfen, China
School of Life Science, Shanxi Normal University, Linfen, China

Yan Gong
Higher Education Key Laboratory of Plant Molecular and Environmental Stress Response (Shanxi Normal University) in Shanxi Province, Linfen, China
School of Life Science, Shanxi Normal University, Linfen, China
School of Chemistry and Material Science, Shanxi Normal University, Linfen, China

Hiroshi Yukawa and Momoko Obayashi
Research Center for Innovative Nanobiodevices, Nagoya University, Furo-cho, Chikusa-ku, Nagoya 464-8603, Japan

Shingo Nakagawa, Yasuma Yoshizumi, Tetsuya Ishikawa and Yumi Hayashi
Department of Medical Technology, Nagoya University, Graduate School of Medicine, Daikominami, Higashi-ku, Nagoya 461-8673, Japan

Masaki Watanabe
Department of Applied Chemistry, Graduate School of Engineering, Nagoya University, Furo-cho, Chikusa-ku, Nagoya 464-8603, Japan

Hiroaki Saito and Ichiro Kato
Nagoya Research Laboratory, MEITO Sangyo Co., Ltd., Kiyosu 452-0067, Japan

Yoshitaka Miyamoto and Shuji Hayashi
Department of Advanced Medicine in Biotechnology and Robotics, Graduate School of Medicine, Nagoya University, Higashi-ku, Nagoya 461-0047, Japan

Hirofumi Noguchi
Department of Regenerative Medicine, Graduate School of Medicine, University of the Ryukyus, 207 Uehara, Nishihara, Okinawa 903-0215, Japan

Koichi Oishi, Kenji Ono and Makoto Sawada
Research Institute of Environmental Medicine, Stress Adaption and Protection, Nagoya University, Furo-cho, Chikusa-ku, Nagoya, 464-8601, Japan

Noritada Kaji
Research Center for Innovative Nanobiodevices, Nagoya University, Furo-cho, Chikusa-ku, Nagoya 464-8603, Japan
Department of Applied Chemistry, Graduate School of Engineering, Nagoya University, Furo-cho, Chikusa-ku, Nagoya 464-8603, Japan

Daisuke Onoshima
Institute of Innovative for Future Society, Nagoya University, Furo-cho, Chikusa-ku, Nagoya 464-8603, Japan

Yoshinobu Baba
Research Center for Innovative Nanobiodevices, Nagoya University, Furo-cho, Chikusa-ku, Nagoya 464-8603, Japan
Department of Applied Chemistry, Graduate School of Engineering, Nagoya University, Furo-cho, Chikusa-ku, Nagoya 464-8603, Japan
Health Research Institute, National Institute of Advanced Industrial Science and Technology (AIST), Hayashi-cho 2217-14, Takamatsu 761-0395, Japan

Andrea Derksen, Andreas Hensel, Fabian Herrmann and Thomas J. Schmidt
Institute of Pharmaceutical Biology and Phytochemistry, University of Münster, Münster, Germany

Wali Hafezi and Joachim Kühn
Institute of Medical Microbiology-Clinical Virology, University Hospital Münster, Münster, Germany

Christina Ehrhardt, Stephan Ludwig
Institute of Molecular Virology, University of Münster, Münster, Germany

Yi Yang, Soonok Oh, Min-Hye Jeong and Jae-Seoun Hur
Korean Lichen Research Institute, Sunchon National University, Sunchon, Republic of Korea

Thanh Thi Nguyen
Korean Lichen Research Institute, Sunchon National University, Sunchon, Republic of Korea
Faculty of Natural Science and Technology, Tay Nguyen University, Buon Ma Thuot, Vietnam

Somy Yoon and Kyung Keun Kim
Medical Research Center for Gene Regulation, Chonnam National University Medical School, Gwangju, Republic of Korea

Hangun Kim, Ho-Bin Lee, Jong-Jin Kim, Sung-Tae Yee and Cheol Moon
College of Pharmacy and Research Institute of Life and Pharmaceutical Sciences, Sunchon National University, Sunchon, Republic of Korea

Florin Crişan
Department of Taxonomy and Ecology, Faculty of Biology and Geology, Babeş-Bolyai University, Cluj-Napoca, Romania

Kwang Youl Lee
College of Pharmacy, Chonnam National University, Gwangju, Korea

Vu T. A. Dang, Kazuaki Tanabe, Yuka Tanaka, Toshihiro Misumi, Yoshihiro Saeki, Nobuaki Fujikuni and Hideki Ohdan
Department of Gastroenterological and Transplant Surgery, Applied Life Sciences, Institute of Biomedical and Health Sciences, Hiroshima University, Hiroshima, Japan

Noriaki Tokumoto
Department of Surgery, Hiroshima City Hospital, Hiroshima, Japan

Diana Mora-Obando, Julián Fernández, José María Gutiérrez and Bruno Lomonte
Instituto Clodomiro Picado, Facultad de Microbiología, Universidad de Costa Rica, San José Costa Rica

Cesare Montecucco
Department of Biomedical Sciences, University of Padova, Padova, Italy

Xingtong Wang, Junjie Wang, He Fang, Zhihong Wang, Yu Sun and Zhaofan Xia
Department of Burn Surgery, the Second Military Medical University affiliated Changhai Hospital, Shanghai, China

Fang Zhang
Department of Burn Surgery, the Second Military Medical University affiliated Changhai Hospital, Shanghai, China
Number 73901 Troop of PLA, Shanghai, China

Xiaochen Qiu
Department of General Surgery, 309th Hospital of PLA, Beijing, China

Jian Jin, Bowen Sui, Jingshuo Liu and Xiangqun Jin
Department of Pharmaceutics, College of Pharmacy Sciences, Jilin University, Changchun, People's Republic of China

Jingxin Gou, Xing Tang, Hui Xu and Yu Zhang
Department of Pharmaceutics, Shenyang Pharmaceutical University, Shenyang, People's Republic of China

Eliška Potůčková, Kateřina Hrušková, Jan Bureš, Petra Kovaříková, Iva A. Špirková, Kateřina Pravdíková, Lucie Kolbabová, Tereza Hergeselová, Pavlína Hašková, Hana Jansová, Miloslav Macháček, Anna Jirkovská, Kateřina Vávrová and Tomáš Šimůnek
Charles University in Prague, Faculty of Pharmacy in Hradec Králové, Hradec Králové, Czech Republic

Vera Richardson, Darius J. R. Lane, Danuta S. Kalinowski and Des R. Richardson
Molecular Pharmacology and Pathology Program, Bosch Institute and Department of Pathology, University of Sydney, Sydney, Australia
Xiaoxi Han and Yifu Guan
Department of Biochemistry and Molecular Biology, China Medical University, Shenyang, China

Shengkun Sun
Department of Urology, The General Hospital of PLA, Beijing, China

Ming Zhao, Xiang Cheng, Guozhu Chen, Song Lin and Xiaodan Yu
Department of Cognitive Science, Institute of Basic Medical Sciences, Cognitive and Mental Health Research Center, Beijing, China

Yongxian Zhuang, Allison B. Haugrud and W. Keith Miskimins
Cancer Biology Research Center, Sanford Research/USD, Sioux Falls, South Dakota, United States of America

Daniel K. Chan
Sanford School of Medicine, The University of South Dakota, Vermillion, South Dakota, United States of America

Bertha Isabel Carvajal-Gamez, Laura Itzel Quintas-Granados, Laura Isabel Vázquez-Carrillo, Eduardo Carrillo-Tapia and María Elizbeth Alvarez- Sánchez
Genomic Sciences Postgraduate, Autonomous University of Mexico City (UACM), Mexico City, Mexico

Rossana Arroyo and Lucero De los Angeles Ramón-Luing
Department of Infectomics and Molecular Pathogenesis, Center for Research and Advanced Studies, IPN, Mexico City, Mexico

XiaoLei Zheng, ZhaoHong Xie, ZhengYu Zhu, Zhen Liu, Yun Wang, LiFei Wei, Hui Yang, HongNa Yang and YiQing Liu
Department of Neural Medicine, Second Hospital of Shandong University, Jinan, China

JianZhong Bi
Department of Neural Medicine, Second Hospital of Shandong University, Jinan, China
Institute of Neurology, Shandong University, Jinan, China
Key Laboratory of Translational Medicine on Neurological Degenerative Disease in Universities of Shandong (Shandong University), Jinan, China

Index

A
Acute Liver Injury, 142-145, 147-149, 151-153
Adipose Tissue, 79-81, 83, 85, 87, 89
Alzheimer's Disease (ad), 221
Aminoglycosides, 12-15, 17, 19-25
Amyloid Precursor Protein (app), 221
Anti-cancer Compound, 1, 3, 5, 7, 9, 11
Anti-inflammatory Agents, 26-27, 29, 31, 33, 35, 37, 39
Anti-influenza Agents, 91, 102-103
Antioxidant Enzyme Metabolism, 66
Astrocytomas, 1, 3, 5, 7, 9-11

B
Biocompatibility, 55, 64, 155, 161
Bone Marrow (bm), 41
Bothrops Asper, 131-133, 137, 140-141
Brain Tumors, 1-2, 10

C
Cadmium Telluride Quantum Dots (cdte-qds), 66-67, 69, 71, 73, 75, 77
Carbon Tetrachloride (ccl4), 142
Cell Adhesion, 55, 57-65
Cellular Uptake, 12-13, 15-19, 21, 23-25, 155, 157, 161, 163-166, 175
Central Nervous System (cns), 79
Cycloheximide Treatment, 213
Cysteine Proteinase, 211, 213, 215, 217, 219-220

D
Dimethyl Sulfoxide (dmso), 13
Dynamic Light Scattering (dls), 155

E
Esculentoside A, 142-143, 145, 147, 149, 151, 153
Extra Cellular Acidification Rate (ecar), 201

F
Flavocetraria Cucullata, 104-105, 107, 109, 111, 113-115, 117
Flow Cytometry, 5, 43, 105, 119-121, 124, 128, 143-144, 188, 191, 193-195, 222, 224-225, 227

G
Glomerular Structures, 12
Gold(i) Complexes, 26-29, 31-33, 35-39

H
Hemagglutinin (ha), 91
Hierarchical Clustering, 41, 43, 45, 48
Human Cancer Cells, 104-105, 107-111, 113, 115, 117
Human Neurodegenerative Diseases, 184
Hydroxyapatite, 55, 57, 59, 61-65
Hydroxyapatite (ha), 55
Hypoxia-inducible Factor 1 (hif-1), 184

I
Immunotherapy, 41, 53
In Vivo Imaging, 79, 81-83, 85, 87, 89
Influenza A Virus, 91-93, 95, 97, 99, 101, 103

L
Lichen Secondary Metabolites, 104-105, 107, 109, 111, 113, 115, 117
Lipopolysaccharides (lps), 142
Low Glucose, 199, 201-207, 209

M
Magnetic Resonance (mr), 79-80
Major Histocompatibility Complex (mhc), 41
Metformin, 25, 199-210
Methyllycaconitine, 221-223, 225, 227, 229
Monodansylcadaverine Staining (mdc), 222

N
N-heterocyclic Carbene (nhc), 26
Nanostructured Hydroxyapatite (nha), 55
Natural Killer (nk), 41, 118, 120-123, 127-129
Nk Cell Differentiation, 41, 43, 45, 47-49, 51-53

O
Ornithine Decarboxylase Enzyme (odc), 211
Oxygen Consumption Rate (ocr), 201, 205

P
Phospholipases A2 (pla2s), 131
Plastic Surgery, 55, 61, 64
Polymeric Micelles, 155, 157, 159, 161, 163, 165-166
Positively Charged Nanoparticle, 79, 81, 83, 85, 87, 89
Programmed Cell, 66-67, 73, 75-78
Prostate Cancer Cells, 109, 116, 155, 157, 159, 161, 163, 165, 210
Prostate Specific Membrane Antigen (psma), 155

Protective Effect, 24, 142-143, 145, 147, 149, 151-153, 221, 225-228
Protein Synthesis, 137, 184, 187, 190, 196, 218
Putrescine, 211-219

R
Rumex Acetosa, 91-93, 95, 97-101, 103

S
Selective Antitumor, 26-27, 29, 31, 33, 35, 37, 39, 183
Signaling Pathway, 9, 48, 53-54, 104, 184, 226, 229
Sillicone Rubber, 55, 57, 59, 61, 63, 65
Specific Membrane Antigen (smlp), 155
Standard Chemotherapy, 1, 209
Stem Cell Transplantation, 79-80, 89
Symbiotic Organisms, 104
Synergism, 131, 133-135, 137-141, 182, 204
Sytox Green Nucleic Acid Stain, 200

T
Temozolomide (tmz), 1
Tissue Filler Material, 55
Transient Receptor Potential (trp), 12
Translational Blockage, 213
Trichomonas Vaginalis, 211, 213, 215, 217, 219-220
Tumorigenic Potentials, 104

U
Ultraviolet-b (uv-b), 66-67, 69, 71, 73, 75, 77

V
Viperid Snake Venom, 131, 133, 135, 137, 139, 141
Von Hippel Lindau Gene (vhl), 184

W
Western Blotting, 121, 185-188, 190-194, 196, 200, 202-203, 205-206, 213
Wheat Seedlings, 66-71, 73, 77

CPSIA information can be obtained
at www.ICGtesting.com
Printed in the USA
BVOW07*0202230218
508872BV00016BA/5/P